चरक संहिता IV

ENGLISH TRANSLATION

डा. जनार्धन वि हेब्बार

Made with ♥ on the Notion Press Platform
www.notionpress.com

क्रम-सूची

क्रम-सूची

चिकित्सास्थानम् Chikitsa Sthanam

1

Chikitsasthana Chapter 18 Kasa Chikitsitam

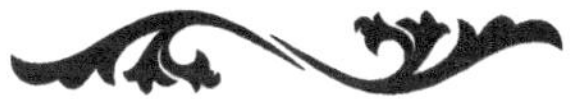

The 18th chapter of Charaka Samhita Chikitsa Sthana is Kasa Chikitsa Adhyaya. It deals with causes, types, treatment and Ayurvedic medicines for cough and associated disorders.

अथातः कास चिकित्सितं व्याख्यास्यामः||१||
इति ह स्माह भगवानात्रेयः||२||
Let us explore the chapter on the treatment on the treatment of Kasa – cough. Thus, said Atreya. [1–2]

Prologue
तपसा यशसा धृत्या धिया च परयाऽन्वितः| आत्रेयः कासशान्त्यर्थं प्राह सिद्धं चिकित्सितम्||३||
Lord Atreya, endowed with the power of Tapas, Yashas – fame, Dhruti – perseverance, and Dhee – intellect expounded the therapies for the treatment of Kasa – cold, cough (bronchitis) [3]

Types of Kasa – Kasa Bheda:
वातादिजास्त्रयो ये च क्षतजः क्षयजस्तथा| पञ्चैते स्युर्नृणां कासा वर्धमानाः क्षयप्रदाः||४||
There are 5 varieties of Kasa – cough. If exacerbated, they may cause cachexia.
These varieties are as follows:
1. Vataja Kasa – caused by Vata Dosha
2. Paittika Kasa – caused by Pitta
3. Kaphaja Kasa – caused by Kapha and
4. Kshayaja Kasa – caused by the diminution of tissues/chest/tuberculosis and
5. Kshataja Kasa – caused by the diminution of tissue elements i.e., tissue depletion or tubercular bronchitis [4]

Kasa Poorvaroopa: Premonitory Signs and Symptoms of Kasa – cold, cough
पूर्वरूपं भवेतेषां शूकपूर्ण गलास्यता|
कण्ठे कण्डूश्च भोज्यानामवरोधश्च जायते||५||
1. Shuka poorna galasyata – Sensation as if the throat and mouth are filled with bristles (a feeling of congestion in the throat)
2. Kante kandu – Itching sensation in throat and
3. Bhojyanam avarodha – Obstruction to the movement of food in the gullet. [5]

Kasa Samprapti: Pathogenesis
अधःप्रतिहतो वायुरूर्ध्वस्रोतःसमाश्रितः| उदानभावमापन्नः कण्ठे सक्तस्तथोरसि||६||
आविश्य शिरसः खानि सर्वाणि प्रतिपूरयन्| आभञ्जन्नाक्षिपन् देहं हनुमन्ये तथाऽक्षिणी||७||

नेत्रे पृष्ठमुरःपार्श्वे निर्भुज्य स्तम्भयंस्ततः| शुष्को वा सकफो वाऽपि कसनात्कास उच्यते||८||

Kasa Samprapti:

Vata Dosha gets obstructed in the lower part of the body. It moves upwards, afflicts the channels of circulation in the upper part of the body, takes over (afflicts) the function of Udana vata (i.e., the function of respiration), and gets lodged in the throat and the chest.

This Vata afflicts and fills up all the channels (cavities) of the head to cause bending (Abhanjan= breaking) and flexing (Akshipan) of the body, jaws, sides of the neck and eyes

Thereafter, this Vata having caused contraction (Nirhujya) and stiffness (Stambhayan) of eyes, back and sides of the chest, gives rise to coughing (Kasanat) which may be dry or with phlegm because of which it is called Kasa – cough. [6–8]

Causes of variation in Pain etc.

प्रतिघात विशेषेण तस्य वायोः सरंहसः| वेदना शब्द वैशिष्ट्यं कासानामुपजायते||९||

Specific varieties in the pain and sound associated with different types of Kasa – cold, cough are caused by the specific nature of the obstruction [by Kapha etc.] to the forcefully moving vata. [9]

Vataja Kasa Nidana:

रूक्ष शीत कषायाल्प प्रमितानशनं स्त्रियः| वेगधारणमायासो वातकास प्रवर्तकाः||१०||

The causative factors of Vatika Kasa are as follows:

1. Ruksha sheeta kashaya anna sevana – Intake of dry, cold and astringent food

2. Pramitashana – Intake of food in less quantity or much less in quantity (Pramita) or not taking food at all (Anasana)

3. Stree vegadharana – Excessive indulgence in sex

4. Vegadharana – Suppression of natural urges and

5. Aayasa – Excessive physical strain

Vatika Kasa Lakshana – signs and symptoms:

हृत्पार्श्वोरःशिरःशूल स्वरभेदकरो भृशम्| शुष्कोरःकण्ठवक्रस्य हृष्टलोम्नः प्रताम्यतः||११||

निर्घोषदैन्यस्तनन दौर्बल्य क्षोभ मोहकृत्| शुष्क कासः कफं शुष्कं कृच्छ्रान्मुक्त्वाऽल्पतां व्रजेत्||१२||

स्निग्धाम्ललवणोष्णैश्च भुक्तपीतैः प्रशाम्यति| ऊर्ध्ववातस्य जीर्णेऽन्ने वेगवान्मारुतो भवेत्||१३||

The signs and symptoms of Vatika Kasa are as follows:

1. Hrit parshva uru shira shula – Excruciating pain in cardiac region, in the sides of the chest and in the chest, headache

2. Svara bheda – Excessive hoarseness of voice

3. Shushka ura kantha vaktra – Dryness in the chest, throat and mouth

4. Hrushtalomnah – Horripilation and fainting

5. Nirghosha dainyastanana – Resonant sound during coughing, feeling of prostration, hollow sound during coughing

6. Daurbalya, ksobha moha – Weakness, agitation and unconsciousness

7. Suska kasa – dry cough

8. Kapham sushka – The phlegm that comes out with pain is semi–solid (dry)

9. Snigdha amla lavana bhukta – The coughing gets alleviated by food and drinks that are unctuous, sour, saline and warm and

10. Urdhva vata jirne anna – The upward moving Vata (which is the cause of this ailment) gets all the more aggravated after the digestion of food. [11–13]

Paittka Kasa Nidana

कटुकोष्ण विदाह्यम्ल क्षाराणामतिसेवनम्| पित्त कासकरं क्रोधः सन्तापश्चाग्निसूर्यजः||१४||

The causative factors of Pittaja Kasa are as follows:

1. Katu ushna vidahi amla kshara ati sevanam – Excessive intake of pungent, hot, Vidahi (which causes burning sensation), sour and Alkaline Food

2. Krodha – Anger and

3. Santapa agni suryajah – Exposure to the heat of the fire and Sun [14]

Pittaj Kasa Lakshana – signs and symptoms:

पीत निष्ठीवनाक्षित्वं तिक्तास्यत्वं स्वरामयः| उरोधूमायनं तृष्णा दाहो मोहोऽरुचिर्भ्रमः||१५||

प्रततं कासमानश्च ज्योतींषीव च पश्यति| श्लेष्माणं पित्तसंसृष्टं निष्ठीवति च पैत्तिके||१६||

The signs and symptoms of Pittaja Kasa are as follows:

1. Peeta nisthivana akshi – Yellowness of the sputum and eyes

2. Tikta aasya – Bitterness in the mouth

3. Svara amayah – impairment of voice

4. Uro dhumayanam – A feeling as if smoke is being vomited out of the chest (smoky eructation)

5. Trushna, Daha, Moha, Aruchi, Bhrama – Morbid thirst, burning sensation, unconsciousness, anorexia and giddiness

6. Jyotimshiva pashyati – Appearance of star like particles in front of the eyes which coughing continuously and

7. Sleshmanam pitta samsrstanam – The patient spits out phlegm mixed with Pitta [15–16]

Kaphaja Kasa Nidana:

गुर्वभिष्यन्दि मधुर स्निग्ध स्वप्नाविचेष्टनैः| वृद्धः श्लेष्माऽनिलं रुद्ध्वा कफकासं करोति हि||१७||

The causative factors of Kaphaja (shlaishmika) Kasa are as follows:

1. Guru, Abhishyandi, Madhura, Snigdha Sevana – Intake of heavy, Abhisyandin (ingredients which cause obstruction to the channels of circulation), sweet and unctuous ingredients [in excess] and

2. Svapna vichesta – Excessive sleep and indolence

3. vṛddhaḥ śleṣmā'nilaṃ ruddhvā – The Kapha gets aggravated because of the above–mentioned regimens and obstructs the movement of vata which gives rise to Kaphaja Kasa. [17]

Kaphaja Kasa Lakshana – signs and symptoms:

मन्दाग्नित्वारुचि च्छर्दि पीनसोत्क्लेश गौरवैः| लोम हर्षास्य माधुर्य क्लेद संसदनैर्युतम्||१८||

बहुलं मधुरं स्निग्धं निष्ठीवति घनं कफम्| कासमानो ह्यरुग् वक्षः सम्पूर्णमिव मन्यते||१९||

The signs and symptoms of Kaphaja Kasa are as follows:

1. Manda agni – – Suppression of the power of digestion

2. Aruchi, Chardi, Pinasa, Utklesha, Gaurava – Anorexia, vomiting, chronic rhinitis, Nausea and feeling of heaviness in the body

3. Loma harsha, madhurya, kleda samsadana, bahulam madhuram snigdha nisthivan ghana kapham –Horripilation, Sweetness and stickiness in the mouth and asthenia, spitting of thick phlegm in large quantity which is sweet in taste and unctuous

4. No feeling of pain in the chest while coughing and

5. Vaksha sampurna – Feeling of fullness in the chest [18–19]

Etiology of Ksataja Kasa

अतिव्यवाय भाराध्वयुद्धाश्वगज विग्रहैः| रूक्षस्योरः क्षतं वायुर्गृहीत्वा कासमावहेत्||२०||

The causative factors of Kshataja Kasa – bronchitis caused by injury are as follows:

1. Ati vyavaya – Excessive indulgence in sex

2. Bharadhva – Carrying excessively heavy load

3. Walking excessively long distance

4. Yudha asva gaja vigraha – Indulgence in fighting and excessive indulgence in restraining the movement of horses and elephants

5. The above–mentioned factors cause injury to the chest (lungs) and bring about dryness in the body.

This, in its turn, causes aggravation of vata, which gives rise to Kshataj Kasa – (bronchitis caused by injury). [20]

Kshataja Kasa laksana:

स पूर्वं कासते शुष्कं ततः ष्ठीवेत् सशोणितम्| कण्ठेन रुजताऽत्यर्थं विरुग्णेनेव चोरसा||२१||

सूचीभिरिव तीक्ष्णाभिस्तुद्यमानेन शूलिना| दुःखस्पर्शेन शूलेन भेदपीडाभितापिना||२२||

पर्वभेद ज्वर श्वास तृष्णा वैस्वर्य पीडितः| पारावत इवाकूजन् कास वेगात्क्षतोद्भवात्||२३||

The signs and symptoms of Ksataja Kasa are as follows:

1. In the beginning, the patient coughs without any phlegm output, but thereafter, he spits out phlegm along with blood.

2. Kanthena rujata – He experiences excessive pain in the throat and feels as if the chest is cracking

3. Suchibhiriva tikshnaabhistudyamanena shulina – He feels pricking pain as if pricked by sharp needles

4. Dukha sparshena shulena – He gets excruciating pain and discomfort by touch

5. He feels miserable because of piercing type of pain

6. Parva bheda –He gets afflicted with pain in the joints of fingers and toes,

7. Jwara – fever,

8. Shvasa – dysponea,

9. Trushna – morbid thirst and

10. Svara bheda – hoarseness of voice and

11. Paravata iva kujan – While coughing he produces cooing sound like that of a pigeon. [21–23]

Kshayaja Kasa Nidana

विषमासात्म्य भोज्यातिव्यवायाद्वेग निग्रहात्| घृणिनां शोचतां नृणां व्यापन्नेऽग्नौ त्रयो मलाः||२४||

कुपिताः क्षयजं कासं कुर्युर्देहक्षयप्रदम्|

The causative factors of Ksayaja Kasa are as follows:

1. Vishama asatmya – Intake of Visama or irregular (vide Cikitsa 15: 236) type of meals and unwholesome food.

2. Ati vyavaya – Excessive indulgence in sex

3. Udvega nigrahat – Suppression of natural urges

4. Ghrininam shocatam nrnam– Immensely hateful disposition and

5. Excessive worry.

Because of the above–mentioned factors, the Agni (Gastric fire) gets adversely affected, and consequently, all the 3 Doshas get aggravated giving rise to Ksayaja Kasa which causes emaciation of the body. [24– 25½]

The first cause – Sahasa, gives rise to signs and symptoms which are similar to Ksataja Kasa which is already explained in the verse no 23 above. The remaining 3 factors give rise to Ksayaja Kasa which is being presently explained.

Kshayaja Kasa Lakshana and Upashaya

दुर्गन्धं हरितं रक्तं ष्ठीवेत् पूयोपमं कफम्||२५||

स्थानादुत्कासमानश्च हृदयं मन्यते च्युतम्| अकस्मादुष्णशीतार्तो बह्वाशी दुर्बलः कृशः||२६||

स्निग्धाच्छमुखवर्णत्वक् श्रीमद्दर्शनलोचनः| पाणिपादतलैः श्लक्ष्णैः सततासूयको घृणी||२७||

ज्वरो मिश्राकृतिस्तस्य पार्श्वरुक् पीनसोऽरुचिः| भिन्नसंहतवर्चस्त्वं स्वरभेदोऽनिमित्ततः||२८||

इत्येष क्षयजः कासः क्षीणानां देहनाशनः| साध्यो बलवतां वा स्याद्याप्यस्त्वेवं क्षतोत्थितः||२९||

नवौ कदाचित् सिध्येतामेतौ पादगुणान्वितौ| स्थविराणां जराकासः सर्वो याप्यः प्रकीर्तितः||३०||

The signs and symptoms of Ksayaja Kasa are as follows:

1. Durgandham haritam raktam sthivana puyopamam – The patient spits phlegm which is foul smelling, green or red

in colour, and which is like pus

2. Hrdayam manyate chyutam – While coughing, he feels as if the heart is displaced (falling down from its normal location)

3. Akasmath ushna shita aarto – He is suddenly afflicted with both hot and cold sensations

4. He consumes food in excessive quantity

5. Bahva durbala krshi – He become weak and emaciated

6. Snigdha mukha varna tvak – His face, complexion and skin become clean and unctuous

7. Darshan lochana– His appearance becomes gracious with his eyes glowing

8. Slakshna pani pada tala – The palms of his hands and soles of his feet become smooth

9. He always rises to find fault with others, and develops immensely hateful disposition

10. He suffers from fever where signs and symptoms of all the aggravated Doshas are manifested.

11. Parshva ruk – He suffers from pain in the sides of the chest,

12. Pinasa – chronic rhinitis, and

13. Aruchi – anorexia

14. Even without any plausible cause, his stool becomes sometimes compact in form and sometimes loose and

15. Svara bheda – His voice becomes hoarse

Prognosis of Kshayaj Kas:

This is called Ksayaja Kasa which leads to the death of the patient if he is already very weak.

If the patient is strong, then the disease can be cured.

Kshataja Kasa [described in the verse nos. 20–23] is palliable if the patient is strong.

If these 2 ailments (Ksataja Kasa and Ksayaja Kasa) are in their initial stage, and if all the 4 limbs of treatment (viz, physician, drugs, attendants and the patient himself) are endowed with efficiency, then both of these are at times curable.

All the types of Kasa are however palliable if the patient is old. [25½ –30]

Kasa Chikitsa Sutra: Line of treatment:

त्रीन्साध्यान्साधयेत्पूर्वान् पथ्यैर्याप्यांश्च यापयेत्| चिकित्सामत ऊर्ध्वं तु शृणु कासनिबर्हिणीम्||३१||

The first 3 types of Kasa [viz, Vatika Kasa, Paittika Kasa, and Shleshmaj Kasa] are curable and should hence be treated. The other types of kasa (kshataja, kshayaja) are palliable and hence shall be palliated/nourished with wholcsome foods and activities/practices. The treatment of different types of Kasa is explained hereafter. [31]

Vatika Kasa – Line of Treatment

रूक्षस्यानिलजं कासमादौ स्नेहैरुपाचरेत्| सर्पिर्भिर्बस्तिभिः पेया यूष क्षीर रसादिभिः||३२||

वातघ्नसिद्धैः स्नेहाद्यैर्धूमैर्लेहैश्च युक्तितः| अभ्यङ्गैः परिषेकैश्च स्निग्धैः स्वेदैश्च बुद्धिमान्||३३||

बस्तिभिर्बद्धविड्वातं शुष्कोर्ध्व चोर्ध्वभक्तिकैः| घृतैः सपितं सकफं जयेत् स्नेहविरेचनैः||३४||

In the event of dryness of body of the patient suffering from Vatika Kasa, a wise physician should first of all treat with Snehana – oleation therapy, Anuvasana basti – Medicated enema, Peya (thin gruel), Yusa (vegetable soup), Ksheera – milk and Rasa (meat soup) prepared by boiling with vata– alleviating drugs.

The patient is given an unctuous diet, Dhuma – smoking, Leha – linctus (medicated recipes), Abhyanga – massage, Pariseka (sprinkling of warm water) and unctuous fomentation appropriately.

Vataja kasa with constipation and flatulence is treated with medicated enema.

If the patient has dryness in the upper part of his body, and the ailment is associated with aggravated Pitta, then he is given medicated ghee after the intake of food (urdhva– bhaktika).

If the patient has dryness of the upper part of the body, and the ailment is associated with aggravated Kapha, then he is given unctuous purgative. [32–34]

Kantakari Ghrita

कण्टकारी गुडूचीभ्यां पृथक् त्रिंशत्पलाद्रसे| प्रस्थः सिद्धो घृताद्वात कासनुद्वह्नि दीपनः||३५||

इति कण्टकारीघृतम्|

1 Prastha (768 g) of Ghee is cooked by adding 30 Palas of each of the juice (or decoction) of

Kantakari – Yellow berried nightshade (whole plant) – Solanum xanthcarpum and

Guduchi –Tinospora cordifolia intake of this medicated ghee cures Vatika kasa. It also promotes the power of digestion. Thus ends the description of Kantakari Ghrita. [35]

Pippalyadi Ghrita

पिप्पली पिप्पलीमूल चव्य चित्रक नागरैः| धान्य पाठा वचा रास्ना यष्ट्याह्व क्षार हिङ्गुभिः||३६||

कोलमात्रैर्घृत प्रस्था ददशमूली रसाढके| सिद्धा च्चतुर्थिकां पीत्वा पेयामण्डं पिबेदनु||३७||

तच्छ्वास कास हृत्पार्श्व ग्रहणीदोष गुल्मनुत्| पिप्पल्याद्यं घृतं चैतदात्रेयेण प्रकीर्तितम्||३८||

इति पिप्पल्यादिघृतम्|

1 Prastha of Ghee is cooked by adding 1 Adhaka of the decoction of Dashamula, and the paste of 1 Kola of each of

Pippali, Pippali Mula, Chavya, Nagara, Dhanya, Patha, Vacha, Rasna, Yasti–Madhu, Ksara, Hingu

After taking 1 Chaturthika (Pala) of this medicated ghee, the patient is given Peya–manda (upper part of the thin gruel).

This recipe called Pippalayadi–Ghrita is propounded by Atreya.

It cures

Shvasa – Asthma, Kasa – cough, Hrud roga – heart diseases, Parshva shula – pain in the sides of the chest, Grahani Dosha – Malabsorption syndrome, Irritable Bowel Syndrome– (sprue syndrome) and Gulma (Phantom tumor)

Thus, ends the description of Pippalyadi ghruta. [36–38]

Trayushanadi Ghrita

त्र्यूषणं त्रिफलां द्राक्षां काश्मर्याणि परूषकम्| द्वे पाठे देवदार्वृद्धिं स्वगुप्तां चित्रकं शटीम्||३९||

ब्राह्मीं तामलकीं मेदां काकनासां शतावरीम्|

त्रिकण्टकं विदारीं च पिष्ट्वा कर्षसमं घृतात्||४०|| प्रस्थं चतुर्गुणे क्षीरे सिद्धं कासहरं पिबेत्|

ज्वर गुल्मारुचि प्लीह शिरो हृत्पार्श्व शूलनुत्||४१|| कामलाशोंऽनिलाष्ठीला क्षत शोष क्षयापहम्|

त्र्यूषणं नाम विख्यातमेतद्घृतमनुत्तमम्||४२||

इति त्र्यूषणाद्यं घृतम्|

1 Prastha of Ghee is cooked by adding 4 Prasthas of milk and the paste of 1 Karsha each of

Sunthi – Zingiber officinale

Pippali – Piper longum, Maricha – Piper nigrum [taken together these three drugs are called Tryusana; hence the title of the recipe is Tryushanadya–Ghrita], Haritaki – Terminalia chebula, Bibhitaka – Terminalia bellerica, Amalaki (Indian gooseberry fruit – Emblica officinalis Gaertn), Draksha – Vitis vinfera, Kashmarya – Gmelina arborea, Parushaka – Grewia asiatica, 2 varieties of Patha – Cyclea peltata, Meda, Shatavari – Asparagus racemosus, Trikantaka, Vidari

This is an effective recipe for the cure of Kasa.

It also cures

Jwara – fever, Gulma – abdominal tumor, distension (phantom tumor), Anoxia, Pliha – splenic disorders, Shiro shula – headache, Hrt parshva shula – pain in the cardiac region and sides of the chest, Kamala –jaundice, Arshas – piles, Vataja Asthila (hard tumor), Phthisis, Kshaya – depletion of body tissues and Yakshma – tuberculosis

This excellent recipe of medicated ghee is well known as Tryusanadya–Ghrita.

Thus, ends the description of Tryusanadya–Ghrita [39–42]

Rasna Ghrita

द्रोणेऽपां साधयेद्द्रास्नां दशमूलीं शतावरीम्| पलिकां माणिकांशांस्तु कुलत्थान्बदरान्यवान्||४३||

तुलार्ध चाजमांसस्य पादशेषेण तेन च| घृताढकं समक्षीरं जीवनीयैः पलोन्मितैः||४४||

सिद्धं तद्दशभिः कल्कैर्नस्यपानानुवासनैः| समीक्ष्य वातरोगेषु यथावस्थं प्रयोजयेत्||४५||
पञ्चकासान् शिरःकम्पं शूलं वङ्क्षण योनिजम्| सर्वाङ्गैकाङ्गरोगांश्च सप्लीहोर्ध्वानिलाञ्जयेत्||४६||
इति रास्नाघृतम्|

In 1 Drona (12.288 liters) of water,

1 Pala (48 g) of each of

Rasna, Bilva, Syonaka, Gambhari, Patala, Ganikarika, Shalaparni, PrsniParni, Brhati, Kantakari, Goksura

1 Manika of each of

Kulatha, Badara

½ tula of Goat–meat is added and boiled till 1/4th of water remains.

To this decoction, 1 Adhaka of each of ghee and milk, and [the paste of] 1 Pala of each of the 10 drugs belonging to the Jivaniya group [vide Sutra 4: 9] is added and cooked.

This medicated ghee is used as Nasya (inhalation therapy), Pana (as drink) and Anuvasana (a type of medicated enema) in the appropriate stage of Vata–roga.

It cures

5 types of Kasa,

Tremor of head,

Colic pain in the inguinal region and genital tract,

Diseases afflicting the whole body or only one limb of the body,

Pliha roga – Splenic disorders and

Urdhva–Vata (upward movement of vata)

Thus, ends, the description of Rasna–Grtha. [43–46]

Vidangadi Churna

विडङ्गं नागरं रास्ना पिप्पली हिङ्गु सैन्धवम्| भार्गी क्षारश्च तच्चूर्णं पिबेद्वा घृतमात्रया||४७||
सकफेऽनिलजे कासे श्वास हिक्काहताग्निषु|

Intake of the powder of

Vidanga, Nagara, Rasna, Pippali, Hingu, Saindhava, Bhargi and Ksara (alkali preparation) along with appropriate quantity of ghee is useful in Vatika Kasa associated with Kapha, Asthma, Hiccup and Suppression of the power of digestion. [47 –1/2 48]

DviKsharadi Churna and Shatyadi–Kalka

द्वौ क्षारौ पञ्चकोलानि पञ्चैव लवणानि च||४८||
शटी नागरकोदीच्य कल्कं वा वस्त्र गालितम्| पाययेत घृतोन्मिश्रं वातकास निबर्हणम्||४९||

The ingredients used:

2 types of Ksara (yava Ksara and Svarji Ksara),

Pippali, Pippali, Chavya, Chitraka, Nagara, Saindhava, Sauvarcala, Vida, Audbhida and Samudra is made of powder.

Intake of this powder along with appropriate quantity of ghee cures Vataja kasa.

The paste of Sati, Nagara and Udichya is squeezed through a cloth, and the paste out of it is added with ghee in appropriate quantity.

Intake of this recipe cures Vatika Kasa. [48 ½ – 49]

Duralabhadi Leha

दुरालभां शटीं द्राक्षां शृङ्गवेरं सितोपलाम्| लिह्यात् कर्कटशृङ्गीं च कासे तैलेन वातजे||५०||

The ingredients used:

Powder of Duralabha, Sati, Raksa, Srngavera, Sitopala (sugar of big crystal) and Karkata–Srngi is mixed with oil, and made to a linctus form. Intake of this recipe cures Vataja Kasa.

Duhsparshadi Leha

दुःस्पर्शी पिप्पली मुस्तं भार्गी कर्कटकीं शटीम्‌। पुराणगुडतैलाभ्यां चूर्णितं वाऽपि लेहयेत्‌।।५१।।

The ingredients used: Powder of

Duhsparsa

Pippali – Piper longum,

Musta – Nut grass (root) – Cyperus rotundus,

Bharangi – Clerodendrum serratum

Karkataki (Karkata– Srngi)

Sati – Hedychium spicatum is mixed with old Jaggery and oil, and made to a linctus form.

Intake of this recipe cures Vatika Kasa. [51]

Vidangadi Leha

विडङ्गं सैन्धवं कुष्ठं व्योषं हिङ्गु मनःशिलाम्‌। मधु सर्पिर्युतं कास हिक्का श्वासं जयेल्लिहन्‌।।५२।।

The powder of Vidanga, Saindhava, Kustha, Sunthi, Pippali, Maricha, Hingu, Manah– Sila is added with honey and ghee, and made to a linctus form.

Intake of this recipe cures Kasa, hiccup and asthma.

Chitrakadi Leha

चित्रकं पिप्पलीमूलं व्योषं हिङ्गु दुरालभाम्‌। शटीं पुष्करमूलं च श्रेयसीं सुरसां वचाम्‌।।५३।।

भार्गीं छिन्नरुहां रास्नां शृङ्गीं द्राक्षां च कार्षिकान्‌। कल्कानर्धतुलाक्वाथे निदिग्ध्याः पलविंशतिम्‌।।५४।।

दत्त्वा मत्स्यण्डिकायाश्च घृताच्च कुडवं पचेत्‌। सिद्धं शीतं पृथक् क्षौद्रपिप्पलीकुडवान्वितम्‌।।५५।।

चतुष्पलं तुगाक्षीर्याश्चूर्णितं तत्र दापयेत्‌। लेहयेत् कास हृद्रोग श्वास गुल्म निवारणम्‌।।५६।।

इति चित्रकादिलेहः।

In ½ Tula of the decoction of Nidigdhika (Kantakari – Yellow berried nightshade (whole plant) – Solanum xanthcarpum)

Powder or paste of 1 Karsa of each of

Chitraka, Pippali– Mula, Sunthi, Pippali, Marica, Hingu, Duralabha, Sati, Puskaramula, Sreyasi, Surasa, Vacha, Bharngi, Chinna–Ruha, Rasna, Srngi and Draksa is added.

To this,

20 Palas of Matsyandika (a sugar –cane preparation) and

1 Kudava of Ghee is added and cooked.

Thereafter, when it becomes cool of its own,

1 Kudava of each

Honey and

Pippali – Long pepper fruit – Piper longum powder, and

4 palas of the powder of Tuga–Ksiri is added.

Intake of this linctus cures

Kasa

Hrud roga – heart diseases,

Shvasa – Asthma and

Gulma – abdominal tumour, distension (phantom tumour)

Thus, ends the description of Chitrakadi leha [53– 56]

Agastya Haritaki

दशमूलीं स्वयङ्गुप्तां शङ्खपुष्पीं शटीं बलाम्‌। हस्तिपिप्पल्यपामार्ग पिप्पलीमूल चित्रकान्‌।।५७।।

भार्गीं पुष्करमूलं च द्विपलांशं यवाढकम्‌। हरीतकी शतं चैकं जले पञ्चाढके पचेत्‌।।५८।।

यवैः स्विन्नैः कषायं तं पूतं तच्चाभयाशतम्‌। पचेद्गुडतुलां दत्त्वा कुडवं च पृथग्घृतात्‌।।५९।।

तैलात् सपिप्पलीचूर्णात् सिद्धशीते च माक्षिकात्| लिह्याद्द्वे चाभये नित्यमतः खादेद्रसायनात्||६०||
तद्वलीपलितं हन्ति वर्णायुर्बलवर्धनम्| पञ्चकासान् क्षयं श्वासं हिक्कां च विषमज्वरम्||६१||
हन्यात्तथाऽशो ग्रहणी हृद्रोगारुचि पीनसान्| अगस्त्यविहितं श्रेष्ठं रसायनमिदं शुभम्||६२||
इत्यगस्त्यहरीतकी|

2 Palas of each of

Dashamoola, Svayangupta, ShankhaPuspi, Shati, Bala, Hasti–Pippali, Apamarga, Pippali, Chitraka, Bharngi and PuskaraMula is added with

1 Adhaka of Yava and

100 fruits of Haritaki – Terminalia chebula

By adding 5 Adhakas of water, these drugs are cooked till the grains of Yava (barley) becomes soft (Svina) and then the decoction is strained out.

These 100 fruits of Abhaya – Harad – Terminalia chebula are then added with the above mentioned decoction, 1 Tula of Jaggery

1 Kudava of each of

Ghee,

Sesame oil and Powder of Pippali

The recipe is then cooked. Thereafter, when it becomes cool, 1 Kuduva of honey is added.

This is a rejuvenating recipe.

Intake of 2 fruits of Abhaya – Harad – Terminalia chebula, thus processed, every day, cures

Wrinkling of the skin and greying of hair (process of aging), and

Promotes complexion, longevity as well as strength

It also cures

5 varieties of Kasa,

Ksaya—depletion of body tissues, Shvasa – Asthma, Hikka – Hiccup, Visama–Jvara – fever (irregular fever), Arshas – Piles, Grahani – Malabsorption syndrome, Hrud roga – heart diseases, Aruchi – anorexia and Pinasa – chronic rhinitis

This excellent rejuvenating recipe propounded by the sage Agastya is auspicious.

Thus, ends the description of Agastya–Haritaki [57–62]

Recipes for Vatika Kasa

सैन्धवं पिप्पलीं भार्गीं शृङ्गवेरं दुरालभाम्| दाडिमाम्लेन कोष्णेन भार्गीनागरमम्बुना||६३||
पिबेत् खदिरसारं वा मदिरादधिमस्तुभिः| अथवा पिप्पलीकल्कं घृतभृष्टं ससैन्धवम्||६४||

Intake of the powder of Saindhava, Pippali, Bharngi, Sringavera – fresh ginger and

Duralabha along with the Luke warm juice of sour dadima – Punica granatum or

The powder of Bhrangi and Nagara – Zingiber officinale should be consumed with hot water.

Intake of powder of Khadirasara –Gum acacia – Acacia catechu along with Madira (alcohol) or curds or supernatant watery portion of curds/butter milk [cures Vatikta Kasa]

Intake of the Paste of Pippali – Long pepper fruit fried (sizzled) with ghee and mixed with a little of Saindhava [cures Vatika kasa] [63–64]

Dhoomapana – Smoking therapy

शिरसः पीडने स्रावे नासाया हृदि ताम्यति| कास प्रतिश्यायवतां धूमं वैद्यः प्रयोजयेत्||६५||
दशाङ्गुलोन्मितां नाडीमथवाऽष्टाङ्गुलोन्मिताम्| शराव सम्पुट च्छिद्रे कृत्वा जिह्मां विचक्षणः||६६||
वैरेचनं मुखेनैव कासवान् धूममा पिबेत्| तमुरः केवलं प्राप्तं मुखेनैवोद्वमेत् पुनः||६७||
स ह्यस्य तैक्ष्ण्यादिवच्छिद्य श्लेष्माणमुरसि स्थितम्| निष्कृष्य शमयेत् कासं वातश्लेष्मसमुद्भवम्||६८||

Dhoomapana – Smoking therapy

If there is headache, running nose and arrhythmia of the heart in a patient suffering from Kasa and Pratishyaya

(Rhinitis), then the physician should administer Dhuma (smoking therapy).

A wise physician should keep the ingredients of the recipe which cause elimination of Doshas from the head (virecana) inside 2 earthen plates with their brims sealed with mud–smeared cloth (sarava– Samputa).

In the upper plate there should be a hole to which a tube, 10 or 8 Angulas in length, is inserted in slightly curved form.

The patient of Kasa should smoke the fume emanating from this tube through his mouth. After the smoke pervades the entire chest (lungs), it is smoked out through the mouth. Because of the sharpness of the ingredients used in this recipe, the phlegm located in the chest gets detached and forcibly thrown out as a result of which Kasa – cold; cough caused by vata and Kapha gets alleviated. [65–68]

Manahsiladi– Dhuma

मनःशिलाल मधुक मांसीमुस्तेड्गुदैः पिबेत्| धूमं तस्यानु च क्षीरं सुखोष्णं सगुडं पिबेत्||६९||

एष कासान् पृथग्दोष सन्निपात समुद्भवान्| धूमो हन्यादसंसिद्धानन्यैर्योगशतैरपि||७०||

After taking the smoke of Manahsila, Ala (Haritala), Madhuka – Madhuca longifolia, Mamsi, Musta – Nut grass (root) – Cyperus rotundus and Ingudi – Balanites aegyptiaca, the patient should take luke–warm milk added with Jaggery.

This cures Kasas caused by the 3 Doshas individually and also jointly (Sannipatika) even if such ailments were not amenable to hundreds of other recipes administered earlier. [69–70]

Prapaundarikadi Dhuma Varti:

प्रपौण्डरीकं मधुकं शाङ्गेष्टां समनःशिलाम्| मरिचं पिप्पली द्राक्षामेलां सुरसमञ्जरीम्||७१||

कृत्वा वर्तिं पिबेद्धूमं क्षौमचेलानुवर्तिताम्| घृताक्तामनु च क्षीरं गुडोदकमथापि वा||७२||

The paste of Prapaundraika,

Madhuka, Sarngesta (Gunja), Manashila, Maricha, Pippali, Draksa, Ela and the inflorescence of Surasa is smeared over a silken cloth, and a varti (cigar) is prepared.

This cigar is smeared with ghee and used for smoking.

The patient should, thereafter, take milk or water mixed with jaggery.

This cures different types of Kasa mentioned in the verse no.70 above. [71–72]

Manashiladi Dhumavarti

मनःशिलैला मरिचक्षाराञ्जनकुटन्नटैः| वंश लेखन सेव्यालक्षौमलक्तक रोहिषैः ||७३||

पूर्वकल्पेन धूमोऽयं सानुपानो विधीयते| मनःशिलाले तद्वच्च पिप्पली नागरैः सह||७४||

According to the procedure laid down in the earlier recipe, smoking therapy is administered with

ManahSila, Ela – Cardamom, Maricha, Kshara – Yavakshar, Anjana, Kutannata, Vamsalochana, Sevya, Ala, Ksauma, Aalaktaka and Rohisa (Gandha–Trna).

After taking this therapy, the patient should use the post–prandial drink as suggested

Similarly, the recipes for smoking therapy can the prepared with Manah Sila, Ala, Pippali – Long pepper fruit and Nagara (ginger). [73–74]

Ingudi Tvagadi Dhuma

त्वगैड्गुदी बृहत्यौ द्वे तालमूली मनःशिला| कार्पासास्थ्यश्वगन्धा च धूमः कास विनाशनः||७५||

The smoking therapy with the recipe containing the

Bark of Ingudi – Balanites aegyptiaca

Brhati – Solanum indicum,

Kantakari – Yellow berried nightshade (whole plant) – Solanum xanthcarpum, Tala–Muli,

Manahsila, Seeds of Karpasa – Gossypium herbaceum and

Asvagandha – Withania somnifera cures [vatika type] Kasa. [75]

Food preparation for Vatika Kasa –

ग्राम्यानूपौदकैः शालि यवगोधूमषष्टिकान्| रसैर्माषात्मगुप्तानां यूषैर्वा भोजयेदिधतान्||७६||

यवानी पिप्पली बिल्वमध्यनागर चित्रकैः| रास्नाजाजी पृथक्पर्णी पलाश शटि पौष्करैः||७७||

स्निग्धाम्ल लवणां सिद्धां पेयामनिलजे पिबेत्| कटी हृत्पार्श्व कोष्ठार्ति श्वास हिक्काप्रणाशिनीम्||७८||

दशमूलरसे तद्वत्पञ्चकोलगुडान्विताम्| सिद्धां समतिलां दद्यात्क्षीरे वाऽपि ससैन्धवाम्||७९||

मात्स्य कौक्कुट वाराहैरामिषैर्वा घृतान्विताम्| सिद्धां ससैन्धवां पेयां वातकासी पिबेन्नरः||८०||

वास्तुको वायसीशाकं मूलकं सुनिषण्णकम्| स्नेहास्तैलादयो भक्ष्याः क्षीरेक्षुरसगौडिकाः||८१||

दध्यारनालाम्लफलप्रसन्नापानमेव च| शस्यते वातकासे तु स्वाद्वम्ललवणानि च||८२||

इति वातकासचिकित्सा|

Diet for Vataja Kasa:

Intake of sali type of rice, barley, wheat and sastika type of rice along with the soup of the meat of animals which are domesticated (gramya) or those which live in marshy lands (Anupa) or aquatic animals, or along with the soup (yusa) of Masa and Atmagupta is useful [for the patient suffering from Vatika Kasa].

Peya (thin gruel) cooked along with – Yavani, Pippali, Bilva, Nagara, Chitraka, Rasna, Prthak, Palasa, Sati and Puskaramula is added with ghee, sour juice and salt.

Intake of this thin gruel cures

Vatika Kasa,

Hrud Shoola – pain in the cardiac region,

Parshva shoola – Sides of the chest, and Koshta (gastro– intestinal tract), Shvasa – Asthma and

Hikka – hiccup.

Intake of the Peya prepared [by boiling rice etc.] with the decoction of Dasamula and added with the powder of Pancha–Kola and Jaggery is useful in Vatika Kasa.

Intake of the Peya prepared with [rice etc.] equal quantity of sesame seed, and boiled by adding milk [is useful in Vatika Kasa].

Similarly, intake of the peya prepared with [rice etc. and] equal quantity of sesame seed, and added with rock –salt (saindhava) [is useful in Vataja Kasa].

Peya prepared by cooking [rice etc.] with the meat of fish, chicken or pig, and by adding ghee and Saindhava is taken [by a person suffering from Vatika Kasa].

Vastuka, leaves of Vayasi (Kakamachi) – Solanum nigrum, Mulaka – Raphanus sativus, Sunisannaka, Unctuous material, Viz oil etc. food preparations made of milk, sugar– cane juice and jaggery, curd, Aranala (a type of Vinegar), sour fruit, Prasanna (a type of Alcoholic drink), and ingredients which are sweet, sour and saline in taste are useful in Vatika type of Kasa. Thus, ends the description of the treatment of Vatika type of Kasa. [76–82]

Treatment of Paittika Kasa:

Vamana – emetic therapy

पैत्तिके सकफे कासे वमनं सर्पिषा हितम्| तथा मदन काश्मर्य मधुक क्वथितैर्जलैः||८३||

यष्ट्याह्वफलकल्कैर्वा विदारीक्षुरसायुतैः| हृतदोषस्ततः शीतं मधुरं च क्रम भजेत्||८४||

If Paittika Kasa is associated with the aggravation of Kapha, then the patient is given emetic therapy with medicated ghee or with the decoction of Madana – Randia dumetroum, Kashmarya – Gmelina arborea and Madhuka – Madhuca longifolia or with the paste of MadhuYasti – Glyccrhiza glabra and MadanaPhala – mixed with the juice of Vidari – Pureria tuberosa and sugar–cane.

After the aggravated Doshas are eliminated, the patient is treated with cooling therapies, and recipes having sweet ingredients. [83–84]

Virechana – Purgation Therapy for Pittaja Kasa

पैत्ते तनुकफे कासे त्रिवृतां मधुरैर्युताम्| दद्याद्घनकफे तिक्तै विरेकार्थ युतां भिषक्||८५||

स्निग्ध शीतस्तनुकफे रूक्षशीतः कफे घने| क्रमः कार्यः परं भोज्यैः स्नेहैर्लेहैश्च शस्यते||८६||

Purgation therapy:

If in Paittika Kasa, the Phlegm is thin, then the patient is given Virechana (purgation) therapy with Trivrt – Operculina turpethum mixed with sweet drugs.

If the phlegm is thick, then Trivrit – Operculina turpethum mixed with bitter drugs is given for purgation.

After the administration of purgation therapy, Peya (thin gruel described above) is given followed by food preparations, medicated ghee and recipes of linctus. [85–86]

Leha Yoga – linctus recipe:

शृङ्गाटकं पद्मबीजं नीलीसाराणि पिप्पली| पिप्पली मुस्त यष्ट्याह्व द्राक्षा मूर्वामहौषधम्||८७||

लाजाऽमृतफला द्राक्षा त्वक्क्षीरी पिप्पली सिता| पिप्पली पद्मक द्राक्षा बृहत्याश्च फलाद्रसः||८८||

खर्जूरं पिप्पली वांशी श्वदंष्ट्रा चेति पञ्च ते| घृतक्षौद्रयुता लेहाः श्लोकार्धैः पित्तकासिनाम्||८९||

Leha Yoga – linctus recipe:

The patient suffering from Paittk Kasa is given the following 5 recipes in the form of Leha (Linctus) by adding ghee and honey:

1. Sringataka, seeds of Padma, solid extract (Sara – laxative, promotes movement of liquids in channels) of Nili and Pippali – Long pepper fruit – Piper longum

2. Pippali, Musta – Nut grass (root) – Cyperus rotundus, Yasti–Madhu – Glyhccrhiza glabra, Draksa – Vitis vinfera, Murva – Marsedenia tenacissima and Sunthi – Zingiber officinale

3. Laja, Amalaki (Indian gooseberry fruit – Emblica officinalis Gaertn), Draksa – Vitis vinfera, Tvakksiri (Vamsa–Locana), Pippali and Sugar

4. Pippali – Padmaka, Draksa – Vitis vinfera and the juice of fruits of Brhati – Solanum indicum and

5. Kharjura – Dates, Pippali, Vamsi (Vamsa–Locana) and Svadamstra. [87–89]

Sharkaradi Leha

शर्करा चन्दन द्राक्षा मधु धात्रीफलोत्पलैः| पैत्ते, समुस्त मरिचः सकफे, सघृतोऽनिले||९०||

If Kasa is caused exclusively by Pitta, then the patient is given the linctus of Sarkara, Chandana – Santalum album, Draksa – Vitis vinfera, Honey, Dhatriphala and Utpala – Water Lily.

If there is association of Kapha, then the patient is given this recipe along with Musta – Nut grass (root) – Cyperus rotundus and Maricha – Piper nigrum. If, however, it is associated with vata, then this recipe is used along with ghee. [90]

मृद्वीकार्धशतं त्रिंशत्पिप्पलीः शर्करापलम्| लेहयेन्मधुना गोर्वा क्षीरपं च शकृद्रसम्||९१||

50 fruits of Mrdvika, 30 fruits of Pippali – Long pepper fruit – Piper longum and 1 Pala of sugar is added with honey and given to the patient suffering from Paittika Kasa.

The juice of cow–dung mixed with honey can also be given to the patient suffering from Paittika Kasa. While taking this recipe, the patient should drink only milk. [91]

Tvagadi Leha

त्वगेला व्योष मृद्वीका पिप्पलीमूल पौष्करैः| लाजा मुस्त शटी रास्ना धात्रीफल बिभीतकैः||९२||

शर्करा क्षौद्र सर्पिर्भिर्लेहः कास विनाशनः| श्वासं हिक्कां क्षयं चैव हृद्रोगं च प्रणाशयेत्||९३||

The linctus prepared of

Tvak, Ela, Shunti, Pippali, Maricha, Mrudvika, Pippali, Puskaramula, Laja, Musta, Sati, Rasna, Dhatri Phala and Bibhitaka –by adding Sugar, honey and ghee

Indicated in –

Kasa – cough

Hikka – Hiccup,

Kshaya – tuberculosis and

Hrud roga – heart diseases [92–93]

Pippalyadi Leha
पिप्पल्यामलकं द्राक्षां लाक्षां लाजां सितोपलाम्| क्षीरे पक्त्वा घनं शीतं लिह्यात् क्षौद्राष्टभागिकम्||९४||

Pippali, Amalaka, Draksa, Laksa, Laja and Sitopala (sugar of big Crystals) is cooked by adding milk. After it becomes cool, 1/8th part of the honey is added.

Intake of these receipes cures Pittaja Kasa [if the Phlegm has become thick] [94]

विदारीक्षुमृणालानां रसान् क्षीरं सितोपलाम्| पिबेद्वा मधुसंयुक्तं पित्तकासहरं परम्||९५||

Intake of the juice of Vidari, Iksu and Mrnala, milk and sitopala mixed with [an appropriate quantity of] honey, cures Paittika Kasa effectively. [95]

मधुरै जाङ्गल रसैः श्यामाक यव कोद्रवाः| मुद्गादियूषैः शाकैश्च तिक्तकै मात्रया हिताः||९६||

Intake of Shyamaka, Yava (barley) and Kodrava along with the Sweetened soup of the meat of the animals inhabiting Jangala (thinly forested) zone or with the soup of Mudga etc. or with the vegetables having bitter taste is useful [in Paittika Kasa] [96]

Management of Thick and Thin Kapha
घनश्लेष्मणि लेहास्तु तिक्तका मधुसंयुताः| शालयः स्युस्तनुकफे षष्टिकाश्च रसादिभिः||९७||

In the Paittika Kasa, if the phlegm is thick, then the patient is given recipes of Leha (linctus) prepared of bitter drugs along with honey.

If the phlegm is thin, then the patient is given Sali and Sastika types of rice along with meat soup, etc. [97]

Anupana – Post–Prandial Drinks
शर्कराम्भोऽनुपानार्थं द्राक्षेक्षूणां रसाः पयः| सर्वं च मधुरं शीतमविदाहि प्रशस्यते||९८||

In the Pittaja Kasa, water mixed with sugar, grape–juice, sugar cane and milk are useful as Anupana (post Prandial drink).

All things which are sweet in taste and cooling in potency but not Vidahi (which cause burning sensation in the abdomen) are useful in this condition. [98]

काकोली बृहती मेदा युग्मैः सवृषनागरैः| पित्तकासे रसान् क्षीरं यूषांश्चाप्युपकल्पयेत्||९९||

For the Pittaj Kasa, Meat–soup, medicated milk and Vegatable–soup, is prepared by adding

Kakoli, Brhati, Meda, Mahameda, Vasaka and Nagara [99]

Ksheerayoga – Medicated Milk
शरादिपञ्चमूलस्य पिप्पली द्राक्षयोस्तथा| कषायेण शृतं क्षीरं पिबेत् स मधु शर्करम्||१००||

The patient suffering from the Paittika Kasa should take milk boiled by adding decoction of either Saradi– Pancamula (trna Panca mula) or the decoction of Pippali and Draksa, after adding honey and sugar. [100]

Ksheera and Guda Yoga – Recipes of medicated Milk and jaggery
स्थिरा सिता पृश्निपर्णी श्रावणी बृहती युगैः| जीवकर्षभ काकोली तामलक्यृद्धि जीवकैः||१०१||
शृतं पयः पिबेत् कासी ज्वरी दाही क्षतक्षयी| तज्जं वा साधयेत् सर्पिः सक्षीरेक्षुरसं भिषक्||१०२||
जीवकाद्यैर्मधुरकैः फलैश्चाभिषुकादिभिः| कल्कैस्त्रिकार्षिकैः सिद्धे पूतशीते प्रदापयेत्||१०३||
शर्करा पिप्पलीचूर्णं त्वक्क्षीर्या मरिचस्य च| शृङ्गाटकस्य चावाप्य क्षौद्र गर्भान्पलोन्मितान्||१०४||
गुडान् गोधूमचूर्णेन कृत्वा खादेद्दिधताशनः| शुक्रासृग्दोष शोषेषु कासे क्षीणक्षतेषु च||१०५||
Recipes of medicated Milk and jaggery
Milk boiled with Sthira, Sita, PrsniParni, Sravani, Brihati, Kantakari, Jivaka, Rishabaka,Kakoli, Tamalaki, Riddhi

Is useful in the treatment of Kasa, fever, Daha – Burning sensation, Phthisis and Kshaya – depletion of body tissues

The ghee collected from the above mentioned milk is added with milk, sugarcane jucie and the paste of 3 Karsas of each of the sweet drugs belonging to Jivaniya group (vide Sutra 4;9), fruits of Abhisuka etc., (Vatama, Aksoda, Mukulaka and Nikocaka–vide Sutra 27; 157) and cooked.

The ghee is then filtered out and made to cool. To this, the powder of Sarkara, Pippali, Tvak–Ksiri, Maricha, Srngataka and honey is added.

This paste is added with wheat–flour, and Gudas (large size Pills) is prepared out of it.

Intake of these Gudas along with wholesome food cures

Seminal and menstrual diseases,

Kshaya – depletion of body tissue,

Kasa – emaciation and Phthisis. [101– 105]

Recipe for Pittaja Kasa –

शर्करा नागरोदीच्यं कण्टकारी शटीं समम्| पिष्ट्वा रसं पिबेत्पूतं वस्त्रेण घृतमूच्छितम्||१०६||

महिष्यजावि गोक्षीर धात्रीफलरसैः समैः| सर्पिः सिद्धं पिबेद्युक्त्या पित्तकास निबर्हणम्||१०७||

इति पित्तकासचिकित्सा|

The paste of Sarkara (Sugar), Nagara – Zingiber officinale, Udicya, Kantakari – Yellow berried nightshade (whole plant) – Solanum xanthocarpum and Sati – Hedychium spicatum, taken in equal quantities, is squeezed through a cloth. This juice is sizzled with ghee. This cures Paittika Kasa.

Ghee is cooked by adding the milk of buffalo, goat, sheep and cow, and the juice of Amalaki (Indian gooseberry fruit – Emblica officinalis Gaertn), all taken in equal quantities.

Intake of this medicated ghee in appropriate quantity cures Paittika Kasa

Thus, ends the treatment of Pitta–Kasa. [106– 107]

Kaphaja Kasa Chikitsa sutra: Line of treatment

बलिनं वमनैरादौ शोधितं कफकासिनम्| यवान्नैः कटुरूक्षोष्णैः कफघ्नैश्चाप्युपाचरेत्||१०८||

पिप्पलीक्षारिकैर्यूषैः कौलत्थैर्मूलकस्य च| लघून्यन्नानि भुञ्जीत रसैर्वा कटुकान्वितैः||१०९||

धान्वबैलरसैः स्नेहैस्तिलसर्षपबिल्वजैः| मध्वम्लोष्णाम्बुतक्रं वा मद्यं वा निगदं पिबेत्||११०||

पौष्करारग्वधं मूलं पटोलं तैर्निशास्थितम्| जलं मधुयुतं पेयं कालेष्वन्नस्य वा त्रिषु||१११||

Line of treatment of Kaphaja Kasa:

If the patient suffering from Kaphaja kasa is strong, then he is given emetic therapy in the beginning. Thereafter, he is given barley and such other Kapha– alleviating is given barley and such other Kapha–alleviating ingredients as pungent, dry and hot in potency, to eat.

The patient should take

• light food with the soup of Kulattha mixed with the powder of Pippali and alkalies (Yava– Ksara) or

• With the juice of Mulaka or

• With the soup of the meat of animals inhabiting arid zone (Dhanva–cari) or burrows (Bilesaya) prepared by adding pungent drugs, or

• With the oil of mustard and Bilva – Bael – Aegle marmelos.

Anupana – water, sour drinks, warm water, buttermilk, or harmless alcoholic drinks.

Puskaramula – Inula racemosa, root of Aragvadha – Cassia fistula and Patola – Pointed Gourd – Trichosanthes dioica is kept in water for the whole night.

Next morning, the water is strained out and added with honey. This is taken before, during and after meals. [108–111]

Decoction etc.,

Katphaladi Kashaya:

कट्फलं कत्तृणं भार्गीं मुस्तं धान्यं वचाभये| शुण्ठीं पर्पटकं शृङ्गीं सुराह्वं च शृतं जले||११२||
मधुहिङ्गुयुतं पेयं कासे वातकफात्मके| कण्ठरोगे मुखे शूने श्वासहिक्काज्वरेषु च||११३||

Katphala, Kattrna, Bharngi, Musta, Dhanya, Vaca, Abhaya, Sunthi, Parpataka, Srngi, Surahva is boiled with water.

This decoction added with honey and hingu is taken if Kasa is caused by vata and Kapha.

It also cures

Kanta roga – throat diseases, Svayathu – oedema in the face, Shvasa – asthma, Hikka – hiccup and Jwara – fever

Pathadi Yoga:

पाठां शुण्ठीं शटीं मूर्वां गवाक्षीं मुस्तपिप्पलीम्| पिष्ट्वा घर्माम्बुना हिङ्गुसैन्धवाभ्यां युतां पिबेत्||११४||
नागरातिविषे मुस्तं शृङ्गीं कर्कटकस्य च| हरीतकीं शटीं चैव तेनैव विधिना पिबेत्||११५||
तैलभृष्टं च पिप्पल्याः कल्काक्षं सितोपलम्| पिबेद्वा श्लेष्मकासघ्नं कुलत्थरससंयुतम्||११६||
कासमर्दाश्वविट्भृङ्गराजवार्ताकजो रसः| सक्षौद्रः कफकासघ्नः सुरसस्यासितस्य च||११७||

Pathadi Yoga:

The patient should take – Patha, Sunthi, Shati, Murva, Gavakshi, Musta

Pippali in paste from along with warm mixed with

Hingu and Saindhava

In the above mentioned manner, the patient should take – Nagara, Ativisa, Musta, Karkata–Sringi, Haritaki and Sati

1 Aksa of the paste of Pippali, fried with oil is added with Sitopala (sugar having large size cerystal).

Intake of this recipe along with the soup of Kulattha – Dolichos biflorus cures kaphaja Kasa.

Intake of the juice of Kasamarda – Cassia occidentalis, stool of horse, Bhrngaraja – Eclipta alba, Vartaka and black variety of Surasa along with honey cures kaphaja Kasa. [112–117]

Leham Yoga: Recipes of Linctus

देवदारु शटी रास्ना कर्कटाख्या दुरालभा| पिप्पली नागरं मुस्तं पथ्या धात्री सितोपलाः||११८||
मधु तैलयुतावेतौ लेहौ वातानुगे कफे| पिप्पली पिप्पलीमूलं चित्रको हस्तिपिप्पली||११९||
पथ्या तामलकी धात्री भद्रमुस्ता च पिप्पली| देवदार्वभया मुस्तं पिप्पली विश्वभेषजम्||१२०||
विशाला पिप्पली मुस्तं त्रिवृता चेति लेहयेत्| चतुरो मधुना लेहान् कफकासहरान् भिषक्||१२१||
सौवर्चलाभया धात्री पिप्पलीक्षार नागरम्| चूर्णितं सर्पिषा वातकफकासहरं पिबेत्||१२२||

Recipes of Linctus (Leha)

Powders of these are mixed with honey and oil and this linctus cures Kaphaja kasa associated with aggravated vata:

Devadaru, Shati, Rasna, Karkata–Srngi, Duralabha

Powders of these mixed with honey cures Kaphaja Kasa:

Pippali, Nagara, Musta, Pathya, Dhatri, Sitopala

These are made into a linctus by adding honey. Intake of this cures Kaphaja Kasa:

Pathya, Tamalaka, Dhatri, Bhadra

Pippali, Deva–Daru, Abhaya, Musta, Pippali, Visva–Bhesaja Trivrta

Intake of the powder of – Sauvarcala, Abhaya, Dhatri, Pippali, Ksara

Nagara alone with ghee cures Kasa caused by Vata and Kapha. [118–122]

Dashamuladi Ghrita

दशमूलाढके प्रस्थं घृतस्याक्षसमैः पचेत्| पुष्कराह्व शटी बिल्व सुरस व्योष हिङ्गुभिः||१२३||
पेयानुपानं तत् पेयं कासे वातकफात्मके| श्वासरोगेषु सर्वेषु कफवातात्मकेषु च||१२४||
इति दशमूलादि घृतम्|

1 Prastha of ghee is cooked by adding 1 Adhaka of the decoction of Dasamula and the paste of one karsha each of Puskaramula, Sati, Bilva, Surasa, Sunthi, Pippali, Maricha, Hingu

Post prandial drink – Peya (Thin gruel)

It cures Kasa caused by vata and Kapha, and all types of Asthma caused by Vata and Kapha.

Thus, ends the description of Dashamuladi– ghrita. [123–124]

Kantakari Gritha:

समूलफलपत्रायाः कण्टकार्या रसाढके| घृतप्रस्थं बला व्योष विडङ्ग शटि चित्रकैः||१२५||

सौवर्चल यवक्षार पिप्पलीमूल पौष्करैः| वृश्चीर बृहती पथ्या यवानी दाडिमर्धिभिः||१२६||

द्राक्षा पुनर्नवा चव्य दुरालम्भाम्लवेतसैः| शृङ्गी तामलकी भार्गी रास्ना गोक्षुरकैः पचेत्||१२७||

कल्कैस्तत् सर्वकासेषु हिक्काश्वासेषु शस्यते| कण्टकारीघृतं ह्येतत् कफव्याधिनिसूदनम्||१२८||

इति कण्टकारीघृतम्|

1 Adhaka (3.072 l)of the decoction of Kantakari – Solanum xanthocarpum along with its root, fruit and leaf, and 1 Prastha (768 g)of ghee are cooked by adding the paste of

Bala, Sunthi, Pippali, Maricha, Vidanga, Sati, Chitraka, Sauvarcala, Yava, Pippali, Puskara Mula, Vrscira, Brihati, Pathya, Yavani, Dadima, Rddhi, Draksha, Punarnava, Chavya, Duralabha, Amlavetasa, Srngi, Tamalaki, Bhargi, Rasana, Goksuraka

Cures:

All types of Kasa,

Hikka – hiccup and

Shvasa – Asthma.

This is called Kantakari Ghrita and it cures all types of diseases caused by Kapha.

Thus, ends the description of Kantakari grtha. [125–128]

Kulatthadi Ghruta

कुलत्थ रसयुक्तं वा पञ्चकोलशृतं घृतम्| पाययेत् कफजे कासे हिक्काश्वासे च शस्यते||१२९||

इति कुलत्थादिघृतम्|

Ghee cooked with the decoction of Kulattha and [the paste] of Pancha–Kola is useful in Kaphaja Kasa, hiccup and asthma.

Thus, end the description of Kulatthandi Ghrita. [129]

Dhumapana for Kaphaja Chikitsa:

धूमांस्तानेव दद्याच्च ये प्रोक्ता वातकासिनाम्| कोशातकीफलान्मध्यं पिबेद्वा समनःशिलम्||१३०||

Recipes for smoking therapy described for the treatment of Vatika Kasa (Shlokas – 65– 75) are used for the treatment of Kaphaja kasa.

This recipe containing the pulp of Kosataki and Manah–Sila is especially useful for smoking in Kaphaja– Kasa [130]

Management of Associated Complications:

तमकः कफकासे तु स्याच्चेत् पित्तानुबन्धजः| पित्तकासक्रियां तत्र यथावस्थं प्रयोजयेत्||१३१||

वाते कफानुबन्धे तु कुर्यात् कफहरीं क्रियाम्| पित्तानुबन्धयोर्वातकफयोः पित्तनाशिनीम्||१३२||

आर्द्रे विरूक्षणं, शुष्के स्निग्धं, वातकफात्मके| कासेऽन्नपानं कफजे सपित्ते तिक्तसंयुतम्||१३३||

इति कफजकासचिकित्सा|

If Kaphaja Kasa is associated with Tamaka (a type of asthma) caused by Pitta, then in this stage of Kasa, the therapies prescribed for Paittika type of Kasa should be administered.

If there is association of Kapha in Vatika Kasa, then therapies for the alleviation of kapha should be planned. In Vata–Kaphaja Kasa if there is association of pitta, treatments to combat the aggravated pitta are adopted.

Thus, ends the description of the treatment of Kaphaja –Kasa. [131–133]

Treatment of Kshataja Kasa

Line of treatment

कासमात्ययिकं मत्वा क्षतजं त्वरया जयेत्| मधुरैर्जीवनीयैश्च बलमांस विवर्धनैः||१३४||

Ksataja Kasa (phthisis) is a serious ailment.

Keeping this in view, the treatment of the patient is initiated instantaneously with sweet drugs and drugs belonging to the Jivaniya group (vide Sutra 4: 9) which are promoters of strength and muscle tissue. [134]

Pippaladi Leha

पिप्पली मधुकं पिष्टं कार्षिकं ससितोपलम्| प्रास्थिकं गव्यमाजं च क्षीरमिक्षुरसस्तथा||१३५||

यवगोधूम मृद्वीकाचूर्णमामलकाद्रसः| तैलं च प्रसृतांशानि तत् सर्वं मृदुनाऽग्निना||१३६||

पचेल्लेहं घृतक्षौद्रयुक्तः स क्षतकासहा| श्वास हृद्रोग कार्श्येषु हितो वृद्धेऽल्परेतसि||१३७||

The paste of 1 karsa of each of Pippali and Madhuka,

1 Karsa (12 g) of– Sitopala (sugar of large size crystal)

1 prastha (768 g) each of – Cow's milk, Goat's milk and Juice of sugar– cane

1 prastha each of the powders of – Yava, Godhuma and Draksha and

1 Prastha each of the Juice of Amalaka and Sesame oil is cooked over a mild fire.

Intake of this linctus along with ghee and honey cures

Ksataja Kasa (phthisis), Asthma, Heart diseases and Emaciation

It is also useful for old persons and those who have less of semen. [135– 137]

Treatment of Associated Complications

क्षत कासाभि भूतानां वृतिः स्यात् पित्तकासिकी| क्षीर सर्पि र्मधुप्राया संसर्गे तु विशेषणम्||१३८||

वातपित्तार्दितेऽभ्यङ्गो गात्रभेदे घृतैर्हितः| तैलैर्मारुतरोगघ्नैः पीड्यमाने च वायुना||१३९||

The regimens prescribed for the Paittika Kasa are useful for the patient suffering from Ksataja kasa (Phthisis). Generally, milk, Ghee and honey are given to such patients.

If 2 of the Doshas are involved in the pathogenesis of this ailment (samsarga), then special therapies are required.

If this ailment is associated with vata and Pitta and the patient has pain all over the body, then massage is given with ghee.

If vata is aggravated in excess causing pain, then massage is given with oil prepared by boiling with vata– alleviating drugs. [138–139]

Medicated Ghee

हृत्पाश्वार्तिषु पानं स्याज्जीवनीयस्य सर्पिषः| सदाहं कासिनो रक्तं ष्ठीवतः सबलेऽनले||१४०||

The patient suffering from Kasa along with Hrt parshva shola – pain in the cardiac region and sides of the chest associated with

Daha – burning sensation,

Rakta sthivana – hemoptysis and aggravation of vata should take Jivaniya grtha [described in the chapter dealing with the treatment of Vata– Rakta–vide Cikitsa 29: 61– 70 [140]

Meat soup etc.

मांसोचितेभ्यः क्षामेभ्यो लावादीनां रसा हिताः| तृष्णार्तानां पयश्छागं शरमूलादिभिः शृतम्||१४१||

रक्ते स्रोतोभ्य आस्याद्वाऽप्यागते क्षीरजं घृतम्| नस्यं पानं यवागूर्वा श्रान्ते क्षामे हतानले||१४२||

स्तम्भायामेषु महतीं मात्रां वा सर्पिषः पिबेत्| कुर्याद्वा वातरोगघ्नं पित्तरक्ताविरोधि यत्||१४३||

If the patient is weak and habituated to taking meat, then the soup of the meat of Lava etc. is useful for him.

If the patient of phthisis is suffering from Trushna (thirst), then he is given goat's milk boiled with the root of Sara, etc., (trna–Pancamula).

If there is bleeding from different channels or from the mouth, then the patient should use ghee extracted from the cream of milk for inhalation therapy and as a drink.

If the patient of Phthisis is fatigued and weak, and if he has low power of digestion, then he is given Yavagu (thick gruel) to eat.

If there is stiffness and contraction of the body, then the patient of Phthisis is given ghee in large doses. Therapies for alleviation of vata which do not aggravate Pitta and Rakta is given to such patients. [141–143]

Dhoomapana for Kshataja Kasa – Smoking Therapy

निवृत्ते क्षतदोषे तु कफे वृद्ध उरः क्षते| दाल्यते कासिनो यस्य स धूमान्ना पिबेदिमान्||१४४||

द्वे मेदे मधुकं द्वे च बले तैः क्षौमलक्तकैः| वर्तितैर्धूममापीय जीवनीयघृतं पिबेत्||१४५||

मनःशिला पलाशाजगन्धा त्वक्क्षीरि नागरैः| भावयित्वा पिबेत् क्षौममनु चेक्षुगुडोदकम्||१४६||

पिष्ट्वा मनःशिलां तुल्यामार्द्रया वटशुङ्गया| ससर्पिष्कं पिबेद्धूमं तित्तिरि प्रतिभोजनम्||१४७||

भावितं जीवनीयैर्वा कुलिङ्गाण्डरसायुतैः| क्षौमं धूमं पिबेत् क्षीरं शृतं चायोगुडैरनु||१४८||

इति क्षतजकासचिकित्सा|

Kshataja Kasa – Smoking Therapy

If the patient suffering from Kshataja Kasa is cured of the Kshata (injury or ulceration in the Uras or Lungs), but there is throbbing type of pain in the place of injury because of aggravation of kapha, then he is given smoking therapy with the recipes described below.

Meda, MahaMeda, Madhuka– Licorice, Bala and MahaBala is made to a paste and smeared over a cloth of silk.

This is then rolled in order to give it the Shape of a cigar.

After smoking this cigar, the patient should drink Jivaniya Ghrita.

A cigar is prepared by smearing (llit. Soaking) a piece of silken cloth with the paste of

Manashila, Palasa, Ajagandha, TvakKsiri and Nagara – Zingiber officinale

After smoking this cigar, the patient should drink sugar– cane juice or water mixed with jaggery.

Manah–Sila is made to a paste by trituring it with the green still root of vata (vata–Sunga).

To this, ghee is added. After taking the smoke of this recipe, the patient should take the soup of the meat of Tittiri.

Smoking with the silken cloth soaked with the decoction of drugs belonging to the Jivaniya group (vide Syutra 4:9) and the sap of the egg of Kulinga, and thereafter, taking the milk immersed with hot iron balls are useful in Ksataja Kasa.

Thus, ends the description of Ksataja Kasa. [144–48]

Treatment of Kshayaja Kasa

Line of Treatment

सम्पूर्णरूपं क्षयजं दुर्बलस्य विवर्जयेत्| नवोत्थितं बलवतः प्रत्याख्यायाचरेत् क्रियाम्||१४९||

तस्मै बृंहणमेवादौ कुर्यादग्नेश्च दीपनम्| बहुदोषाय सस्नेहं मृदु दद्यादिवरेचनम्||१५०||

Line of treatment for Kshayaja Kasa:

If the Ksayaja Kasa is manifested with all the signs and symptoms, and the patient is weak, then he should not be treated.

However, if the disease has recently occurred (navotitha) and if the patient is strong, then such a patient may be treated even though the disease is incurable (because, occasionally such a patient may be cured).

In the beginning, such a patient is given nourishing therapy, and his Agni (power of digestion and metabolism) is stimulated.

If the Doshas are over aggravated, then he may be given mild purgative along with unctuous ingredients (medicated ghee). [149– 150]

Ghrita for Mrudu Virechana: Medicated Ghee for Mild Purgation

शम्पाकेन त्रिवृतया मृद्वीका रसयुक्तया| तिल्वकस्य कषायेण विदारी स्वरसेन च||१५१||

सर्पिः सिद्धं पिबेद्युक्त्या क्षीणदेहो विशोधनम् (हितं तद्देहबलयोरस्य संरक्षणं मतम्)||१५२||

Ghrita for Mrudu Virechana: Medicated Ghee for Mild Purgation

Ghee is cooked with the decoction of Sampaka (fruit–pulp of Aragvadha (Cassia fistula)) and Trivrt – Operculina turpethum, the juice of grape.

The decoction of Tilvaka, and (or) the juice of Vidari (Ipomoea paniculata/Pueraria tuberosa) is given in appropriate dose for the elimination (Sodhana of Doshas) to the patient whose body is weak.

This is a mild purgative. It is useful for the protection of the body and strength of the patient and also eliminates the morbid doshas. [151–152]

Recipe of Medicated Ghee
पित्ते कफे च सङ्क्षीणे परिक्षीणेषु धातुषु| घृतं कर्कटकी क्षीरदिवबलासाधितं पिबेत्||१५३||

When because of the administration of the above–mentioned purgation therapy] Pitta and kapha become reduced in quantity, the patient, whose tissue elements are already denuded, should take the ghee prepared by boiling with

KarkataSrngi – Rhus succadenea,

Milk,

Bala – Country mallow (root) – Sida cordifolia and

Atibala – Abutilon indicum [153]

Medicated Ghee and medicated Milk:
विदारीभिः कदम्बैर्वा तालसस्यैस्तथा शृतम्| घृतं पयश्च मूत्रस्य वैवर्ण्ये कृच्छ्रनिर्गमे||१५४||

If there is discoloration of the urine or if there is dysuria, the patient is given milk and ghee boiled by adding Vidari – Pueraria tuberosa or Kadamba or the pulp of tender fruits of Tala. [154]

Recipe for Anuvasana Basti – fat enema:
शूने सवेदने मेढ्रे पायौ सश्रोणिवङ्क्षणे|

घृतमण्डेन मधुनाऽनुवास्यो मिश्रकेण वा||१५५||

If there is swelling and pain in the phallus, Anus, hips and Pelvic region, the patient is given Anuvasana Basti (fat enema) with the scum of ghee (Ghrita Manda) or honey or with ghee and oil mixed together (Misraka). [155]

Diet after Anuvasana Therapy
जाङ्गलैः प्रतिभुक्तस्य वर्तकाद्या बिलेशयाः| क्रमशः प्रसहाश्चैव प्रयोज्याः पिशिताशिनः||१५६||

औष्ण्यात् प्रमाथिभावाच्च स्रोतोभ्यश्च्यावयन्ति ते| कफं, शुद्धेश्च तैः पुष्टिं कुर्यात्सम्यग्वहन्नसः||१५७||

After the administration of Anuvasana type of enema, the patient is given the soup the meat of animals and birds which arc Jangalas (those living in this forests), Vartaka, etc., those which are Bileshaya (those living in burrows) and meat– eating Prasahas (those eating by snatching their food).

Because of their hot potency and Pramathi attribute (ingredients which help in the exudation of Doshas from the channels), these ingredients cause exudation of Kapha accumulated in the channels of circulation.

After the body is cleansed of this aggravated Kapha, these meat– soups, while flowing appropriately in the channels of circulation, cause nourishment of tissues [156– 157]

DviPanchaMuladi Ghruta
द्विपञ्चमूली त्रिफला चविका भार्गि चित्रकैः| कुलत्थ पिप्पलीमूल पाठा कोलयवैर्जले||१५८||

शृतैर्नागर दुःस्पर्शा पिप्पली शटि पौष्करैः| कल्कैः कर्कटशृङ्ग्या च समैः सर्पिर्विपाचयेत्||१५९||

सिद्धेऽस्मिंश्चूर्णितौ क्षारौ द्वौ पञ्च लवणानि च| दत्त्वा युक्त्या पिबेन्मात्रां क्षयकास निपीडितः||१६०||

इति द्विपञ्चमूलादिघृतम्|

Decoction is prepared of Dvi panchamoola (Dashamoola), Triphala, Cavika, Bhargi, Chitraka, Kulattha, Pippalimula, Patha, Kola and Yava by boiling with water.

To this decoction, ghee and the paste of

Nagara, Duhsparsa, Pippali, Sati, Puskaramula, Karkata Srngi is added, and cooked.

After the medicated ghee is prepared,

Yava Ksara, Svarji–Ksara, Saindhava–Lavana, Samudra–Lavana, Sauvarcala Lavana, Vida–Lavana

Audbhida–Lavana is added in powder form [only in small quantiies].

Intake of this medicated ghee in appropriate dose cures Ksayaja Kasa.

Thus ends the description of DviPancamuladi Ghrita [158–160]

Guduchyadi Ghrita

गुडूची पिप्पली मूर्वा हरिद्रां श्रेयसीं वचाम्| निदिग्धिकां कासमर्दं पाठां चित्रक नागरम्||१६१||

जले चतुर्गुणे पक्त्वा पादशेषेण तत्समम्| सिद्धं सर्पिः पिबेद्गुल्म श्वासार्ति क्षय कासनुत्||१६२||

इति गुडूच्यादिघृतम्|

Guduci, Pippali, Murva, Haridra, Sreyasi, Vacha, Nigdighika, Kasamarda, Patha, Chitraka, Nagara is added with 4 times water, and boiled till 1/4th remains.

To this decoction, equal quantity of ghee is added and cooked.

Intake of this medicated ghee cures

Gulma (Phantom tumour),

Asthma and

Kshayaj Kasa

Thus, ends the description of Guducyadi Ghrita. [161– 162]

Recipes of Medicated Ghee

कासमर्दाभया मुस्त पाठा कट्फल नागरैः| पिप्पली कटुका द्राक्षा काश्मर्य सुरसैस्तथा||१६३||

अक्षमात्रैर्घृतप्रस्थं क्षीर द्राक्षा रसाढके| पचेच्छोष ज्वर प्लीहसर्वकासहरं शिवम्||१६४||

धात्रीफलैः क्षीरसिद्धैः सर्पिर्वाऽप्यवचूर्णितम्| द्विगुणे दाडिमरसे विपक्वं व्योषसंयुतम्||१६५||

पिबेदुपरि भक्तस्य यवक्षारघृतं नरः| पिप्पलीगुड सिद्धं वा च्छागक्षीरयुतं घृतम्||१६६||

एतान्यग्निविवृद्ध्यर्थ सर्पींषि क्षयकासिनाम्| स्युर्दोषबद्धकोष्ठोरःस्रोतसां च विशुद्धये||१६७||

1 Prastha (768 g)of ghee is cooked by adding the paste of 1 Aksa of each of

Kasamarda, Abhaya, Musta, Patha, Katphala, Nagara, Pippali, Katuka, Draksha, Kasmarya, Surasa

1 Adhaka (3.072 l) of milk and

1 Adhaka of Grape– Juice

This recipe of medicated ghee is auspicious, and it cures

Shosha – emaciation,

Jwara – fever,

Pliha – spleen–diseases and

All the types of Kasa

Fruits of amalaki are boiled in milk and made into powder. Ghee sprinkled with this powder is taken by the patient suffering from Ksayaja Kasa, among others.

Yava – Ksara–Ghrita prepared by cooking with double the quantity of Dadima – Pomegranate – Punica granatum–Jucice and added with powder of Sunthi, Pippali – Long pepper fruit – Piper longum and Maricha – Black pepper fruit – piper nigrum is taken at the end of the meal by the patient suffering from Kasayaja Kasa among others

Ghee cooked with the paste of Pippali and Jaggery, and goat milk is similarly useful

All the above–mentioned recipes of medicated ghee promote Agni (power of digestion and medicated metabolism) of the patient suffering from Ksayaja Kasa. These recipes also cleanse the Adhered Doshas from the channels of Kostha (gastro Intestinal Tract) and Chest. [163– 167]

Haritaki Leha

हरीतकीर्यवक्वाथद्व्याढके विंशतिं पचेत्| स्विन्ना मृदित्वा तास्तस्मिन् पुराणं गुडषट्पलम्||१६८||

दद्यान्मनःशिलाकर्ष कर्षार्धं च रसाञ्जनात्| कुडवार्धं च पिप्पल्याः स लेहः श्वासकासनुत्||१६९||

इति हरीतकीलेहः|

20 fruits of Haritaki are boiled in 1 Adhaka of the decoction of Yava – Barley (Hordeum vulgare) (barley).

These boiled and softened fruits of Haritaki are smashed, [their seeds are removed] and the pulp is made to a paste.
In this paste,
6 Palas of old jaggery,
1 Karsa of Manah–Sila,
½ Karsa of Rasanjana (Aqueous extract of Berberis aristata) and
½ Kudava of Pippali is added and cooked. This preparation of linctus cures Asthma and Kasa
Thus, ends the description of Haritaki–Leha. [168–169]

Churna – Leha Yoga: Recipes of powders and Linctus
श्वाविधः सूचयो दग्धाः सघृत क्षौद्र शर्कराः| श्वास कासहरा बर्हिपादौ वा क्षौद्रसर्पिषा||१७०||
एरण्डपत्रक्षारं वा व्योषतैलगुडान्वितम्| लिह्यादेतेन विधिना सुरसैरण्डपत्रजम्||१७१||
द्राक्षा पद्मक वार्ताक पिप्पलीः क्षौद्र सर्पिषा| लिह्यात्र्यूषणचूर्णं वा पुराणगुड सर्पिषा||१७२||
चित्रकं त्रिफलाजाजी कर्कटाख्या कटुत्रिकम्| द्राक्षां च क्षौद्र सर्पिभ्यां लिह्यादद्यादगुडेन वा||१७३||
Recipes of powders and Linctus
Intake of the ashes of Quills of Svavidha along with ghee, honey and sugar cures asthma and kasa.
Intake of the ashes of Peacock legs along with honey and ghee cures asthma and Kasa.
Intake of this linctus cures asthma and Kasa:
Eranda Ksara (alkali preparation) is added with
Sunthi, Pippali, Maricha, Oil and Jaggery
The kshara of the leaves of
Surasa and Eranda is mixed with Sunthi, Pippali, Maricha, Oil and Jaggery, Intake of this linctus cures asthma and Kasa
The powder of – Draksha, Vartaka and Pippali is added with honey and ghee. Intake of this linctus cures asthma and kasa.
The powder of – Sunthi, Pippali, and Maricha is added with old jaggery and ghee.
Intake of this recipe cures Asthma and Kasa.
The powder of Chitraka, Haritaki, Bibhitaka, Amalaka, Ajaji, Karkata–Srngi, Sunthi, Pippali, Maricha, Draksha is mixed with honey and ghee or with jaggery. Intake of these two recipes cures Asthma and kasa.

Padmakadi Leha
पद्मकं त्रिफलां व्योषं विडङ्गं सुरदारु च| बलां रास्नां च तुल्यानि सूक्ष्मचूर्णानि कारयेत्||१७४||
सर्वैरभिः समं चूर्णैः पृथक् क्षौद्रं घृतं सिताम्| विमथ्य लेहयेल्लेहं सर्वकासहरं शिवम्||१७५||
इति पद्मकादिलेहः|
Recipes of powders and Linctus
These are taken in equal quantities (1 Part of each) and made to fine powder:
Padmaka, Haritaki, Bibhitaka, Amalaki, Sunthi, Pippali, Maricha, Vidanga, Suradaru, Bala, Rasna
To this powder, equal quantities (eleven parts) each of honey, ghee and sugar is added and mixed well.
This recipe of linctus is auspicious and it cures all types of kasa.
Thus, ends the description of Padmakadi Leha. [174–175]
Jivantyadi – Leha
All these are taken in equal quantities and made to a powder:
Jivanti MadhukaPatha Tvak–Ksiri, Haritaki, Bibhitaka, Amalaki, Sati, Musta, Ela, Padmaka, Draksha, Brihati, Kantakari, Itunnaka, Sariva, Puskaramula, Karkata–Sringi, Rasanjana (Aqueous extract of Berberis aristata), Punarnava, LohaRajata (bhasma), Trayamana, Yavanika, Bhargi, Tamalaki, Rddhi, Vidanga, Dhanvayasaka, Ksara (Alkali preparation), Chitraka, Chavya, Amla–Vetasa, Sunthi, Pippali, Maricha and
Deva–Daru
Dosage: 1 Panitala

Adjuvant: Honey and ghee
Cures: all the 5 varieties of Kasa [176–179]

Recipes

लिह्यान्मरिचचूर्णं वा सघृत क्षौद्र शर्करम्| बदरीपत्र कल्कं वा घृतभृष्टं ससैन्धवम्||१८०||

स्वरभेदे च कासे च लेहमेतं प्रयोजयेत्|

The powder of Maricha – Black pepper fruit – piper nigrum is mixed with ghee, honey and sugar.

This preparation of linctus is taken by the patient.

The paste of the leaves of Badari is sizzled with ghee and mixed with Saindhava (rock–salt).

This is given to the patient, suffering from hoarseness of voice (Svara– Bheda) and kasa. [180– 181½]

Tilvakadi Utkarika

पत्रकल्कं घृतैभृष्टं तिल्वकस्य सशर्करम्||१८१||

पेया चोत्कारिका च्छर्दितृट्कासामातिसारनुत्|

The paste of the leaves of Tilvaka is sizzled with ghee and made into an Utkarika (food preparation in paste form) by adding sugar.

Intake of this cure:

Chardi – vomiting,

Trut – morbid thirst,

Kasa and

Atisara – diarrhea associated with Ama (product of improper digestion). (181 ½– ½ 182)

गौर सर्षप गण्डीर विडङ्ग व्योष चित्रकान्| साभयान् साधयेत्तोये यवागूं तेन चाम्भसा||१८२||

ससर्पिर्लवणां कासे हिक्काश्वासे सपीनसे| पाण्ड्वामये क्षये शोथे कर्णशूले च दापयेत्||१८३||

These drugs are boiled with water and the decoction is prepared:

White variety of Sarshapa, Gandira, Vidanga, Sunthi, Pippali, Maricha, Chitraka, Abhaya

With this decoction, yavagu (thick gruel) is prepared.

To this Yavagu, some ghee and salt is added.

This medicated Yavagu is administered to a patient suffering from

Hikka – hiccup, Shvasa –asthma, Pinasa – chronic Rhinitis, Pandu – Anaemia, Kshaya – tissue depletion, Shotha – oedema and Karna shoola – earache [½ 182– 183]

कण्टकारी रसे सिद्धो मुद्गयूषः सुसंस्कृतः| सगौरामलकः साम्लः सर्वकासाभिषग्जितम्||१८४||

Soup of Mudga prepared by adding the juice (decoction) of Kantakari – Solanum xanthocarpum is properly sizzled.

Intake of this soup by adding green Amalaki (Gauramalaka) and sour ingredients cures all types of kasa [184]

वातघ्नौषध निष्क्वाथं क्षीरं यूषान् रसानपि| वैष्किर प्रतुदान् बैलान् दापयेत् क्षयकासिने||१८५||

The patient suffering from Kshayaja Kasa is given

Ksheeram – milk,

Yusha – vegetable–soup and meat–soup prepared of the meat of birds/animals belonging to Viskira who collect food by scratching), Pratuda (who collect food by Pricking) and Bilesaya (who dwell in burrows) groups.

These foods– preparations are made by boiling with the decoction of vata– alleviating drugs. [185]

Smoking therapy for Kshataja kasa:

क्षतकासे च ये धूमाः सानुपाना निदर्शिताः| क्षयकासेऽपि तानेव यथावस्थं प्रयोजयेत्||१८६||

Recipes for smoking therapy prescribed for the treatment of Ksataja Kasa along with the Anupanas (post– Prandial drinks) (vide verse nos. 144–148) should also be administered to patients suffering from Ksataja kasa in appropriate stages of the disease. [186]

Management of kasa in general

दीपनं बृंहणं चैव स्रोतसां च विशोधनम्| व्यत्यासात्क्षयकासिभ्यो बल्यं सर्वं हितं भवेत्||१८७||

सन्निपातभवोऽप्येष क्षयकासः सुदारुणः| सन्निपातहितं तस्मात् सदा कार्यं भिषग्जितम्||१८८||

दोषानुबलयोगाच्च हरेद्रोगबलाबलम्| कासेष्वेषु गरीयांसं जानीयादुत्तरोत्तरम्||१८९||

To the patient suffering from Ksayaja Kasa

Dipana (digestive stimulants)

Brmhana (nourishing therapy) and

Srotas– Sodhana (therapies which cleanse the channels of circulation) is given alternatively.

All the therapies that promote strength (balya) are useful in this condition.

Ksayaja Kasa is caused by Sannipata (simultaneous aggravation of all 3 Doshas). Therefore, therapies which alleviate all the associated Doshas keeping this in view, treatment are administered.

The physician should know that among Vatika Kasa, Paittika Kasa, Kaphaja Ksataja and Ksayaja Kasa, the succeeding ones are more serious than the preceding. [187– 189]

Different Categories of Therapies:

भोज्यं पानानि सर्पींषि लेहाश्च सह पानकैः| क्षीरं सर्पिर्गुडा धूमाः कास भैषज्य सङ्ग्रहः||१९०||

For the treatment of Kasa the following categories of therapies are described to be administered:

1. Bhojya (food preparation)
2. Pana (drinks)
3. Sarpis (medicated ghee)
4. Leha (recipes of linctus) along with post– pradial drinks
5. Ksira (milk boiled with medicines)
6. Sarpirguda (preparation containing ghee, jaggery, etc.), which are used either in linctus from or in the form of pills and
7. Dhuma (recipes for smoking) [190]

तत्र श्लोकः–

सङ्ख्या निमित्तं रूपाणि साध्यासाध्यत्वमेव च| कासानां भेषजं प्रोक्तं गरीयस्त्वं च कासिनः||१९१||

In this chapter, the following topics are discussed:

The number or types of kasa

Etiological factors of different types of Kasa

Signs and symptoms of different types of Kasa

Curability and incurability of different types of Kasa

Recipes for the treatment of different types of Kasa and

Comparative seriousness of different types of Kasa. [191]

इत्यग्निवेशकृते तन्त्रे चरक प्रतिसंस्कृतेऽप्राप्ते दृढबल सम्पूरिते चिकित्सा स्थाने कास चिकित्सितं नामाष्टादशोऽध्यायः||१८||

Thus, ends the 18th chapter in Chikitsasthana dealing with the treatment of Kasa in the work of Agnivesa which was redacted by Charaka and supplemented by Drudhabala.

2

Chikitsasthana Chapter 19 Atisara Chikitsitam

The 19th chapter of Charaka Samhita Chkitsa Sthana is Atisara Chikitsa Adhyaya. It deals with symptoms, types and treatment of diarrhoea and dysentery.

अथातोऽतीसार चिकित्सितं व्याख्यास्यामः||१||

इति ह स्माह भगवानात्रेयः||२||

We shall now explore the chapter on the treatment of Atisara (diarrhoea, dysentery). Thus said Lord Atreya [1-2]

Prologue

भगवन्तं खल्वात्रेयं कृताह्निकं हुताग्निहोत्रमासीनमृषिगण परिवृतमुत्तरे हिमवतः पार्श्वे विनयादुपेत्याभिवाद्य चाग्निवेश उवाच- भगवन्! अतीसारस्य प्रागुत्पत्ति निमित्त लक्षणोपशमनानि प्रजानुग्रहार्थमाख्यातुमर्हसीति||३||

Lord Atreya was sitting on the northern slope of Himalayas surrounded by sages, after completing his daily worship and oblations to the fire, Agnivesha approached him, offered his salutations and asked him to kindly expound the origin, aetiology, signs and symptoms, and treatment of Atisara for the well-being of humanity. [3]

Mythological origin of Atisara:

अथ भगवान् पुनर्वसुरात्रेयस्तदग्निवेश वचन मनुनिशम्योवाच- श्रूयतामग्निवेश! सर्वमेतदखिलेन व्याख्यायमानम्|

आदिकाले खलु यज्ञेषु पशवः समालभनीया बभूवुर्नालम्भाय प्रक्रियन्ते स्म|

ततो दक्षयज्ञं प्रत्यवरकालं मनोः पुत्राणां नरिष्यन्नाभागेक्ष्वाकुनृगशर्यात्यादीनां क्रतुषु पशूनामेवाभ्यनुज्ञानात् पशवः प्रोक्षणमवापुः|

अतश्च प्रत्यवरकालं पृषध्रेण दीर्घसत्रेण यजता पशूनामलाभाद्गवामालम्भः प्रवर्तितः|

तं दृष्ट्वा प्रव्यथिता भूतगणाः, तेषां चोपयोगादुपाकृतानां गवां गौरवादौष्ण्यादसात्म्यत्वादशस्तोपयोगाच्चोपहताग्नीनामुपहतमनसां चातीसारः पूर्वमुत्पन्नः पृषध्रयज्ञे||४||

Mythological origin of Atisara:

Hearing the plea of Agnivesha, Lord Punarvasu said "O! Agnivesha, hear me. I shall explain every topic of your query in detail".

In ancient times, the sacrificial animals were released soon after the recitation of the Sacrificial Mantras, and these animals were not actually killed during the course of the sacrifice (yajna).

However, in later times, Daksha Prajapati, the sons of Manu, like Narisyan, Nabhaga, Iksvaku, Nrga and Saryathi started actually killing these sacrificial animals during the performance of Yajna (Sacrificial ritual) thinking that it was so ordained in the Shastras (Scriptures) or being pressed by the animals themselves [as it was felt that the animals associated during the sacrifice will directly attain heaven].

Subsequently, it became quite impossible to get other animals in the required number, and Prushadhra who was performing a sacrifice (Yajna) for a long duration, started sacrificing even bulls and cows. After observing this, the living creatures were bewildered. The meat of the sacrificed bulls and cows proved to be too heavy, too hot and too harmful. Person par-taking that meat started suffering from the loss of the power of digestion and loss of mental equilibrium. Thus, Atisara (diarrhoea) originated from the sacrifice (Yajna) performed by Prushadhra. [4]

Vataja Atisara: Nidana, Samprapti, Lakshana:
अथावरकालं वातलस्य वातातप व्यायामातिमात्र निषेविणो रूक्षाल्प प्रमिताशिनस्तीक्ष्णमद्य व्यवाय नित्यस्योदावर्तयतश्च वेगान् वायुः प्रकोपमापद्यते, पक्ता चोपहन्यते; स वायुः कुपितोऽग्नावुपहते मूत्रस्वेदौ पुरीषाशयमुपहृत्य, ताभ्यां पुरीषं द्रवीकृत्य, अतीसाराय प्रकल्पते| तस्य रूपाणि- विज्जलमामं विप्लुतमवसादि रूक्षं द्रवं सशूलमामगन्धमीषच्छब्दमशब्दं वा विबद्धमूत्र वातमतिसार्यते पुरीष, वायुश्चान्तःकोष्ठे सशब्दशूलस्तिर्यक् चरति विबद्ध इत्यामातिसारो वातात्|
पक्वं वा विबद्धमल्पाल्पं सशब्दं सशूल फेन पिच्छा परिकर्तिकं हृष्टरोमा विनिःश्वसत्र् शुष्कमुखः कट्यूरु त्रिक जानु पृष्ठ पार्श्वशूली भ्रष्टगुदो मुहुर्मुहु विग्रथितमुपवेश्यते पुरीषं वातात्; तमाहुरनु ग्रथितमित्येके, वातानु ग्रथित वर्चस्त्वात्||५||
Causes for Vataja Atisara:
As a consequence of the above mentioned primordial causative factor, at later stage [Vatika type of Atisara is manifested] if a person having Vatika type of constitution resorts to the following factors:
Vatala vata aatapa vyayama atimatra- Exposure to the excessively strong wind, hot sun and physical exercise
Ruksha alpa – Indulgence in dry food or pramitasana- less quantity of food or irregular meals or Teekshna madya – strong alcoholic drinks or Vyavaya – excessive sexual intercourse and
Suppression of natural urges
Vataja Atisara Samprapti: Pathogeneisis:
Because of the aforementioned factors, Vata Dosha gets aggravated and the power of digestion (Agni) gets afflicted.
The aggravated Vata, forcefully brings down the urine and sweat (moistness in the body) to the colon (Purishashaya), and with the help of these (urine and sweat) liquefies the stool, causing diarrhoea thereby.
The signs and symptoms of the Vata type of Atisara, when associated with Ama
1. Vit jalam amam – The stool is slimy and mixed with Mucus (Ama)
2. The stool floats on water
3. The stool when placed over the earth gets soaked
4. Ruksham dravam – The stool is rough and liquid
5. Sa shula aamagandha – defecation is associated with colic pain
6. The stool smells like undigested food
7. Defecation is associated with less of sound or no sound at all
8. It is associated with non-voiding of flatus and urine and
9. The aggravated Vayu (flatus) moves in the Kostha (gastrointestine tract) obliquely along with gurgling sound, while causing colic pain.

Signs and symptoms of Pakwa Vataja Atisara:
1. the patient voids hard stool in small quantities
2. The voiding of stool is associated with sound and colic pain
3. The stool is frothy and slimy
4. The patient suffers from griping pain, horrification, groaning, dryness of the mouth, pain in the lumbar region, thighs, sacral region, knees, back and sides of the chest, and prolapse of the rectum and
5. He voids granular (grathita) / pellet like stool frequently.
According to some physicians, this type of diarrhoea is also called Anugrathita-Atisara because of the voiding of the Scybalous stool. [5]

Pittaja Atisara Nidana, Samprapti, Lakshana:
पित्तलस्य पुनरम्ल लवण कटुक क्षारोष्ण तीक्ष्णातिमात्र निषेविणः प्रतताग्निसूर्य सन्तापोष्ण मारुतोपहतगात्रस्य क्रोधेष्र्याबहुलस्य पित्तं प्रकोपमापद्यते|
तत् प्रकुपितं द्रवत्वादूष्माणमुपहृत्य पुरीषाशय विसृतमौष्ण्याद् द्रवत्वात् सरत्वाच्च भित्वा पुरीषमतिसाराय प्रकल्पते|

तस्य रूपाणि- हारिद्रं हरितं नीलं
कृष्णं रक्तपित्तोपहितमतिदुर्गन्धमतिसार्यते पुरीषं, तृष्णा दाह स्वेद मूच्छर्छा शूल ब्रध्न सन्तापपाकपरीत इति पित्तातिसारः||६||

Causes for Pittaja Atisara:

A person of Paittika constitution indulging in the following factors gets Pittaja type of Atisara (Diarrhoea):

1. Excessive intake of Amla (sour), Lavana (salt), Katu (pungent), Kshara (alkaline) Ushna (hot) and Teekshna (sharp) ingredients.

2. Pratata Agni Surya Santapa ushna marutopahata gatrasya – Affliction of the body by excessive exposure to the heat of strong (pratata) fire, hot rays of the sun and hot wind and

3. Krodha irshya bahula – Excessively wrathful and jealous disposition

By the above mentioned factors, Pitta gets aggravated.

Paittika Atisara Samprapti: pathogenesis:

This aggravated Pitta on account of its liquidity suppresses the power of Agni (power of digestion), and having arrived at the colon, disintegrates the stool because of its heat, liquidity and mobility thereby causing Paittika type of Atisara (Diarrhoea).

The signs and symptoms of Paittika Atisara:

1. Haridram, haritam, nilam, krshnam purisham -The patient voids frequent loose motions which are either yellow, green, blue or black in colour

2. Rakta pitta upahita, ati durgandha purisham – The stool is mixed with blood and bile, and it is excessively foul smelling and

3. The patient suffers from Trishna (excess thirst), Daha (burning sensation), Ati sweda (excessive sweating), Murcha (fainting), Shula (colic pain) and Santapa (hot sensation) and

4. There is suppuration of the anus [6]

Kaphaja Atisara Nidana, Samprapti, Lakshana:

श्लेष्मलस्य तु गुरु मधुर शीत स्निग्धोप सेविनः सम्पूरकस्याचिन्तयतो दिवास्वप्न परस्यालसस्य श्लेष्मा प्रकोपमापद्यते|
स स्वभावाद् गुरु मधुर शीत स्निग्धः स्रस्तोऽग्निमुपहत्य सौम्यस्वभावात् पुरीषाशयमुपहत्योपक्लेद्य पुरीषमतिसाराय कल्पते|
तस्य रूपाणि- स्निग्धं श्वेतं पिच्छिलं तन्तुमदामं गुरु दुर्गन्धं श्लेष्मोपहितमनुबद्धशूलमल्पाल्पमभीक्ष्णमतिसार्यते सप्रवाहिकं, गुरूदर गुद बस्ति वङ्क्षणदेशः कृतेऽप्यकृतसञ्ज्ञः सलोमहर्षः सोत्क्लेशो निद्रालस्यपरीतः सदनोऽन्नद्वेषी चेति श्लेष्मातिसारः||७||

Causes for Kaphaja Atisara:

A person of Kapha type of constitution indulging in the following factors gets Kaphaja type of Atisara (diarrhoea)

1. Guru madhura shita snigdha ahara sevana – Intake of heavy, sweet, cold and unctuous ingredients in excess

2. Inactivity of the mind, lethargy and

3. Diva swapna – Habitually sleeping during the day time

Kaphaja Atisara Samprapti: Pathogenesis:

Because of the above mentioned factors, Kapha gets aggravated. By nature, Kapha is heavy, sweet, cold and unctuous. It moves downwards (because of its heaviness, etc) and afflicts the agni (power of digestion) because of its natural cooling property. Thereafter, having arrived at the colon, it liquefies the stool to cause diarrhoea.

The signs and symptoms of Kaphaja Atisara:

1. The patient voids stool which is Snigdha (unctuous), Shvetam (white), Picchila (slimy), fibrous, mixed with mucus as well as undigested food particles, Guru (heavy), Durgandham (foul- smelling) and mixed with phlegm

2. Badhha shoola – The patient suffers from continuous pain.

3. Alpam abhikshnam atisara – He voids stool, frequently in small quantities

4. Pravahikam – The voiding of stool is associated with griping pain

5. Guru udara guda basti vankshana shoola- The patient suffers from heaviness in the abdomen, in the region of urinary bladder and in the pelvic region

6. The patient feels the urge for passing another bout of stool even after evacuation and

7. He suffers from Loma harsha (horripilation), Utklesha (Nausea), Ati nidra (excessive sleep), Aalasya (indolence), Sadana (prostration) and Anna dveshi (dislike for food). [7]

Sannipatik Atisar Nidana, Samprapti:

अतिशीत स्निग्ध रूक्षोष्ण गुरु खर कठिन विषम विरुद्धा सात्म्य भोजनादभोजनात् कालातीतभोजनाद् यत्किञ्चिदभ्यवहरणात् प्रदुष्ट मद्यपानीयपानादतिमद्यपानाद् संशोधनात् प्रतिकर्मणां विषम गमनादनुपचाराज्ज्वलनादित्य पवन सलिलातिसेवनाद स्वप्ना-दतिस्वप्नाद्वेग विधारणादृतु विपर्ययादयथाबलमारम्भाद्भय शोक चित्तोद्वेगातियोगात् कृमि शोष ज्वरार्शोविकारातिकर्षणाद्वा व्यापन्नाग्नेस्त्रयो दोषाः प्रकुपिता भूय एवाग्निमुपहत्य पक्वाशयमनु प्रविश्यातीसारं सर्वदोष लिङ्गं जनयन्ति॥८॥

Causes for Sannipatika Atisara (diarrhoea caused by the simultaneous vitiation of all the 3 Doshas)

1. Intake of Ati sheeta (excessive cold), Snigdha (unctuous), Ruksha (dry), Ushna (hot) Guru (heavy), Khara (coarse) and Kathina (hard) ingredients

2. Intake of Vishama aahar (irregular meals), Viruddha (ingredients of food having mutually contracting properties) and unwholesome food,

3. Abhojana – Avoiding intake of food.

4. Kalaateeta bhojana – Intake of food long after the scheduled time

5. Yat kinchat abhyavaranat – Intake of food wsithout caring for its wholesomeness or otherwise

6. Pradusta madya paniya pana – Drinking of alcohol and other drinks which are polluted

7. Ati madyapana – Drinking of alcohol in excess

8. Samshodhana pratikarma – Not resorting to elimination therapies [in appropriate seasons]

9. Inappropriate administration or non-administration of therapies

10. Vishama gamana, anupa chara jvala aditya pavana salila sevana – Excessive exposure to fire, hot rays of the sun, strong wind and bath, etc., in strong current of water

11. Ati svapna vega – Not sleeping or sleeping in excess

12. Vega vidharana – Suppression of natural urges

13. Not resorting to appropriate regimens during different seasons.

14. Excessively daring attitude

15. Shoka, udvega – Excessive exposure to fear, grief and anxiety and

16. Krsha due to Krimi, Jvara, sosha – Excessive emaciation due to worm- infection, consumption, fever and piles bleeding

Because of the above-mentioned causative factors, the Agni (power of digestion) gcts vitiated as a result of which all the 3 Doshas get aggravated. These aggravated Doshas, in their turn, further afflict the Agni, and having entered into Pakvashaya (colon), cause Atisara (diarrhoea) in which the signs and symptoms of all the 3 types of Atisara (viz, Vatika, Paittika and kaphaja Atisara, described before) are manifested. [8]

Signs and symptoms of Sannipatika Atisara

अपि च शोणितादीन् धातूनतिप्रकृष्टं दूषयन्तो धातु दोष स्वभावकृतानतीसारवर्णानुप दर्शयन्ति।

तत्र शोणितादिषु धातुष्वतिप्रदुष्टेषु हारिद्र हरित नील माञ्जिष्ठ मांसधावन सन्निकाशं रक्तं कृष्णं श्वेतं वराहभेदःसदृशमनुबद्ध वेदनमवेदनं वा समास व्यत्यासादुपवेश्यते शकृद् ग्रथितमामं सकृत्, सकृदपि पक्वमनतिक्षीण मांस शोणित बलो मन्दाग्नि विहत मुखरसश्च; तादृशमातुरं कृच्छसाध्यं विद्यात्।

एभिर्वर्णैरतिसार्यमाणं सोपद्रवमातुरमसाध्योऽयमिति प्रत्याचक्षीत; तद्यथा- पक्वशोणिताभं यकृत्खण्डोपमं मेदो मांसोदक सन्निकाशं दधि घृत मज्ज तैल वसा क्षीर वेसवाराभमतिनीलमतिरक्तमतिकृष्णमुदकमिवाच्छं पुनर्मेचकाभमतिस्निग्धं हरित नील कषाय वर्णं कर्बुरमाविलं पिच्छिलं तन्तुमदामं चन्द्रकोपगतमतिकुणप पूतिपूय गन्ध्यामाम मत्स्यगन्धि मक्षिकाकान्तं कुथित बहुधातु स्रावमल्प पुरीषमपुरीष वाऽतिसार्यमाणं तृष्णा दाह ज्वर भ्रम तमक हिक्का श्वासानुबन्धमतिवेदनमवेदनं वा स्रस्त पक्व गुदं पतित गुदवलिं मुक्तनालमतिक्षीणबलमांस शोणितं सर्व पर्वास्थिशूलिनमरोचकारति प्रलाप सम्मोह परीतं सहसोपरतविकारमतिसारिणम चिकित्स्यं विद्यात्; इति सन्निपातातिसारः॥९॥

The 3 aggravated Doshas (referred to above) cause excessive vitiation of Dhatus (Tissue elements) like Rakta (blood)

resulting in the manifestation of different colours [in the stool]. The nature of these colours depends upon the nature of the vitiated Dhatus and Doshas. If the Dhatus like Rakta are excessively vitiated, then the following signs and symptoms are manifested

1. The patient voids stool having yellow (like the colour of turmeric), green, blue, reddish (like the meat is Manjistha), pink (like the colour of water in which meat is washed), red black, white and yellowish (like the colour of the pig-fat) in colour.

2. The patient suffers from continuous pain or he may be free from any pain [in the abdomen]

3. Sometimes, the patient may avoid scybalous stool, sometimes it may be mixed with mucus (Ama) and sometimes, the stool may be free from Mucus (Pakva).

4. There is diminution of the muscle tissue, blood and strength

5. The power of digestion (Agni) of the patient is suppressed and

6. There is impairment of the taste in the mouth of the patient.

Such a patient is Kricchra-Sadhya (difficult to cure).

The patient becomes Asadhya (incurable) if the Diarrhoea is associated with the colours and complications as follows:

1. The patient voids stool having the colour of digested blood, (Malena), piece of liver, washing of fat or flesh, curd, ghee, bone- marrow, oil, muscle fat (Vasa) milk and Vesavara (minced meat).

2. The colour of the stool is excessively blue, red, black, transparent like water or tar-colored

3. The stool is exceedingly greasy

4. The colour of the stool is a mixture of green, blue and brown (Kasaya) colours

5. The stool is variegated in colour (Karbura), dirty, slimy, fibrous, mixed with mucus and spotted with Candraka (coloured patches circular in shape like moon)

6. The stool has exceedingly bad smell like that of a dead body or it is exceedingly putrid in smell or the stool bears the smell of undigested products or it is like (raw) fish

7. The stool attracts flies in excess

8. The stool contains sloughs (Kuthita) and tissue elements in excess

9. The stool contains less or no faecal matter

10. The patient continuously suffers from Trshna (excess thirst), Daha (burning sensation), Jwara (fever), Pralapa (giddiness), Murcha (fainting), Hikka (hiccup), Shvasa (asthma), Tivra shoola (excessive pain) or no pain

11. There is prolapse and inflammation of the anal canal or the rectum sphincters come out of their sites or the whole of the rectum comes out (mukta- Nala)

12. There is excessive loss of strength, muscle tissue and blood,

13. Parva asthi shoola – There is pain in all the joints and bones

14. The patient suffers from excessive form of Aruchi (anorexia), Arati (dislike for everything), Pralapa (Delirium) and Sammoha (unconsciousness), and

15. There is sudden cessation of the signs and symptoms of the disease.

Such a patient is rejected.

These are the characteristic features of Sanipatika type of Atisara (Diarrhoea). [9]

Atisara Chikitsa – Treatment

तमसाध्यतामसम्प्राप्तं चिकित्सेद् यथा प्रधानोपक्रमेण हेतूपशय दोष विशेष परीक्षया चेति||१०||

The patient who has not yet reached the state of absolute incurability is properly treated after the examination of causative factors, Upashaya (treatability) and nature of the aggravation of specific Doshas.

In this condition, the most aggravated Dosha is treated in the beginning followed by the treatment of the less aggravated Doshas. [10]

Agantuja Atisara

आगन्तू द्वावतीसारौ मानसौ भय शोकजौ| ततयोर्लक्षणं वायोर्यदतीसार लक्षणम्||११||

The exogenous type of Atisara (Diarrhea) is of mental origin, and is of 2 types.

1. Bhayaja – fear and

2. Shokaja – grief

Their signs and symptoms are similar to those of the Vatika type of Atisara. [11]

Management of Exogenous (mental) Diarrhea:

मारुतो भयशोकाभ्यां शीघ्रं हि परिकुप्यति| तयोः क्रिया वातहरी हर्षणाश्वासनानि च||१२||

इत्युक्ताः षडतीसाराः, साध्यानां साधनं त्वतः| प्रवक्ष्याम्यनुपूर्वेण यथावत्तन्निबोधत||१३||

Because of fear and grief, Vayu gets aggravated instantaneously. Therefore, for the treatment of these 2 varieties of Diarrhea, Vayu alleviating drugs and therapies are administered.

The patient suffering from diarrhoea caused by fear (Bhayaja) is exhilarated, and the patient suffering from Diarrhoea caused by Shoka (grief) is consoled for their cure.

Thus, 6 types of Atisara (Diarrhoea) are described above, the curable varieties of these are treated. Therefore, the methods of their treatment will be described seriatim. You (addressed to the disciples) should understand these methods appropriately. [12-13]

Atisara Chikitsa Sutra: Line of treatment

दोषाः सन्निचिता यस्य विदग्धाहार मूर्च्छिताः| अतीसाराय कल्पन्ते भूयस्तान् सम्प्रवर्तयेत्||१४||

न तु सङ्ग्रहणं देयं पूर्वमामातिसारिणे| विबध्यमानाः प्रागदोषा जनयन्त्यामयान् बहून्||१५||

दण्डकालसकाध्मान ग्रहण्यर्शो गदांस्तथा| शोथ पाण्ड्वामय प्लीह कुष्ठ गुल्मोदर ज्वरान्||१६||

तस्मादुपेक्षेतोत्क्लिष्टान् वर्तमानान् स्वयं मलान्| कृच्छ्रं वा वहतां दद्यादभयां सम्प्रवर्तिनीम्||१७||

तया प्रवाहिते दोषे प्रशाम्यत्युदरामयः| जायते देह लघुता जठराग्निश्च वर्धते||१८||

प्रमथ्यां मध्यदोषाणां दद्याद्दीपन पाचनीम्| लङ्घनं चाल्पदोषाणां प्रशस्तमतिसारिणाम्||१९||

Atisara Line of treatment:

When the diarrhoea is caused by the aggravated Doshas impelled by Vidagdha (Undigested) food, the patient is given laxative to eliminate these Doshas. It is not desirable to give laxatives in the beginning, in the Ama (primary or immature) stage of Diarrhoea.

When ama is not there in the initial stage, administration of such bowel-binding therapies (Sangrahana chikitsa) obstructs the movement and elimination of the already aggravated Doshas which gives rise to several diseases (complications) like

Dandakalasaka (obstruction to intestinal peristalsis), Adhmana (flatulence), Grahani (sprue syndrome), Arshas (Piles), Bhagandara (Fistula- in Ano), Shotha (Oedema), Pandu (Anaemia), Pliha (Splenic disorders), Kushta (skin diseases including leprosy), Gulma (phantom tumour),

Udara (obstinate abdominal diseases including ascites) and Jwara – fever.

Therefore, the physician should ignore the downward movement of the already detached (Utklista) morbid matter which is moving downwards on its own.

By implication, diarrhoea is allowed to continue and should not be stopped by medicines which cause constipation.

If the Diarrhea is associated with griping pain (difficulty in voiding), then Haritaki – Harad is given as a mild laxative.

When the morbid matter is eliminated through downward movement [as suggested above], then it gets cured, the body becomes light and the abdominal Agni (power of digestion) becomes strong.

If the Doshas are moderately aggravated, then Pramathya (a type of decoction of drugs) which simulates the power of digestion (Dipana) and which is carminative (Pachana) is administered.

If the Doshas are only slightly aggravated and causing Diarrhoea, then Langhana (fasting therapy) is very useful. [14-19]

Recipes of Pramathya

पिप्पली नागरं धान्यं भूतीकमभया वचा| ह्रीवेरं भद्रमुस्तानि बिल्वं नागर धान्यकम्||२०||

पृश्निपर्णी श्वदंष्ट्रा च समङ्गा कण्टकारिका| तिस्रः प्रमथ्या विहिताः श्लोकार्धैरतिसारिणाम्||२१||

वचा प्रतिविषाभ्यां वा मुस्त पर्पटकेन वा| ह्रीवेर शृङ्गवेराभ्यां पक्वं वा पाययेज्जलम्||२२||

These recipes of Pramathya which are useful in the treatment of Diarrhoea are as follows:

1. Pippali – Piper longum, Nagara – Zingiber officinale, Dhanya, Bhutika, Abhaya – Terminalia chebula and Vacha – Acorus calamus [According to the commentary, the decoction or Pramathya prepared of these herbs is useful for Vatika Diarrhoea]

2. Hrivera – Pavonia odorata, Bhadramusta, Bilva – Aegle marmelos, ginger and coriander [According to the commentary, the pramathya prepared of these herbs is useful in Paittika type of Diarrhoea] and

3. Prishniparni – Uraria picta, Svadamshtra – tribulus terrestris, Samanga – Rubia cordifolia and Kantakari – Solanum xanthocarpum [According to the commentary, the Pramathya prepared of these herbs is useful in Kaphaja Diarrhoea].

The decoctions of the following ingredients are also useful for the treatment of Diarrhoea:

1. Vacha (Acorus calamus Linn.) and Prativisha [According to the commentary, the decoction of these herbs is useful in Vatika Diarrhoea]

2. Musta – Cyperus rotundus and Parpataka [According to the commentary, the decoction of these herbs is useful in Paittika Diarrhoea] and

3. Hrivera – Pavonia odorata and Shringavera – Ginger – Zingiber officinale [According to the commentary, the decoction of these herbs is useful for Kaphaja Diarrhoea]. [20-22]

Diet for Atisara:

युक्तेऽन्नकाले क्षुत्क्षामं लघून्यन्नानि भोजयेत्| तथा स शीघ्रमाप्नोति रुचिमग्निबलं बलम्||२३||

तक्रेणावन्तिसोमेन यवाग्वा तर्पणेन वा| सुरया मधुना चादौ यथा सात्म्यमुपाचरेत्||२४||

यवागूभिर्विलेपीभिः खडै यूषै रसौदनैः| दीपन ग्राहि संयुक्तैः क्रमश्च स्यादतः परम्||२५||

At appropriate meal time, when the patient is hungry, he is given light food to eat. By this, he develops appetite for food, his Agni (power of digestion) gets stimulated, and his strength is promoted immediately.

In the beginning, depending upon the wholesomeness (Satmya), the patient is given [the above mentioned light food] along with butter-milk, Avanti-Soma or Kanji (a sour drink), Yavagu (thick Gruel), Tarpana (Roasted flour of cereals mixed with water), alcoholic drink.

Thereafter, the patient is gradually given Yavagu (thick gruel), Vilepi (a sticky gruel), Khada (a sour appetiser), Yusha (vegetable soup) and boiled rice mixed with meat soup which is prepared by doing digestive stimulants and astringent (constipative) herbs. [23-25]

Group of herbs Useful in Diarrhea

शालपर्णी पृश्निपर्णी बृहतीं कण्टकारिकाम्| बलां श्वदंष्ट्रां बिल्वानि पाठां नागर धान्यकम्||२६||

शटीं पलाशं हपुषां वचां जीरक पिप्पलीम्| यवानीं पिप्पलीमूलं चित्रकं हस्तिपिप्पलीम्||२७||

वृक्षाम्लं दाडिमाम्लं च सहिङ्गु बिड सैन्धवम्| प्रयोजयेदन्नपाने विधिना सूप कल्पितम्||२८||

वातश्लेष्महरो ह्येष गणो दीपन पाचनः| ग्राही बल्यो रोचनश्च तस्माच्छस्तोऽतिसारिणाम्||२९||

Shala-Parni Prsni Parni, Brihati Kantakari Bala Svadamstra Bilva PathaNagara Dhanyaka Sati Palasha Hapusa Vacha Jiraka Pippali Yavani Pippali Chitraka Hasti-Pippali Vrikshamla Sour Dadima Hingu Vida

Saindhava - these ingredients are appropriately used in processing food preparation. Herbs belonging to this group alleviate Vata and Kapha.

These are

Dipana (digestive stimulant)

Pachana (carminative)

Grahi (constipating)

Balya (Promoter of strength)

Rocana (Appetiser). Therefore, these herbs are useful for the patient suffering from Atisara (Diarrhoea). [26-29]

Management of Diarrhea Associated with griping Pain

आमे परिणते यस्तु विबद्धमतिसार्यते| सशूलपिच्छमल्पाल्पं बहुशः सप्रवाहिकम्||३०||
यूषेण मूलकानां तं बदराणामथापि वा| उपोदिकायाः क्षीरिण्या यवान्या वास्तुकस्य वा||३१||
सुवर्चलायाश्चञ्चोर्वा शाकेनावल्गुजस्य वा| शट्याः कर्करुकाणां वा जीवन्त्याश्चिर्भटस्य वा||३२||
लोणिकायाः सपाठायाः शुष्क शाकेन वा पुनः| दधि दाडिम सिद्धेन बहु स्नेहेन भोजयेत्||३३||

After the maturity of Ama (product of indigestion), if the patient voids loose motions along with scybalous stool associated with colic pain and mucus very frequently in small quantities, and if there is griping pain, then he is given food along with the soup of

Mulaka, Badara, Upodika, Ksheerini, Yavani, Vastuka, Suvarcala, Cancu, Leaves of Avalguja, Sati, Karkaruka, Jivanti, Cirbhata, Linika Patha or Suska-saka.

These soups are cooked along with curd (yoghurt) and Dadima – Pomegranate – Punica granatum, are added with ghee (fat) in the profuse quantity. [30-33]

Treatment of Pravahika

कल्कः स्याद्बाल बिल्वानां तिलकल्कश्च तत्समः| दध्नः सरोऽम्ल स्नेहाद्यः खडो हन्यात् प्रवाहिकाम्||३४||

Khada (a type of soup) is prepared by adding the paste of tender fruits of Bilva – Aegle marmelos, equal quantity of the paste of Tila – Sesame - Sesamum indicum, cream of sour curd and profuse quantity of ghee. Intake of this Khada cures Pravahika (griping pain) [34]

Treatment of Varcah-Ksaya (Scanty Formation of Stool)

यवानां मुद्ग माषाणां शालीनां च तिलस्य च| कोलानां बाल बिल्वानां धान्य यूषं प्रकल्पयेत्||३५||
एकध्यं यमके भृष्टं दधि दाडिम सारिकम्| वर्चःक्षये शुष्कमुखं शाल्यन्नं तेन भोजयेत्||३६||

If there is Varcah Ksaya (scanty stool) and Sushka mukha (dryness of the mouth), then the patient is given
Dhanya- Yusha (a type of soup prepared of cereals and Pulses) made of
Yava – Barley (Hordeum vulgare),
Mudga – Vigna radiata
Masha
Shali type of rice,
Sesame seeds
Kola and
Tender fruits of Bilva, sizzled with Yamaka (ghee and oil) taken together, curd and the extract of Dadima – Pomegranate Along with this soup he should take boiled Shali type of Rice [35- 36]

दध्नः सरं वा यमके भृष्टं सगुड नागरम्| सुरां वा यमके भृष्टां व्यञ्जनार्थे प्रदापयेत्||३७||
फलाम्लं यमके भृष्टं यूष गृञ्जनस्य वा| लोपाक रसमम्लं वा स्निग्धाम्लं कच्छपस्य वा||३८||
बर्हि तितिरि दक्षाणां वर्तकानां तथा रसाः| स्निग्धाम्लाः शालयश्चाग्र्या वर्चःक्षय रुजापहाः||३९||
अन्तराधिरसं पूत्वा रक्तं मेषस्य चोभयम्| पचेद्दाडिम साराम्लं सधान्य स्नेह नागरम्||४०||
ओदनं रक्तशालीनां तेनाद्यात् प्रपिबेच्च तत्| तथा वर्चःक्षय कृतै र्व्याधिभि विप्रमुच्यते||४१||

If there is Varcah-kshaya (Scanty stool), then the patient is given the following:
1. Cream of curd sizzled with ghee and oil, and mixed with Jaggery and Sunthi – Zingiber officinale. This is used as Vyanjana (a side dish)
2. Alcohol sizzled with ghee and oil. This is given as Vyanjana (side-dish)
3. Sour fruits sizzled with ghee and oil. This is used as Vyanjana (side-dish)
4. Soup of Grnjanaka, soup of the meat of Kacchapa added with ghee and sour ingredients or the soup of the meat of Barhi, Tittiri, Daksha or Vartaka. These soups is used as Vyanjana (side- dish)
5. Red variety of Shali (rice) boiled by adding ghee and sour ingredients and

6. The decoction of the meat taken from the trunk of sheep is added with its blood, and sizzled by saddling the extract of Dadima – Pomegranate, Dhanya, ghee and Nagara . This soup is used for boiling red varieties of Shali rice. Intake of this cooked rice and drinking this soup make the patient free from the ailments caused by varcah- Ksaya (scanty stool). [37-41]

Prolapse of Rectum

गुदनिःसरणे शूले पानमम्लस्य सर्पिषः| प्रशस्यते निरामाणामथवाऽप्यनुवासनम्||४२||

If there is prolapse of rectum and colic pain, and if the Diarrhoea is free from Ama, then the patient is given sour-ghee (medicated ghee to be described below). Such a patient may also be given Anuvasana type of medicated enema [with this type of sour ghee].

Changeri Ghrita and Chavyadi Ghrta

चाङ्गेरी कोल दध्यम्ल नागर क्षार संयुतम्| घृतमुत्क्वथितं पेयं गुदभ्रंश रुजापहम्||४३||

इति चाङ्गेरीघृतम्|

सचव्य पिप्पलीमूलं सव्योष विड दाडिमम्| पेयमम्लं घृतं युक्त्या सधान्याजाजि चित्रकम्||४४||

इति गुदभ्रंशे चव्यादिघृतम्|

Ghee is cooked with the juice of Changeri, decoction of Kola and sour curd, and the paste of Nagara and Ksara (alkali preparation). Intake of this medicated ghee cures ailments caused by prolapse of rectum.
Thus, ends the description of Changeri-Ghrta.
Ghee is cooked with the sour ingredients (juice of Changeri- Oxalis corniculata, decoction of Kola and sour curd), and the paste of Chavya – Piper retrofractum, Pippali – Long pepper fruit – Piper longum, Maricha – Black pepper fruit – piper nigrum, Vida and Dadima – Pomegranate – Punica granatum. Intake of this medicated ghee along with Dhanya, Ajaji and Chitraka – Leadwort – Plumbago zeylanica in appropriate quantity [cures prolapse of rectum].
Thus, ends the description of Chavyadi- Ghrta for prolapsed rectum. [43- 44]

Anuvasana Type of enema for Prolapse Rectum

दशमूलोपसिद्धं वा सबिल्वमनुवासनम्| शटी शताह्वा बिल्वैर्वा वचया चित्रकेण वा||४५||

इति गुदभ्रंशेऽनुवासनम्|

For the treatment of Prolapse rectum, Anuvasana therapy is administered with the following recipes:
1. Dashamula cooked with fat
2. Bilva – Aegle marmelos cooked with fat
3. Sati – Hedychium spicatum, Shatahva or Bilva cooked in fat
4. Vacha (Acorus calamus Linn.) cooked with fat
5. Chitraka – Plumbago zeylanica cooked with fat
Thus ends the description of the Anuvasana type of enema for prolapsed rectum. [45]

Management of Strangulated Prolapse Rectum

स्तब्ध भ्रष्टगुदे पूर्वं स्नेह स्वेदौ प्रयोजयेत्| सुस्विन्नं तं मृदूभूतं पिचुना सम्प्रवेशयेत्||४६||

If the prolapse rectum becomes stiff or strangulated, and does not go inside of its own, then oil is applied over it and fomentation is given. Thereafter, when the prolapsed rectum is well fomented and it has become soft, then with the help of a cotton pad (or pad made of thick cloth), it is pushed inside and restored to its original place. [46]

Ksheera yoga – Use of Medicated Milk

विबद्ध वात वर्चास्तु बहुशूल प्रवाहिकः| सरक्त पिच्छस्तृष्णार्तः क्षीर सौहित्यमर्हति||४७||

यमकस्योपरि क्षीरं धारोष्णं वा पिबेन्नरः| शृतमेरण्डमूलेन बाल बिल्वेन वा पयः ||४८||

एवं क्षीर प्रयोगेण रक्तं पिच्छा च शाम्यति| शूलं प्रवाहिका चैव विबन्धश्चोपशाम्यति||४९||

If the movement of flatus and stool is arrested, if the patient suffers from acute colic pain or griping pain, if the patient voids blood and mucus, and if the patient is thirsty, then a profuse quantity of milk is administered. Such a patient is given Yamaka (ghee and oil mixed together), and thereafter, lukewarm milk collected directly from the udder (dharosna) is given.

Milk boiled with the root of Eranda – Ricinus communis or tender fruit of Bilva – Aegle marmelos may also be given in the above-mentioned condition.

By the intake of the recipes of medicated ghee mentioned above, bleeding mucus discharge from the anus stops. These recipes also cure colic pain, griping pain and constipation. [47-49]

Treatment of Paittika Atisara

पित्तातिसारं पुनर्निदानोपशयाकृतिभिरामान्वयमुपलभ्य यथाबलं लङ्घन पाचनाभ्यामुपाचरेत्|

तृष्यतस्तु मुस्त पर्पटकोशीर सारिवा चन्दन किराततिक्तकोदीच्यवारिभिरुपचारः|

लङ्घितस्य चाहारकाले बलातिबलासूर्पपर्णी शालपर्णी पृश्निपर्णी बृहती कण्टकारिका शतावरी श्वदंष्ट्रा निर्यूह संयुक्तेन यथासात्म्यं यवागू मण्डादिना तर्पणादिना वा क्रमेणोपचारः|

मुद्ग मसूर हरेणुमकुष्ठकाढकी यूषैर्वा लावक पिञ्जल शश हरिणैणकालपुच्छकरसैरीषदम्लैरनम्लैर्वा क्रमशोऽग्निं सन्धुक्षयेत्|

अनुबन्धे त्वस्य दीपनीय पाचनीयोपशमनीय सङ्ग्रहणीयान् योगान् सम्प्रयोजयेदिति||५०||

If Paittika type of Atisara (Diarrhoea) is associated with Ama which can be determined by causative factors, Upashaya (homologation), signs and symptoms, then the patient is given Langhana (fasting therapy) and Pachana (carminative therapy) appropriate to the strength of the patient.

If he is thirsty, then such a patient is given the decoction of

Musta (Cyperus rotundus),

Parapataka, Ushira, Sariva, Chandana, Kirata tiktaka and Udicya to drink

After the fasting therapy is administared, during meal time, the patient is gradually given Yavagu (thick gruel), manda (a type of thin gruel) and the Niryuha (decoction prepared according to the procedure suggested for Sadanga-Paniya (vide commentary on Chikitsa 3 : 145-146] of Bala – Country mallow (root) – Sida cordifolia, Atibala – Abutilon indicum, Surpa-parni (mudgaparni and Mashaparni), shalaparni – Desmodium gangeticum, Prsniparni – Uraria picta, Brihati – Solanum indicum, Kantakari – Solanum xanthocarpum, Shatavari – Asparagus racemosus and Svadamstra – Tribulus terristeris

His Agni (power of digestion) is stimulated gradually with the vegetable soup of

Mudga, Masura, Harenu, Makustha and Adhaki or

With the soup of the meat of

Lava, Kapinjala, Sasa, Harina, Ena and Kalapuccha

These vegetable soups and meat soups may be slightly sour or may not be sour.

If the Paittika type of Diarrhoea continues in site of the above mentioned measures, then the patient is treated with recipes which are

Dipaniya (digestive stimulant),

Pacaniya (carminative),

Upasamaniya (Dosha- alleviator) and

Sangrahaniya (constipating) [50]

Ayurvedic Medicines for Paittika Atisara

सक्षौद्रातिविषं पिष्ट्वा वत्सकस्य फल त्वचम्| पिबेत् पित्तातिसारघ्नं तण्डुलोदक संयुतम्||५१||

किरात तिक्तको मुस्तं वत्सकः सरसाञ्जनः| बिल्वं दारुहरिद्रा त्वक् ह्रीबेरं सदुरालभम्||५२||

चन्दनं च मृणालं च नागरं लोध्रमुत्पलम्| तिला मोचरसो लोध्रं समङ्गा कमलोत्पलम्||५३||

उत्पलं धातकीपुष्पं दाडिमत्वइमहौषधम्| कट्फलं नागरं पाठा जम्ब्वामास्थि दुरालभाः||५४||

योगाः षडेते सक्षौद्रास्तण्डुलोदक संयुताः| पेयाः पित्तातिसारघ्नाः श्लोकार्धेन निर्दिशिताः||५५||

जीर्णौषधानां शस्यन्ते यथायोगं प्रकल्पितैः| रसैः साङ्ग्राहिकैर्युक्ताः पुराणा रक्तशालयः||५६||

The following recipes are useful for the patient suffering from Paittika type of Atisara (diarrhoea)

1. The fruit and bark of Vatsaka (Holarrhena antidysenterica Wall.) is added with Ativisa—Aconitum heterophyllum and honey. Intake of this along with rice-water (tandulodaka) cures Paittika atisara.

2. Powder of Kiratatiktaka – Swertia chirata, Musta (Cyperus rotundus), Vatsaka (Holarrhena antidysenterica) and Rasanjana (Aqueous extract of Berberis aristata)

3. Powder of Bilva – Aegle marmelos, Daru-Haridra (turmeric – Curcuma longa), Tvak, Hribera – Pavonia odorata and Duralabha – Fagonia arabica

4. Powder of Chandana (Sandalwood – Santalum album), Mrnala, Nagara – Zingiber officinale, Lodhra (Symplocos racemosa) and Utpala (Nymphaea alba)

5. Powder of tila, mocha-Rasa, Lodhra (Symplocos racemosa), Samanga – Rubia cordifolia, kamala and Utpala (Nymphaea alba)

6. Powder of Utpala (Nymphaea alba), Dhataki – Woodfordia fruticosa (flower), Dadima – Pomegranate – Punica granatum, Tvak and Mahausadha and Katphala – Myrica nagi, Nagara – Zingiber officinale, Patha- Cissampelos pareira, seed-pulp of Jambu – syzygium cumini and Amra – mango – Mangifera indica and Duralabha

The above mentioned 6 recipes (nos- 2-7) are taken along with appropriately cooked meat-soup added with constipating herbs.

Administration of milk

पित्तातिसारो दीपाग्नेः क्षिप्रं समुपशाम्यति| अजाक्षीर प्रयोगेण बलं वर्णश्च वर्धते||५७||

बहुदोषस्य दीप्ताग्नेः सप्राणस्य न तिष्ठति| पैत्तिको यद्यतीसारः पयसा तं विरेचयेत्||५८||

पलाशफल निर्यूहं पयसा सह पाययेत्| ततोऽनुपाययेत् कोष्णं क्षीरमेव यथाबलम्||५९||

प्रवाहिते तेन मले प्रशाम्यत्युदरामयः| पलाशवत् प्रयोज्या वा त्रायमाणा विशोधिनी||६०||

Administration of goat-milk to the patient having strong digestion cures the Paittika type of Atisara (Diarrhoea), and promotes strength as well as complexion.

If because of excessively aggravated Doshas, the Paittika type of Diarrhoea is not cured and if the patient has strong power of digestion and vitality, then he is given laxative therapy with milk.

He is given the decoction of the fruits of Palasa – Butea monosperma along with milk. Thereafter, depending upon the strength of the patient, he is given lukewarm milk to drink. This will restore bowel movement as a result of which Diarrhoea will be controlled.

On the above lines Trayamana – Gentiana kurroo can also be administered for the cleansing of the bowel. [57-60]

Anuvasana type of medicated Enema

सांसर्ग्यां क्रियमाणायां शूलं यद्यनुवर्तते| सुतदोषस्य तं शीघ्रं यथावदनुवासयेत्||६१||

शतपुष्पावरीभ्यां च पयसा मधुकेन च| तैलपादं घृतं सिद्धं सबिल्वमनुवासनम्||६२||

If in the course of Samsarjana- Karma (gradual administration of light to heavy food) [after the administration of the laxative therapy], the colic pain recurs, then to such a patient (from whose body the morbid matter is already eliminated) appropriate Anuvasana (a type of medicated enema) therapy is administered immediately.

Ghee is cooked by adding 1/4th (in quantity) of oil, decoction of Shatavari – Asparagus racemosa and Madhuka– Licorice – Glycyrrhiza glabra, and [the paste of] Bilva – Aegle marmelos. This medicated ghee is used for giving Anuvasana type of medicated enema. [61- 62]

Piccha-Basti (Mucilaginous Enema)

कृतानुवासनस्यास्य कृत संसर्जनस्य च| वर्तते यद्यतीसारः पिच्छाबस्तिरतः परम्||६३||

परिवेष्ट्य कुशैरार्द्रैरार्द्रवृन्तानि शाल्मलेः| कृष्ण मृतिकयाऽऽलिप्य स्वेदयेद्गोमयाग्निना||६४||

सुशुष्कां मृतिकां ज्ञात्वा तानि वृन्तानि शाल्मलेः| शृते पयसि मृदनीयादापोथ्योलूखले ततः||६५||

पिण्डं मुष्टिसमं प्रस्थे तत् पूतं तैलसर्पिषोः| स्नेहितं मात्रया युक्तं कल्केन मधुकस्य च||६६||

बस्तिमभ्यक्तगात्राय दद्यात् प्रत्यागते ततः| स्नात्वा भुञ्जीत पयसा जाङ्गलानां रसेन वा||६७||

पित्तातिसार ज्वर शोथ गुल्म जीर्णातिसार ग्रहणी प्रदोषान्| जयत्ययं शीघ्रमति प्रवृद्धान् विरेचनास्थापनयोश्च बस्तिः ||६८||

If Diarrhoea persists in spite of the administration of Anuvasana type of medicated enema and the administration of Samsarjana karma (gradual administration of lighter to heavier food), then Piccha-Basthi (Mucilaginous type of medicated enema) is given thereafter.

Green stalks of Salmali – Salmalia malabarica are covered with green Kusa (Desmostachya bipinnata), and tied. This bundle is smeared with the mud of black soil and placed over cow dung fire. After the mud is dried up, the stalks of Shalmali – Salmalia malabarica are removed. These stalks are then triturated in a pestle and mortar. One Musti (ala or handful) of this paste is mixed with 1 Prastha of boiled milk and filtered. In this milk, oil and ghee, and the paste of Madhuka– Licorice – Glycyrrhiza glabra is added in adequate quantities. This recipe is used for medicated enema to be given to the patient after his body is massaged with oil. After the ingredients of enema come out of the rectum, the patient should take a bath, and thereafter, take food along with either milk or the soup of the meat of animals inhabiting the jangala area (thin forest).

This Piccha-basthi (mucilaginous enema) cures

Paittika type of Diarrhoea,

Jwara – fever

Shotha – oedema

Gulma (phantom tumour), chronic Diarrhoea,

Grahani (sprue syndrome) and the acute complications of Purgation as well as Asthapana (a type of medicated enema containing decoction etc) therapies [63-68]

Raktatisara (Hemorrhagic Diarrhea)

पित्तातिसारी यस्त्वेतां क्रियां मुक्त्वा निषेवते| पित्तलान्यन्नपानानि तस्य पित्तं महाबलम्||६९||

कुर्याद्रक्तातिसारं तु रक्तमाशु प्रदूषयेत्| तृष्णां शूलं विदाहं च गुदपाकं च दारुणम्||७०||

If the patient suffering from Paittika diarrhoea does not follow the above mentioned therapeutic measures, and on the other hand, resorts to such food and drinks which cause aggravation of pitta, then the exceedingly aggravated Pitta causes Raktatisara (haemorrhagic Diarrhoea) and instantaneous vitiation of Rakta (blood). This leads to serious complications like excessive thirst, colic pain, burning sensation and suppuration of the anus. [69- 70]

Raktatisara Chikitsa: Treatment of Haemorrhagic Diarrhoea

तत्र च्छागं पयः शस्तं शीतं समधु शर्करम्| पानार्थं भोजनार्थं च गुद प्रक्षालने तथा||७१||

ओदनं रक्तशालीनां पयसा तेन भोजयेत्| रसैः पारावतादीनां घृतभृष्टैः सशर्करैः||७२||

शशपक्षि मृगाणां च शीतानां धन्वचारिणाम्| रसैरनम्लैः सघृतैर्भोजयेत् सशर्करैः||७३||

रुधिरं मार्गमाजं वा घृतभृष्टं प्रशस्यते| काश्मर्यफल यूषो वा किञ्चिदम्लः सशर्करः||७४||

नीलोत्पलं मोचरसं समङ्गा पद्मकेशरम्| अजाक्षीर युतं दद्याज्जीर्णे च पयसौदनम्||७५||

दुर्बलं पाययित्वा वा तस्यैवोपरि भोजयेत्| प्राग्भक्तं नवनीतं वा दद्यात् समधु शर्करम्||७६||

Treatment of Haemorrhagic Diarrhoea

In haemorrhagic Diarrhoea, goat's milk is very useful. It is used, when cooled, with honey and sugar for drink, along with food, and for washing the anal region.

Boiled rice of red variety of Shali is given to the patient to eat along with the Goat's milk.

The boiled rice may also be given along with the soup of the meat of Paravata etc. sizzled with ghee and mixed with sugar. The soup of the meat, having a cooling effect like those of rabbits, birds and deer inhabiting deserts, is sizzled with ghee, mixed with sugar and given to such patients. It may be ensured that these soups are free from any sour ingredients.

For these ailments the blood of deer or goat, sizzled with ghee is also very useful.

The soup of the fruits of kashmarya, made slightly sour and mixed with sugar is also useful in this condition.

The powder of Nilotpala, Mocharasa, Samanga and Padmakesara is administered along with the goat's milk. After the digestion of this potion, the patient is given rice with milk. If the patient is weak, then food can be given to him even before the above-mentioned potion is digested.

To the patient suffering from haemorrhagic dirrhoea, butter along with honey and sugar may be given before meals. [71-76]

Recipes for haemorrhagic Diarrhoea

प्राश्य क्षीरोत्थितं सर्पिः कपिञ्जलरसाशनः| त्र्यहादारोग्यमाप्नोति पयसा क्षीरभुक् तथा||७७||

पीत्वा शतावरी कल्कं पयसा क्षीरभुग्जयेत्| रक्तातिसारं पीत्वा वा तया सिद्धं घृतं नरः||७८||

घृतं यवागू मण्डेन कुटजस्य फलैः शृतम्| पेयं तस्यानु पातव्या पेया रक्तोप शान्तये||७९||

After taking ghee collected from the cream of milk along with milk, the patient is given with the soup of Kapinjala. During this therapy, he should take milk [in adequate quantity]. This cures hemorrhagic diarrhoea in the 3 days. While taking milk as food (drink), the patient should take the paste of Shatavari – Asparagus racemosus mixed with milk. He may also take milk boiled with Shatavari paste. Both these recipes cure haemorrhagic Diarrhoea.

Intake of ghee cooked by adding the paste of the fruits of Kutaja (Holarrhena antidysenterica Wall.), along with the scum (upper part) of the Yavagu and intake of Peya (thin gruel) thereafter, alleviates Rakta or blood (stops bleeding). [77-79]

Darvyadi- Ghrita

त्वक् च दारुहरिद्रायाः कुटजस्य फलानि च| पिप्पली शृङ्गवेरं च द्राक्षा कटुकरोहिणी||८०||

षड्भिरेतैर्घृतं सिद्धं पेया मण्डावचारितम्| अतीसारं जयेच्छीघ्रं त्रिदोषमपि दारुणम्||८१||

Ghee is cooked by adding the 6 herbs, viz, the bark of Daru-haridra – Berberis aristata, fruits of Kutaja Pippali, Shringavera, Draksha and Kutuka-Katukarohini . Intake of Peya (thin gruel) and Manda (very thin gruel) along with this medicated ghee cures serious types of Diarrhoea even if caused by Sannipata (simultaneous aggravation of all the 3 Doshas). [80-81]

Hemostatic Recipes

कृष्णमृन्मधुकं शङ्खं रुधिरं तण्डुलोदकम्| पीतमेकत्र सक्षौद्रं रक्त सङ्ग्रहणं परम्||८२||

पीतः प्रियङ्गुका कल्कः सक्षौद्रस्तण्डुलाम्भसा| रक्त स्रावं जयेच्छीघ्रं धन्वमांसरसाशिनः||८३||

कल्कस्तिलानां कृष्णानां शर्करा पञ्चभागिकः| आजेन पयसा पीतः सद्यो रक्तं नियच्छति||८४||

Medicines and herbs to stop bleeding:

Intake of Krsna-Mrt (black earth), Madhuka– Licorice – Glycyrrhiza glabra, Sankha, Rudhira (blood or Kesara) and rice- water mixed with honey can stop bleeding instantaneously.

The paste of Priyangu (Callicara macrophylla) is added with rice- water (Tandulambu). Intake of this, while taking the soup of the meat of animals inhabiting arid zones, in food, stops bleeding instantaneously.

1 part of the paste of the black variety of Tila – Sesame (Sesamum indicum) is added with 4 parts of sugar. Intake of this potion along with the goat's milk stops bleeding instantaneously. [82-84]

पलं वत्सकबीजस्य श्रपयित्वा रसं पिबेत्| यो रसाशी जयेच्छीघ्रं स पैत्तं जठरामयम्||८५||

पीत्वा सशर्करा क्षौद्रं चन्दनं तण्डुलाम्भसा| दाह तृष्णा प्रमेहेभ्यो रक्तस्रावाच्च मुच्यते||८६||

Intake of the decoction of the seeds of Vatsaka (Holarrhena antidysenterica Wall) while taking meat-soup as food cures Paittika type of Diarrhoea (Jatharamaya- abdominal diseases).

Intake of Chandana along with rice-water, mixed with sugar and honey cures burning sensation, excess thirst, Prameha (obstinate urinary diseases including diabetes) and bleeding [85- 86]

Treatment of Gudapaka – Anal Suppuration

गुदो बहुभिरुत्थानैर्यस्य पित्तेन पच्यते| सेचयेतं सुशीतेन पटोल मधुकाम्बुना||८७||

पञ्चवल्क मधूकानां रसैरिक्षुरसैर्घृतैः| छागैर्गव्यैः पयोभिर्वा शर्कराक्षौद्रसंयुतैः||८८||

Treatment of Gudapaka – Anal Suppuration

The Anus may get suppurated by the aggravated Pitta on account of the frequent voidance of stool. The anus of such a patient is sprinkled with the following recipes:

1. Exceeding cold decoction of Patola – Trichosanthes dioica and Madhuka- Madhuca longifolia
2. Decoction of Pancha-Valkala (barks of Nyagrodha – Ficus bengalensis,Udumbara – Ficus racemosa, Asvattha – Ficus religiosa, Parisa - Thespesia populnea and Plaksa – Ficus lacor or sugar cane juice and
3. Milk or ghee of goat or cow mixed with sugar and honey. [87- 88]

प्रक्षालनानां कल्कैर्वा ससर्पिष्कैः प्रलेपयेत्| एषां वा सुकृतैश्चूर्णैस्तं गुदं प्रतिसारयेत्||८९||

धातकी लोध्र चूर्णैर्वा समांशैः प्रतिसारयेत्| तथा स्रवति नो रक्तं गुदं तैः प्रतिसारितम्||९०||

पक्वता प्रशमं याति वेदना चोपशाम्यति| यथोक्तैः सेचनैः शीतैः शोणितेऽतिस्रवत्यपि||९१||

गुद वङ्क्षण कट्यूरु सेचयेद्घृतभावितम्| चन्दनाद्येन तैलेन शतधौतेन सर्पिषा||९२||

कार्पास सङ्गृहीतेन सेचयेद्गुद वङ्क्षणम्|९३|

The paste of herbs mentioned above for washing (sprinkling over) the anus may be mixed with ghee and applied over the suppurated anus

The powder of the above mentioned herbs may also be used for Pratisarana (dusting) over the suppurated anus.

The powder of Dhataki – Woodfordia fruticosa and Lodhra (Symplocos racemosa), taken in equal quantities, may be used for dusting over the suppurated Anus.

The bleeding stops, and the suppuration as well as pain subside soon after the anal region is dusted with the above recipes.

If there is excessive bleeding (from the anus), the cold decoction of the above mentioned herbs is impregnated with ghee, and sprinkled over the anal region, pelvic region, lumbar region and thighs.

To stop excessive bleeding, a cotton pad is soaked with Chandanadya-Taila (described in Chikitsa3; 258) or Shatadhauta Grtha (ghee washed with cold water for 100 times), and the oil or ghee is sprinkled by squeezing this pad over the Anal and pelvic regions. [89- ½ 93]

Picchabasti for griping Pain

अल्पाल्पं बहुशो रक्तं सशूलमुपवेश्यते||९३||

यदा वायु र्विबद्धश्च कृच्छ्रं चरति वा न वा| पिच्छा बस्तिं तदा तस्य यथोक्तमुपकल्पयेत्||९४||

प्रपौण्डरीक सिद्धेन सर्पिषा चानुवासयेत्| प्रायशो दुर्बल गुदाश्चिरकालातिसारिणः||९५||

तस्मादभीक्ष्णशस्तेषां गुदे स्नेहं प्रयोजयेत्|९६|

When the movement of the aggravated Vata (Flatus) gets obstructed or its movements are not smooth or when there is absolutely no movement of this Vata, then the patient voids blood frequently in small quantities which is associated with pain. To such a patient, Piccha-Basthi (Mucilaginous enema) is administered. Recipes of this type of medicated enema are already described (in the verse nos. 63-68)

The above-mentioned type of patient is given Anuvasana type of medicated enema with the medicated ghee prepared by cooking with Prapaundarika – red variety.

Because of chronic Diarrhoea, the Anus of the patient generally becomes weak. Therefore, (cotton soaked in) medicated ghee (described above) is inserted into his anus frequently (or may be given Anuvasana type of medicated enema with this medicated ghee.). [93 ½ – ½ 96]

Basti, Lehayoga: Medicated Enema and Recipes of Linctus

पवनोऽतिप्रवृत्तो हि स्वे स्थाने लभतेऽधिकम्||९६||

बलं तस्य सपितस्य जयार्थे बस्तिरुत्तमः| रक्तं विट्सहितं पूर्वं पश्चाद्वा योऽतिसार्यते||९७||

शतावरी घृतं तस्य लेहार्थमुपकल्पयेत्| शर्कराऱ्धांशिकं लीढं नवनीतं नवोद्धृतम्||९८||

क्षौद्रपादं जयेच्छीघ्रं तं विकारं हिताशिनः| न्यग्रोधोदुम्बराश्वत्थ शुङ्गानापोथ्य वासयेत्||९९||

अहोरात्रं जले तप्ते घृतं तेनाम्भसा पचेत्| तदर्ध शर्करायुक्तं लिह्यात् सक्षौद्रपादिकम्||१००||

अधो वा यदि वाऽप्यूर्ध्वं यस्य रक्तं प्रवर्तते|१०१|

Basti, Lehayoga: Medicated Enema and Recipes of Linctus

The Vata aggravated in the above said way becomes stronger in its own location, (i.e colon which is afflicted by Diarrhoea). For the alleviation of this aggravated Vayu associated with Pitta (which takes place in hemorrhagic diarrhoea), Basti or medicated enema (both the Anuvasana and Niruha types) is the best therapy.

If bleeding takes places along with the stool before voiding stool or after voiding stool in hemorrhagic type of Diarrhoea, then the patient is given Shatavari-Ghrta (vide Cikista 30 : 64-69) in the form of a Linctus.

Intake of freshly collected butter along with ½ quantity of sugar and 1/4th in quantity of honey cures the above mentioned ailments. While taking this potion, the patient should take wholesome food.

Adventitious roots of Nyagrodha – Ficus bengalensis, Udumbara – Ficus racemosa and Asvattha- Ficus religiosa are crushed and kept soaked in hot water for 24 hours. Ghee is cooked along with this water. This medicated ghee is added with ½ the quantity of sugar and 1/4th in quantity of honey, and taken in the form of linctus. This cures hemorrhagic Diarrhoea associated with bleeding either before or after the voiding of stool. [96 ½ – ½ 101]

Suppuration of Anal Sphincters

यस्त्वेवं दुर्बलो मोहात् पित्तलान्येव सेवते||१०१||

दारुणं स वलीपाकं प्राप्य शीघ्रं विपद्यते|१०२|

If the patient who has become weak because of hemorrhagic diarrhea indulges in Pitta-aggravating ingredients / foods out of ignorance, then the anal sphincters get suppurated. This is a serious condition leading to instantaneous death [101 ½ – ½ 102]

Treatment of Kaphaja Atisara:

श्लेष्मातिसारे प्रथमं हितं लङ्घन पाचनम्||१०२||

योज्यश्चामातिसारघ्नो यथोक्तो दीपनो गणः| लङ्घितस्यानुपूर्व्या च कृतायां न निवर्तते||१०३||

कफजो यद्यतीसारः कफघ्नैस्तमुपाचरेत्|१०४|

For the treatment of Kaphaja type of Diarrhea, in the beginning, fasting (langhana) and carminative (Pachana) therapies are administered.

Similarly, the group of herbs which stimulates the power of digestion (Dipana- Gana) as described earlier (in verse nos- 26-29), and which are prescribed for the treatment of Ama- Atisara is given.

If, in spite of the Dipana and Pachana therapies, and despite administration of Langhana therapy, Kaphaja type of atisara does not subside, then the patient is given Kapha- alleviating therapies. [102 ½- ½ 104]

Recipes for Kaphaja Atisara

बिल्वं कर्कटिका मुस्तमभया विश्वभेषजम्||१०४||

वचा विडङ्गं भूतीकं धान्यकं देवदारु च| कुष्ठं सातिविषा पाठा चव्यं कटुकरोहिणी||१०५||

पिप्पली पिप्पलीमूलं चित्रकं हस्तिपिप्पली| योगाञ्छलोकार्धविहितांश्चतुरस्तान् प्रयोजयेत्||१०६||

शृताञ्छलेष्मातिसारेषु कायाग्नि बल वर्धनान्|

Administration of the decoction of the following 4 recipes cures Kaphaja type of Atisara:

1. Bilva – Aegle marmelos, Karkatika, Musta (Cyperus rotundus), Abhaya – Terminalia chebula and VisvaBheshaja – ginger

2. Vacha (Acorus calamus Linn.),Vidanga – Embelia ribes, Bhutika, coriander and Devadaru – Cedrus deodara

3. Kushta, Ativisa – Aconitum heterophyllum,Patha – cissampelos pareira, Chavya – Piper retrofractum and Katuka- Katukarohini – Picrorhiza kurroa and

4. Pippali, Pippali Mula, Chitraka – Leadwort and Gaja-Pippali

The above-mentioned 4 recipes also promote Kayagni (the power of digestion and metabolism). [104 ½ – 107 ½]

अजाजीमसितां पाठां नागरं मरिचानि च||१०७||

धातकी द्विगुणं दद्यान्मातुलुङ्गरसाप्लुतम्|

Administration of the recipe containing 1 part each of black variety of Patha – Cissampelos parriera, nagara –

Zingiber officinale and Maricha – Black pepper fruit – piper nigrum, and 2 parts of Dhataki – Woodfordia fruticosa, along with profuse quantity of lime- juice cures Kaphaja type of Atisara. [107 ½ – ½ 108]

रसाञ्जनं सातिविषं कुटजस्य फलानि च||१०८||
धातकी द्विगुणं दद्यात् पातुं सक्षौद्र नागरम्|

1 part each of Rasanjana (Aqueous extract of Berberis aristata), Ativisha – Aconitum heterophyllum and fruits of Kutaja – Connessi (Holarrhena antidysenterica Wall.), and 2 parts of Dhataki – Woodfordia fruticosa is added with honey and ginger. This potion is given to a patient suffering from Kaphaja Atisara to drink. [108 ½ – ½ 109]

Khada preparation:
धातकी नागरं बिल्वं लोध्रं पद्मस्य केशरम्||१०९||
जम्बू त्वङ्नागरं धान्यं पाठा मोचरसो बला| समङ्गा धातकी बिल्वमध्यं जम्ब्वाम्रयोस्त्वचः||११०||
कपित्थानि विडङ्गानि नागरं मरिचानि च| चाङ्गेरी कोल तक्राम्लांश्चतुरस्तान् कफोत्तरे||१११||
श्लोकार्धं विहितान् दद्यात् सस्नेह लवणान् खडान्|

For the treatment of Kaphaja Atisara, the following 4 recipes are given in the form of Khada (a type of sour drink which stimulates the power of digestion):
1. Dhataki – Woodfordia fruticosa, Nagara, Bilva – Aegle marmelos, Lodhra (Symplocos racemosa) and Padma-Kesara
2. Bark of Jambu – Syzygium cumini, Nagara – Zingiber officinale, Dhanya, Patha – cissampelos pareira, Mocarasa and Bala – Country mallow (root) – Sida cordifolia:
3. Samanga, Dhataki – Woodfordia fruticosa, Pulp of Bilva and bark of Jambu and Amra – mango – Mangifera indica and
4. Kapittha, Vidanga – Embelia ribes, Nagara and Maricha
The above-mentioned recipes are added with the sour juice of Changeri and kola and buttermilk and given to the patient after adding ghee and salt. [109 ½ – 1/ 112]

Leha for diarrhea:
कपित्थ मध्यं लीढ्वा तु सव्योष क्षौद्र शर्करम्||११२||
कट्फलं मधुयुक्तं वा मुच्यते जठरामयात्|११३|

Intake of the pulp of Kapittha (Feronia limonia) along with Ginger, long pepper, black pepper, honey and sugar, or Katphala – Myrica nagi along with honey cures abdominal diseases (Kaphaja type of Diarrhea) [112 ½- ½ 113]

Long pepper with honey and buttermilk:
कणां मधुयुतां पीत्वा तक्रं पीत्वा सचित्रकम्||११३||
जग्ध्वा वा बाल बिल्वानि मुच्यते जठरामयात्|

Intake of Pippali – Piper longum along with honey, or butter-milk added with the powder of Chitraka – Leadwort – Plumbago zeylanica or the powder of the fruits of Bilva cures abdominal diseases (diarrhoea). [113 ½ – ½ 114]

Bael fruit:
बाल बिल्वं गुडं तैलं पिप्पली विश्वभेषजम्|
लिह्याद्वाते प्रतिहते सशूलः सप्रवाहिकः||११४||
भोज्यं मूलकषायेण वातघ्नैश्चोपसेवनैः| वातातिसार विहितै यूषैर्मांसरसैः खडैः||११५||
पूर्वोक्तमम्ल सर्पिर्वा षट्पलं वा यथाबलम्| पुराणं वा घृतं दद्याद्यवागूमण्डमिश्रितम्||११६||

If the movement of Vayu (flatus) is obstructed resulting in colic pain and griping pain, then the patient is given tender fruits of Bilva – Aegle marmelos, Jaggery, oil, Pippali – Piper longum and Sunthi – Zingiber officinale. He is given a diet prepared with Vayu- Alleviating ingredients along with the vegetable soup, meat soup and Khada (a type of sour drink) described earlier for the treatment of Vatika Atisara.

Similarly, this patient is given the sour medicated ghee described earlier (in verse no. 43 with the title) Changeri ghrta or Satpala Ghrta (vide Chikitsa 5: 147) or (ten years) old ghee mixed with Yavagu (thick gruel) and (thin gruel). [½ 114- 116]

Piccha Basti and Anuvasana basti:

वातश्लेष्म विबन्धे वा कफे वाऽतिस्रवत्यपि| शूले प्रवाहिकायां वा पिच्छा बस्तिं प्रयोजयेत्||११७||

पिप्पली बिल्व कुष्ठानां शताह्वावचयोरपि| कल्कैः सलवणैर्युक्तं पूर्वोक्तं सन्निधापयेत्||११८||

प्रत्यागते सुखं स्नातं कृताहारं दिनात्यये| बिल्वतैलेन मतिमान्सुखोष्णेनानुवासयेत्||११९||

वचान्तैरथवा कल्कैस्तैलं पक्त्वाऽनुवासयेत्| बहुशः कफवातार्तस्तथा स लभते सुखम्||१२०||

Piccha Basti and Anuvasana basti: (enema therapy) –

If Vayu and Kapha are obstructed [in the colon], if there is excessive voiding of Kapha (mucus) and if there is colic pain as well as griping pain, then Piccha- basti (mucilaginous enema) is administered. This Piccha- Basti is prepared with the paste of pippali – Piper longum, Bilva – Aegle marmelos, Kushta – Saussurea lappa, Shatahva and Vacha (Acorus calamus Linn.) by adding salt. After the ingredients of this Piccha-basti come out of the anus and the patient feels comfortable, he is given a bath. Thereafter, he is given food. In the afternoon, he is given Anuvasana type of enema with lukewarm Bilva Taila (Vide Siddhi 4: 4-7).

The Anuvasana type of medicated enema can also be given frequently with the oil cooked with the paste of Pippali, Bilva, Kushta Shatahva and Vacha

Administration of the above-mentioned recipes cures the ailments (Diarrhoea) abused by Kapha and Vata. [117-120]

Need for Immediate Treatment

स्वे स्थाने मारुतोऽवश्यं वर्धते कफ सङ्क्षये|

स वृद्धः सहसा हन्यात्तस्मात्तं त्वरया जयेत्||१२१||

When Kapha gets reduced because of the above mentioned therapies / measures, the Vayu undoubtedly gets aggravated in its own location (colon), this aggravated Vayu may cause instantaneous death: hence its treatment is attempted without delay. [121]

Line of treatment of Sannipatika Atisara

वातस्यानु जयेत् पित्तं, पित्तस्यानु जयेत् कफम्|

त्रयाणां वा जयेत् पूर्वं यो भवेद्बलवत्तमः||१२२||

If it is caused by sannipata (simulataneous aggravation of all the 3 Doshas), then in the beginning, the aggravated Vayu is alleviated followed by the alleviation of the aggravated Pitta, and thereafter, alleviation of kapha. Alternatively, of the 3 Doshas, the most aggravated one is treated (alleviated) first of all (which is to be followed by the treatment of the remaining 2 Doshas). [122]

To sum up

तत्र श्लोकः:-

प्रागुत्पत्ति निमित्तानि लक्षणं साध्यता न च| क्रिया चावस्थिकी सिद्धा निर्दिष्टा ह्यतिसारिणाम्||१२३||

In this chapter, the following topics in respect of the patient suffering from Atisara (Diarrhoea) are described:

1. Mythological origin of Atisara

2. Etiology of different types of Atisara

3. Signs and symptoms of Atisara

4. Curability and incurability of Atisara and

5. Effective treatment for different stages of Atisara. [123]

इत्यग्निवेशकृते तन्त्रे चरक प्रतिसंस्कृते चिकित्सा स्थानेऽतिसार चिकित्सितं नामैकोनविंशोऽध्यायः||१९||

Thus, ends the nineteenth chapter in chikitsa—Sthana (section on the treatment of diseases) dealing with the treatment of Atisara (Diarrhoea) in the work of Agnivesha as redacted by Master Charaka.

3

Chikitsasthana Chapter 20 Chardi Chikitsitam

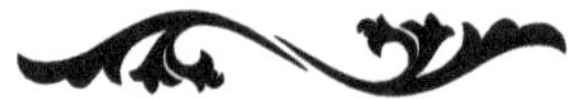

The 20th chapter of Charaka Samhita, Chikitsa Sthana is called Chardi Chikitsa Adhyaya. It deals with causes, types and Ayurvedic treatment for vomiting.

अथातश्छर्दि चिकित्सितं व्याख्यास्यामः||१||

इति ह स्माह भगवानात्रेयः||२||

We shall now expound the chapter on the Treatment of Chardi (vomiting). Thus, said Lord Atreya [1-2]

Prologue

यशस्विनं ब्रह्मतपोद्युतिभ्यां ज्वलन्तमग्न्यर्क समप्रभावम्| पुनर्वसुं भूतहिते निविष्टं पपच्छ शिष्योऽत्रिजमग्निवेशः||३||

Agnivesha, the disciple, asked Punarvasu Atreya, a reputed physician, dazzling with lustre of divine knowledge and penance, who was endowed with the brilliance like that of fire and the sun, and who was dedicated to the well-being of all living beings, as follows: [3]

Dialogue:

याश्छर्दयः पञ्च पुरा त्वयोक्ता रोगाधिकारे भिषजां वरिष्ठ! | तासां चिकित्सां स निदान लिङ्गां यथावदाचक्ष्व नृणां हितार्थम्||४||

तदग्निवेशस्य वचो निशम्य प्रीतो भिषक्श्रेष्ठ इदं जगाद| याश्छर्दयः पञ्च पुरा मयोक्तास्ता विस्तरेण ब्रुवतो निबोध||५||

Oh! Revered Physician, please let us know the treatment of the 5 types of Chardi (vomiting) described by you earlier, while discussing the classification of diseases (in Charaka Sutrasthana 19/3-4) together with their aetiology, signs and symptoms comprehensively, for the well-being of human beings.

After hearing this query of Agnivesha, the eminent physician (Punarvasu Atreya) was pleased and said, "I shall explain in detail the five kinds of chardi – vomiting which had been mentioned earlier. Listen". [4-5]

Types of Chardi:

दोषैः पृथक्त्रिप्रभवाश्चतस्रो द्विष्टार्थ योगादपि पञ्चमी स्यात्|६|

Chardi is of 5 types as follows:

1. Vatika Chardi (vomiting caused by Vata)

2. Paittika Chardi (caused by Pitta)

3. Kaphaja Chardi (caused by Kapha)

4. Sannipatika chardi (caused by vitiation of all the 3 Doshas) and

5. Dvishtartha -yojana-Chardi (vomiting caused due to unwanted objects i.e., coming into contact with the sight, sounds, taste, feel and smell of things which are unpleasant to the mind) [½ 6]

Chardi Purvaroopa:

तासां हृदुत्क्लेश कफप्रसेकौ द्वेषोऽशने चैव हि पूर्वरूपम्||६||

Premonitory Signs and Symptoms of Chardi:

1. Hrudaya utklesha – Nausea with uneasy feeling in the cardiac region

2. Kapha praseka – Excessive Salivation and

3. Ashana dvesha – Hateful disposition toward food [6 ½]

Vataja Chardi – Nidana, Samprapti, Lakshana:

व्यायाम तीक्ष्णौषध शोक रोगभयोपवासाद्यति कर्शितस्य| वायुर्महास्रोतसि सम्प्रवृद्ध उत्क्लेश्य दोषांस्तत ऊर्ध्वमस्यन्||७||

आमाशयोत्क्लेशकृतां च मर्म प्रपीडयंश्छर्दिमुदीरयेत्तु| हृत्पार्श्वपीडा मुखशोष मूर्धनाभ्यर्ति कास स्वरभेद तोदैः||८||

उद्गार शब्द प्रबलं सफेनं विच्छिन्न कृष्णं तनुकं कषायम्| कृच्छ्रेण चाल्पं महता च वेगेनार्तोऽनिलाच्छर्दयतीह दुःखम्||९||

Aetiology, Pathogenesis, signs and Symptoms of Vatika Chardi:

In a person, emaciated because of

Ati vyayama (excessive exercise)

Tikshna aushadha sevana (intake of medicines having sharp attributes)

Shoka (Grief)

Bhaya (fear)

Upavasa (fasting) etc

Vata gets aggravated in the gastrointestinal tract (Maha- srotas or Kostha), incites the local Doshas and pushes them upward. These Doshas cause agitation in the stomach (Amashaya), and after afflicting the vital organs (Marma) (viz heart) gives rise to Chardi (vomiting).

Vatika Chardi – Lakshana – signs and symptoms:

Hrit parshva peeda – Pain in the cardiac region and sides of the chest

Mukha shosha – Dryness of the mouth

Murdha nabhya arti – Pain in the head and umbilical region

Kasa – Coughing

Svara bheda -hoarseness of the voice and

Toda – pricking pain

Udgara shabda prabala – Eructation with loud noise

Sa phena, vicchinna, krshna, tanu kashayam – Vomiting of material which is frothy, scattered, black in colour, thin and astringent in taste.

Krchrena alpam – The urge for vomiting is forceful, but the patient vomits only in small quantities with pain and The patient feels miserable. [7-9]

Pittaja Chardi Nidana, Samprapti, Lakshana:

अजीर्ण कट्वम्ल विदाह्य शीतैरामाशये पित्तमुदीर्ण वेगम्| रसायनीभिर्विसृतं प्रपीड्य मर्मोर्ध्वमागम्य वमिं करोति||१०||

मूर्च्छा पिपासा मुखशोष मूर्धताल्वक्षि सन्ताप तमो भ्रमार्तः| पीतं भृशोष्णं हरितं सतिक्तं धूम्रं च पित्तेन वमेत् सदाहम्||११||

Because of the intake of food before the previous meal is digested, and because of the intake of Katu (pungent), Amla (sour), Vidahi (which cause burning sensation) and Ushna ahara (hot foods and drinks), Pitta Dosha in the Amashaya (stomach) gets aggravated. This aggravated Pitta circulates through the channels (Rasayani) and afflicts the vital organs located in the upper part of the body giving rise to vomiting:

Signs and symptoms of this Paittika Chardi

1. Moorcha – Fainting, Pipasa – Morbid thirst and Mukha shosha – dryness of the mouth

2. Santapa – Burning (or heating) sensation in the head, Palates and eyes

3. Tamo pravesha- A feeling as if the entering into darkness

4. Bhrama – Giddiness

5. Pitam bhrsoshanam haritam satiktam dhumram-Vomiting of material which is yellow, excessively hot, green, bitter and smoky in appearance and

6. Sa daham – Vomiting takes place with burning sensation [10-11]

Kaphaja Chardi Nidana, Samprapti, Lakshana:

स्निग्धातिगुर्वाम विदाहि भोज्यैः स्वप्नादिभिश्चैव कफोऽतिवृद्धः| उरः शिरो मर्म रसायनीश्च सर्वाः समावृत्य वमिं करोति||१२||

तन्द्रास्यमाधुर्य कफप्रसेक सन्तोष निद्रारुचि गौरवार्तः| स्निग्धं घनं स्वादु कफादिविशुद्धिं सलोमहर्षोऽल्परुजं वमेत्||१३||

Etiology, Pathogenesis, Signs and symptoms of Kaphaja Chardi:

Because of the intake of food, the ingredients of which are

Snigdha (unctuous), Ati guru (excessively heavy),

Aama (uncooked) and Vidahi anna and

sleeping in the day time and such other factors,

Kapha Dosha gets excessively aggravated. This aggravated Kapha afflicts (occludes) the chest, head, vital organs and all the (concerned) channels to cause Chardi (vomiting).

Signs and symptoms of this Kaphaja type of Chardi:

1. Tandra – Drowsiness, Madhura aasya – sweet taste in the mouth and Kapha praseka – Salivation

2. Santosha – Sense of satisfaction, Nidra – sleep, Aruchi – anorexia and Gauravam – heaviness of the body

3. Vomiting of material which is Snigdha – unctuous, Ghana – thick, Svadu – sweet and free from any undesirable smell and

4. Loma harsha – Horripilation and Alpa ruja – less of pain [12- 13]

Sannipatika Chardi Nidana, Samprapti, Laskhana:

समशनतः सर्वरसान् प्रसक्तमाम प्रदोषर्तु विपर्ययैश्च| सर्वे प्रकोपं युगपत् प्रपन्नाश्छर्दिं त्रिदोषां जनयन्ति दोषाः||१४||

शूलाविपाकारुचि दाह तृष्णाश्वास प्रमोह प्रबला प्रसक्तम्| छर्दिस्त्रिदोषाल्लवणाम्लनीलसान्द्रोष्णरक्तं वमतां नृणां स्यात्||१५||

Etiology, Pathogenesis, signs and Symptoms of Sannipatika Chardi:

Because of the habitual intake of wholesome and unwholesome ingredients together, having all the different tastes, because of Ama- dosha (ailments caused by improper digestion) and because of seasonal perversions, all the 3 Doshas get simultaneously aggravated to cause Sannipatika type of Chardi.

Signs and symptoms:

1. Shula – Colic pain, Avipaka – indigestion, Aruchi – Anorexia, Daha – burning sensation, Trshna – morbid thirst, Shvasa – dyspnoea and fainting which are of serious nature and persistent and

2. Vomiting of material which is Lavana – saline, amla-sour, Anila – blue, Sandra -dense, Ushna -hot and Rakta – red (mixed with blood). [14- 15]

Complications leading to Incurability of Chardi:

विट्स्वेद मूत्राम्बु वहानि वायुः स्रोतांसि संरुध्य यदोर्ध्वमेति| उत्सन्न दोषस्य समाचितं तं दोषं समुद्धूय नरस्य कोष्ठात्||१६||

विण्मूत्रयोस्तत् समवर्णगन्धं तृट्श्वास हिक्कार्तियुतं प्रसक्तम्| प्रच्छर्दयेद्दुष्टमिहातिवेगात्तयाऽदितश्चाशु विनाशमेति||१७||

When the aggravated Vata Dosha occludes the channels carrying stool, sweet, urine and ambu (aqueous material) and moves upwards, then the morbid matter (dosha) from the gastro- intestinal tract (kostha) of the person in whom the Doshas are aggravated, gets incited to cause vomiting. This type of vomiting has the following signs and symptoms:

1. Vin mutra sama varna – Vomiting of the material having the same colour and smell of the urine and stool

2. Trut – Persistent thirst, Shvasa – dyspnoea and Hikka – hiccup

3. Vomiting of foul smelling or putrid material (Dusta) and

4. Prachardana – Bouts of vomiting with great force

Such a patient succumbs to death instantaneously. [16-17]

Dvistartha Yogaja Chardi

द्विष्ट प्रतीपाशुचिपूत्यमेध्य बीभत्स गन्धाशन दर्शनैश्च|

यच्छर्दयेत्तप्तमना मनोध्नैर्दिर्वष्टार्थसंयोगभवा मता सा||१८||

Smelling, eating and seeing despicable, antagonistic, unclean, putrid, unholy and gruesome ingredients and objects afflict the mind. This mental disgust gives rise to vomiting which is called Dvistartha- Yogaja Chardi or vomiting caused by the contact with the unwanted objects. [18]

Incurability of Chardi

क्षीणस्य या छर्दिरतिप्रवृद्धा सोपद्रवा शोणित पूययुक्ता| सचन्द्रिकां तां प्रवदन्त्यसाध्यां साध्यां चिकित्सेदनुपद्रवां च||१९||

If in an emaciated person, vomiting continues incessantly, if there are complications, and if the vomited material is associated with blood, pus and Chandrika (circular patches with variegated colour like the one at the top of peacock feather) then the patient is incurable (Asadhya).

The physician should treat only curable types of vomiting which are not associated with any complications. [19]

Chardi Chikitsa Sutra – Line of treatment

आमाशयोत्क्लेशभवा हि सर्वाश्छर्द्यो मता लङ्घनमेव तस्मात्| प्राक्कारयेन्मारुतजां विमुच्य संशोधनं वा कफपित्तहारि||२०||

चूर्णानि लिह्यान्मधुनाऽभयानां हृद्यानि वा यानि विरेचनानि| मद्यैः पयोभिश्च युतानि युक्त्या नयन्त्यधो दोषमुदीर्णमूर्ध्वम्||२१||

वल्लीफलाद्यैर्वमनं पिबेद्वा यो दुर्बलस्तं शमनैश्चिकित्सेत्| रसैर्मनोज्ञैर्लघुभिर्विशुष्कैर्भक्ष्यैः सभोज्यैर्विविधैश्च पानैः||२२||

Chardi Chikitsa Sutra – Line of treatment

Langhana therapy – All except Vatika chardi (Because the Doshas are caused by the agitation of Doshas in the stomach)

Samshodhana therapy – Kapha and Pitta chardi (Because the Doshas are aggravated in excess)

Along with honey, the powder of Abhaya – Terminalia chebula is given in a linctus form for the purpose of purgation. Such other purgative drugs which are cardio-tonics may also be given appropriately along with alcohol or milk. These recipes cause downward movement of the aggravated Doshas having the tendency to move upwards.

Such patients may also be given Vamana therapy, with the recipes containing Valli-Phala etc.

If the patient is weak, then he is treated with Shamana or alleviation therapy for which delicious soups and light as well as dry food is given for eating along with different types of drinks. [20-22]

Vataja Chardi Chikitsa:

सुसंस्कृतास्तित्तिरि बर्हि लावरसा व्यपोहन्त्यनिलप्रवृत्ताम्| छर्दि तथा कोल कुलत्थ धान्य बिल्वादिमूलाम्लयवैश्च यूषः||२३||

वातात्मिकायां हृद्यद्रवार्तो नरः पिबेत् सैन्धववद्घृतं तु| सिद्धं तथा धान्यक नागराभ्यां दध्ना च तोयेन च दाडिमस्य||२४||

व्योषेण युक्तां लवणैस्त्रिभिश्च घृतस्य मात्रामथवा विदध्यात्| स्निग्धानि हृद्यानि च भोजनानि रसैः सयूषैर्दधि दाडिमाम्लैः||२५||

Treatment of Vatika Chardi:

The following cure Vatika type of Chardi (vomiting):

1. The well sizzled soup of the meat of Tittiri, Barhi and Lava

2. Vegetable soup of Kola, Kulattha, Dhanya, Bilva – Aegle marmelos, Syonaka – Oroxylum indicum, Gambhari – Gmelina arborea, Patali – Stereospermum suaveolens, Ganikarika – Clerodendrum phlomidis, Mulamla (sour drink prepared of radish) and yava;

3. Ghee with rock- salt (cooked with rock salt). This recipe is given to the patient of Vatika Chardi, associated with the palpitation of the heart.

4. Ghee cooked with Dhanyaka –Coriandrum sativum, Nagara – Zingiber officinale, Yoghurt and the juice of Dadima – Pomegranate – Punica granatum and

5. Ghee added with the powder of Sunthi, Pippali , Maricha and Saindhava, Sauvarchala and Vida type of salt;

The patient of Vatika Chardi is given food which is unctuous and pleasing to the heart along with meat- soup, vegetable- soup, yogurt and sour pomegranate. [23-25]

Pittaja Chardi Chikitsa:

पित्तात्मिकायामनुलोमनार्थं द्राक्षा विदारीक्षुरसैस्त्रिवृत् स्यात्| कफाशयस्थं त्वतिमात्रवृद्धं पित्तं हरेत् स्वादुभिरूर्ध्वमेव||२६||

शुद्धाय काले मधु शर्कराभ्यां लाजैश्च मन्थं यदि वाऽपि पेयाम्| प्रदापयेन्मुद्गरसेन वाऽपि शाल्योदनं जाङ्गलजै रसैर्वा||२७||

सितोपला माक्षिक पिप्पलीभिः कुल्माष लाजा यव सक्तुगृञ्जान्| खर्जूर मांसान्यथ नारिकेलं द्राक्षामथो वा बदराणि लिह्यात्||२८||

स्रोतोजलाजोत्पल कोल मज्जचूर्णानि लिह्यान्मधुनाऽभयां च| कोलास्थिमज्जाञ्जन मक्षिका विड्लाजासितामागधिकाकणान् वा||२९||

द्राक्षारसं वाऽपि पिबेत् सुशीतं मृद्भृष्टलोष्टप्रभवं जलं वा| जम्ब्वाम्रयोः पल्लवजं कषायं पिबेत् सुशीतं मधुसंयुतं वा||३०||

निशि स्थितं वारि समुद्ग कृष्णं सोशीरधान्यं चणकोदकं वा| गवेधुकामूलजलं गुडूच्या जलं पिबेदिक्षुरसं पयो वा||३१||

सेव्यं पिबेत् काञ्चन गैरिकं वा सबालकं तण्डुल धावनेन| धात्री रसेनोतमचन्दनं वा तृष्णावमिघ्नानि समाक्षिकाणि||३२||

कल्कं तथा चन्दन चव्य मांसी द्राक्षोत्तमाबालक गैरिकाणाम्| शीताम्बुना गैरिक शालि चूर्ण मूर्वा तथा तण्डुलधावनेन||३३||

Treatment of Paittika Chardi:

In the Paittika type of Chardi, the patient is given the powder of Trivrt – Operculina turpethum along with the juice of Draksha – Raisin – Vitis vinifera, Vidari (Pueraria tuberosa) and sugarcane for causing Anulomana or downward movement of the morbid matter, i.e. purgation. When Pitta is over-aggravated in the chest (in the region above the abode of the kapha- stomach), then (emetic therapy with the help of) drugs having sweet taste is administered.

After the body is cleansed of morbid matter, the patient is given during meal- time the Laja-mantha (flour of popped-rice, diluted in water) or Laja-Peya (thin gruel made of popped- rice) along with honey and sugar. The patient may also be given boiled Shali- rice along with the soup of Mudgaa or the soup of the meat of animals inhabiting an arid zone.

Kulmasha (the paste of boiled green gram), Masura (red lentil) etc.,) Laja (popped paddy), Yava – Barley (Hordeum vulgare) – Saktu (flour of roasted barley), Grnja (boiled barley along with its scum), or the pulp of Kharjura – Phoenix dactyliera, Coconut, Draksha – Raisin or Kola is made to a linctus by adding Sitopala (sugar having big crystals), honey and Pippali . These recipes are given to the patient suffering from Paittika type of vomiting.

The powder of Srotonjana Laja (popped paddy), Utpala (Nymphaea alba), the seed- pulp of Kola (ber fruit) and Abhaya – Terminalia chebula is made to a linctus by adding honey, and given to the patient. Similarly, the seed- pulp of Kola, Anjana, and stool of fly, Laja (popped paddy), sugar and grains of Pippali – Piper longum mixed with honey may be given to the patient.

The patient may drink cooled juice of Draksha – Raisin – Vitis vinifera or the leaves of jambu –Syzygium cumini and Amra by adding honey (after the decoction is cooled).

Water is added with the powder of mudga – Vigna radiate, Pippali, Ushira – Vetiver – Vetiveria zizanioides and Dhanya – Coriandrum sativum and kept overnight. In the morning the powder is strained out and the filtered water is taken by the patient. Similarly, the water added with the powder of chanaka (bengal gram) or Gavedhuka- root or Guduchi – Tinospora cordifolia, kept overnight can be given to the patient.

The patient may be given sugarcane juice or milk to drink.

Recipes useful for curing Trishna (excess thirst) and Chardi:

1. The powder of Sevya and Balaka along with rice- water (tandulodaka) and honey);

2. Powder of Kancana- Gairika and Balaka along with rice- water and honey and

3. The paste of white variety of Chandana – Santalum album mixed with the juice of Amalaki – Emblica officinalis along with honey.

The following recipes also cure Paittika type of vomiting:

1. The paste of Chandana – Santalum album, Chavya – Piper retrofractum, Mamsi – Nardostachys jatamamsi, Draksha – Raisin – Vitis vinifera of good quantity,

2. Powder of Gairika and Shali along with cold water and honey

3. Powder of Murva – Marsedenia tenacissima along with rice- water (Tandulodaka) and honey.

Kaphaja Chardi Chikitsa:

कफात्मिकायां वमनं प्रशस्तं सपिप्पली सर्षप निम्ब तोयैः| पिण्डीतकैः सैन्धव सम्प्रयुक्तैर्वम्यां कफामाशय शोधनार्थम्||३४||

गोधूमशालीन् सयवान् पुराणान् यूषैः पटोलामृत चित्रकाणाम्| व्योषस्य निम्बस्य च तक्र सिद्धैर्यूषैः फलाम्लैः कटुभिस्तथाऽद्यात्||३५||

रसांश्च शूल्यानि च जाङ्गलानां मांसानि जीर्णान्मधु सीध्वरिष्टान्| रागांस्तथा षाडव पानकानि द्राक्षा कपित्थैः फलपूरकैश्च||३६||

मुद्गान्मसूरांश्चणकान् कलायान् भृष्टान् युतान्नागर माक्षिकाभ्याम्| लिह्यात्तथैव त्रिफला विडङ्गचूर्णं विडङ्ग प्लवयोरथो वा||३७||

सजाम्बवं वा बदराम्लचूर्णं मुस्तायुतां कर्कटकस्य शृङ्गीम्| दुरालभां वा मधु सम्प्रयुक्तां लिह्यात् कफच्छर्दि विनिग्रहार्थम्||३८||

मनःशिलायाः फलपूरकस्य रसैः कपित्थस्य च पिप्पलीनाम्| क्षौद्रेण चूर्णं मरिचैश्च युक्तं लिहञ्जयेच्छर्दिमुदीर्णवेगाम्||३९||

Treatment of kaphaja Chardi:

In Kaphaja type of Chardi (vomiting), emetic therapy gives the best results. For this purpose, the patient is given the decoction of Pippali , Sarsapa – Brassica campestris and Nimba – Neem (Azadirachta indica) added with the powder of Pinditaka (Madana-Phala – Randia dumetorum) and rock salt. This cleanses (eliminates) Kapha from Amashaya (stomach).

The patient is given wheat, rice and barley which are old (more than 6 months old after harvesting) as food. Along with this food, he is given the following side –dishes and drinks

1. Vegetables soup of Patola – Trichosanthes dioica, Amrta and Chitraka – Leadwort – Plumbago zeylanica

2. Butter-milk or soup cooked by adding Sunthi , Pippali, and Maricha – Black pepper fruit

3. Water / Butter- milk cooked by adding Nimba – Neem (Azadirachta indica)

4. Soup of sour fruits along with pungent drugs (pepper)

5. Soup of the meat of animals and birds inhabiting arid zone (Jangala) or roasted meat of these animals may also be given along with food.

6. Old honey, Sidhu (alcohol prepared of sugar-cane- juice) and Arista (a type of alcoholic drink) and

7. Raga (condiments), sadava (pickles) and Panaka (syrup) prepared with Draksha – Vitis vinfera, Kapittha (Feronia limonia) and Phala- Puraka (bija-Puraka) – Citrus medica.

The following recipes are useful for the patient suffering from kaphaja type of vomiting:

1. Linctus is prepared with the powder of the roasted Mudga – green gram, Masura – Lens esculenta (red lentil), Chanaka (bengal gram) and kalaya (peanut) mixed with the powder of Sunthi and honey.

2. Linctus prepared of the powder of Haritaki – Terminalia chebula, Bibhitaka – Terminalia bellerica, Amalaki – Emblica officinialis and Vidanga – Embelia ribes mixed with the powder of Sunthi – Zingiber officinale and honey.

3. Linctus prepared of the powder of Vidanga and Plava (Kaivarta mustaka) mixed with the powder of sunthi and honey.

4. Powder of Jambu (Jamun seed) and sour fruits of Badara – Zizyphus jujuba mixed with honey

5. Powder of Musta and Karkatasrngi mixed with honey and

6. Powder (or juice) of Duralabha – Fagonia cretica mixed with honey.

The following recipes subside the forcefully generated urge for vomiting:

Powder of (purified) Manahsila with the juice of Bija-Puraka – Citrus medica, Honey and powder of Maricha and Powder of Pippali mixed with the juice of Kapittha honey and the powder of Maricha. [34-39]

Treatment of Sannipatika Chardi:

यैषा पृथक्त्वेन मया क्रियोक्ता तां सन्निपातेऽपि समस्य बुद्ध्या| दोषर्तुरोगाग्निबलान्यवेक्ष्य प्रयोजयेच्छास्त्रविदप्रमत्तः||४०||

Various types of treatment suggested by me (by Atreya) for the treatment of different types of Chardi, (Viz, Vatika,pattika and Kaphaja Chardi) is appropriately and judiciously combined, and given by the physician to the patient suffering from Sannipatika type of Chardi. The physician well versed in ayurvedic scriptures is (specially) vigilant (with regard to the Sannipatika type of Chardi) keeping in view the relative preponderance of the Doshas involved, the season when the disease has occurred, the stage of the disease and the power of digestion of the patient [40]

Treatment of Dvistartha Yogaja Chardi

मनोभिघाते तु मनोनुकूला वाचः समाश्वासन हर्षणानि| लोक प्रसिद्धाः श्रुतयो वयस्याः शृङ्गारिकाश्चैव हिता विहाराः||४१||

गन्धा विचित्रा मनसोऽनुकूला मृत्पुष्पशुक्ताम्लफलादिकानाम्| शाकानि भोज्यान्यथ पानकानि सुसंस्कृताः षाडव राग लेहाः||४२||

यूषा रसाः काम्बलिका खडाश्च मांसानि धाना विविधाश्च भक्ष्याः| फलानि मूलानि च गन्ध वर्ण रसैरुपेतानि वमिं जयन्ति||४३||

गन्धं रसं स्पर्शमथापि शब्दं रूपं च यद्यत् प्रियमप्यसात्म्यम्| तदेव दद्यात् प्रशमाय तस्यास्तज्जो हि रोगः सुख एव जेतुम्||४४||

Treatment of Dvistartha Yogaja Chardi

For the treatment of vomiting caused by the mental disgust or affliction of the mind (Manobhighata), the following steps are taken:

• Mano anukula – The patient is made to hear pleasing talks

• Ashvasana – He is consoled and encouraged.

• Loka prasiddha sruta – He is made to hear reputed folk tales including mythological stories

• He is attended to by congenial companions and he should resort to amorous and wholesome regimes (games)

• He is made to smell various types of pleasing perfumes emanating from the earth, flowers, Sukta (vinegar) and Sour fruits

• He is given to eat well prepared vegetables, eatables, syrups, Shadavas (Pickles), raga (condiments) and Lehas (preparations in the form of linctus or jam).

• Eatables like vegetable- soup, meat- soups, Kambalika (sour curry of fish and meat), Khada (sour drinks prepared of fruits), meat preparations, popped cereals, different food preparations, fruits and roots having pleasing smell, colour and taste cure vomiting caused by mental disgust and

• In general, whatever smell, taste, touch, sound or vision is pleasing to such patients is administered even though some of these might be unwholesome, because the ailments caused by such unwholesome contacts can be treated easily. [41-44]

Upadrava Chikitsa:

छर्द्युत्थितानां च चिकित्सितात् स्वाच्चिकित्सितं कार्यमुपद्रवाणाम्| अतिप्रवृत्तासु विरेचनस्य कर्मातियोगे विहितं विधेयम्||४५||

Treatment of Complications:

Complications associated with the disease (vomiting) are treated on the lines suggested in respect of each of these ailments. If there is excess vomiting, then the therapeutic measures suggested in Siddhi 6: 52- 56 is administered to the patient. [45]

Management of Chronic Chardi:

वमि प्रसङ्गात् पवनोऽप्यवश्यं धातु क्षयाद्धृद्धिमुपैति तस्मात्| चिर प्रवृत्तास्वनिलापहानि कार्याण्युपस्तम्भन बृंहणानि||४६||

सर्पिर्गुडाः क्षीरविधिर्घृतानि कल्याणक त्र्यूषण जीवनानि| वृष्यास्तथा मांसरसाः सलेहाश्चिरप्रसक्तां च वमिं जयन्ति||४७||

If vomiting persists continuously for a long time, then because of the diminution of tissue elements (Dhatus), the Vata Dosha certainly gets aggravated. Therefore, if the vomiting has become chronic, then therapeutic measures which are upastambhana (anti- emetic) and Brmhana (nourishing) is administered.

Recipes like Sarpirguda (vide Chikitsa 11: 50- 77), Ksira-Vidhi (milk boiled by adding Vata balancing herbs), Kalyanaka Ghrta (vide Chikitsa 9: 33-42), Tryushana- Ghrita (vide Chikitsa 18: 39- 42), Jivaniya –ghrita (vide Chikitsa 29: 55- 57), meat- soup and different types of linctus cure chronic type of Chardi (vomiting). [46-47]

तत्र श्लोकः:-

हेतुं सङ्ख्यां लक्षणमुपद्रवान् साध्यतां न योगांश्च| छर्दीनां प्रशमार्थं प्राह चिकित्सितं मुनिवर्यः||४८||

In this chapter, the reputed saint (lord Atreya) propounded the following topics:

Etiology of Chardi

Enumeration of different varieties of Chardi

Signs and symptoms of different types of Chardi

Complications of Chardi

Curability and incurability of different types of Chardi and

Recipes for the treatment of different types of Chardi

इत्यग्निवेशकृते तन्त्रे चरक प्रतिसंस्कृतेऽप्राप्ते दृढबल सम्पूरिते चिकित्सा स्थाने छर्दि चिकित्सितं नाम विंशोऽध्यायः||२०||

Thus, ends the 20th chapter in Chikitsa- Sthana (section on the treatment of diseases) dealing with the treatment of Chardi (vomiting) in the work of Agnivesha which was redacted by Charaka, and because of its non- availability (subsequently) supplemented by Dridhabala.

4

Chikitsasthana Chapter 21 Visarpa Chikitsitam

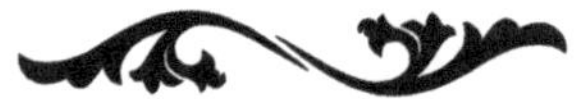

The 21st Chapter of Charaka Samhita Chikitsa Sthana is called Visarpa Chikitsa. It deals with the symptoms, types, curability and treatment for herpes disease.

अथातो विसर्प चिकित्सितं व्याख्यास्यामः||१||

इति ह स्माह भगवानात्रेयः||२||

Let us explore the chapter on the treatment of Visarpa (erysipelas, herpes, spreading type of skin disease). Thus, said Lord Atreya [1-2]

Prologue:

कैलासे किन्नराकीर्णे बहु प्रस्रवणौषधे| पादपै विविधैः स्निग्धैं नित्यं कुसुम सम्पदा||३||

वमद्भिर्मधुरान् गन्धान् सर्वतः स्वभ्यलङ्कृते| विहरन्तं जितात्मानमात्रेयमृषिवन्दितम्||४||

महर्षिभिः परिवृतं सर्वभूतहिते रतम्| अग्निवेशो गुरुं काले विनयादिदमुक्तवान्||५||

भगवन्! दारुणं रोगमाशीविषविषोपमम्| विसर्पन्तं शरीरेषु देहिनामुपलक्षये||६||

सहसैव नरास्तेन परीताः शीघ्रकारिणा| विनश्यन्त्यनुपक्रान्तास्तत्र नः संशयो महान्||७||

स नाम्ना केन विज्ञेयः सज्ज्ञितः केन हेतुना| कतिभेदः कियद्धातुः किन्निदानः किमाश्रयः||८||

सुखसाध्यः कृच्छ्रसाध्यो ज्ञेयो यश्चानुपक्रमः| कथं कैर्लक्षणैः किं च भगवन्! तस्य भेषजम्||९||

तदग्निवेशस्य वचः श्रुत्वाऽऽत्रेयः पुनर्वसुः| यथावदखिलं सर्व प्रोवाच मुनिसत्तमः||१०||

Lord Punarvasu Atreya, who was self-controlled, who was being worshiped by the sages of eminence, and who was dedicated to the welfare of all living beings, was walking around Mount Kailasa, the abode of Kinnaras (celestial musicians) and several springs, which was aromatic all around because of the sweet fragrance emitting from the blossoming flowers. Agnivesha approached him (the preceptor) with queries regarding the ailment 'terrific like cobra venom' spreading to various body parts. Agnivesha inquired – "People get afflicted with this serious disease instantaneously, and if not properly treated, succumb to death. So we are seriously concerned about this ailment. Kindly enlighten us on the following aspects of this disease:

1. What is the name of this ailment?

2. Why is the name given to the disease?

3. What are the different varieties of this disease?

4. Which are the Dhatus (tissue elements, Doshas and waste products) involved in the causation of this disease?

5. What are the etiological factors of this disease?

6. Where is this disease located?

7. How to identify the varieties of this disease which are easily curable, which are difficult of cure and which are incurable?

8. What are the signs and symptoms (of different varieties) of this disease?

9. What is the treatment of this disease?"
Having heard the above queries of Agnivesha Lord Punarvasu Atreya, the sage of eminence, explained all the relevant details of this disease" Visarpa "as follows: [3-10]

Name of the Ailment and Its Justification:
विविधं सर्पति यतो विसर्पस्तेन स स्मृतः| परिसर्पोऽथवा नाम्ना सर्वतः परिसर्पणात्||११||
This ailment is called Visarpa because it spreads (Sarpana) in different directions (vide i.e. Vividha). This is also called Parisarpa because it spreads (Sarpana) all over the body (Pari i.e Paritah). [11]

Visarpa Bheda – types:
स च सप्तविधो दोषैर्विज्ञेयः सप्तधातुकः| पृथक् त्रयस्त्रिभिश्चैको विसर्पो द्वन्द्वजास्त्रयः||१२||
वातिकः पैत्तिकश्चैव कफजः सान्निपातिकः| चत्वार एते विसर्पा वक्ष्यन्ते द्वन्द्वजास्त्रयः||१३||
आग्नेयो वातपित्ताभ्यां ग्रन्थ्याख्यः कफवातजः| यस्तु कर्दमको घोरः स पित्तकफ सम्भवः||१४||
Types of Visarpa:
Visarpa which is caused by the vitiation of 7 Dhatus (4 tissue elements and 3 Doshas to be explained in the subsequent verse no. 15), is of 7 types, viz
1. Vatika
2. Paittika
3. Kaphaja
4. Sannipatika
5. Vata-Pittaja
6. Kapha-Vataja and
7. Pitta- Kaphaja.
The type of Visarpa caused by:
Vata- Pitta is called Agneya Visarpa.
Kapha-Vata is called Granthi Visarpa.
Pitta-Kapha is called Kardamaka Visarpa which represents a serious condition. [12-14]

7 Elements Involved in the Pathogenesis of Visarpa:
रक्तं लसीका त्वङ्मांसं दूष्यं दोषास्त्रयो मलाः| विसर्पाणां समुत्पत्तौ विज्ञेयाः सप्त धातवः||१५||
The 7 Dhatus (elements) which give rise to Visarpa are:
1. Rakta (blood)
2. Lasika (Lymph)
3. Tvak (skin)
4. Mamsa (Muscle tissue) and
Doshas, viz
5. Vata,
6. Pitta and
7. Kapha [15]

Visarpa Nidana – Causes:
लवणाम्ल कटूष्णानां रसानामतिसेवनात्| दध्यम्ल मस्तु शुक्तानां सुरासौवीरकस्य च||१६||
व्यापन्नबहुमद्योष्णरागषाडवसेवनात्| शाकानां हरितानां च सेवनाच्च विदाहिनाम्||१७||
कूर्चिकानां किलाटानां सेवनान्मन्दकस्य च| दध्नः शाण्डाकिपूर्वाणामासुतानां च सेवनात्||१८||
तिल माष कुलत्थानां तैलानां पैष्टिकस्य च| ग्राम्यानूपौदकानां च मांसानां लशुनस्य च||१९||
प्रक्लिन्नानामसात्म्यानां विरुद्धानां च सेवनात्| अत्यादानादिदिवास्वप्नादजीर्णाध्यशनात् क्षतात्||२०||
क्षत बन्ध प्रपतनाद्धर्मकर्मातिसेवनात् | विषवाताग्निदोषाच्च विसर्पाणां समुद्भवः||२१||

एतैर्निदानैर्व्यामिश्रैः कुपिता मारुतादयः| दूष्यान् सन्दूष्य रक्तादीन् विसर्पन्त्यहिताशिनाम्||२२||

Visarpa is caused by the following factors:

1. Lavaṇāmla kaṭūṣṇānāṃ rasānāmatisevanāt – Excessive intake of hot ingredients having Saline, sour and pungent tastes.

2. Intake of Dadhi (sour curd), Mastu (the liquid in the upper part of curd), Sukta (vinegar), Sura (alcoholic drinks) and Sauvira (a sour drink prepared of dehusked barley)

3. Excessive intake of Madya (a type of alcoholic drink), and intake of polluted Madya, Raga (condiments) and Shadava (pickles) prepared of excessively hot ingredients.

4. Intake of Haritas (ingredients eaten in raw form described in Sutrasthana 27: 166- 177), Vidahis (ingredients causing burning sensation), Kurchika (curdled milk preparation), Kilata (cheese), Mandaka (Immature curd) Sandaki (a type of fermented wine) and such other fermented drinks, Tila – Sesame (Sesamum indicum), Masha (black gram), Kulattha (horse gram), different types of oil and pastries

5. Intake of meat of animals which are domesticated and which inhabit marshy land and water

6. Intake of Lashuna (garlic)

7. Intake of Praklinna (putrefied), Asatmya (unwholesome) and Viruddha ahara (mutually contradictory) ingredients

8. Intake of food in large quantity, Diva swapna (sleeping during day time), intake of food before the previous meals digested and intake of food immediately after the meal (Adhyasana)

9. Affliction by Kshaya (depletion of body tissues), Injury, Bandha (being tied with ropes, etc) and falls:

10. Excessive exposure to hot sun and excessive physical work and

11. Exposure to poisons, strong wind and fire.

Because of the contribution of the above mentioned causative factors, Vata, etc get aggravated to vitiate the Dushyas (tissue elements), Viz Rakta (blood) etc. to cause Visarpa in a person who indulges in unwholesome food. [16-22]

Visarpa Adhishtana – Location:

बहिःश्रितः श्रितश्चान्तस्तथा चोभयसंश्रितः| विसर्पो बलमेतेषां ज्ञेयं गुरु यथोत्तरम्||२३||

बहिर्मार्गाश्रितं साध्यमसाध्यमुभयाश्रितम्| विसर्प दारुणं विद्यात् सुकृच्छ्रं त्वन्तराश्रयम्||२४||

अन्तःप्रकुपिता दोषा विसर्पन्त्यन्तराश्रये| बहिर्बहिःप्रकुपिताः सर्वत्रोभयसंश्रिताः||२५||

Depending upon the location, Visarpa is of 3 types as follows:

1. Bahih-Srita (Visarpa located in the periphery)
2. Antah-Srita (Visarpa located in the interior part of the body) and
3. Ubhaya-Samsrita (Visarpa located in both the periphery and the interior part of the body)

The above mentioned 3 types of Visarpa are consecutively more and more serious.

Curability: The Visarpa located in the periphery of the body is curable. The Visarpa located in the interior part of the body represents a serious condition which is difficult to cure. When the Doshas spread in the internal organs of the body, they cause the interior type of Visarpa. When they spread in the exterior part of the body, they cause peripheral type of Visarpa. If, however, they spread all over the body, they cause Visarpa located in both the Periphery and the interior part of the body. [23-25]

Signs and Symptoms of Antar Visarpa:

मर्मोपघातात् सम्मोहादयनानां विघट्टनात्| तृष्णातियोगाद्वेगानां विषमाणां प्रवर्तनात्||२६||

विद्यादिवसर्पमन्तर्जमाशु चाग्निबलक्षयात्| अतो विपर्ययाद्बाह्यमन्यैर्विद्यात् स्वलक्षणैः||२७||

The signs and symptoms of internal Visarpa:

• Marma upaghata – Affliction of Marma (vital organs, specially heart),
• Sammoha – unconsciousness,
• Vighattana – obstruction to the channels of circulation,
• Trshna – excessive thirst

• Udvega vishamanam pravartanat – irregular manifestation of normal urges and

• Agni bala kshyat – instantaneous diminution of the power of digestion

The external type of Visarpa is characterized by the signs and symptoms related to the respective Doshas (which are to be described hereafter). [26-27]

Asadhya Visarpa – incurable:

यस्य सर्वाणि लिङ्गानि बलवद्यस्य कारणम्| यस्य यस्य सर्वाणि लिङ्गानि बलवद्यस्य कारणम्|

Characteristics of Incurable Visarpa:

If Visarpa is associated with all the signs and symptoms (described in respect of each variety), if it is caused by strong causative factors, if it is associated with painful complications, and if it is located in the vital organs, then this leads to death. [28]

Vataja Visarpa Nidana, Samprapti:

रूक्षोष्णैः केवलो वायुः पूरणैर्वा समावृतः| प्रदुष्टो दूषयन् दूष्यान् विसर्पति यथाबलम्||२९||

Vata aggravated by its own causative factors like un-unctuous and hot ingredients or being occluded [by Kapha and Pitta] because of over-nourishment, vitiates the Dushyas (Tissue elements), and spreads in accordance with its own strength [to cause Vatika type of Visarpa]. [29]

Vataja Visarpa Lakshana:

तस्य रूपाणि- भ्रम दवथु पिपासा निस्तोद शूलाङ्गमर्दा द्वेष्टन कम्प ज्वर तमक- कासास्थिसन्धिभेद विश्लेषण वेपनारोचकाविपाकाश्चक्षुषोराकुलत्वमस्त्रागमनं पिपीलिका सञ्चार इव चाङ्गेषु, यस्मिंश्चावकाशे विसर्पो विसर्पति सोऽवकाशः श्यावारुणाभासः श्वयथुमान् निस्तोद भेद शूलायामसङ्कोच हर्ष स्फुरणैरतिमात्रं प्रपीड्यते, अनुपक्रान्तश्चोपचीयते शीघ्रभेदैः स्फोटकैस्तनुभिररुणाभैः श्यावैर्वा तनु विशदारुणाल्पास्त्रावैः, विबद्ध वातमूत्रपुरीषश्च भवति, निदानोक्तानि चास्य नोपशेरते विपरीतानि चोपशेरत इति वातविसर्पः||३०||

Signs and symptoms of Vatika type of Visarpa:

1. Bhrama – dizziness, Davathu (burning sensation in eyes etc.,) Pipasa – thirst,

2. Nistoda – Pricking pain, Shoola – colic pain, Anga marda – Malaise, Udvestana – Cramps, Kampa – Tremors

3. Jwara – fever, Tamaka (a type of Asthma), Kasa -bronchitis,

4. Asthi sandhi bheda – pain in the bones and joints and their dislocation, Vepana – Shivering

5. Aruchi – anorexia, Avipaka – Indigestion

6. Chakshushoh akulatvam – cloudiness of the eyes, Asru agamanam – lachrymation, and Pipilika – a feeling as if ants are crawling over the body

7. The space through which the Visarpa spreads becomes Shyava aruna bhasa – greyish or Pinkish in colour and Shvayathu – oedematous.

8. That space becomes excessively afflicted with Nistoda – pricking pain, Bheda – breaking pain, Shoola – colic pain, Sankocha – expansion, Harsha – contraction, Sphurana – tingling sensation and Prapidyate – throbbing sensation.

9. If not treated, the space becomes replete (accumulated) with instantaneous cracking, pustules which are small in size and pink or greyish in colour, and secretion of liquid which is thin, transparent, and pink and in small quantity

10. Vibaddha vata mutra purisha – Arrest of flatus, urine and stool and

11. Factors described to cause vata- visarpa are not homologatory to such a patient. On the other hand, the patient feels comfortable with ingredients having opposite attributes. [30]

Pittaja Visarpa Nidana and Samprapti:

पित्तमुष्णोपचारेण विदाह्यम्लाशनैश्चितम्| दूष्यान् सन्दूष्य धमनीः पूरयन् वै विसर्पति||३१||

Etiology and Pathogenesis of Paittika visarpa:

Pitta, accumulated because of hot regimens, and by the intake of Vidahi (which cause burning sensation) and sour food, vitiates the Dushyas (tissue elements), fills up (obstructs) the Dhamanis (Channels of blood circulation) and spreads which gives rise to Paittika type of Visarpa. [31]

Paittika Visarpa Lakshana:
तस्य रूपाणि- ज्वरस्तृष्णा मूच्छ मोहश्छर्दिररोचकोऽङ्गभेदः स्वेदोऽतिमात्रमन्तर्दाहः प्रलापः शिरोरुक् चक्षुषोराकुलत्वमस्वप्नमरतिर्भ्रमः शीतवातवारितर्षोऽतिमात्रं हरित हारिद्रनेत्र मूत्रवर्चस्त्वं हरितहारिद्ररूपदर्शनं च, यस्मिंश्चावकाशे विसर्पोऽनुसर्पति सोऽवकाशस्ताम्र हरित हारिद्र नील कृष्ण रक्तानां वर्णानामन्यतमं पुष्यति, सोत्सेधैश्चातिमात्रं दाह सम्भेदनपरीतैः स्फोटकैरुपचीयते तुल्यवर्णासावैश्चिरपाकैश्च, निदानोक्तानि चास्य नोपशेरते विपरीतानि चोपशेरत इति पित्तविसर्पः॥३२॥
Signs and symptoms of Paittika type of Visarpa:

1. Jwara – Fever, Trushna – morbid thirst
2. Murchha – fainting, Moha – unconsciousness
3. Chardi – vomiting, Aruchi – anorexia
4. Anga bheda – breaking pain in the body, Ati matra sveda – excessive sweating and Antar daha- burning sensation in the interior part of the body
5. Pralapa – Delirium, Shiro ruk – headache, turbidity of the eyes, Asvapna – sleeplessness
6. Arati – dislike for everything, Bhrama – giddiness and Shita vata aavarita – excessive longing for cold wind and cold water
7. Harita (Green) and Haridra (yellow) coloration of the Akshi (eyes), Mutra (urine) and stool
8. Harita haridra rupa darshana – Green and yellow vision of objects
9. The space in which this disease spreads, becomes either Tamra (coppery colored), Harita (green), Haridra (yellow), Nila (blue), Krishna (black) or Rakta (red)
10. This space becomes full of pustules which are excessively swollen and associate with excessive burning sensation and breaking pain
11. The exudates from these pustules have the colours like those of the pustules
12. These pustules get suppurated very quickly and
13. Factors described to cause Pitta-Visarpa are not homogatory to such a patient. On the other hand, the patient feels comfortable with the ingredients, having the opposite attributes. [32]

Kaphaja Visarpa Nidana, Samprapti:
स्वाद्वम्ल लवण स्निग्ध गुर्वन्न स्वप्न सञ्चितः| कफः सन्दूषयन् दूष्यान् कृच्छ्रमङ्गे विसर्पति॥३३॥
Etiology and Pathogenesis of Kaphaja Visarpa:
Kapha accumulated because of the intake of ingredients which are

• Madhura (sweet)
• Amla (sour)
• Lavana (Saline)
• Snigdha (unctuous) and
• Diva swapna – heavy sleep [during day time] vitiates the Dushyas (tissue elements) and spreads slowly which gives rise to Kaphaja type of Visarpa. [33]

Signs and Symptoms of Kaphaja Visarpa:
तस्य रूपाणि- शीतकः शीतज्वरो गौरवं निद्रा तन्द्राऽरोचको मधुरास्यत्वमास्योपलेपो निष्ठीविका छर्दिरालस्यं स्तैमित्यमग्निनाशो दौर्बल्यं च, यस्मिंश्चावकाशे विसर्पोऽनुसर्पति सोऽवकाशः श्वयथुमान् पाण्डुर्नातिरक्तः स्नेह सुप्ति स्तम्भ गौरवैरन्वितोऽल्पवेदनः कृच्छ्रपाकैश्चिरकारिभिर्बहुलत्वगुपलेपैः स्फोटः श्वेतपाण्डुभिरनुबध्यते, प्रभिन्नस्तु श्वेतं पिच्छिलं तन्तुमद्घनमनुबद्धं स्निग्धमास्रावं स्रवति, ऊर्ध्वं च गुरुभिः स्थिरैर्जालावततैः स्निग्धै बहुलत्वगुपलेपैर्व्रणैरनुबध्यतेऽनुषङ्गी च भवति, श्वेत नख नयन वदन त्वङ्मूत्रवर्चस्त्वं, निदानोक्तानि चास्य नोपशेरते विपरीतानि चोपशेरत इति श्लेष्म विसर्पः॥३४॥
The following are the signs and symptoms of Kaphaja type of Visarpa:

• Sheeta – Feeling of chill, Shita jvara – cold-fever
• Gauravam – heaviness, Ati nidra – excessive sleep, Tandra – drowsiness

• Aruchi -anorexia, Madhura aasya – sweet taste in the mouth, Aasya aalepa – adherence of sticky material in the mouth, spitting of Saliva, Chardi -vomiting

• Aalasya – laziness, Staimityam – timidity, Agni nasha -diminution of the power of digestion (Agni) and Daurbalyam – weakness

• The space in which the disease (Visarpa) spreads, becomes Shyvathuman – oedematous, pāṇḍurnātiraktaḥ sneha – Pale- yellow, not very red and unctuous;

• There is Supti (numbness), Stambha (stiffness), Gauravam (heaviness) and Alpa vedana (less of pain in the body)

• The pustules in this space get suppurated very late, they become chronic, they appear in large number; the skin over these pustules gets covered with sticky material, and these pustules are either white or pale- yellow in colour

• When there is eruption of these pustules, then exudates which is white, slimy, fibrous, dense, knotty and unctuous, comes out

• After the eruption of these pustules, the space is covered with ulcers which are heavy (deep- seated) stable, surrounded by the capillary network, unctuous and covered with many skin scabs (sticks skins)

• These ulcers continue to stay for a long time

• The nails, eyes, face, skin, urine and stool of the patient are white in colour and

The factors described to cause Kaphaja Visarpa are not liked by the patient. On the other hand, the patient feels comfortable with the ingredients having opposite attributes. [34]

Agnivisarpa – Nidana, Samprapti:

वातपित्तं प्रकुपितमतिमात्रं स्वहेतुभिः| परस्परं लब्धबलं दहद्गात्रं विसर्पति||३५||

Etiology and Pathogenesis of Agni- Visarpa:

Vata Dosha and Pitta Dosha are simultaneously aggravated because of their respective causative factors, gain strength from each other and spread over the body along with burning sensation which is called Agni- Visarpa. [35]

Agni Visarpa Lakshana:

तदुपतापादातुरः सर्वशरीरमङ्गारैरिवाकीर्यमाणं मन्यते, छर्द्यतीसार मूर्च्छा दाह मोह ज्वर तमकारोचकास्थिसन्धिभेद तृष्णाविपाकाङ्गभेदादिभिश्चाभिभूयते, यं यं चावकाशं विसर्पोऽनुसर्पति सोऽवकाशः शान्ताङ्गारप्रकाशोऽतिरक्तो वा भवति, अग्निदग्ध प्रकारैश्च स्फोटैरुपचीयते, स शीघ्रगत्वादाश्वेव मर्मानुसारी भवति, मर्मणि चोपतप्ते पवनोऽतिबलो भिनत्यङ्गान्यतिमात्रं प्रमोहयति सञ्ज्ञां, हिक्काश्वासौ जनयति, नाशयति निद्रां, स नष्टनिद्रः प्रमूढसञ्ज्ञो व्यथितचेता न क्वचन सुखमुपलभते, अरतिपरीतः स्थानादासनाच्छय्यां क्रान्तुमिच्छति, क्लिष्टभूयिष्ठश्चाशु निद्रां भजति, दुर्बलो दुःखप्रबोधश्च भवति; तमेवंविधमग्निविसर्प परीतम चिकित्स्यं विद्यात्||३६||

Signs and symptoms of Agni visarpa:

1. Being afflicted by this type of Visarpa, the patient feels as if his whole body is sprinkled with live charcoal

2. Affliction by Chardi (vomiting), Atisara (Diarrhoea), Murccha (Fainting), Daha (burning sensation), Moha (unconsciousness), Jwara (fever), Tamaka (a feeling as if entering into darkness), Aruchi (anorexia), Asthi bheda (pain in the bones and joints), Trushna (morbid thirst), Avipaka (indigestion), Anga bheda (breaking pain all over the body), etc

3. The space in which the Visarpa spreads appears likes the extinguished charcoal (bark) or excessively red

4. The space becomes surrounded with pustules like those accused by burns

5. If afflicts the Marmas (vital organs) because of its nature to spread rapidly

6. Because of the affliction of the vital organs, the Vata Dosha gets excessively aggravated to cause breaking pain in the limbs in excess and unconsciousness

7. This aggravated Vata Dosha causes Hikka (hiccup), Shvasa (Asthma) and Insomnia;

8. Because of lack of sleep, his mind becomes dull, he feels miserable and he never feels happy anywhere

9. Because of this disposition of disliking for everything, he is always disturbed and confused and would wish to leave his place, seat or cot and run away.

10. Being afflicted with miseries, he gets sleep quickly and

11. He becomes so weak that it becomes very difficult to awaken him from sleep

The patient suffering from Agni- Visarpa like this (with the above mentioned signs and symptoms) is incurable. [36]

Kardama Visarpa Nidana Samprapti:

कफपित्तं प्रकुपितं बलवत् स्वेन हेतुना| विसर्पत्येकदेशे तु प्रक्लेदयति देहिनम्||३७||

Kapha and Pitta get simultaneously aggravated because of their respective etiological factors, and spread in a localized manner, giving rise to softening of the tissues of the locality. This is called Kardama- Visarpa [37]

Kardama Visarpa Lakshana:

तद्विकाराः- शीतज्वरः शिरोगुरुत्वं दाहः स्तैमित्यमङ्गावसदनं निद्रा तन्द्रा मोहोऽन्नद्वेषः प्रलापोऽग्निनाशो दौर्बल्यमस्थिभेदो मूर्च्छा पिपासा स्रोतसां प्रलेपो जाड्यमिन्द्रियाणां प्रायोपवेशनमङ्गविक्षेपोऽङ्गमर्दोऽरतिरौत्सुक्यं चोपजायते, प्रायश्चामाशये विसर्पत्यलसक एकदेशग्राही च, यस्मिंश्चावकाशे विसर्पो विसर्पति सोऽवकाशो रक्तपीत पाण्डुपिडकावकीर्ण इव मेचकाभः कालो मलिनः स्निग्धो बहूष्मा गुरुः स्तिमितवेदनः श्वयथुमान् गम्भीरपाको निरास्रावः शीघ्रक्लेदः स्विन्नक्लिन्नपूतिमांसत्वक् क्रमेणाल्परुक् परामृष्टोऽवदीर्यते कर्दम इवावपीडितोऽन्तरं प्रयच्छत्युपक्लिन्नपूतिमांसत्यागी सिरास्नायुसन्दर्शी कुणपगन्धी च भवति सञ्ज्ञास्मृतिहन्ता च; तं कर्दमविसर्पपरीतमचिकित्स्यं विद्यात्||३८||

Signs and symptoms of Kardama Visarpa:

1. Sheeta jvara – Cold fever, Shiro ruk – heaviness of the head, Daha – burning sensation
2. Staimitya (timidity), Anga avasada – Prostration of the limbs
3. Nidra – sleep, Tandra – drowsiness, Moha – Unconsciousness
4. Anna dvesha – dislike for food, Pralapa – delirium, Agni nasha – diminution of the power of digestion
5. Daurbalya -weakness, Asthi bheda – breaking pain in the bones, Murcha – fainting
6. Pipasa – morbid thirst, Srotasam pralepa – adhesion of sticky material in the channels of circulation, insensibility (jadya) of sense organs, constant feeling for voiding stool
7. Anga-Viksepa (stretching of limbs), Angamarda -Malaise
8. Arti – disliking for everything and Utsukya – anxiety
9. This disease generally spreads in slow spread in the Amashaya (region of the stomach) and gets localized there
10. The space in which this type of Visarpa spreads, becomes as if studded with eruptions of Rakta pita pandu pidaka - red, yellow and pale- yellow colour
11. The space looks muddy, black, dirty and unctuous, and it is excessively hot, Gaurava (heavy), with dull pain, oedema and deep-seated suppuration
12. These eruptions are free from any exudation and become sloughy very quickly.
13. The skin and muscle tissue over these eruptions are shriveled, sticky and suppurated.
14. The pain over this space is less and it appears gradually
15. By rubbing, these eruptions get cracked, and when pressed, sticky and putrefied muscle tissue comes out of these eruptions
16. In the space at the bottom of these eruptions (after taking out the slough), one can visualize vessels and ligaments, and smell like that of a dead body is emitted from this space and
17. The patient loses consciousness and memory.

This is called Kardama- Visarpa, and it is incurable. [38]

Granthi Visarpa Nidana, Lakshana:

स्थिर गुरु कठिन मधुर शीत स्निग्धान्नपानाभिष्यन्दि सेविनाम् व्यायामादिसेविनाम् प्रतिकर्म शीलानां श्लेष्मा वायुश्च प्रकोपमापद्यते, तावुभौ दुष्ट प्रवृद्धावतिबलौ प्रद्रष्य दूष्यान् विसर्पाय कल्पेते; तत्र वायुः श्लेष्मणा विबद्धमार्गस्तमेव श्लेष्माणमनेकधा भिन्दन् क्रमेण ग्रन्थिमालां कृच्छ्रपाकसाध्यां कफाशये सञ्जनयति, उत्सन्नरक्तस्य वा प्रद्रष्य रक्तं सिरास्नायुमांसत्वगाश्रितं ग्रन्थीनां मालां कुरुते तीव्ररुजानां स्थूलानामणूनां वा दीर्घवृत्तरक्तानां, तदुपतापाज्ज्वरातिसार कास हिक्का श्वास शोष- प्रमोह वैवर्ण्यारोचकविपाक प्रसेक च्छर्दि मूर्च्छाऽङ्ग भङ्ग निद्रातिसदनाद्याः प्रादुर्भवन्त्युपद्रवाः; स एतैरुपद्रुतः सर्वकर्मणां विषयमतिपतितो विवर्जनीयो भवतीति ग्रन्थिविसर्पः||३९||

Etiology, Pathogenesis, Signs and Symptoms of Granthi- Visarpa:

Kapha and Vata get aggravated because of the following:

1. Intake of food and drinks which are Sthira (having the attribute of stability), Guru (heavy), Kathina (hard), Madhura (sweet), Shita (cold), Snigdha (unctuous) and Abhisyandi (ingredients which cause obstruction to the channels of circulation)

2. Avyayama – Lack of exercise etc and

3. Habitually avoiding administration of elimination therapies (panca-karma) at the appropriate time

Both these vitiated Doshas get excessively aggravated and vitiate the Dushyas (tissue elements) giving rise to Visarpa. The channel of circulation of Vata gets obstructed by the aggravated Kapha (which causes further aggravation of Vata). This aggravated Vata, on its turn, causes splitting of the Kapha into several parts gradually giving rise to a series of Granthis (glandular enlargements) in the abodes of Kapha. These enlarged glands get suppurated very slowly and the ailment becomes difficult to cure.

Besides, in a person having excess blood, [aggravated Vata and Kapha] vitiate the blood giving rise to a series of glandular enlargements located in vessels, ligaments (or nerves), muscles and skin. These enlarged glands are extremely painful; some of these might be big in size and some others small; and some of these might be elongated, some round in shape and some of these are red in color.

Being afflicted by this type of Visarpa, the patient may get complications like

Jwara – fever, Atisara – diarrhoea, Kasa – bronchitis, Hikka – hiccup, Tamaka shvasa – asthma, Kshaya – consumption, Sammoha – unconsciousness, Vaivarnya – Discoloration of the skin, Aruchi – anorexia,

Avipaka – indigestion, Praseka – Salivation, Chardi – vomiting, Murchha – fainting,

Anga bheda – splitting pain in the body parts / Fractures in the limbs, Ati nidra – excessive sleep, Arati (dislike for everything) and Anga sada – prostration.

The patient having all these complications transcends all the therapeutic measures. Therefore, treatment of such patients is not attempted since it is incurable. [39]

Complications (Upadrava):

उपद्रवस्तु खलु रोगोत्तरकालजो रोगाश्रयो रोग एव स्थूलोऽणुर्वा, रोगात् पश्चाज्जायत इत्युपद्रवसञ्ज्ञः।

तत्र प्रधानो व्याधिः, व्याधेर्गुणभूत उपद्रवः, तस्य प्रायः प्रधानप्रशमे प्रशमो भवति।

स तु पीडाकरतरो भवति पश्चादुत्पद्यमानो व्याधि परिक्लिष्ट शरीरत्वात्; तस्मादुपद्रवं त्वरमाणोऽभिबाधेत॥४०॥

The ailment which is associated with a disease, and is manifested after the manifestation of the main disease is called Upadrava (complication). It may be a major or minor ailment.

It is called Upadrava because it occurs after the manifestation of the disease. It is the main disease which is predominant, and the ailment which appears as a complication is of secondary nature. The complication generally gets subsided when the main disease is cured. But the complication which is already very weak due to its earlier affliction by the main disease Therefore, the treatment of such complications is undertaken expeditiously. [40]

Sannipatika Visarpa

सर्वायतन समुत्थं सर्व लिङ्ग व्यापिनं सर्वधात्वनुसारिणमाशुकारिणं महात्ययिकमिति सन्निपात विसर्पमचिकित्स्यं विद्यात्॥४१॥

The Sannipatika type of Visarpa is caused by all the etiological factors [described in respect of each of the earlier varieties of Visarpa]. All the signs and symptoms described in respect of each of the earlier varieties of Visarpa are manifested in this type of Visarpa. It pervades all the Dhatus (tissue elements). It spreads instantaneously, and it is a serious ailment. This Sannipatika type of Visarpa is incurable [41]

Prognosis:

तत्र वात पित्त श्लेष्म निमित्ता विसर्पास्त्रयः साध्या भवन्ति; अग्निकर्दमाख्यौ पुनरनुपसृष्टे मर्मणि अनुपगते वा सिरा स्नायु मांस क्लेदे साधारण क्रियाभिरुभावेवाभ्यस्यमानौ प्रशान्तिमापद्येयाताम्, अनादरोपक्रान्तः पुनस्तयोरन्यतरो हन्याद्देहमाश्वेवाशीविषवत्; तथा ग्रन्थिविसर्पमजातोपद्रवमारभेत चिकित्सितुम्, उपद्रवोपद्रुतं त्वेनं परिहरेत्; सन्निपातजं तु सर्वधात्वनुसारित्वादाशुकारित्वादिविरुद्धोपक्रमत्वाच्चासाध्यं विद्यात्॥४२॥

Vatika-Visarpa, Paittika-Visarpa and Kaphaja-Visarpa- these 3 types are curable.

Agni-Visarpa and Kardama-Visarpa can be alleviated by the habitual (constant) use of general therapeutic measures (to counteract the respective etiological factors) only when the vital organs (like heart, etc) are not afflicted, and when there is no softening of the vessels, ligaments and muscle tissue. If not properly treated, any one of these two may cause instant death like snake poison.

The patient of Granthi-Visarpa is treated only if its complications are not manifested. If the complications are already manifested, then the patient should not be treated.

Sannipatika type of Visarpa is incurable because it pervades all the tissue elements, it spreads instantaneously and its treatment involves mutually contradictory therapeutic measures. [42]

Visarpa Chikitsa Sutra: Line of treatment

तत्र साध्यानां साधनमनुव्याख्यास्यामः||४३||

लङ्घनोल्लेखने शस्ते तिक्तकानां च सेवनम्| कफस्थानगते सामे रूक्षशीतैः प्रलेपयेत्||४४||

पित्तस्थानगतेऽप्येतत् सामे कुर्याच्चिकित्सितम्| शोणितस्यावसेकं च विरेकं च विशेषतः||४५||

मारुताशयसम्भूतेऽप्यादितः स्याद्विरूक्षणम्| रक्तपित्तान्वयेऽप्यादौ स्नेहनं न हितं मतम्||४६||

वातोल्बणे तिक्तघृतं पैत्तिके च प्रशस्यते| लघुदोषे, महादोषे पैत्तिके स्याद्विरेचनम्||४७||

न घृतं बहुदोषाय देयं यन्न विरेचयेत्| तेन दोषो ह्युपष्टब्धस्त्वङ्मांसरुधिरं पचेत्||४८||

तस्मादि्वरेकमेवादौ शस्तं विद्यादि्वसर्पिणः| रुधिरस्यावसेकं च तदध्यस्याश्रयसञ्ज्ञितम्||४९||

Visarpa Chikitsa Sutra: Line of treatment

If the Doshas causing Visarpa are of Ama (uncooked) nature and if these Doshas are located in the abode of:

Kapha (upper part of the body, i.e. chest, neck and head) – Langhana (fasting) and Vamana (emetic) therapies are useful. Such a patient is given ingredients having Katu (bitter) taste. The affected part of the body is anointed with the paste of the ingredients having un-unctuousness and cooling effect.

Pitta (i.e., Middle part of the body), - then also the therapeutic measures suggested above is administered. In addition, bloodletting and purgation therapies are specifically administered to such patients.

Vata (lower part of the body), - then Rookshana therapy is administered in the beginning. Since the disease involves the vitiation of Rakta (blood) and Pitta (in the Samanya Samprapti or general Pathogenesis), in the beginning, oleation therapy is not useful.

If Vata is aggravated in excess and Pitta is less aggravated to cause Visarpa, then Tiktaka Ghrta (Charaka Chikitsasthana 7: 140- 150) is useful. However, if Pitta is aggravated in excess, then the patient is treated with purgation therapy.

If the Doshas causing Visarpa are aggravated in excess then recipes of medicated ghee which do not cause purgation are not administered. Otherwise, these recipes of medicated ghee (which are not purgatives) occlude the Doshas resulting in the sloughing / suppuration (Paka) of the skin, muscle tissue and blood. Therefore, in the beginning the Visarpa patient is given purgation therapy. This patient is administered bloodletting therapy because the vitiated blood is the Asraya (main supporting factor) in the pathogenesis of Visarpa [43- 49]

इति वीसर्पनुत् प्रोक्तं समासेन चिकित्सितम्| एतदेव पुनः सर्वं व्यासतः सम्प्रवक्ष्यते||५०||

In the above verses, the treatment of Visarpa is described only in brief. The treatment in detail will be spelt out hereafter. [50]

Vamana Yoga – Emetic Recipes:

मदनं मधुकं निम्बं वत्सकस्य फलानि च| वमनं सम्प्रदातव्यं विसर्पे कफपित्तजे||५१||

पटोल पिचुमर्दाभ्यां पिप्पल्या मदनेन च| विसर्पे वमनं शस्तं तथा चेन्द्रयवैः सह||५२||

यांश्च योगान् प्रवक्ष्याभि कल्पेषु कफपित्तिनाम्| विसर्पिणां प्रयोज्यास्ते दोषनिर्हरणाः शिवाः||५३||

Vamana Yoga – Emetic Recipes:

If Visarpa is caused by either Kapha or Pitta or both Kapha and Pitta, then the patient is given emetic therapy with the following recipes:

1. Madana – Randia dumetorum, Madhuka– Licorice – Glycyrrhiza glabra, Nimba – Neem (Azadirachta indica) and Fruits of Vatsaka (Holarrhena antidysenterica Wall.)

2. Patola – Trichosanthes dioica, Picumarda, Pippali – Long pepper fruit – Piper longum, madana and Indrayava – seeds of Holarrhena antidysenterica. [51- 53]

Kashaya Yogas – Herbal decoction:

मुस्त निम्ब पटोलानां चन्दनोत्पलयोरपि| सारिवामलकोशीर मुस्तानां वा विचक्षणः||५४||

कषायान् पाययेद्वैद्यः सिद्धान् वीसर्पनाशनान्| किराततिक्तकं लोध्रं चन्दनं सदुरालभम्||५५||

नागरं पद्म किञ्जल्कमुत्पलं स बिभीतकम्| मधुकं नागपुष्पं च दद्याद्वीसर्प शान्तये||५६||

प्रपौण्डरीकं मधुकं पद्मकिञ्जल्कमुत्पलम्| नागपुष्पं च लोध्रं च तेनैव विधिना पिबेत्||५७||

द्राक्षां पर्पटकं शुण्ठीं गुडूचीं धन्वयासकम्| निशापर्युषितं दद्यात्तृष्णा वीसर्प शान्तये||५८||

पटोलं पिचुमर्दं च दार्वीं कटुकरोहिणीम्| यष्ट्याह्वां त्रायमाणां च दद्याद्वीसर्पशान्तये||५९||

पटोलादिकषायं वा पिबेत्त्रिफलया सह| मसूर विदलै र्युक्तं घृतमिश्रं प्रदापयेत्||६०||

पटोलपत्र मुद्गानां रसमामलकस्य च| पाययेत घृतोन्मिश्रं नरं वीसर्प पीडितम्||६१||

The following decoctions are useful for the treatment of Visarpa:

1. Decoction of Musta (Cyperus rotundus), Nimba – Neem (Azadirachta indica) and Patola – Trichosanthes dioica

2. Decoction of Chandana (Sandalwood – Santalum album) and Utpala (Nymphaea alba) Sariva – Indian Sarsaparilla – Hemidesmus indicus, Amalaka, Ushira – Vetiver – Vetiveria zizanioides and Musta (Cyperus rotundus)

A wise physician should administer these (above mentioned therapeutically effective decoctions for the cure of Visarpa.

1. Decoction of Kiratatikta – Swertia chirata, Lodhra -Symplocos racemosa, Chandana (Sandalwood – Santalum album), Duralabha, Nagara – Zingiber officinale, Androciums of Padma – Lotus (Nelumbo nucifera), Utpala (Nymphaea alba), Bibhitaka – Terminalia bellerica, Madhuka– Licorice – Glycyrrhiza glabra, and Naga-Puspa

2. Decoction of Prapaundarika (Nymphaea lotus) – red variety, Madhuka– Licorice – Glycyrrhiza glabra, Androceums of Padma – Lotus (Nelumbo nucifera), Utpala (Nymphaea alba), Nagapuspa and Lodhra (Symplocos racemosa)

3. The Sita – white variety of Cynodon dactylon - Kasaya (cold decoction) prepared of Draksha – Raisin – Vitis vinifera, Parpataka, Sunthi – Zingiber officinale, Guduchi – Tinospora cordifolia and Dhanvasaka this is useful for the cure of morbid thirst and Visarpa

4. The cold decoction of Patola – Trichosanthes dioica, Picumarda, Darvi, Katuka-Katukarohini – Picrorhiza kurroa, Yastimadhu – Glycyrrhiza glabra and Trayamana – Gentiana kurroo

5. To the above mentioned recipe of Patola – Trichosanthes dioica, etc. Triphala and De-husked seeds of masura may be added, and made to a decoction. This decoction is added with ghee and

6. Decoction of the leaves of Patola – Trichosanthes dioica, Mudga and the juice of Amalaki – Emblica offcinalis. This decoction is administered by adding ghee. [54-61]

Recipes of Medicated Ghee

यच्च सर्पिर्महातिक्तं पित्त कुष्ठ निबर्हणम्| निर्दिष्टं तदपि प्राज्ञो दद्याद्वीसर्पशान्तये||६२||

त्रायमाणाघृतं सिद्धं गौल्मिके यदुदाहृतम्| विसर्पाणां प्रशान्त्यर्थं दद्यातदपि बुद्धिमान्||६३||

त्रिवृच्चूर्णं समालोड्य सर्पिषा पयसाऽपि वा| घर्माम्बुना वा संयोज्य मृद्वीकानां रसेन वा||६४||

विरेकार्थं प्रयोक्तव्यं सिद्धं वीसर्पनाशनम्| त्रायमाणाशृतं वाऽपि पयो दद्यादिवरेचनम्||६५||

त्रिफलारस संयुक्तं सर्पिस्त्रिवृत्या सह| प्रयोक्तव्यं विरेकार्थं विसर्प ज्वरनाशनम्||६६||

रसमामलकानां वा घृतमिश्रं प्रदापयेत्| स एव गुरुकोष्ठाय त्रिवृच्चूर्णयुतो हितः||६७||

दोषे कोष्ठगते भूय एतत् कुर्याच्चिकित्सितम्|६८|

MadhuTiktaka Ghrita described earlier (in Chikitsa 7: 144-150) for the treatment of Paittika Kushta is used by a wise physician to cure of Visarpa.

The reputed Trayamana Ghruta described earlier (in Chikitsa 5: 128- 129) for the treatment of Gulma (tumour) also is used by a wise physician for the treatment of Visarpa.

The powder of Trivrt – Operculina turpethum is boiled by adding ghee or milk, and administered along with warm water or the juice of Mrdvika for purgation. This is a reputed recipe for the cure of Visarpa.

Similarly, milk boiled by adding Trayamana is administered to cause purgation in a patient suffering from Visarpa.

The decoction of Triphala is added with ghee and Trivrt – Operculina turpethum and given for purgation to the patient of Visarpa associated with fever.

Similarly, the decoction or juice of Amalaki – Emblica officinalis is administered for purgation, by adding ghee. If the patient of Visarpa had costive bowel, then the powder of Trivrt – Operculina turpethum is added to this recipe.

If the Doshas in the patient of visarpa are located in the Kostha (Gastro- Intestinal tract) then also the above mentioned recipes are to be administered. [62- ½ 68]

Raktamokshana – Blood- letting Therapy for Bahi Visarpa:

शाखादुष्टे तु रुधिरे रक्तमेवादितो हरेत्||६८||

भिषग्वातान्वितं रक्तं विषाणेन विनिर्हरेत्| पित्तान्वितं जलौकोभिः, कफान्वितमलाबुभिः||६९||

यथासन्नं विकारस्य व्यधयेदाशु वा सिराम्| त्वङ्मांसस्नायुसङ्क्लेदो रक्तक्लेदादिध जायते||७०||

Raktamokshana – Bloodletting Therapy for Bahi Visarpa:

If the blood in the periphery is vitiated to cause Visarpa, then in the beginning, bloodletting therapy is administered by the physician.

Vatanvita Rakta – Shrunga (Vishaana) – If the vitiated Rakta is associated with aggravated Vata, then the vitiated blood is taken out through the help of horn.

Pittanvita Rakta – Jalauka – If there is association of aggravated Pitta, then the blood is taken out with the help of leeches.

Kaphanvita Rakta – Alabu – If there is association of aggravated Kapha, then the vitiated blood is taken out with the help of alabu (the outer shell of the fruit with the pulp removed).

In addition, Venesection is performed to take out the vitiated blood from the adjacent vein. This bloodletting therapy is essential], without which the vitiated blood gives rise to the sloughening of the skin, muscle tissue and ligaments. [68½ – 70]

External therapies

अन्तःशरीरे संशुद्धे दोषे त्वङ्मांस संश्रिते| आदितो वाऽल्पदोषाणां क्रिया बाह्या प्रवक्ष्यते||७१||

Even after the interior of the body is cleansed [by the above mentioned elimination therapies], the residual Doshas remain in the exterior of the body, i.e. in the skin and muscle tissue. To remove these morbid Doshas, external therapies are administered. Such external therapies can also be administered in the beginning, if the Doshas causing Visarpa are less aggravated.

Udumbaradi Pradeha:

उदुम्बर त्वङ्मधुकं पद्म किञ्जल्कमुत्पलम्| नागपुष्पं प्रियङ्गुश्च प्रदेहः सघृतो हितः||७२||

The paste of the bark of Udumbara – Ficus racemosa, Madhuka– Licorice – Glycyrrhiza glabra, Padma – Lotus (Nelumbo nucifera)- kinjalka, Utpala (Nymphaea alba), Naga puspa and Priyangu (Callicara macrophylla) is added with Ghee and applied externally (Pradeha) for the cure of Visarpa. [72]

Nyarodhadya Lepa

न्यग्रोधपादास्तरुणाः कदली गर्भे संयुताः| बिसग्रन्थिश्च लेपः स्याच्छतधौतघृताप्लुतः||७३||

The paste of the tender adventitious roots of Nyagrodha – Ficus bengalensis, Pith of Kadali and Bisa- Granthi (rhizome of lotus) is mixed with Shata- Dhauta- Ghrta (ghee washed with water for 100 times) and applied externally. [73]

Kaliyadi Pralepa

कालीयं मधुकं हेम वन्यं चन्दन पद्मकौ| एला मृणालं फलिनी प्रलेप: स्याद्धृताप्लुत:||७४||

The paste of Kaliya, Madhuka– Licorice – Glycyrrhiza glabra, Hema (Mesua ferrea), Vanya, Chandana (Sandalwood – Santalum album), Padmaka – Prunus cerasoides, Ela (Elettaria cardamomum Maton) Mrnala and Phalini is mixed with ghee and applied externally. [74]

Shadvaladi –Pradeha:

शाद्वलं च मृणालं च शङ्खं चन्दनमुत्पलम्| वेतसस्य च मूलानि प्रदेह: स्यात् सतण्डुल:||७५||

The paste of Shadvala (Durva (Cynodon dactylon), Mrunala, Shankha, Chandana (Sandalwood – Santalum album), Utpala (Nymphaea alba), root of Vetasa and Tandula (rice) is applied externally. [75]

Sarivadya-Pralepa:

सारिवा पद्मकिञ्जल्कमुशीरं नीलमुत्पलम्| मञ्जिष्ठा चन्दनं लोध्रमभया च प्रलेपनम्||७६||

The paste of Sariva – Indian Sarsaparilla – Hemidesmus indicus, Padma – Lotus (Nelumbo nucifera)- Kinjalka, Ushira – Vetiver – Vetiveria zizanioides, nila- Utpala (Nymphaea alba), Manjistha – Rubia cordifolia, Chandana – Santalum album, Lodhra (Symplocos racemosa) and Abhaya – Terminalia chebula is applied externally. [76]

Naladadi Pralepa

नलदं च हरेणुश्च लोध्रं मधुक पद्मकौ | दूर्वा सर्जरसश्चैव सघृतं स्यात् प्रलेपनम्||७७||

The paste of Nalada, Harenu, Lodhra (Symplocos racemosa), Madhuka– Licorice – Glycyrrhiza glabra, Padmaka – Prunus cerasoides, Durva – Cynodon dactylon and Sarja (Vateria indica)-Rasa is mixed with ghee and applied externally. [77]

यावका: सक्तवश्चैव सर्पिषा सह योजिता:| प्रदेहो मधुकं वीरा सघृता यव सक्तव:||७८||

Yavaka (gruel prepared of barley) or Saktu (roasted flour of cereals) is mixed with ghee and applied externally.
The paste of Madhuka, Vara and Yava – Barley -Saktu (Flour prepared of roasted barley) is mixed with ghee and applied externally. [78]

Baladi Lepa

बलामुत्पल शालूकं वीरामगुरु चन्दनम्| कुर्यादालेपनं वैद्यो मृणालं च बिसान्वितग्ग||७९||

The physician should apply externally the paste of Bala – Country mallow (root) – Sida cordifolia, Utpala (Nymphaea alba) - Saluka (rhizome of lotus), Vira Kanda Vidari Pueraria tuberosa), Aguru – Aquallaria agallocha and Chandana (Sandalwood – Santalum album).
Similarly, the paste of Mrnala (root of lotus) & Bisa (stem of lotus) is applied externally. [79]

यवचूर्ण समधुकं सघृतं च प्रलेपनम्|

The paste of the powder of barley and Madhuka– Licorice – Glycyrrhiza glabra is mixed with ghee and applied externally. [½ 80]

हरेणवो मसुराश्च समुद्गा: श्वेत शालय:||८०||
पृथक् पृथक् प्रदेहा: स्यु: सर्वे वा सर्पिषा सह|

Harenu, Masura, Mudga and white variety of Shali-rice- – these drugs taken individually or all together is made to a paste, mixed with ghee and applied externally [80 ½ –81½]

पद्मिनी कर्दमः शीतो मौक्तिकं पिष्टमेव वा||८१||
शङ्खः प्रवाल: शुक्तिर्वा गैरिकं वा घृताप्लुतम्|

(पृथग्गेते प्रदेहाश्च हिता ज्ञेया विसर्पिणाम्)।

The cooling mud from a lotus pond or the paste of pearl, or the paste of Sankha, or the paste of Pravala, or the paste of Sukti, or the paste of Gairika is mixed with ghee and applied externally which is useful for the patient suffering from Visarpa. [81 ½ – ½ 82]

Prapanudarikadi Pralepa
प्रपौण्डरीकं मधुकं बला शालूकमुत्पलम्॥८२॥
न्यग्रोध पत्रदुग्धीके सघृतं स्यात् प्रलेपनम्।

The paste of Prapaundarika (Nymphaea lotus) – red variety, Madhuka– Licorice – Glycyrrhiza glabra, Bala – Country mallow (root) – Sida cordifolia, Saluka, Utpala (Nymphaea alba), leaves of Nyagrodha – Ficus bengalensis and Dugdhika is mixed with ghee and applied externally. [82 1/2 – ½ 83]

बिसानि च मृणालं च सघृताश्च कशेरुकाः॥८३॥
शतावरी विदार्योश्च कन्दौ धौतघृताप्लुतौ।

The paste of Bisa (Lotus Root), Mrinala (lotus stalk) or Kasheru is mixed with ghee and applied externally.
Similarly, the paste of Shatavari – Asparagus racemosus and Vidari - Pueraria tuberosa mixed with Shata-Dhauta-Ghrta (Ghee washed with water 100 times) may be used externally. [83 ½- 84½]

शैवालं नलमूलानि गोजिह्वा वृष कर्णिका॥८४॥
इन्द्राणिशाकं सघृतं शिरीषत्वग्बलाघृतम् ।

The paste of Saivala, the root of Nava (Nala), Gojihva, Vrsa- Karnika (Musika-Parnika) and leaves of Indrani (Nirgundi (Vitex negundo) is mixed with ghee and applied externally. Similarly, the paste of the bark of Sirisha (Albizia lebbeck Benth.) mixed with root bark of Bala – Country mallow – Sida cordifolia mixed with Ghrta – ghee may be applied externally. [84 ½ –85½]

न्यग्रोधोदुम्बर प्लक्ष वेतसाश्वत्थ पल्लवैः॥८५॥
त्वक्कल्कैर्बहुसर्पिर्भिः शीतैरालेपनं हितम्।

The paste of the leaves and barks of Nyagrodha – Ficus bengalensis, Udumbara – Ficus racemosa, Plaksa – Ficus lacor, vetasa and Asvattha – Ficus religiosa is mixed with profuse quantity of ghee and applied externally after making them cool. [85 ½- 86½]

प्रदेहाः सर्व एवैते वात पित्तोल्बणे शुभाः॥८६॥
सकफे तु प्रवक्ष्यामि प्रदेहानपरान् हितान्।

All the above mentioned Pradehas (recipes used externally in paste form) are useful in the Visarpa caused by the aggravation of Vata and Pitta. Other recipes, in addition to the above mentioned ones, which are useful in the treatment of Visarpa caused by aggravated Kapha, will be described hereafter. [86 ½ –86½]

Triphala Pradeha
त्रिफलां पद्मकोशीरं समङ्गां करवीरकम्॥८७॥
नलमूलान्यनन्तां च प्रदेहमुपकल्पयेत्।

The paste of Triphala, Padmaka – Prunus cerasoides, Ushira – Vetiver – Vetiveria zizanioides, Samanga – Rubia cordifolia, Karaviraka, root of Nala and Ananta mixed with a small quantity of ghee is useful in Kaphaja type of Visarpa. [87 ½ –88½]

Khadiradya lepana:
खदिरं सप्तपर्णं च मुस्तमारग्वधं धवम्॥८८॥
कुरण्टकं देवदारु दद्यादालेपनं भिषक्।

The paste of Khadira – Acacia catechu, Saptaparna – Alstonia scholaris, Musta (Cyperus rotundus), Aragvadha (Cassia fistula), Dhava, Kurantaka and Devadaru (Cedrus deodara) mixed with a small quantity of ghee is useful in kaphaja type of Visarpa. [88 ½ –89½]

Kaphaja Visarpa Yogas:
आरग्वधस्य पत्राणि त्वचं श्लेष्मातकस्य च||८९||
इन्द्राणि शाकं काकाह्वां शिरीष कुसुमानि च| शैवालं नलमूलानि वीरां गन्ध प्रियङ्गुकाम्||९०||
त्रिफलां मधुकं वीरां शिरीष कुसुमानि च| प्रपौण्डरीकं ह्रीबेरं दार्वी त्वङ्मधुकं बलाम्||९१||
पृथगालेपनं कुर्याद्द्वन्द्वशः सर्वशोऽपि वा|
The following recipes are useful in the kaphaja type of Visarpa:
1. Paste of the leaves of Aragvadha (Cassia fistula) and the bark of Slesmataka
2. Paste of the leaves of Indrani, Kakahva and flowers of Sirisha (Albizia lebbeck Benth.)
3. Paste of Saivala, root of Nala, Vira and Gandha-Priyangu (Callicarpa macrophylla)
4. Paste of Triphala, Madhuka– Licorice – Glycyrrhiza glabra,Vira and flowers of Sirisha (Albizzi lebbeck Benth.) and
5. Paste of Prapaundrarika – Nymphaea lotus, Hribera, bark of Darvi – Berberis aristata, Madhuka– Licorice – Glycyrrhiza glabra and Bala – Sida cordifolia
The above mentioned recipes may be used individually or two of these may be combined or all of these may be used together externally by adding a small quantity of ghee for the cure of Kaphaja type of Visarpa. [89 ½ –92½]

Use of ghee in Recipes:
प्रदेहाः सर्व एवैते देयाः स्वल्प घृता प्लुताः||९२||
वातपित्तोल्बणे ये तु प्रदेहास्ते घृताधिकाः| घृतेन शतधौतेन प्रदिह्यात् केवलेन वा||९३||
All the recipes described above for external application to treat Kaphaja type of Visarpa are mixed with ghee only in small quantities. The recipes described earlier for the treatment of Vatika and Paittika types of Visarpa should however, be added with ghee in profuse quantity.
Even Shata Dhauta ghrita (ghee washed with water 100 times) also can be used externally for the treatment of Visarpa. [92 ½ – 93]

Recipes to cleanse the skin lesions: – Seka Yogas
घृतमण्डेन शीतेन पयसा मधुकाम्बुना| पञ्चवल्ककषायेण सेचयेच्छीतलेन वा||९४||
वातासृक्पित्तबहुलं विसर्पं बहुशो भिषक्|
If the Visarpa is caused by the excessive aggravation or vitiation of Vata, Rakta and Pitta, then the Physician should effuse (Seka) the ulcers frequently with the supernatant part of ghee or cooled milk or cooled decoction of Madhuka– Glycyrrhiza glabra or the cooled decoction of Pancha-Valkala. [94 –95½]

Recipes Used in different other Forms:
सेचनास्ते प्रदेहा ये त एव घृतसाधनाः||९५||
ते चूर्णयोगा वीसर्पव्रणानामवचूर्णनाः|
The recipes described above for effusion (secana) and for external application (Pradeha) may also be used for cooking medicated ghee. Similarly, these ingredients (recipes) can also be used for dusting (Avachurnna). Application of this medicated ghee and dusting the powders of these recipes help in the healing of the ulcers of Visarpa.

Durvadi –Ghrta and Darvyadi Avachurna
दूर्वा स्वरस सिद्धं च घृतं स्याद्व्रणरोपणम्||९६||
दार्वीत्वङ्मधुकं लोध्रं केशरं चावचूर्णनम्|
Ghee cooked with the juice of Durva (Cynodon dactylon) is applied externally which helps in the healing of the

ulcers caused by Visarpa.

Avachurnana – dusting – Similarly, the powder of the bark of Darvi – Berberis aristata, madhuka, Lodhra (Symplocos racemosa) and Kesara may be used for dusting over these ulcers. [96 ½ –97½]

Recipe for Washing the Ulcers

पटोलः पिचुमर्दश्च त्रिफला मधुकोत्पले||९७||

एतत् प्रक्षालनं सर्पिर्व्रणचूर्ण प्रलेपनम्|९८|

Decoction of Patola – Trichosanthes dioica, Picumarda, Triphala, Madhuka– Licorice – Glycyrrhiza glabra and Utpala (Nymphaea alba) may be used for washing ulcers of Visarpa. Medicated ghee prepared of the above mentioned ingredients may be applied over these ulcers. Similarly, the powder of these ingredients may be used for dusting over these ulcers of Visarpa. [97 ½ –98½]

Method of Using Ointments (Pradeha or lepa)

प्रदेहाः सर्व एवैते कर्तव्याः सम्प्रसादनाः||९८||

क्षणे क्षणे प्रयोक्तव्याः पूर्वमुद्धृत्य लेपनम्| अधावनोद्धृते पूर्व प्रदेहा बहुशोऽघनाः||९९||

देयाः प्रदेहाः कफजे पर्याधानोद्धृते घनाः| त्रिभागाङ्गुष्ठमात्रः स्यात् प्रलेपः कल्कपेषितः||१००||

नातिस्निग्धो न रूक्षश्च न पिण्डो न द्रवः समः| न च पर्युषितं लेपं कदाचिदवचारयेत्||१०१||

न च तेनैव लेपेन पुनर्जातु प्रलेपयेत्| क्लेदवीसर्पशूलानि सोष्णाभावात् प्रवर्तयेत्||१०२||

लेपो ह्युपरि पट्टस्य कृतः स्वेदयति व्रणम्| स्वेदजाः पिडकास्तस्य कण्डूश्चैवोपजायते||१०३||

उपर्युपरि लेपस्य लेपो यद्यवचार्यते| तानेव दोषाञ्जनयेत् पट्टस्योपरि यान् कृतः||१०४||

अतिस्निग्धोऽतिद्रवश्च लेपो यद्यवचार्यते| त्वचि न श्लिष्यते सम्यङ्न दोषं शमयत्यपि||१०५||

तन्वालिप्तं न कुर्वीत संशुष्को ह्यापुटायते| न चौषधिरसो व्याधिं प्राप्नोत्यपि च शुष्यति||१०६||

तन्वालिप्तेन ये दोषास्तानेव जनयेद्भृशम्| संशुष्कः पीडयेद्व्याधिं निःस्नेहो ह्यवचारितः||१०७||

Method of Using Ointments (Pradeha or lepa)

All the above mentioned ointments cure Samprasadana (which brings back the natural colour of the skin or which cause alleviation of Rakta and Pitta). These are to be used repeatedly after removing the previously applied ointment. The earlier used ointment is removed without washing with water, and thereafter, fresh ointment which is not very thick is applied. This process is repeated several times.

In Kaphaja Visarpa, thick ointment is used after the previously applied ointment is dried up and removed. The triturated paste is used externally in the form of ointment, and the thickness of this paste is 3/4th of the thickness of the thumb.

The paste is neither too unctuous nor too un-unctuous / dry. The paste is neither in a bolus form nor should it be too thin. The paste is of moderate consistency.

The paste which has become stale should never be used over the ulcers of Visarpa. The same paste which was used earlier and removed should not be applied again.

The paste smeared over a piece of cloth is used (tied as a bandage) over these ulcers because this arrests the evaporation of heat from these ulcers thereby causing sloughing, spread of the ulcers (Visarpa) and Pain. It produces more heat as a result of which pimples appear in the skin giving rise to itching.

If the paste is applied over the earlier one (without removing the earlier paste), then the same ailments arise as are described above (application of the paste by smearing over a cloth).

If the paste is applied in a thin layer, then while drying, the layer of the paste develops cracks, and it gets dried up before the medicinal value penetrates into the skin to cure the ailment

If the paste is applied without adding ghee, it produces the same adverse effects as those produced by the application of a thin layer of the paste (described above). While getting dried up, this paste causes more pain or aggravates the disease [98- 107]

Wholesome Food and Drinks

अन्नपानानि वक्ष्यामि विसर्पाणां निवृत्तये| लङ्घितेभ्यो हितो मन्थो रूक्षः सक्षौद्रशर्करः||१०८||
मधुरः किञ्चिदम्लो वा दाडिमामलकान्वितः| सपरूषक मृद्वीकः सखर्जूरः शृताम्बुना||१०९||
तर्पणैर्यवशालीनां सस्नेहा चावलेहिका| जीर्णे पुराणशालीनां यूषैर्भुञ्जीत भोजनम्||११०||
मुद्गान्मसूरांश्चणकान् यूषार्थमुपकल्पयेत्| अनम्लान् दाडिमाम्लान् वा पटोलामलकैः सह||१११||
जाङ्गलानां च मांसानां रसांस्तस्योपकल्पयेत्| रूक्षान् परूषक द्राक्षा दाडिमामलकान्वितान्||११२||
रक्ताः श्वेता महाह्वाश्च शालयः षष्टिकैः सह| भोजनार्थे प्रशस्यन्ते पुराणाः सुपरिस्रुताः||११३||
यवगोधूमशालीनां सात्म्यान्येव प्रदापयेत्| येषां नात्युचितः शालिर्नरा ये च कफाधिकाः||११४||

Wholesome food and drinks useful for curing Visarpa

The patient in the beginning should observe fast. Thereafter, he is given Mantha (roasted flour of cereals added with water in profuse quantity).This drink is free from any unctuous material, but is added with Dadima – Pomegranate, Amalaka, Parushaka, Mrudvika and Kharjura – dates. The above mentioned flour of roasted cereals and other ingredients is mixed with boiled water.

The roasted flour of barley and Shali type of rice may be added with ghee, and given to the patient to eat in the form of linctus.

When the above mentioned recipe is digested the patient is given boiled old rice along with vegetable soup. Mudga, Masura and Chanaka are used for the preparation of this vegetable soup. To these Yusha, patola – Trichosanthes dioica and Amalaka may also be added for the preparation of the soup. This soup may not be made sour. But if the patient so desires, the soup can be made sour by adding sour Dadima – Pomegranate.

The patient is given the soup of the meat of animals inhabiting an arid zone. The meat-soup is added with any unctuous material like ghee. Parusaka – Grewia asiatica, Draksha – Raisins, Dadima – Pomegranate – Punica granatum and Amalaka may be added while preparing the meat soup.

Red, white Mahahva types of Shali rice, and Sastika type of rice, which are old and which are boiled with the residual water completely removed, is given to the patient as food.

Depending upon the eating habit (wholesomeness), the patient may be given either barley or wheat or Shali type of rice to eat. If Shali type of rice is not very homologatory, and if kapha is aggravated in excess, (then barley and wheat is used as food). [108- 114]

Unwholesome Diet, Drinks and Regimens

विदाहीन्यन्नपानानि विरुद्धं स्वपनं दिवा| क्रोध व्यायाम सूर्याग्निप्रवातांश्च विवर्जयेत्||११५||

The patient suffering from Visarpa should avoid the following:

1. Food and drinks which are Vidahi (causing burning sensation)
2. Viruddha ahara – Mutually contradictory ingredients of food and drinks;
3. Diva svapna – Sleep during the day time
4. Krodha – Anger,Vyayama – Physical exercise and envy and
5. Exposure to hot rays of the sun, fire and strong wind [115]

General Line of Treatment:

कुर्याच्चिकित्सितादस्माच्छीतप्रायाणि पैत्तिके| रूक्षप्रायाणि कफजे स्नैहिकान्यनिलात्मके||११६||
वातपित्त प्रशमनमग्निवीसर्पणे हितम्| कफपित्त प्रशमनं प्रायः कर्दमसञ्ज्ञिते||११७||

From the above mentioned recipes, the cooling ones are to be used for Paittika type of Visarpa. The un-unctuous type of recipe is used for Kaphaja type of Visarpa. For the treatment of Vatika type of Visarpa, unctuous type of recipe is used.

Agni- Visarpa is treated with recipes which alleviate Vata and Pitta.

Kardama- Visarpa is treated with recipes which generally alleviate kapha and Pitta.

Treatment of Granthi- Visarpa:

रक्त पित्तोत्तरं दृष्ट्वा ग्रन्थि वीसर्पमादितः| रूक्षणै लंघनैः सेकैः प्रदेहैः पाञ्चवल्कलैः||११८||

सिरा मोक्षै र्जलौकोभि र्वमनैः सविरेचनैः| घृतैः कषाय तिक्तैश्च कालज्ञः समुपाचरेत्||११९||

If granthi- Visarpa is dominated by Rakta and Pitta, then in the beginning, the patient is given

Ruksana (drying therapy),

Langhana (fasting therapy),

Seka (affusion) with the decoction of Panca- valkala,

Sira-Moksa (venesection),

Jalaukavacarana (blood- letting therapy with leech),

Vamana (emetic therapy),

Virecana (Purgation therapy) and medicated ghee prepared of Astringent and bitter drugs.

The physician should administer these therapies in appropriate time. [118- 119]

ऊर्ध्वं चाधश्च शुद्धाय रक्ते चाप्यवसेचिते| वातश्लेष्महरं कर्म ग्रन्थिवीसर्पिणे हितम्||१२०||

After the body is cleansed through upward tract (by emetic therapy) and through downward tract (by purgation therapy) and after the administration of bloodletting therapy, the patient suffering from granthi-Visarpa is given external therapies, etc for the alleviation of Vata and kapha. [120]

External Therapy for Granthi Visarpa:

उत्कारिकाभिरुष्णाभिरुपनाहः प्रशस्यते| स्निग्धाभिर्वेशवारैर्वा ग्रन्थि वीसर्प शूलिनाम्||१२१||

The patient suffering from Granthi- Visarpa associated with colic pain is given external application of Upanaha (thick layer of paste applied when it is warm) with Utkarika (Pancaka) or Vesavara (Minced meat) which are warm and which are mixed with fat (ghee or oil). [121]

Affusion for Granthi Visarpa:

दशमूलोपसिद्धेन तैलेनोष्णेन सेचयेत्| कुष्ठतैलेन चोष्णेन पाक्यक्षारयुतेन च||१२२||

गोमूत्रैः पत्रनिर्यूहैरुष्णैर्वा परिषेचयेत्|

The nodules of Granthi- Visarpa are sprinkled with warm oil medicated by boiling with Dashamula. The oil cooked with Kushta and added with Pakva- Ksara (an Alkali preparation details of which are described in Susruta- Samhita) may also be used, when warm, for the affusion of these nodules. Similarly, affusion could be made with warm cow's urine or warm juice of the leaves (which alleviate Vata and Kapha, but do not cause vitiation of Rakta and Pitta). [122 - 123½]

Paste of External Application:

सुखोष्णया प्रदिह्याद्वा पिष्टया चाश्वगन्धया||१२३||

शुष्क मूलक कल्केन नक्तमालत्वचाऽपि वा| बिभीतक त्वचां वाऽपि कल्केनोष्णेन लेपयेत्||१२४||

बलां नागबलां पथ्यां भूर्जग्रन्थिं बिभीतकम्| वंशपत्राण्यग्निमन्थं कुर्याद्ग्रन्थिप्रलेपनम्||१२५||

दन्ती चित्रक मूलत्वक् सुधार्कपयसी गुडः| भल्लातकास्थि कासीसं लेपो भिन्द्याच्छिलामपि||१२६||

बहिर्मार्गस्थितं ग्रन्थिं किं पुनः कफसम्भवम्|

The warm paste of either Ashwagandha – Withania somnifera or dried radish or the bark of Naktamala - Karanja (Pongamia pinnata) is applied over the nodules.

The paste of Bala – Country mallow (root) – Sida cordifolia, Nagabala, Pathya, Bhurja granthi, Vibhitaka, leaves of Vamsa (Bamboo) and Agnimantha – Clerodendrum phlomidis is useful for the application over these nodules of Granthi- Visarpa.

Application of the paste of Danti – Baliospermum montanum, bark of the root of Chitraka – Leadword – Plumbago zeylanica, latex of Sudha, Latex of Arka – Calotropis procera, Jaggery, seed of Bhallataka (Semecarpus anacardium Linn.) and Kasisa breaks even a stone, what to speak of the nodules caused by Kapha which are located in the exterior of the body. [123 ½- 127½]

Recipes for external Application over Chronic Nodules:

दीर्घकाल स्थितं ग्रन्थिं भिन्द्याद्वा भेषजैरिमैः||१२७||

मूलकानां कुलत्थानां यूषैः सक्षारदाडिमैः| गोधूमान्नैर्यवान्नैर्वा ससीधुमधुशर्करैः||१२८||

सक्षौद्रैर्वारुणीमण्डै र्मातुलुङ्ग रसान्वितैः| त्रिफलायाः प्रयोगैश्च पिप्पलीक्षौद्र संयुतैः||१२९||

मुस्तभल्लातशक्तूनां प्रयोगैर्माक्षिकस्य च| देवदारु गुडूच्योश्च प्रयोगैर्गिरिजस्य च||१३०||

धूमैर्विरेकैः शिरसः पूर्वोक्तैर्गुल्मभेदनैः| अयो लवण पाषाण हेम ताम्र प्रपीडनैः||१३१||

For breaking open chronic nodules, the following recipes and therapies is administered

1. The patient should use the soups of Mulaka – Raphanus sativus and Kulattha – Dolichos biflorus along with Alkalies and Dadima – Pomegranate – Punica granatum

2. The patient may take boiled wheat or barley along with Sidhu (a type of wine), honey and sugar.

3. The patient should drink supernatant part of Varuni (a type of alcoholic drink) along with honey and the juice of Matulunga – Lemon variety – Citrus decumana / Citrus limon

4. Triphala along with Pippali and honey is administered to the patient

5. The roasted flour of Musta (Cyperus rotundus) or Bhallataka – Semecarpus anacardium is given to him

6. Maksika (iron pyrite) or Devadaru (Cedrus deodara) and Guduchi – Tinospora cordifolia or Shilajatu is administered to the patient

7. The patient is given Dhuma (smoking therapy) and Siro- Virecana (inhalation therapy) for the elimination of morbid matter from the head

8. Recipes described earlier (in Chikitsa ; 5) for breaking open the growth of Gulma (Phantom tumor) and

9. Putting pressure on the nodules with (hot) iron, bolus of salt, stone, gold, or copper [127 ½ – 131]

Agnikarma and Shastrakarma for Granthi Visarpa treatment: Cauterization and Surgical Intervention

आभिः क्रियाभिः सिद्धाभिर्विविधाभिर्बली स्थिरः| ग्रन्थिः पाषाणकठिनो यदा नैवोपशाम्यति||१३२||

अथास्य दाहः क्षारेण शरैर्हेम्नाऽथ वा हितः| पाकिभिः पाचयित्वा वा पाटयित्वा समुद्धरेत्||१३३||

मोक्षयेद्बहुशश्चास्य रक्तमुत्क्लेशमागतम्| पुनश्चापहृते रक्ते वातश्लेष्मजिदौषधम्||१३४||

धूमो विरेकः शिरसः स्वेदनं परिमर्दनम्| अप्रशाम्यति दोषे च पाचनं वा प्रशस्यते||१३५||

प्रक्लिन्नं दाहपाकाभ्यां भिषक् शोधनरोपणैः| बाह्यैश्चाभ्यन्तरैश्चैव व्रणवत् समुपाचरेत्||१३६||

कम्पिल्लकं विडङ्गानि दार्वीं कारञ्जकं फलम्| पिष्ट्वा तैलं विपक्तव्यं ग्रन्थिव्रणचिकित्सितम्||१३७||

द्विव्रणीयोपदिष्टेन कर्मणा चाप्युपाचरेत्| देशकालविभागज्ञो व्रणान् वीसर्पजान् बुधः||१३८||

इति ग्रन्थिविसर्पचिकित्सा|

Cauterization and Surgical Intervention

If these nodules have become strong, stabilized, and hard like stone, and therefore, not amenable to the above mentioned therapeutic measures, then their cauterization with the help of Alkalis or hot rod of gold is useful.

These nodules are suppurated by the external application of suppurating ointments. Thereafter, these suppurated nodules are incised and removed. The blood from this location which is already incited is taken out frequently. After the vitiated blood is removed, medicines for the alleviation of Vata and kapha are given to the patient.

He is given Dhuma (smoking therapy), Shiro- virecana (inhalation therapy for the elimination of morbid from the head), Svedana (fermentation therapy), and Parimardana (rubbing therapy). If by the above mentioned therapeutic measures, the vitiated Doshas do not get alleviated, then the patient is given Pacana (recipes to bring about maturity of the Ama or immature metabolic product) therapy.

When these nodules have become soft because of cauterization and application of suppuration recipes, the physician should treat these nodules of Granthi- Visarpa like an ulcer with the cleansing and healing therapies both externally and internally. [132- 136]

With fruit of Kampillaka, vidanga, daruharidra and karanja made in to paste and can be used to prepare oil. That is indicated in the treatment of granthi vrina. The physician who is well versed in the knowledge of Desa and Kala should administered the same measures explanied in Dvi vranya chapter (To treat Vranas - Ulcers) for the treatment of Ulcers caused by Visarpa also. (137- 138)

Treatment of Ulcers

य एव विधिरुद्दिष्टो ग्रन्थीनां विनिवृत्तये| स एव गलगण्डानां कफजानां निवृत्तये||१३९||

गलगण्डास्तु वातोत्था ये कफानुगता नृणाम्| घृत क्षीर कषायाणामभ्यासान्न भवन्ति ते||१४०||

The therapeutic measures described above for the treatment of the nodules of Granthi- Visarpa are useful for the treatment of Gala-Ganda (goiter) caused by the aggravation of kapha. Habitual intake of ghee, milk and decoctions, prevent the occurrence of Gala Ganda or goiter (including Ganda-Mala or cervical adenitis) caused by aggravation of Vata in association of Kapha. [139- 140]

Treatment of Galaganda (Goiter)

यानीहोक्तानि कर्माणि विसर्पाणां निवृत्तये| एकतस्तानि सर्वाणि रक्त मोक्षणमेकतः||१४१||

विसर्पो न ह्यसंसृष्टो रक्तपित्तेन जायते| तस्मात् साधारणं सर्वमुक्तमेतच्चिकित्सितम्||१४२||

विशेषो दोषवैषम्यान्न च नोक्तः समासतः| समासव्यासनिर्दिष्टां क्रियां विद्वानुपाचरेत्||१४३||

Importance of Bloodletting Therapy

Since Visarpa is never manifested without the vitiation of Rakta and Pitta, blood letting therapy (which is the most effective measure to correct this morbidity) can match all the other modes of treatment described above for curing Visarpa.

Therefore, the therapeutic measures to alleviate the fundamental causative factors, viz; Rakta and Pitta are described in this chapter. It is not that the therapeautic measures for the alleviation of other causative factors in specific cases viz. Vata and Kapha are not explained here. Thus, the therapeutic measures both in general (for the alleviaton of Rakta and Pitta) and in specific cases (for the alleviation of other causative factors like Vata and Kapha) are described both in brief and in detail. A wise physician should administer these therapies appropriately (with desecration). [141-143]

तत्र श्लोकाः-

निरुक्तं नाम भेदाश्च दोषा दूष्याणि हेतवः| आश्रयो मार्गतश्चैव विसर्प गुरु लाघवम्||१४४||

लिङ्गान्युपद्रवा ये च यल्लक्षण उपद्रवः| साध्यत्वं, न च, साध्यानां साधनं च यथाक्रमम्||१४५||

इति पिप्रक्षवे सिद्धिमग्निवेशाय धीमते| पुनर्वसुरुवाचेदं विसर्पाणां चिकित्सितम्||१४६||

Thus, Punarvasu (Atreya) explained the perfect treatment of Visarpa to Agnivesha, the learned inquie with reference to the following topics:

1. Derivation of the Visarpa
2. Synonyms of Visarpa
3. Doshas, Dushyas (tissue elements) and other causative factors of Visarpa
4. The Asraya (location) of Visarpa in different channels viz exterior or interior part of the body
5. The seriousness and non- seriousness of different types of Visarpa
6. Signs and symptoms and complications of different types of Visarpa
7. Nature of Upadrava (complication)
8. Curability and incurability of different types of Visarpa and
9. Appropriate therapeutic for the treatment of curable varieties of Visarpa. [144-146]

Colophon

इत्यग्निवेशकृते तन्त्रे चरक प्रतिसंस्कृते चिकित्सा स्थाने विसर्प चिकित्सितं नामैकविंशोऽध्यायः||२१||

Thus, ends the 21st chapter in Chikitsa Sthana (section on treatment of diseases) dealing with the treatment of visarpa (erysiples and herpes) in Agnivesha's work as redacted by Charaka.

5

Chikitsasthana Chapter 22 Trishna Chikitsitam

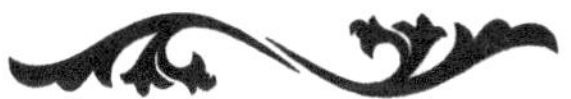

The 22nd Chapter of Charaka Samhita Chikitsa Sthana deals with Trishna Chikitsa – treatment for dry mouth or excessive thirst. The chapter is called Trishna Chikitsa Adhyaya.

अथातस्तृष्णा चिकित्सितं व्याख्यास्यामः||१||

इति ह स्माह भगवानात्रेयः||२||

Let us explore the chapter on the treatment of Trishna (morbid thirst). Thus said Lord Atreya [1-2]

Prologue:

ज्ञान प्रशमतपोभिः ख्यातोऽत्रिसुतो जगद्धितेऽभिरतः| तृष्णानां प्रशमार्थं चिकित्सितं प्राह पञ्चानाम्||३||

The son of Atri (Lord Punarvasu) reputed as an abode of knowledge, peace and penance, and deeply interested in the well-being of the world, explained the treatment for the alleviation of the 5 categories of Trishna (excess thirst). [3]

Topics covered in this chapter:

Trishna Nidana and Samanya Samprapti:

क्षोभाद्भयाच्छ्रमादपि शोकात्क्रोधादिवलङ्घनान्मद्यात्| क्षाराम्ल लवण कटुकोष्ण रूक्ष शुष्कान्न सेवाभिः||४||

धातुक्षयगदकर्षणवमनाद्यतियोग सूर्य सन्तापैः| पितानिलौ प्रवृद्धौ सौम्यान्धातूंश्च शोषयतः||५||

रसवाहिनीश्च नाडौ जिह्वामूल गलतालुक क्लोम्नः | संशोष्य नृणां देहे कुरुतस्तृष्णां महाबलायेतौ||६||

पीतं पीतं हि जलं शोषयतस्तावतो न याति शमम्| घोर व्याधि कृशानां प्रभवत्युपसर्गभूता सा||७||

Causes of Morbid Thirst / dryness of mouth:

Vata and Pitta get excessively aggravated because of the following:

1. Ksobha – Irritation, Bhaya -fear, Shrama – fatigue, Shoka – grief, Krodha – anger and Langhana – fasting

2. Madyapana – Intake of alcohol

3. Consumption of food ingredients of which are Ksara (alkaline), Amla (sour), Lavana (Saline) Katu (pungent), Ushna (hot), Ruksha (un-unctuous) and Sushka (dry)

4. Dhatu kshaya – Diminution of tissue elements

5. Gada karshana – Emaciation of the body because of suffering from chronic diseases

6. Ati vamana – Excessive administration of emetic therapy etc and

7. Surya santapa – Excessive exposure to the rays of the sun.

General Pathogenensis of mouth dryness:

These excessively aggravated Vata and Pitta cause dehydration of the tissue elements of the body which are liquid in nature (like Kapha, Rasa (taste) or Plasma and Udaka or Lymph) and the channels carrying Rasa (taste) or Plasma, at the root of the tongue, throat, Palate and Kloma (lungs). As a result of this, morbid thirst is manifested in the body because of these 2 powerful Doshas (excessively aggravated Vata and Pitta).

The patient afflicted with this ailment drinks water very frequently which gets dried up. As a result of this, his thirst is never quenched. This type of morbid thirst also occurs as a complication in a patient who is emaciated because of his suffering from serious diseases. [4-7]

Trushna Purvaroopa:

प्रागूपं मुखशोषः, स्वलक्षणं सर्वदाऽम्बुकामित्वम्|
तृष्णानां सर्वासां लिङ्गानां लाघवमपायः||८||

Premonitory Signs and Symptoms of morbid thirst:

Mukha shosha (Dryness of the mouth).

Constant desire to drink water is the invariable characteristic feature of this ailment.

The signs and symptoms are manifested in a lighter or less prominent form at the premonitory stage, and at times, some of these signs and symptoms are not manifested at all at this stage. [8]

Trushna Samanya Lakshana:

मुखशोष स्वरभेद भ्रम सन्ताप प्रलाप संस्तम्भान्| ताल्वोष्ठ कण्ठ जिह्वा कर्कशतां चित्तनाशं च||९||
जिह्वा निर्गममरुचिं बाधिर्य मर्मद्यनं सादम्| तृष्णोद्भूता कुरुते, पञ्चविधां लिङ्गतः शृणु ताम्||१०||

General signs and symptoms of excess thirst:

Mukha shosha – Dryness of the mouth

Svara bheda – Hoarseness of the voice

Bhrama – giddiness

Santapa – burning sensation

Pralapa – delirium

Stambha- stiffness

Talu ostha kantha jihva karkasha – roughness of the palate, lips, throat and tongue

Chitta nasham – unconsciousness

Jihva nirgaman – Protrusion of the tongue

Aruchi – anorexia

Badhirya – Deafness

Marma anga sada – pain in the vital parts of the body and prostration

Hereafter, the signs and symptoms of each of the 5 varieties of morbid thirst will be described. [9-10]

Vatika Trushna Nidana, Samanya Samprapti:

अब्धातुं देहस्थं कुपितः पवनो यदा विशोषयति| तस्मिन्नशुष्के शुष्यत्यबलस्तृष्यत्यथ विशुष्यन्||११||
निद्रानाशः शिरसो भ्रमस्तथा शुष्क विरसमुखता च स्रोतोऽवरोध इति च स्याल्लिङ्गं वात तृष्णायाः||१२||

Pathogenesis, Signs and symptoms of the Vatika Trishna:

When the aggravated Vata absorbs the tissue elements in the body which are liquid in nature, the patient becomes dehydrated by their diminution. Such a dehydrated patient suffers from Trushna (morbid thirst).

The signs and symptoms of Vatika type of Trushna (morbid thirst):

Nidra nasha – Insomnia

Shirasha bhrama – Giddiness in the head

Sushka virasa mukha – dryness as well as distaste in the mouth, and

Sroto rodha – obstruction to the channels of circulation [11- 12]

Paittika Trushna Nidana, Samprapti:

पित्तं मतमाग्नेयं कुपितं चेतापयत्यपां धातुम्| सन्तप्तः स हि जनयेत्तृष्णां दाहोल्बणां नृणाम्||१३||
तिक्तास्यत्वं शिरसो दाहः शीताभिनन्दता मूर्च्छा| पीताक्षि मूत्रवर्चस्त्वमाकृतिः पित्त तृष्णायाः||१४||

Pathogenesis, Signs and Symptoms of Paittika Trushna:

Pitta is dominated by Agni- mahabhuta (having heating effect).

Therefore, its aggravation causes heating of the liquid tissue elements of the body. Because of this hot attribute, these tissue elements produce Trushna (morbid thirst) dominated by burning sensation in human beings.

The signs and symptoms of Paittika type of Trushna (morbid thirst):

Tiktasyatvam - bitter taste in the mouth

Shiraso daha - burning sensation in the head

Shitabhinandata - liking towards cold things and comforts

Murcha - fainting, loss of consciousness

Pitakshimutravarchastvam - yellowish discoloration of eyes, urine and faeces [13-14]

Signs and Symptoms of Amaja Trishna:

तृष्णा याऽऽम प्रभवा साऽप्याग्नेयाऽऽमपित जनितत्वात् | लिङ्गं तस्याश्चारुचिराध्मान कफप्रसेकौ च||१५||

Amaja Trishna is caused by Ama (a product of undigested food) and Pitta. Therefore, it is also Agneya (caused by Heat) in nature. Its signs and symptoms are

Aruchi – anorexia

Aadhmana – flatulence and

Kapha praseka – excessive salivation [15]

Pathogenesis, Signs and Symptoms of Kshayaja Trishna:

देहो रसजोऽम्बुभवो रसश्च तस्य क्षयाच्च तृष्येदि्ध| दीन स्वरः प्रताम्यन् संशुष्कहृदयगलतालुः ||१६||

The body is made of Rasa (plasma), and this Plasma is made of aqueous elements (Ambu). Thus, the diminution of Rasa gives rise to (Ksayaja type of) Trishna or morbid thirst. In such patients, the voice becomes low; he trembles; and his heart, throat and palate become parched (dry) [16]

Upasargaja Trishna (Thirst Manifested as Complication):

भवति खलु योपसर्गातृष्णा सा शोषिणी कष्टा| ज्वर मेहक्षय शोष श्वासाद्युपसृष्ट देहानाम् ||१७||

Trushna (Thirst) is manifested as an Upasarga (complication) in a patient afflicted with diseases like

Jwara – fever,

Meha (obstinate urinary disorders including diabetes),

Kshaya (Phthisis),

Sosha (consumption) and

Svasa (Asthma).

This causes emaciation (dehydration) of the body, and this ailment is difficult to cure. [17]

Prognosis of Trushna:

सर्वास्त्वतिप्रसक्ता रोगकृशानां वमि प्रसक्तानाम्| घोरोपद्रवयुक्तास्तृणा मरणाय विज्ञेयाः||१८||

If morbid thirst persists for a long time in a patient emaciated because of his suffering from other diseases, if vomiting persists along with morbid thirst, and if thirst is associated with serious types of complications, then this leads to the death of the patient. [18]

Important role of Pitta and Vata Dosha in the Pathogenesis of Thirst:

नाग्निं विना हि तर्षः पवनाद्वा तौ हि शोषणे हेतू| अब्धातोरतिवृद्धावपां क्षये तृष्यते नरो हि||१९||

गुर्वन्नपयःस्नेहैः सम्मूर्च्छद्दिभिर्विदाहकाले च| यस्तृष्येद्वृतमार्गे तत्राप्यनिलानलौ हेतू||२०||

तीक्ष्णोष्ण रूक्ष भावान्मद्यं पित्तानिलौ प्रकोपयति| शोषयतोऽपां धातुं तावेव हि मद्य शीलानाम्||२१||

तप्तास्विव सिकतासु हि तोयमाशु शुष्यति क्षिप्तम्| तेषां सन्तप्तानां हिम जलपानाद्भवति शर्म||२२||

Thirst is never manifested without Agni (pitta) and Vata Dosha, because these 2 are responsible for absorption of liquids in the body. When these 2 Doshas are excessively aggravated, then a person suffers from morbid thirst.

Even when a person taking heavy food, milk and fat, suffers from thirst during digestion because of obstruction of the channels by their digestion because of obstruction of the channels by their mixture, it is the Vata Dosha and Pitta which are responsible for the manifestation of this ailment.

Alcohol, because of its sharpness, heat and un-unctuousness, aggravates Pitta and vata leading to the absorption of the aqueous elements or to dehydration resulting in morbid thirst in a habitual drunkard.

Sprinkling of water over hot sand gets dried up soon. Likewise, the tissue elements which are hot [because of affliction by aggravated Pitta and vata], get pacified by the drinking of ice- cold water. [19-22]

Prohibition of Cold water bath:

शिशिर स्नातस्योष्मा रुद्धः कोष्ठं प्रपद्य तर्षयति| तस्मान्नोष्ण क्लान्तो भजेत सहसा जलं शीतम्||२३||

However, a bath with exceedingly cold water obstructs the dissipation of heat. The heat thus enters the Kostha (gastrointestinal tract) and causes thirst. Therefore, a person fatigued by exposure to heat should not instantaneously resort to cold water (bath). [23]

Trushna Samanya Chikitsa Sutra:

लिङ्गं सर्वास्वेतास्वनिलक्षय पित्तजं भवत्यथ तु| पृथगागमाच्चिकित्सितमतः प्रवक्ष्यामि तृष्णानाम्||२४||

General line of treatment:

In all the varieties of Trushna, aggravation of vata, diminution of aqueous elements and aggravation of Pitta take place. But these are caused by different etiological factors (Agama). Therefore, treatment of all these varieties of Trushna will be described separately hereafter. [24]

Use of Rainwater:

अपां क्षयादिध तृष्णा संशोष्य नरं प्रणाशयेदाशु| तस्मादैन्द्रं तोयं समधु पिबेतद्गुणं वाऽन्यत्||२५||

किञ्चित्तुवरानुरसं तनु लघु शीतलं सुगन्धि सुरसं च| अनभिष्यन्दि च यत्तत्क्षितिगतमप्यैन्द्रवज्ज्ञेयम्||२६||

Since Trushna causes death by dehydration because of the diminution of aqueous elements in the body, the patient is given Aindra type of water (rain- water which is collected from the sky before it falls on the earth) by adding honey. Other types of water [collected from the ground] having properties of Aindra or rain water may also be used by the patient.

This water should be slightly astringent in Anurasa (sub-taste), thin, light, cold, free from any bad smell or taste and Anabhisyandi (which does not cause obstruction to the channels of circulation). The groundwater having the above mentioned properties are like Aindra water (rain –water collected from the sky before it falls on the earth). [25-26]

Recipes of Medicated Drinks

शृतशीतं ससितोपलमथवा शर पूर्व पञ्चमूलेन| लाजा सक्तु सिताह्वा मधुयुतमैन्द्रेण वा मन्थम्||२७||

वाट्यं वाऽस्मयवानां शीतं मधु शर्करायुतं दद्यात्| पेयां वा शालीनां दद्याद्वा कोरदूषाणाम्||२८||

पयसा शृतेन भोजनमथवा मधु शर्करायुतं योज्यम्| पारावतादिकरसैर्घृतभृष्टैर्वाऽप्यलवणाम्लैः||२९||

तृणपञ्चमूलमुञ्जातकैः प्रियालैश्च जाङ्गला: सुकृता:| शस्ता रसाः पयो वा तैः सिद्धं शर्करा मधुमत्||३०||

शतधौत घृतेनाक्तः पयः पिबेच्छीततोयमवगाह्य| मुद्ग मसूर चणकजा रसास्तु भृष्टा घृते देयाः||३१||

मधुरैः सजीवनीयैः शीतैश्च सतिक्तकैः शृतं क्षीरम्| पानाभ्यञ्जनसेकेष्विष्टं मधु शर्करायुक्तम्||३२||

तज्जं वा घृतमिष्टं पानाभ्यङ्गेषु नस्यमपि च स्यात्|नारी पयः सशर्करमुष्ट्रया अपि नस्यमिक्षुरसः||३३||

The patient suffering from morbid thirst is given the following recipes:

1. Water boiled by adding Shara-Pancha-Mula (the roots of Sara, Iksu – Saccharum officinarum, Darbha – Demostachya bipinnata, kasa and Shali (rice). This boiled water is cooled after boiling and added with sitopala (large crystal sugar).

2. Mantha (demulcent drink) prepared of the flour of laja (propped paddy), in rain water by adding sugar and honey

3. The Cooled Vatya (paste) prepared of immature barley grains (by slightly roasting and then smashing) is given along with honey and sugar

4. The Peya (thin gruel) prepared of Shali rice or Koradusa

5. Food prepared by boiling with milk along with honey and sugar

6. The soup of the meat of Paravata etc, sizzled with ghee, and not added with salt and sour ingredients

7. Soup of the meat of animals inhabiting arid zone well prepared by boiling with the roots of Kusa (Desmostachya bipinnata), Kasa, Sara, Darbha – Demostachya bipinnata and iksu – Saccharum officinarum , or Munjataka or Priyala

8. Milk boiled with the roots of Kusha , kasa Sara, Darbha and Iksu – Saccharum officinarum, or with Munjataka or with Priyalaby adding sugar and honey.

9. Milk mixed with Shata Dhauta-Ghrta (ghee washed for one hundred times). This is taken after taking a bath in cold water.

10. The soup of Mudga (green gram), Masura (lentil) and Chanaka (Bengal gram) sizzled with ghee.

11. Milk is boiled by adding ingredients which are sweet in taste, which belong to the Jivaniya group, which are cooling in potency, and which are bitter in taste. This milk is added with honey and sugar, and used for drinking, massage and sprinkling over the body of the patient.

12. The ghee collected from the above mentioned milk is also useful for drinking, massage and inhalation therapy and

13. The women's milk or camel milk mixed with sugar or the sugar cane juice may also be used for Nasya (inhalation therapy) [27-33]

Recipes and Regimens for Trushna:

क्षीरेक्षुरस गुडोदक सितोपला क्षौद्र सीधु माद्र्वीकैः | वृक्षाम्ल मातुलुङ्गैर्गण्डूषास्तालुशोषघ्नाः||३४||

जम्ब्वाम्रातक बदरी वेतस पञ्चवल्क पञ्चाम्लैः| हृन्मुख शिरःप्रदेहाःसघृता मूर्च्छा भ्रम तृष्णाघ्नाः स्युः||३५||

दाडिम दधित्थ लोधैः सविदारी बीजपूरकैः शिरसः| लेपो गौरामलकैर्घृतारनालायुतैश्च हितः||३६||

शैवल पङ्काम्बुरुहैः साम्लैः सघृतैश्च शक्तुभिर्लेपः| मस्त्वारनालार्द्रवसनकमलमणिहार संस्पर्शाः||३७||

शिशिराम्बु चन्दनार्द्रस्तनतट पाणितल गात्र संस्पर्शाः| क्षौमार्द्रनिवसनानां वराङ्गनानां प्रियाणां च||३८||

हिमवद्दरीवनसरित्सरोऽम्बुजपवनेन्दुपाद शिशिराणाम्| रम्य शिशिरोदकानां स्मरणं कथाश्च तृष्णाघ्नाः||३९||

Gargling with milk, sugarcane- juice, jaggery mixed with water, solution of Sitopala (sugar of large crystal), honey, Sidhu (a type of alcoholic drink), Mardvika (drink prepared of Grapes), juice of Vrikshamla – Garcinia morella and juice of Matulunga – Lemon variety –Citrus limon cures dryness of the Palate.

Paste is prepared of Jambu – Sygyzium cumini, Amrataka Badari, Vetasa, Pancha-Valkala (bark of 5 trees). Viz Nyagrodha – Ficus bengalensis, Udumbara – Ficus racemosa, Asvattha – Ficus religiosa, Vetasa and Plaksa and Panchamla (5 sour preparations Viz., Kolamla, Cukrikamla, Matulunga – Lemon variety – Citrus decumana / Citrus limon, Amla-Vetasa – Garcinia pedunculata and Dadima – Pomegranate), and mixed with ghee. Application of this paste in the cardiac region, face and head causes fainting, giddiness and morbid thirst.

Paste is prepared of Dadima – Pomegranate, Dadhittha, Lodhra (Symplocos racemosa) and Vidari Pueraria tuberosa) by triturating with the juice of Bijapuraka – Citrus medica. Application of this paste on the head cures morbid thirst.

Similarly, application of the paste of Saivala (Vallisneria spiralis), Panka (mud) and lotus along with sour juice and ghee or the paste of Saktu (roasted corn- flour) mixed with sour juice and ghee cures morbid thirst.

Touching the body of the patient with a cloth soaked with Mastu (upper part of the curd) or Aranala (a sour drink) or with a necklace made of gems cures morbid thirst.

Touch of the breasts, Palms, and bodies of beautiful and lovable ladies who are made wet by cold water or the paste of Chandana (Sandalwood – Santalum album) and who have worn wet silken cloth cures morbid thirst.

Thinking of the caves of the Himalayas, forests, rivers, ponds, lotus, wind, cooling moon- rays and beautiful lakes having cold water, and hearing talks about them cures morbid thirst. [34-39]

Vataja Trushna Chikitsa:

वातघ्नमन्नपानं मृदु लघु शीतं च वात तृष्णायाम्| क्षय कासनुच्छृतं क्षीर घृतमूर्ध्ववात तृष्णाघ्नम् ||४०||

स्याज्जीवनीय सिद्धं क्षीरघृतं वात पित्तजे तर्ष|४१|

Treatment of Vatika Trushna:

For the treatment of Vatika Trushna, food and drinks which would alleviate vata and which are soft, light and cooling are useful.

Milk and ghee which are boiled with drugs used for the treatment of Ksayaja- Kasa, cure Urdhva-Vata (Svasa or asthma) and morbid thirst

Milk and ghee boiled with drugs belonging to the Jivaniya group cure thirst caused by vata and Pitta. [40- 41½]

Pittaja Trisna Chikitsa:

पैत्ते द्राक्षा चन्दन खर्जूरोशीर मधुयुतं तोयम्||४१||

लोहित शालि तण्डुल खर्जूर परूषकोत्पल द्राक्षाः| मधु पक्वलोष्टमेव च जले स्थितं शीतलं पेयम्||४२||

लोहित शालि प्रस्थः सलोध्र मधुकाञ्जनोत्पलः क्षुण्णः| पक्वामलोष्ट जल मधु समायुतो मृन्मये पेयः||४३||

वट मातुलुङ्ग वेतस पल्लव कुश काश मूल यष्ट्याह्वैः| सिद्धेऽम्भस्यग्निनिभां कृष्णमृदं कृष्णसिकतां वा||४४||

तप्तानि नवकपालान्यथवा निर्वाप्य पाययेताच्छम्| आपाक शर्करं वाऽमृतवल्ल्युदकं तृषां हन्ति||४५||

क्षीरवतां मधुराणां शीतानां शर्करा मधु विमिश्राः| शीत कषाया मृद्भृष्टसंयुताः पित्त तृष्णाघ्नाः||४६||

Treatment of Paittika Trushna:

For the cure of Paittika type of Trushna the following recipes are useful:

1. Intake of water boiled with Raisin, sandalwood, dates and Ushira – Vetiver – Vetiveria zizanioides and added with honey

2. Intake of cold water is added with a red variety of Shali- rice, Kharjura – dates, Parusaka – Grewia asiatica, Utpala (Nymphaea alba), Draksha – Raisin, honey and baked cl0d of earth.

3. 1 Prastha (768 g) of red variety of Shali-rice and (1 Pala each of), Lodhra (Symplocos racemosa), Madhuka – Madhuka longifolia, Rasanjana (Aqueous extract of Berberis aristata) and Utpala (Nymphaea alba) is made to a coarse powder. Water is added to this powder. A freshly baked clod of earth is immersed into it. By adding (1/4th in quantity of) honey, this water is taken in an earthen beaker.

4. Decoction is prepared by boiling water with Vata – Ficus bengalensis, Matulunga – Citrus medica, leaves of vetasa, Roots of Kusa (Desmostachya bipinnata) and Kasa, and Yastimadhu – Glycyrrhiza glabra. Black soil or black sand are heated till they become red. This soil or sand or heated Kapala (pieces of earthen pot) is immersed in the decoction. The water is then filled and given to the patient suffering from Trushna

5. The decoction of Amrta-Valli (Guduchi – Tinospora cordifolia) is cooked with sugar till it becomes a syrup cures Trushna and

6. The cold infusion (Hima) of ingredients having milky- latex, sweet taste and cold potency is immersed with a roasted cold of earth. This decoction should then be added with sugar and honey. Intake of this cures Paittika type of Trushna. [44 ½ – 46]

Treatment of Amaja Trushna:

व्योष वचा भल्लातक तिक्त कषायास्तथाऽऽमतृष्णाघ्नाः| यच्चोक्तं कफजायां वम्यां तच्चैव कार्य स्यात्||४७||

स्तम्भारुच्य विपाकालस्यच्छर्दिषु कफानुगां तृष्णाम्| ज्ञात्वा दधि मधु तर्पण लवणोष्ण जलै वमनमिष्टम्||४८||

दाडिममम्लफलं वाऽप्यन्यत् सकषायमथ लेहम्| पेयमथवा प्रदद्याद्रजनी शर्करायुक्तम्||४९||

The decoction of Sunthi – Zingiber officinale, Pippali – Long pepper fruit – Piper longum, Maricha – Black pepper fruit – piper nigrum, Vacha (Acorus calamus Linn.), Bhallataka and Tiktaka (Kirata- Tikta – Swertia chirata) cures Amaja type of Trushna. Therapies prescribed for the treatment of Kaphaja type of Chardi (vomiting) are also useful for the treatment of Amaja type of Trushna.

Association of aggravated kapha in Trushna is to be determined from the signs and symptoms like

Stambha – stiffness

Aruchi – anorexia

Vipaka – indigestion

Laziness and

Chardi – vomiting

In such a condition, emetic therapy is administered with the recipe containing curd, honey, tarpana (demulcent drink containing roasted corn- flour), salt and warm water. Such emetic therapies should also be given with the recipes of decoction and linctus (described in the kapha section) by adding Dadima – Pomegranate or sour Fruit- Juice.

The patient suffering from Amaja type of Trushna may also be given a drink added with sugar and Rajani (haridra) [47- 49]

Treatment of Kshayaja Trushna

क्षय कासेन तु तुल्या क्षय तृष्णा सा गरीयसी नृणाम्| क्षीण क्षत शोष हितैस्तस्मातां भेषजैः शमयेत्||५०||

Kshayaja Trushna like Ksayaja kasa is a serious ailment. Therefore, such a patient is given the therapies prescribed for the treatment of Ksina (ksayaja Kasa), Ksata (urah-Ksata or Phthisis) and Sosha (consumption). [50]

Treatment of Upasargaja Trushna:

पान तृषार्तः पानं त्वर्धोदकमम्ल लवण गन्धाढ्यम्| शिशिर स्नातः पानं मद्याम्बु गुडाम्बु वा तृषितः||५१||

भक्तोपरोध तृषितः स्नेह तृषार्तोऽथवा तनु यवागूम्| प्र पिबेद्गुरुणा तृषितो भुक्तेन तदुद्धरेद्भुक्तम्||५२||

मद्याम्बु वाऽम्बु कोष्णं बलवांस्तृषितः समुल्लिखेत् पीत्वा| मागधिका विशद मुखः सशर्करं वा पिबेन्मन्थम्||५३||

बलवांस्तु तालु शोषे पिबेद्धृतं तृष्यमद्याच्च| सर्पिर्भृष्टं क्षीरं मांस रसांश्चाबलः स्निग्धान्||५४||

अतिरूक्ष दुर्बलानां तर्ष शमयेन्नृणामिहाशु पयः| छागो वा घृतभृष्टः शीतो मधुरो रसो हृदयः||५५||

स्निग्धेऽन्ने भुक्ते या तृष्णा स्यातां गुडाम्बुना शमयेत्| तर्ष मूर्च्छाभिहतस्य रक्तपित्तापहैर्हन्यात्||५६||

[Morbid thirst may be caused as a complication of inappropriate food, drinks or regimens. Treatments of such types of morbid thirst is as follows]

If Trishna is caused by the intake of alcohol in excess, then the patient is given alcohol drinks diluted with half the quantity of water, and added profusely with ingredients which are sour, Saline or aromatic.

If it is caused by a bath with excessively cold water, then the patient is given Madyambu (alcohol diluted with water) or Gudambu (Jaggery made to a solution by adding water) to drink.

If it is caused by Bhaktoparodha (fasting) or if it is caused by the inappropriate administration of Sneha (ghee, oil etc) then the patient is given thin gruel to drink.

If it is caused by the intake of heavy food, the ingested food is made to be vomited out. If the patient is physically strong, then he is given Madyambu (alcohol diluted with water) or tepid water to cause emesis. Alternately, he is given Magadhika (Pippali) to chew for the cleansing of his mouth, and thereafter, he is given Mantha (demulcent drink) along with sugar to drink.

If the patient, suffering from the parching of the palate, is strong, then he is given (medicated) ghee to drink, and is given such foods to eat which would alleviate thirst. If however, he is weak, he is given milk sizzled with ghee or the soup of the meat of fatty animals.

The thirst of excessively un-unctuous and weak patients is quenched immediately by milk. The soup of the goat meat which is sizzled with ghee, which is sweet and which is cool works as a cardiac tonic for such patients.

If the morbid thirst is caused by the excessive intake of unctuous food, then it is alleviated by Gudambu (jaggery solution made by adding water).

The thirst of the patient afflicted with Murccha (fainting) is cured by the administration of therapies prescribed for the treatment of Rakta-Pitta (a condition characterized by bleeding from different parts of the body). [51-66]

Usage of different Types of water

तृट्दाह मूर्च्छा भ्रम क्लम मदात्ययास्र विष पित्ते | शस्तं स्वभाव शीतं, शृतशीतं सन्निपातेऽम्भः||५७||

हिक्का श्वास नवज्वर पीनस घृत पीत पार्श्व गल रोगे| कफवातकृते स्त्याने सद्यःशुद्धे च हितमुष्णम्||५८||

पाण्डूदर पीनस मेह गुल्म मन्दानलातिसारेषु| प्लीहिन च तोयं न हितं कामममसह्ये पिबेदल्पम्||५९||

पूर्वामयातुरः सन् दीनस्तृष्णार्दितो जलं काङ्क्षन्| न लभेत स चेन्मरणमाश्वेवाप्नुयाद्दीर्घरोगं वा||६०||

तस्माद्धान्याम्बु पिबेत्तृष्यन् रोगी सशर्करा क्षौद्रम्| यद्वा तस्यान्यत्स्यात् सात्म्यं रोगस्य तच्चेष्टम्||६१||

तस्यां विनिवृत्तायां तज्जन्य उपद्रवः सुखं जेतुम्| तस्मात्तृष्णां पूर्वं जयेद्बहुभ्योऽपि रोगेभ्यः||६२||

Usage of different Types of water:

Naturally, cold water is useful in morbid thirst, burning syndrome, fainting, giddiness, mental fatigue, alcoholism, bleeding, poisoning and ailments caused by aggravated Pitta. The water cooled after boiling is useful in Sannipatika (a type of fever).

Hot Water is useful in hiccup, in Asthma, in freshly occurring (at the first stage of) fever and in Pinasa (Rhinitis), after the intake of ghee, in the diseases of the sides of the chest and throat, diseases caused by Kapha and vata, when the Doshas have become Styana (thick) and immediately after the administration of elimination therapies.

Intake of water is not useful for the patient suffering from

Pandu – Anemia

Udara (obstinate abdominal diseases including ascites)

Pinasa (chronic Rhinits) at its later stage

Meha (obstinate urinary disorders including diabetes)

Gulma (Phantom Tumour)

Suppression of power of digestion

Atisara – Diarrhoea and

Pliha – splenic disorders.

However, if there is intolerable thirst in this patient, then water may be given only in small quantities. If the patients, suffering from the above mentioned diseases, become dehydrated because of morbid thirst, and because of not getting water even when they intensely need it, then this may cause instant death or may lead to long- standing diseases. Therefore such a thirsty patient is given water boiled by adding dhanyaka, and thereafter, by adding other ingredients which are wholesome for the disease. After overcoming the thirst, the complications caused by the intake of water can be cured easily.

Thereafter, treatment of the thirst is given priority over the treatment of several other diseases. [57-62]

तत्र श्लोकः:-

हेतू यथाऽग्निपवनौ कुरुतः सोपद्रवां च पञ्चानाम्| तृष्णानां पृथगाकृतिरसाध्यता साधनं चोक्तम्||६३||

In this chapter on the treatment of Trisna (morbid thirst), the following topics are discussed:

1. The manner in which Agni and Pavana cause Trusna (morbid thirst) along with its complications

2. Signs and symptoms of 5 varieties of Trusna separately

3. The signs and symptoms indicating the incurability of the disease and

4. Treatment of different types of Trisna (Morbid thirst) [63]

इत्यग्निवेशकृते तन्त्रे चरक प्रति संस्कृतेऽप्राप्ते दृढबल सम्पूरिते चिकित्सा स्थाने तृष्णा रोग चिकित्सितं नाम द्वाविंशोऽध्यायः||२२||

Thus ends the 22nd chapter of Chikitsa sthana (section on the treatment of diseases) dealing with the treatment of Trsihna in the work of Agnivesha, which was redacted by Charaka, and supplemented by Dridhabala.

6

Chikitsasthana Chapter 23 Visha Chikitsitam

The 23rd Chapter of Charaka Samhita ChikitsaSthana is called VishaChikitsa. It deals with symptoms and Ayurvedic treatment of poisoning due to snake bite, scorpion bite, food poisoning etc.

अथातो विष चिकित्सितं व्याख्यास्यामः||१||
इति ह स्माह भगवानात्रेयः||२||

Let us explore the treatment of Visha (poisoning). Thus, said Lord Atreya. [1-2]

Topics to be discussed:

प्रागुत्पत्तिं गुणान् योनिं वेगाॅल्लिङ्गान्युपक्रमान्| विषस्य ब्रुवतः सम्यगग्निवेश निबोध मे||३||

O! Agnivesha, hear me carefully. I shall describe Visha (poison) and the following aspects related to it.

1. Mythological origin of poison
2. Properties of poison
3. Source of poison
4. The stage of virulence of poison
5. Signs and symptoms of poisoning and
6. Therapeutic measures to prevent poisoning. [3]

Mythological Origin of Visha:

अमृतार्थं समुद्रे तु मथ्यमाने सुरासुरैः| जज्ञे प्रागमृतोत्पत्तेः पुरुषो घोरदर्शनः||४||
दीप्त तेजाश्चतुर्दंष्ट्रो हरिकेशोऽनलेक्षणः| जगद्विषण्णं तं दृष्ट्वा तेनासौ विष सञ्ज्ञितः||५||
जङ्गम स्थावरायां तद्योनौ ब्रह्मा न्ययोजयत्| तदम्बु सम्भवं तस्मादिद्विविधं पावकोपमम्||६||
अष्टवेगं दशगुणं चतुर्विंशत्युपक्रमम्|७|

Mythological Origin of poison:

In the days of Yore, while the ocean was being churned by the Gods and the demons for obtaining Amrutha – ambrosia, even prior to the production of Ambrosia, a ferocious- looking person who came with Aura, and who had 4 fangs, tawny hair and fiery eyes emerged. The world became despaired (Vishanna) at his sight because of which he was called Visha or poison.

Lord Brahma deposited this poison in Jangama (mobile) and Sthavara (immobile) things. Therefore, poison which originated from water is of 2 types – JangamaVisha and SthavaVisha. It resembles fire.

Its action is manifested in 8 virulent stages, it has 10 attributes and the ailments caused by its affliction can be treated by 24 categories of therapeutic measures. [4- 7½]

Normal aggravation and Alleviation of Visha:

तद्वर्षास्वम्बुयोनित्वात् सङ्क्लेदं गुडवद्गतम्||७||
सर्पत्यम्बुधरापाये तदगस्त्यो हिनस्ति च| प्रयाति मन्दवीर्यत्वं विषं तस्माद्धनात्यये||८||

The poison originates from water, and becomes sticky like jaggery when it comes in contact with water, and spreads during the rainy season. However, the star Agastya (canopos) at the end of the rainy season counteracts the effects of this poison. Therefore, the effects of poison become milder after the rains are over. [7 ½ – 8]

JangamaVisha (poison of Mobile Origin):
सर्पाः कीटोन्दुरा लूता वृश्चिका गृहगोधिकाः|
जलौका मत्स्य मण्डूकाः कणभाः सकृकण्टकाः||९||
श्वसिंह व्याघ्र गोमायुतरक्षुनकुलादयः| दंष्ट्रिणो ये विष तेषां दंष्ट्रोत्थं जङ्गमं मतम्||१०||

The poison of these creatures constitutes animal poisons (poison of mobile origin):
Sarpa – Snakes, Keeta – insects, Luta – spiders, Vrschika – scorpions, Grhagodhika – house lizards, Jalauka – leeches, Matsya – fish, Manduka – frogs, Kanabha or Salabha – locusts, Krkantaka (Chamelion), Shvana – dogs, Simha – lion, Vyaghra – tiger, Gomaya (jackal), Taraksu (hyena), Mongoose, etc., are the fanged animals through whose fangs the poison is transmitted. [9- 10]

Sthavara Visha (poison of Immobile Origin):
मुस्तकं पौष्करं क्रौञ्चं वत्सनाभं बलाहकम्| कर्कटं कालकूटं च करवीरक सञ्ज्ञकम्||११||
पालकेन्द्रायुधं तैलं मेघकं कुश पुष्पकम्| रोहिष पुण्डरीकं च लाङ्गलक्यञ्जनाभकम्||१२||
सङ्कोचं मर्कटं शृङ्गीविषं हालाहलं तथा| एवमादीनि चान्यानि मूलजानि स्थिराणि च||१३||

The poisons of immobile origin are: the roots (including Rhizomes) of
Mustaka, Pushkara, Krauncha, Vatsanabha, Balahaka, Karkata, Kalakuta, Karavira, Palaka, Indrayudha, Taila, Meghaka, Kusha, Rohisha, Pundarika, Langalika, Anjanabhaka, Sankocha, MarkkataSrungi -Visha Halahala and Such other poisonous roots [11- 13]

Garavisha (Artificial Poisons):
गर संयोगजं चान्यद्गरसञ्ज्ञं गद प्रदम्| कालान्तर विपाकित्वान्न तदाशु हरत्यसून्||१४||

There is another variety of poison called Garavisha which is prepared artificially by the mixture of various substances. It produces diseases. Since it takes some time for this type of poison to get metabolised and to produce its toxic effects, it does not cause instantaneous death of a person. [14]

Effects of Sthavara and Jangama Visha:
निद्रां तन्द्रां क्लमं दाहं सपाकं लोमहर्षणम्| शोफं चैवातिसारं च जनयेज्जङ्गमं विषम्||१५||
स्थावरं तु ज्वरं हिक्कां दन्तहर्ष गलग्रहम्| फेनवम्यरुचि श्वास मूर्च्छाश्च जनयेदिषम्||१६||
जङ्गमं स्यादधोभागमूर्ध्वभागं तु मूलजम्| तस्माद्दंष्ट्राविषं मौलं हन्ति मौलं च दंष्ट्रजम्||१७||

JangamaVisha Lakshana:
JangamaVisha (poison of mobile origin or normal poison) produces
• Nidram – somnolence, excess sleep
• Tandram – drowsiness
• Klamam – mental fatigue
• Daha – burning sensation
• Sa pakam – inflammation
• Loma harshanam – horripilation
• Sopham – edema and
• Atisara – diarrhoea

Sthavara Visha Lakshana
(poison of immobile origin or vegetable poison) produces

• Jwara – fever
• Hikka – hiccup
• Dantaharsham – tingling sensation in the teeth
• Gala graham – obstruction in the throat
• Phenavamya – vomiting of frothy materials,
• Aruchi – anorexia
• Shvasa – dyspnoea and
• Murccha – fainting

The animal poison moves downwards whereas the vegetable poison moves upwards in the alimentary canal. Therefore, the animal-poison cures poisoning by vegetable- poison, and the poisoning caused by animal- poison is cured by vegetable – poison. [15-17]

Visha Vega –

तृण्मोह दन्तहर्ष प्रसेक वमथक्लमा भवन्त्याद्ये| वेगे रस प्रदोषादसृक्प्रदोषादिद्वतीये तु||१८||
वैवर्ण्य भ्रम वेपथु मूर्च्छा जृम्भाङ्ग चिमिचिमातमकाः | दुष्ट पिशितात्तृतीये मण्डल कण्डू श्वयथु कोठाः||१९||
वातादिजाश्चतुर्थे दाह च्छर्द्यङ्गशूल मूर्च्छाद्याः| नीलादीनां तमसश्च दर्शनं पञ्चमे वेगे||२०||
षष्ठे हिक्का, भङ्गः स्कन्धस्य तु सप्तमेऽष्टमे मरणम्| नृणां, चतुष्पदां स्याच्चतुर्विधः, पक्षिणां त्रिविधः||२१||
सीदत्याद्ये भ्रमति च, चतुष्पदो वेपते, ततः शून्यः | मन्दाहारो म्रियते श्वासेन हि चतुर्थवेगे तु||२२||
ध्यायति विहगः प्रथमे वेगे, प्रभ्राम्यति द्वितीये तु| स्रस्ताङ्गश्च तृतीये विषवेगे याति पञ्चत्वम्||२३||

Stages of Poisoning in Human beings, Animals and Birds:

In human beings, the effects of poisons are manifested in 8 different stages as follows:

1st stage – Prathama Visha Vega:

In the first stage because of the vitiation of Rasa (chyle or Plasma), the patient suffers from
• Trut – morbid thirst
• Moha – unconsciousness
• Dantaharsha – tingling sensation in teeth
• Praseka – salivation
• Vamathu – vomiting and
• Klama – mental fatigue.

2nd stage – DvitiyaVisavega:

. In the second stage because of the vitiation of blood, the patient suffers from
• Vaivarnya – discoloration of the skin
• Bhrama – giddiness
• Vepathu -Tumbling
• Bhrama – fainting
• Jrmbha – Yawning
• Bhanga – tingling sensation in the limbs and
• Shvasa -dyspnoea

3rd Visa vega

In the third stage, because of the vitiation of Mamsa (muscle tissue), the patient suffers from
• Mandala (circular eruptions)
• Kandu – Pruritus
• Shyvathu – oedema and
• Kotha – Urticaria

4th stage:

. In the fourth stage, because of the vitiation of Vata, etc. The patient suffers from
• Chardi – vomiting

• Daha – burning sensation
• Angashula – pain in the limbs
• Murccha – Fainting etc.

5. In the fifth stage, the patient suffers from
• Neeladarshana – blue vision or
• Tamadarshana – dark vision etc.

6. In the sixth stage, the patient suffers from
• Hikka – hiccup

7. In the seventh stage, the patient suffers from
• SkandhaBhanga (Paralysis of the muscles in the shoulder girdle) and

8. In the eighth stage the patient succumbs to death.

The above mentioned 8 stages of poisoning are manifested in human beings.

Effect of poisoning on quadruped animals –

The effects of poisoning are manifested in 4 different stages and in birds, it is manifested in three stages.

The 4 stages of poisoning in animals are follows:

1. In the first stage, the animal gets depression and giddiness

2. In the second stage, the animal trembles

3. In the third stage, the animal feels emptiness (Sunya) , and it stops eating and {the term" Suna" in the first line of the verse no. 22 has a variant reading as 'Suna' meaning oedema. By implication, the animal gets swollen during the third stage of poisoning, and this appears to be more appropriate].

4. In the fourth stage, the animal dies because of the obstruction to respiration.

Effect of poisoning on birds:

1. In the first stage, the bird gets depressed

2. In the second stage, the bird gets giddiness and

3. In the third stage, the bird develops smoothness of the limbs resulting in death. [18- 23]

Visha Guna – qualities of poison:

लघु रूक्षमाशु विशदं व्यवायि तीक्ष्णं विकासि सूक्ष्मं च| उष्णमनिर्देश्य रसं दशगुणमुक्तं विषं तज्ज्ञैः||२४||

रौक्ष्याद्वातम शैत्यात्पित्तं सौक्ष्म्यादसृक् प्रकोपयति| कफमव्यक्तरसत्वादन्नरसांश्चानुवर्तते शीघ्रम्||२५||

शीघ्रं व्यवायिभावादाशु व्याप्नोति केवलं देहम्| तीक्ष्णत्वान्मर्मघ्नं प्राणघ्नं तद्विकासित्वात्||२६||

दुरुपक्रमं लघुत्वाद्वैशद्यात् स्यादसक्तगतिदोषम्| दोष स्थान प्रकृतीः प्राप्यान्यतमं ह्युदीरयति||२७||

Visha qualities:

The 10 attributes of poison according to the expert toxicologists:

• Laghu – Lightness
• Ruksha – dryness
• Asu – quickness
• Vishada – non-sliminess
• Vyavayi – which pervades the whole body before getting digested
• Tikshna – Sharpness
• Vikasi – which causes looseness of joints by the diminution of Ojas or vital essence
• Sukshma – Subtleness
• Ushna – heat and
• Anirdesya Rasa – indistinct taste

Aggravating factors: Because of
• Ruksha (dryness) – aggravates Vata;

• Ushna (heat) it causes aggravation of Pitta;
• Sukshma (Subtleness), it vitiates Rakta (blood);
• Ashu (quickness) quickly permeates through (lit. Follows) the Anna Rasa (Chyle);
• Vyavayi- Attribute, it spreads throughout the body instantaneously;
• Tikshna (sharpness) it causes injury to the Marmas (vital organs)
• Vikasi- attribute, it causes death;
• Laghu (lightness) it becomes difficult of therapeutic management; and
• Vaisadya (no sliminess), it pervades all the Doshas circulates along with them constantly.
Depending upon the location of the Doshas and the contribution of the patient, poisons produce several other complications. [24- 27]

Dosha based symptoms of Visha:
स्याद्वातिकस्य वात स्थाने कफ पित्त लिङ्गमीषत्| तृण्मोहारति मूर्च्छा गलग्रह च्छर्दि फेनादि ||२८||
पित्ताशय स्थितं पैत्तिकस्य कफवातयोर्विषं तद्वत्| तृट्कास ज्वर वमथु क्लम दाह तमोतिसारादि ||२९||
कफदेशं कफस्य च दर्शयेद्वातपित्तयोश्चेषत्| लिङ्गं श्वास गलग्रह कण्डू लाला वमथ्वादि||३०||
Dosha based symptoms of Visha:
If the poison gets lodged in the habitat of Vata (i.e Colon) in a person having a Vatika type of constitution, then the patient suffers from:
• Trut – morbid thirst
• Moha – unconsciousness
• Arati (dislike for everything)
• Murchha – fainting
• Gala graha – obstruction in the throat,
• Chardi – vomiting
• Phenadipraseka – foamy salivation etc.,
There will be less manifestation of the signs and symptoms of kaphaja and Pittaja.

If the poison gets lodged in the habitat of Pitta, in a person having a pattika type of constitution, then the patient suffers from:
• Trut – morbid thirst
• Kasa – coughing
• Jwara – fcvcr
• Chardi – vomiting
• Klama – mental fatigue
• Daha – burning sensation
• Tamas (appearance of darkness before the eyes)
• Atisara – Diarrhoea etc.
There will be less manifestation of the signs and symptoms of Kapha and Pitta.

If the poison gets lodged in the habitat of Kapha, in a person having a Kapha type of constitution, then the patient suffers from:
• Shvasa – Dyspnoea
• Gala graha – obstruction to the throat
• Kandu – itching
• Praseka – excessive salivation
• Chardi – vomiting Etc.
There will be less manifestation of the signs and symptoms of Vata and Pitta [28- 30]

Signs of DushiVisha (Artificial Poison):
दूषी विषं तु शोणितदुष्ट्याः:किटिम कोठ लिङ्गं च| विषमेकैकं दोषं सन्दूष्य हरत्यसूनेवम्||३१||

Dusi- Visha (a type of artificial poison) vitiates blood and produces symptoms like Aru (eczema in the head), Kitibha (Psoriasis) and Kotha (urticaria). This type of poison afflicts each one of the Doshas and causes death of the patient. [31]

The cause of Death by Poison:
क्षरति विषतेजसाऽसृक् तत् खानि निरुध्य मारयति जन्तुम्| पीतं मृतस्य हृदि तिष्ठति दष्टविद्धयोर्दंशदेशे स्यात्||३२||
Because of the power of the poison, the [vitiated] blood transudes to obstruct the channels of circulation leading to the death. If the poison is taken orally, then it gets lodged in the Hrdaya or heart (stomach according to some scholars), and if the poison is transmitted by bite or puncture (as in case of being stung by a poisoned arrow), it gets lodged in the place of the bite (at the time of the death of the patient). [32]

Visha Marana Linga:
नीलौष्ठ दन्त शैथिल्य केशपतनाङ्गभङ्ग विक्षेपाः| शिशिरैर्न लोमहर्षो नाभिहते दण्डराजी स्यात्||३३||
क्षतजं क्षताच्च नायात्येतानि भवन्ति मरण लिङ्गानि| एभ्योऽन्यथा चिकित्स्यास्तेषां चोपक्रमाञ्छृणु मे||३४||
The signs indicating (imminent) death of a poisoned patient:
• Niloshta – Blueness of the lips
• Dantashaitilya – looseness of the teeth
• Kesha patana – falling of the hair
• Angabhanga – breaking of the limbs
• Vikshepa – Rigor mortis / convulsions?
• Shishirainalomaharsha – Absence of horrification / horripilation even if touched by cold things
• Na abhi hate – non- formation of contusion marks in the body in reaction to blows
• Dandaraji hate – absence of bleeding from ulcers
Listen to their line of treatment as being explained by me (hereafter).

24 VishaUpakrama – Therapeutic Measures:
मन्त्रारिष्टोत्कर्तन निष्पीडन चूषणाग्नि परिषेकाः| अवगाह रक्तमोक्षण वमन विरेकोपधानानि||३५||
हृदयावरणाञ्जन नस्यधूम लेहौषध प्रशमनानि | प्रतिसारणं प्रतिविषं सञ्ज्ञा संस्थानपनं लेपः||३६||
मृतसञ्जीवनमेव च विंशतिरेते चतुर्भिरधिकाः| स्युरुपक्रमा यथा ये यत्र योज्याः शृणु तथा तान्||३७||
24 ways of treating poisoning:
In order to cure the patient afflicted with poison, the 24 therapeutic measures to be adopted are as follows:
1. Mantra recitation
2. Arista (Tying an amulet impregnated with Mantra or tying a bandage above the place of bite)
3. Utkartana (excision of the part afflicted with the poisonous bite).
4. Nispidana (squeezing out blood from the place of the bite)
5. Cusana (sucking out the poison from the place of the bite)
6. Agni (cauterization)
7. Pariseka (bath / shower with medicated water)
8. Avagaha (tub bath with medicated water)
9. RaktaMokshana (bloodletting)
10. Vamana (emesis)
11. Virechana (Purgation)
12. Upadhana (application of medicine after making an incision over the scalp)
13. Hrdayavarana (giving medicines to protect the heart);
14. Anjana (application of collyrium)
15. Nasya (inhalation of medicated oil. Etc)
16. Dhuma (smoking Therapy)

17. Leha (drugs in the form of linctus given for licking)

18. Ausadha (administration of anti- toxic drugs or wearing as an amulet)

19. Prashamana (sedatives)

20. Pratisarana (application of Alkalies)

21. Prativisha (administration of poisons as medicines to counteract the original poison);

22. Sanjna – Samsthapana (administration of medicines for the restoration of consciousness);

23. Lepa (application of medicines in the form of a paste or ointment) and

24. Mruta Sanjivana (measures for the revival of life of an apparently dead person).

Now listen to the details of these therapeutic measures with reference to the mode and place of their application (as described hereafter) [35- 37].

Details of Therapeutic Measures (Arista, Utkartana, Nispidana&Cusana):

दंशात् तु विष दष्टस्याविसृतं वेणिकां भिषग्बद्ध्वा| निष्पीड्येद्भृशं दंशमुद्धरेन्मर्मवर्ज वा||३८||

तं दंशं वा चूषेन्मुखेन यवचूर्ण पांशु पूर्णेन|३९|

Before the spreading of the poison from the place of the bite, the venika (string or rope) is tied (at the proximal part of the bite), the site of the bite is excised unless it is a vital part (marma) and the poison is sucked out with the help of mouth filled with the flour of barely or dust. [38- ½ 39]

Bloodletting therapy Etc:

प्रच्छन शृङ्गजलौका व्यधनैः स्राव्यं ततो रक्तम्||३९||

रक्ते विष प्रदुष्टे दुष्येत् प्रकृतिस्ततस्त्यजेत् प्राणान्| तस्मात् प्रघर्षणैरसृगवर्तमानं प्रवर्त्यं स्यात्||४०||

त्रिकटु गृहधूम रजनी पञ्चलवण रोचनाः सवार्ताकाः| घर्षणमतिप्रवृत्ते वटादिभिः शीतलै लेपः||४१||

रक्तं हि विषाधानं वायुरिवाग्नेः प्रदेह सेकैस्तत्| शीतैः स्कन्दति तस्मिन् स्कन्ने व्यपयाति विषवेगः||४२||

विषवेगान्मद मूर्च्छा विषाद हृदय द्रवाः प्रवर्तन्ते| शीतै निवर्तयेतान् वीज्यश्चा लोमहर्षात् स्यात्||४३||

Thereafter, bloodletting is performed by

• Pracchana (Scratching with the rough- surfaced instruments)

• Srunga (application of horn)

• Jalauka (application of Leeches) or

• Sira Vyadhana (Venesection)

The blood afflicted by poison causes vitiation of other tissue elements in the body leading to death therefore, if the blood does not come out of the site of bite, then Praharsana (rubbing therapy) is employed to cause the blood to flow out. For this purpose, rubbing is done with the help of the powder of

Shunthi – Ginger

Pippali – Long pepper fruit – Piper longum

Maricha – Black pepper fruit – piper nigrum

GrihaDhuma – suit

Rajani (Turmeric) – Curcuma longa

5 types of salt (Saindhava, Samudra, Sauvarcala, Bida and Audbhida) and

Vartaka (seeds)

If there is excess bleeding, then cooling paste of vata, etc is applied externally.

The blood is the vehicle of poison as the wind is of fire. With the help of Pradeha (application of ointment) and Seka (Effusion) which are cooling in effect, the blood etc gets coagulated and so it arrests the virulent spread of the poison.

As a result of the spreading of the poison, the patient suffers from

Mada – intoxication

Murccha – fainting

Vishada – depression and

Hrdaya Drava – Tachycardia

Application of cooling therapies alleviates such complications. The patient is fanned till horrification takes place because of its cooling effect. [½ 39- 43]

Cheda (Excision):

तरुरिव मूलच्छेदाद्दंशच्छेदान्न वृद्धिमेति विषम्| आचूषणमानयनं जलस्य सेतुर्यथा तथाऽरिष्टाः||४४||

त्वङ्मांसगतं दाहो दहति विषं स्रावणं हरति रक्तात्| पीतं वमनैः सद्यो हरेद्विरेकैर्द्वितीये तु||४५||

As a tree stops growing as soon as its root is cut, similarly, the (effect of) poison does not grow or spread (get aggravated) as soon as its site (of bite) is excised. The process of Suction induces the poison mixed with blood to flow out.

Simily: As the flow of water is arrested by a dam, so also the flow and spread of poison is arrested by the tying of Aristas. Cauterization causes burning of the poison located in the skin and the flesh Srvana (drugs used to cause exudation of liquids from the body) helps the flowing out of poison from the blood.

Emesis helps in the instantaneous elimination of poison taken orally. In the second stage of poisoning, purgation therapy helps in its elimination. [44-45]

Hrudayavarana (Protection of Heart)

आदौ हृदयं रक्ष्यं तस्यावरणं पिबेद्यथालाभम्| मधु सर्पि मज्जपयो गैरिकमथ गोमयरसं वा||४६||

इक्षुं सुपक्वमथवा काकं निष्पीड्य तद्रसं वरणम्| छागादीनां वाऽसृग्भस्म मृदं वा पिबेदाशु||४७||

क्षारागदस्तृतीये शोफहरैर्लेखनं समध्वम्बु| गोमय रसश्चतुर्थे वेगे सकपित्थ मधु सर्पिः||४८||

काकाण्ड शिरीषाभ्यां स्वरसेनाश्च्योतनाञ्जने नस्यम्| स्यात्पञ्चमेऽथ षष्ठे सञ्ज्ञायाः स्थापनं कार्यम्||४९||

गोपित्तयुता रजनी मञ्जिष्ठा मरिच पिप्पली पानम्| विषपानं दष्टानां विषपीते दंशनं चान्ते||५०||

In the beginning, the heart of the patient is protected, and whatever is available for the protection of the heart is administered to him. Honey, Ghee, Bone marrow, Milk, red juice squeezed out of the meat of cow is given to him for the protection of the heart. He is given the blood of goat, etc Ashes or mud diluted with water to drink immediately. In the third stage of the spread of the poison, the patient is given Ksharagada (recipe of which will be described in the verses 101- 104) along with honey and water. This recipe removes oedema, and it is lekhana (which scrapes out unwanted waste products from the body).

During the fourth stage of the spread of the poison, the patient should take the juice of cow dung along with the juice of Kapittha (Feronia limonia), Honey and ghee.

During the fifth stage of the spread of poison, the patient is given therapies for the revival of his consciousness. For this purpose, the patient is given to drink the potion prepared of

Rajani (Turmeric) – Curcuma longa

Manjistha – Rubia cordifolia,

Maricha – Black pepper fruit – piper nigrum and

Pippali – Long pepper fruit – Piper longum added with cow's bile. [According to Chakrapani, Rajani (turmeric) added with cow's bile is to be used for Aschyottana etc]

At the end the patient is given a potion containing poison to drink if he is afflicted by the poison caused by bite (Damsa). If he is afflicted by the poison taken orally, then he is made to be bitten by a poisonous animal. [46- 50]

Revival of an apparently dead person:

शिखि पित्तार्धयुतं स्यात् पलाशबीजमगदो मृतेषु वरः| वार्ताकुफाणितागार धूमगोपित्त निम्बं वा||५१||

गोपित्तयुतै गुटिकाः सुरसाग्रन्थिद्विव रजनी मधुक कुष्ठैः | शस्ताऽमृतेन तुल्या शिरीष पुष्पकाकाण्डकरसैर्वा||५२||

काकाण्डसुरस गवाक्षी पुनर्नवा वायसी शिरीष फलैः| उद्बन्ध विष जल मृते लेपौपधि नस्य पानानि ||५३||

If the Patient appears to bleed on account of Poisoning, then he is given the powder of the seed of Palasha – Butea monosperma mixed with 1/2 the quantity of the bile of Peacock.

Alternatively, he may be given Vartaku (Seeds), Phanita (a preparation of Jaggery), Agara Dhuma (Kitchen soot), cow's bile and Nimba – Neem (Azadirachta indica) (in powder form).

The pill made of Surasa (Tulsi), Granthi (Vacha), Haridra (turmeric – Curcuma longa), Daruharidra – Berberis aristata, Madhuka– Licorice and Kushta – Saussurea lappa mixed with cow's bile is useful like Amrta (Ambrosia), and it is given to the patient for his revival.

Alternatively, this pill is prepared of Surasa, granthi, Haridra (turmeric – Curcuma longa), Daru Haridra – Berberis aristata,Madhuka– Licorice – Glycyrrhiza glabra and Kushta – Saussurea lappa by triturating with the juice of the flower of Sirisha and the juice of kakandaka.

If the patient appears to be dead because of hanging (Udbandhana), Poisoning or drowning in water (Jala Mruta), then the potion comprising Kakanda, Surasa, gavaksi, Punarnava – boerhaviadiffusa, Vayasi and Fruits of Sirisha (Albizia lebbeck) is administered in the form of Lepa (ointment) along with Ausadhi (application of the paste over the head after making incisions in the form of Kakapada or the paw of a crow), Nasya (inhalation therapy) and Pana (drink), for his revival [51-53]

Mrita Sanjivana Agada:

स्पृक्का प्लव स्थौणेय काङ्क्षी शैलेय रोचनातगरम्| ध्यामक कुङ्कुम मांसी सुरसाग्रैलाल कुष्ठघ्नम्||५४||

बृहती शिरीष पुष्पं श्रीवेष्टक पद्म चारटि विशालाः| सुरदारु पद्म केशर सावरक मनःशिला कौन्त्यः||५५||

जात्यर्क पुष्प रस रजनी द्वयहिङ्गु पिप्पली लाक्षाः| जल मुद्गपर्णि चन्दन मधुक मदन सिन्धुवाराश्च||५६||

शम्पाक लोध्र मयूरक गन्धफलाना कुली विडङ्गाश्च| पुष्ये संहृत्य समं पिष्ट्वा गुटिका विधेयाः स्युः||५७||

सर्व विषघ्नो जयकृद्विष मृतसञ्जीवनो ज्वरनिहन्ता| घ्रेय विलेपन धारण धूमग्रहणे गृहस्थश्च||५८||

भूतविषजन्त्व लक्ष्मीकार्मणमन्त्राग्न्यशन्यरीन् हन्यात्| दुःस्वप्न स्त्रीदोषानकालमरणाम्बु चौर भयम्||५९||

धन धान्यकार्य सिद्धिः श्रीपुष्ट्यायु विवर्धनो धन्यः| मृत सञ्जीवन एष प्रागमृताद्ब्रह्मणा विहितः||६०||

इति मृतसञ्जीवनोऽगदः|

Taken in equal quantities, these herbs are to be triturated, made to a paste, and pills are made out of this paste:

Sprukka, Plava, Sthauneyaka , Kanksi (Saurastrika), Saileya , Rocana, Tagara Valeriana wallichii

Dhyanaka – Coriandrum sativum

Kunkuma – Crocus sativus

Mamsi – Nardostachys jatamansi

Agara (inflorescence) of Surasa

Ela – Elettaria cardamomum

Ala (Haritala)

Kusthaghna (Khadira (Acacia catechu)

Brihati – Solanum indicum

Flower of Sirisha (Albizia lebbeck .)

Srivestaka –

Padama- Carati,

Vishala,

Suradaru (Cedrus deodara),

Padma – Lotus (Nelumbo nucifera)- Kesara,

Savaraka (a type of Lodhra (Symplocos racemosa),

Manahshila – realgar

Kaunti (Renuka)

Juice of the flowers of Jati – Jasminum grandiflorum and

Arka – Calotropis gigantea,

Haridra (turmeric – Curcuma longa),

Daruharidra – Berberis aristata

Hingu,

Pippali – Piper longum,

Laksha,

Jaa (Haridra),

Mudgaparni – Phaseolus trilobus

Chandana (Sandalwood – Santalum album),

Madhuka– Licorice – Glycyrrhiza glabra,

Madana – Randia dumetorum

Sindhuvara (Vitex negundo),

Sampaka

Lodhra (Symplocos racemosa),

Mayuraka (Apamarga – Achyranthes aspera),

Gandhaphala (Priyangu (Callicara macrophylla),

Nakuli

Rasna (Pluchea lanceolata) and

Vidanga – Embelia ribes are collected in Pushya constellation.

It cures all types of poison, makes a person victorious, revives a person who is apparently dead because of poisoning and cures fever.

If inhaled, applied externally as an ointment, carried in the body as an amulet, smoked or kept in the house, it annihilates the afflictions by evil spirits, poisons, germs, Alaksmi (inauspiciousness), karmana (black Magic), Mantra (incantations recited to inflict injury to others), fire, thunderbolt and enemies.

It counteracts the evil effects of bad dreams and Stri Dosha (poisons secretly given by women) it prevents untimely death, fear of water and fear of thieves.

It endows a person with wealth, food grains and success in all tasks undertaken. It promotes auspiciousness, nourishment and longevity. This excellent recipe is called Mrita Sanjivana (a recipe that helps in the revival of a dead person). Lord Brahma rounded this recipe prior to the discovery of Amrita (ambrosia).

Thus, ends the description of the recipe called Mritsanjivani Agad. [54-60]

Treatment of Poisoning according to Locations:

मन्त्रैर्ध मनीबन्धोऽवमार्जनं कार्यमात्म रक्षा च| दोषस्य विषं यस्य स्थाने स्यात्तं जयेत्पूर्वम्||६१||

वातस्थाने स्वेदो दध्ना नत कुष्ठ कल्कपानं च| घृत मधुपयोऽम्बुपानावगाह सेकाश्च पित्तस्थे||६२||

क्षारागदः कफस्थानगते स्वेदस्तथा सिरा व्यधनम्| दूषी विषेऽथ रक्त स्थिते सिराकर्म पञ्चविधम्||६३||

भेषजमेवं कल्प्यं भिषग्विदाऽऽलक्ष्य सर्वदा सर्वम्| स्थानं जयेदिद्ध पूर्व स्थान स्थस्याविरुद्धं च||६४||

Dhamani Bandha (application of tourniquet)

Avamarjana (causing downward movement of poison) and

AtmaRaksa (protection of the patient from the attacks of evil spirits including microbes) is done with the help of Mantras.

In the beginning, the Dosha in whose place the poison is located is treated.

If the poison is located in the site of

• Vata Dosha – drink the paste of Nata (Valeriana wallicii) and Kushta added with curd.

• Pitta – ghee, honey, milk and water to drink. He should also be given a bath and affusion (with cold water).

• Kapha – Ksaragada (Antidotes of Poisons containing alkalies), fomentation therapy and venesection therapy.

If dushivisha is located in the blood, bloodletting through venesection and panchakarma should be administered. This will help in removing the dushivisha located in the blood. For this one vein should be cut for bloodletting – in 2 veins in the upper limbs (one each in each upper limb), in 2 veins of the lower limbs (one each in each limb) and one in the trunk (middle portion of the body). In this way the physician should skilfully adopt these principles (of treatment) in dealing with all kinds of poisonings and firstly remove the poison. Firstly, the poisons located in specific locations (localized poisons) should be initially dealt with and removed / destroyed. Care also should be taken that the dosha or doshas in that locality (place of the body afflicted by poisons) should not be aggravated or imbalanced / vitiated. [61-64]

Nasya and Anjana Therapies:

विषदूषित कफमार्गः स्रोतःसंरोधरुद्ध वायुस्तु| मृत इव श्वसेन्मर्त्यः स्याद साध्यलिङ्गै विर्हीनश्च||६५||

चर्म कषायाः कल्कं बिल्व समं मूर्धिन काकपदमस्य| कृत्वा दद्यात्कटभी कटुकट्फल प्रधमनं च||६६||

छागं गव्यं माहिषं वा मांसं कौक्कुटमेव वा| दद्यात् काकपदे तस्मिंस्ततः सङ्क्रमते विषम्||६७||

नासाक्षि कर्ण जिह्वा कण्ठ निरोधेषु कर्म नस्तः स्यात्| वार्ताकु बीजपूर ज्योतिष्मत्यादिभिः पिष्टैः||६८||

अञ्जनमक्ष्युपरोधे कर्तव्यं बस्तमूत्रपिष्टैस्तु| दारु व्योष हरिद्रा करवीर करञ्ज निम्ब सुरसैस्तु||६९||

When the channel of circulation of Kapha gets vitiated by poison, then this causes obstruction in the channel because of which the movement of Vata Dosha gets obstructed. As a result of this, the patient breathes as if he is going to die very soon. If he is free from signs and symptoms of incurability, then incisions are made on his scalp resembling the paw of the crow (Kakapada), and 1 Bilva of paste of Carmakasa (Saptala – Ophiorrhiza mungos – Mongoose plant) is applied over it he may also be given pradhamana (a type of inhalation therapy in which the recipe in powder from is blown into the nostrils) with Katabhi, Trikatu (Sunthi – Zingiber officinale, pippali – Piper longum and Maricha – Black pepper fruit – piper nigrum) and Kathala. Over the Kaka-Pada (incisions in the scalp), the meat of goat, cow, buffalo or cock is applied which will absorb the poison from the body.

If there is obstruction to the nose, eyes (vision), ears, tongue and throat, then the patient is given Nasya (inhalation therapy) with the help of the paste of Vartaku, Beejapoora – Citrus medica, Jyotismati – Celastruspaniculatus, etc

If there is obstruction to the eyes (vision), then the collyrium prepared of Devadaru – Cedrus deodara, Sunthi – Zingiber officinale, Pippali – Long pepper fruit – Piper longum, Maricha – Black pepper fruit – piper nigrum, Haridra (turmeric – Curcuma longa), Karavira – Nerium indicum, Karanja (Pongamia pinnata), Nimba – Neem (Azadirachta indica) and Surasa by Triturating with goat's urine is applied over the eyes.[65- 69]

GandhaHasti Agada:

श्वेता वचाऽश्वगन्धा हिङ्गमृता कुष्ठ सैन्धवे लशुनम्| सर्षप कपित्थ मध्यं टुण्टुक करञ्जबीजानि ||७०||

व्योष शिरीष पुष्पं द्विरजन्यौ वंशलोचनं च समम्| पिष्ट्वाऽजस्य मूत्रेण गोश्व पितेन सप्ताहम्||७१||

व्यत्यासभावितोऽयं निहन्ति शिरसि स्थितं विष क्षिप्रम्| सर्व ज्वर भूतग्रह विसूचिकाजीर्ण मूच्छार्तीः||७२||

उन्मादापस्मारौ काच पटल नीलिका शिरो दोषान्| शुष्काक्षिपाक पिल्लार्बुदार्म कण्डू तमो दोषान्||७३||

क्षय दौर्बल्य मदात्यय पाण्डु गदांश्चाञ्जनात्तथा मोहान्| लेपादिविषदिग्ध क्षत लीढ दष्टपीत विषघाती||७४||

अर्शःस्वानद्दधेषु च गुदलेपो योनिलेपनं स्त्रीणाम्| मूढे गर्भे दुष्टे ललाटलेपः प्रतिश्याये||७५||

वृद्धौ किटिमे कुष्ठे श्वित्र विचर्चिकादिषु लेपः| गज इव तरून् विष गदान्निहन्त्यगदगन्धहस्त्येषः||७६||

इति गन्ध हस्ती नामाऽगदः|

GandhaHasti Agada:

Sveta Katabhi – Clitoria ternatea), Vacha – Acorus calamus, Ashwagandha – Winter Cherry / Indian ginseng (root), Hingu, Amrta, Kushta – Saussurea lappa, Saindhava, Lasuna – Garlic, Sarsapa – Brassica campestris, Pulp of Kapittha (Feronia limonia), Tuntuka, seeds of Haridra (turmeric – Curcuma longa) and Vamsalocana is taken in equal quantities, and impregnated as well as triturated with goat's urine, cow's bile and horse bile alternatively for 7 days each. Its application as a collyrium instantaneously cures the poison located in the head.

This collyrium also cures all types of fever, afflictions by evil spirits and Graha (supernatural bodies), Apasmara (epilepsy), different eye- diseases like Kaca, patala and Nilika, diseases of the head, other eye-diseases like Suskaksipaka, Pilla, Arbuda, Arma, Kandu and Tamas, Ksaya (consumption), Asthenia, alcoholism, anaemia and unconsciousness.

External application of this recipe cures ulcers caused by a poisonous arrow, ailments caused by poisons transmitted through licking and bite or by poisons taken orally.

To cure swollen piles, its paste is applied over the anus. If there is obstructed labour or if the foetus is dead, its paste is applied in the vagina of women to cure coryza, its paste is applied over the forehead.

Application of its paste cures:

Vruddhi (enlargement of scrotum),

Kitibha (a type of skin) disease,

Kushta (skin diseases),

Shvitra (leucoderma),

Vicharchika (Eczema) etc

This recipe which is an antidote of poisons is called Gandhahasti.

Simile given: As trees are destroyed by an elephant, so also all the ailments caused by poisoning are cured by this recipe.

Thus ends the descriptions of the recipe called GandhaHasti. [70- 76]

MahaGandhaHasti Agada:

पत्रागुरुमुस्तैला निर्यासाः पञ्च चन्दनं स्पृक्का| त्वइनलदोत्पल बालक हरेणुकोशीर वन्य नखाः||७७||

सुरदारु कनक कुङ्कुमध्यामक कुष्ठ प्रियङ्गवस्तगरम्| पञ्चाङ्गानि शिरीषाद्व्योषालमनःशिलाजाज्यः||७८||

श्वेत कटभी करञ्जौ रक्षोघ्नी सिन्धु वारिका रजनी| सुरसाञ्जन गैरिक मञ्जिष्ठा निम्ब निर्यासाः||७९||

वंशत्वगश्वगन्धा हिङ्गु दधित्थाम्लवेतसं लाक्षा| मधु मधुक सोमराजी वचारुहारोचना तगरम्||८०||

अगदोऽयं वैश्रवणायाख्यातस्त्रयम्बकेण षष्ट्यङ्गः| अप्रतिहत प्रभावः ख्यातो महागन्धहस्तीति||८१||

पित्तेन गवां पेष्यो गुटिकाः कार्यास्तु पुष्ययोगेन| पानाञ्जन प्रलेपैः प्रसाधयेत् सर्व कर्माणि||८२||

पिल्लं कण्डूं तिमिरं रात्र्यान्ध्यं काचमर्बुदं पटलम्| हन्ति सतत प्रयोगादिधतमितपथ्याशिनां पुंसाम्||८३||

विषमज्वरानजीर्णान्दद्रुं कण्डूं विसूचिकां पामाम्| विष मूषिकलूतानां सर्वेषां पन्नगानां च|

आशु विषं नाशयति समूलजमथ कन्दजं सर्वम्||८४||

एतेन लिप्तगात्रः सर्पान् गृह्णाति भक्षयेच्च विषम्| कालपरीतोऽपि नरो जीवति नित्यं निरातङ्कः||८५||

आनद्धे गुदलेपो योनौ लेपश्च मूढगर्भाणाम्| मूर्छार्तिषु च ललाटे प्रलेपनमाहुः प्रधानतमम्||८६||

भेरी मृदङ्ग पटहाञ्छत्राण्यमुना तथा ध्वजपताकाः| लिप्त्वाऽहि विषनिरस्त्यै प्रध्वनयेद्दर्शयेन्मतिमान्||८७||

यत्र च सन्निहितोऽयं न तत्र बालग्रहा न रक्षांसि| न च कार्मणवेताला वहन्ति नाथर्वणा मन्त्राः||८८||

सर्वग्रहा न तत्र प्रभवन्ति न चाग्निशस्त्रनृपचौराः| लक्ष्मीश्च तत्र भजते यत्र महागन्धहस्त्यस्ति||८९||

पिष्यमाण इमं चात्र सिद्धं मन्त्रमुदीरयेत्| 'मम माता जया नाम जयो नामेति मे पिता||९०||

सोऽहं जय जयापुत्रो विजयोऽथ जयामि च| नमः पुरुषसिंहाय विष्णवे विश्वकर्मणे||९१||

सनातनाय कृष्णाय भवाय विभवाय च| तेजो वृषाकपेः साक्षात्तेजो ब्रह्मेन्द्रयोर्यमे||९२||

यथाऽहं नाभिजानामि वासुदेवपराजयम्| मातुश्च पाणि ग्रहणं समुद्रस्य च शोषणम्||९३||

अनेन सत्यवाक्येन सिध्यतामगदो ह्ययम्| हिलिमिलि संस्पृष्टे रक्ष सर्व भेषजोत्तमे स्वाहा ||९४||'

इति महागन्धहस्तीनामाऽगदः|

The recipe called MahaGandhahasti comprises 60 ingredients viz

Patra – Cinnamomum tamala

Musta (Cyperus rotundus), Ela (Elettaria cardamomum Maton)

5 types of exudates

Chandana (Sandalwood – Santalum album) Sprka , Tvak – Cinnamonum zeylanica,Nalada, Utapala , Balaka, Harenuka

Ushira – Vetiver – Vetiveria zizanioides

Vanya-Nakha (Sen's edition reads Vayahra-Nakha)

Deva daru – Cedrus deodara

Kanaka – Datura metel

Kunkuma – Crocus sativus

Dhyanaka – Coriandrum sativum

Kustha –Sausserea lappa

Priyangu - Callicara macrophylla

Tagara – Valeriana wallichii

(26-30) 5 parts of Sirisha (Albizia lebbeck .) (Viz flower, fruit, leaf, root and bark)

Sunthi – Zingiber officinale

Pippali – Piper longum

Maricha – Black pepper fruit – piper nigrum

Haritala

Manashila

Ajaji – Cuminum cyminum

Sveta (white variety of aparajita) – Clitoria ternatea

Katabhi

Karanja – Pongamia pinnata

Lata Karanja

Raksoghni – Acorus calamus

Sindhu- varika

Rajani (turmeric) – Curcuma longa

Surasa – Cinnamonum zeylanica

Anjana, Gairika

Manjistha – Rubia cordifolia

Resin of nimba – Azadirachta indica

Vamsatvak

Ashwagandha – Winter Cherry / Indian ginseng (root) – Withania somnifera

Hingu – Asa foetida

Dadhittha

Amlavetasa – Garcinia pedunculata

Laksa

Madhu

Madhuka – Madhuca longifolia

Somaraji – Psoralea corylifolia

Vacha – Acorus calamus

Ruha and

Rochana

Tagara

This recipe having infallible effect was taught to Varisravana or Kubera (the celestial treasurer) by lord Tryambaka (Siva). During Pushya constellation, these ingredients are to be ground by adding cow's bile, and pills are made out of this paste.

This recipe can be taken internally in the form of a drink (by diluting with liquids) or applied in the form of a collyrium in the eyes or applied externally in the form of a paste to achieve success in all therapeutics.

If used constantly (regularly) along with a wholesome diet of useful ingredients in appropriate quantities.

It cures eye diseases like Pilla, Kandi, Timira, Ratryandha, Kaca, Arbuda, and Patala. It cures

Vishama Jvara (irregular fever),

Avipaka – indigestion,

Dadru (ringworm),

Kandu (Pruritus),

Atisara – chronic diarrhoea and

Pama (scabies)

It instantaneously cures the ailments caused by the poisons of rats, spiders, all types of snakes, and poisons from all types of roots and rhizomes.

A person having smeared his body with the Paste of this poison can catch a (Poisonous) snake and drink its venom with the help of this recipe. A person facing death also would regain life and live till the end of his span of life, free from any disease.

In anaha (constipation or obstruction in rectum), the paste of this recipe is applied over the anus. In Mudha Garbha (obstructed labour), this paste is applied over the vagina. Application of its paste over the forehead of a patient with poisonous fainting brings about quick results.

For curing ailments caused by poisoning, a wise physician should smear musical instruments like Bheri, Mrdanga and Pataha with the paste of this recipe and make sounds with them. He should also smear this paste over the umbrellas, banners and flags, and exhibit them before the patient suffering from poisoning.

The ace where this recipe is kept becomes absolutely inaccessible to Bala Grahas (celestial bodies afflicting children), Rakshas (evil creatures), karmana (black magic of enemies), Vetala (hobgoblins) and Atharvana Mantras (Spells of evil charms).

The person with this recipe cannot be adversely affected by any of the lantes (positioned in the antagonistic houses of the zodiac sign), fire, weapons, kings (with evil motives) and thieves.

The place where this recipes called MahaGandhaHasti is kept becomes the abode of Lakshmi (Goddess of wealth)

While triturating the ingredients of this recipe, the following Mantra should be recited:

"mama mātā jayā nāma jayo nāmeti me pitā||90||

so'haṃ jaya jayāputro vijayo'tha jayāmi ca| namaḥ puruṣasiṃhāya viṣṇave viśvakarmaṇe||91||

sanātanāya kṛṣṇāya bhavāya vibhavāya ca| tejo vṛṣākapeḥ sākṣāttejo brahmendrayoryame||92||

yathā'haṃ nābhijānāmi vāsudevaparājayam| mātuśca pāṇi grahaṇaṃ samudrasya ca śoṣaṇam||93||

anena satyavākyena sidhyatāmagado hyayam| hilimili saṃspṛṣṭe rakṣa sarva bheṣajottame svāhā ||94||"

The name of my mother is Jaya, and that of my father is Jaya. Since I am the son of jaya and jaya, I am called Vijaya, and I shall become victorious. I offer prayers to Narasimha, Vishnu who is VisvaKarma (the builder of the universe), Sanatana (eternal), Krsna, Bhava (one who endows auspiciousness) and Vidhava (one who endows wealth). I am the glory of VrushaKay (agni) and I am the direct glory of Brahma, Indra and Yama. I never knew the defeat of Vasudeva, or the marriage of my mother or the drying of the ocean by these statements of truth, let this recipe of antidote achieve its success. Hilimili is the Beeja mantra (seed) of this incantation, and its association may protect this recipe which is the best among the remedies. "

Thus, ends the description of the recipe called MahaGandhaHastiAgad. [77- 94]

Treatment of Complications Caused by poisoning:

ऋषभक जीवक भार्गी मधुकोत्पल धान्य केशराजाज्यः| ससित गिरि कोल मध्याः पेयाः श्वास ज्वरादिहराः||९५||

हिङ्गु च कृष्णायुक्तं कपित्थ रस युक्तमग्र्य लवणं च| समधुसितौ पातव्यौ ज्वर हिक्का श्वास कासघ्नौ||९६||

लेहः कोलास्थ्यञ्जन लाजोत्पल मधु घृतै र्वम्याम्| बृहतीद्वयाढकी पत्रधूम वर्तिस्तु हिक्काघ्नी||९७||

शिखि बर्हि बलाकास्थीनि सर्षपाश्चन्दनं च घृतयुक्तम्| धूमो गृहशय नासन वस्त्रादिषु शस्यते विषनुत्||९८||

घृतयुक्ते नतकुष्ठे भुजगपतिशिरः शिरीष पुष्पं च| धूमागदः स्मृतोऽयं सर्व विषघ्नः श्वयथुहृच्च||९९||

जतुसेव्यपत्र गुग्गुलु भल्लातक ककुभपुष्प सर्जरसाः| श्वेता च धूम उरगाखुकीटवस्त्रक्रिमिनुदग्र्यः||१००||

Treatment for breathing difficulty and fever caused due to poisoning:

Intake of Rishabhaka – Manilkara hexandra, Jivaka – Malaxis acuminata, Bharngi, Madhuka– Licorice, Utpala (Nymphaea alba), Dhanya – Coriandrum sativum, Kesara, Ajaji, Sitagiri (Sveta-Aaparajita) and the pulp of kola in the form of a drink cures Svasa (dyspnoea), fever, etc, caused by poisoning.

Treatment for hiccup caused by poisoning:

Intake of Hingu – Asafoetida and Krsna along with honey and sugar, or the juice of Kapittha (Feronia limonia) and Saindhava along with honey and sugar cures fever, hiccup, dyspnoea and cough caused by poisoning.

Intake of the seed-pulp of Kola, Anjana, Laja, Utpala (Nymphaea alba) Honey and ghee in the form of a linctus cures hiccups caused by poisoning.

Treatment for Edema:

DhumaVarti (inhalation of the fume an incense stick) of Brihati – Solanum indicum, Kantakari – Solanum xanthocarpum and Leaves of Adhaki—Cajanus cajan cures hiccup caused by poisoning

The fumigation with Nata i, Kushta – Saussurea lappa, head of Bhujagaati (snake having two heads or fangs) and flower of Sirisha (Albizia lebbeck .) by adding ghee is called 'Dhumagada', and it cures all types of poison and oedema. The fumigation with Jatu (Shilajatu), Sevya, Patra – Cinnamomum tamalaNees and Eberum., Guggulu (Commiphora mukul Engl.), Bhallataka (Semecarpus anacardium Linn.), flower of Kakubha, Sarja (Vateria indica)-Rasa and Sveta is an excellent remedy for curing poisoning by snake and rat bite it also helps in destroying the insects (counteracting their poison) and Vastra- Krimi (Yuka or lice). [95-100]

Ksharagada:

तरुण पलाश क्षारं सुतं पचेच्चूर्णितैः सह समांशैः| लोहित मृद्रजनी द्वय शुक्ल सुरसमञ्जरी मधुकैः||१०१||

लाक्षा सैन्धव मांसी हरेणु हिङ्गु द्विव सारिवा कुष्ठैः| सव्योषै बाह्लीकैर्दर्वीविलेपनं घट्टयेद्यावत्||१०२||

सर्व विष शोथ गुल्मत्वग्दोषार्शोभगन्दर प्लीह्नः| शोथापस्मार क्रिमि भूत स्वरभेद पाण्डु गदान्||१०३||

मन्दाग्नित्वं कासं सोन्मादं नाशयेयुरथ पुंसाम्| गुटिकाश्छाया शुष्काः कोल समास्ताः समुपयुक्ताः||१०४||

इति क्षारागदः|

Kshara derived by decanting the ashes of a tender tree of palasha – Butea monosperma is added with equal quantities of

• Lohitamrit (Gairika),
• Haridra (turmeric – Curcuma longa),
• Daru Haridra – Berberis aristata,
• Manjari (inflorecense) of the white variety of Surasa,
• Madhuka– Licorice – Glycyrrhiza glabra,
• Laksha,
• Saindhava – rock salt
• JataMamsi – Nardostachys jatamansi ,
• Harenu
• Hingu – Asa foetida,
• Sariva – Indian Sarsaparilla – Hemidesmus indicus,
• Ananta Mula
• Kushta – Saussurea lappa
• Sunthi – Zingiber officinale,
• Pippali – Long pepper fruit – Piper longum,
• Maricha – Black pepper fruit – piper nigrum and
• Bahlika (Kunkuma kesara).

This recipe is made out of this paste and dried in shade.

Intake of this cures:

• Sarvavisha shotha – inflammation caused by all types of poisoning
• Gulma – phantom tumour
• Tvak dosha – skin diseases
• Arsha – piles
• Bhagandara – Fistula- in- ano
• Pleeha – splenic disorders
• Shotha – oedema
• Apasmara – epilepsy
• Krimiroga – parasitic infestation
• Bhutaroga – affliction by evil spirits
• Svarabheda – hoarseness of voice
• Pandu – anaemia
• Manda agni – suppression of the power of digestion

• Kasa – cough and

• Unmada – insanity

Thus ends, the description of Ksharagad [101- 104]

Precautions for the King:

विष पीतदष्ट विद्धैष्वेतदि्दिग्धे च वाच्यमुद्दिष्टम्| सामान्यतः, पृथक्त्वान्निर्देशमतः शृणु यथावत्||१०५||

रिपु युक्तेभ्यो नृभ्यः स्वेभ्यः स्त्रीभ्योऽथवा भयं नृपते| आहार विहार गतं तस्मात् प्रेष्यान् परीक्षेत||१०६||

The Statements made in brief above pertain to the treatment of ailments caused by the poisons taken orally, transmitted through bites and stings, and applied externally in general. Now, the same will be separately elaborated. The king is exposed to danger of being poisoned through food and regimens by the attendants secretly employed in his palace by another king having enmity, and also form his own wives. Therefore, the residues are carefully examined. [105- 106]

Signs of a Poison- Giver:

अत्यर्थ शङ्कितः स्याद्बहुवागथवाऽल्पवाग्विगत लक्ष्मीः| प्राप्तः प्रकृति विकारं विष प्रदाता नरो ज्ञेयः||१०७||

A person who behaves in an extremely suspicious manner, who speaks too much or who speaks very little, who has lost luster of his face and who exhibits changes in his characteristic features is a poison giver. [107]

Visha Ahara Pareeksha:

दृष्ट्वैवं न तु सहसा भोज्यं कुर्यातदन्नमग्नौ तु| सविष हि प्राप्यान्नं बहून्विकारान् भजत्यग्निः||१०८||

शिखि बर्हिव चित्रार्चिस्तीक्ष्णाक्षम रूक्ष कुणप धूमश्च | स्फुटति च सशब्दमेकावर्तो विहतार्चिरपि च स्यात्||१०९||

पात्रस्थं च विवर्ण भोज्यं स्यान्मक्षिकांश्च मारयति| क्षामस्वरांश्च काकान् कुर्यादिवरजेच्चकोराक्षि||११०||

पाने नीला राजी वैवर्ण्य स्वां च नेक्षते छायाम्| पश्यति विकृतामथवा लवणाक्ते फेनमाला स्यात्||१११||

Examination of poisoned food:

When a person exhibiting the characteristic features of a poison- giver is located then the food etc served by him should not be taken immediately, but a part of it is thrown over fire.

If the food is poisoned, then the flame of the fire exhibits abnormal characteristics like different colours of peacock feather.

The smoke which comes out of such a fire is sharp, intolerable and dry. The smoke smells like a corpse. The flame makes a cracking noise, it moves spirally or it gets extinguished.

The poisoned food when kept in a pot gets discoloured, and flies sitting on it succumb to death. When this poisoned food is seen by crows, their voice becomes feeble, and when the chakora bird sees it, its eyes become discoloured.

If the poison is added to drinks like alcohol, then blue lines appear over its surface or it becomes discoloured.

A person's own shadow is not reflected through such drinks or the shadow is reflected in a distorted manner. If such drinks are added with salt, then there is effervescence. [108- 111]

Other Characteristics of Poisoned food, Drinks etc

पानान्नयोःसविष योगर्गन्धेन शिरोरुग्घृदि च मूर्च्छा च| स्पर्शन पाणि शोथः सुप्त्यङ्गुलि दाह तोद नख भेदाः||११२||

मुखगे त्वोष्ठ चिमिचिमा जिह्वा शूना जडा विवर्णा च| द्विज हर्ष हनुस्तम्भास्य दाह लालागल विकाराः||११३||

आमाशयं प्रविष्टे वैवर्ण्य स्वेद सदनमुत्क्लेदः| दृष्टि हृदयोपरोधो बिन्दु शतैश्चीयते चाङ्गम्||११४||

पक्वाशयं तु याते मूर्च्छामद मोह दाह बल नाशाः| तन्द्रा कार्श्य च विषे पाण्डुत्वं चोदरस्थे स्यात्||११५||

दन्त पवनस्य कूर्चा विशीर्यते दन्तौष्ठ मांस शोफश्च| केशच्युतिः शिरोरुग्ग्रन्थयश्चसविषेऽथ शिरोभ्यङ्गे||११६||

दुष्टेऽञ्जनेऽक्षि दाह स्रावात्युपदेह शोथ रागाश्च| खाद्यैरादौ कोष्ठः स्पृश्यैस्त्वग्दूष्यते दुष्टैः||११७||

स्नानाभ्यङ्गोत्सादन वस्त्रालङ्कारवर्णकैर्दुष्टैः| कण्डवर्ति कोठ पिडकारोमोद्गम चिमिचिमा शोथाः||११८||

एते कर चरण दाह तोद क्लमाविपाकाश्च| भूपादुकाश्वगजवर्मकेतुशयनासनैर्दुष्टैः||११९||

माल्यमगन्धं म्लायति शिरोरुजा लोमहर्ष करम्| स्तम्भयति खानि नासामुपहन्ति दर्शनं च धूमः||१२०||

कूप तडागादिजलं दुर्गन्धं सकलुषं विवर्णं च| पीतं श्वयथुं कोठान् पिडकाश्च करोति मरणं च||१२१||

आदावामाशयगे वमनं त्वक्स्थे प्रदेह सेकादि| कुर्याद्भिषक् चिकित्सां दोषबलं चैव हि समीक्ष्य||१२२||

इति मूलविष विशेषाः प्रोक्ताः ...|१२३|

Other Characteristics of Poisoned food, Drinks etc

The smell of poisoned food and drinks causes

• Shiro ruk (headache)

• Hrudiruk (pain in the cardiac region) and

• Murcha (fainting)

If touched, such poisoned food and drinks cause

• Shotha – oedema and

• Suptaanguli – numbness in the hands,

• Daha – burning sensation and

• Toda nakha – pinching pain in the fingers, and

• Nakhabheda – cracking of the nails

When put into mouth, these poisoned food and drinks cause

• Ostachimchima – tingling sensation in lips

• Jada – swelling, stiffness

• Shuna – numbness and

• Osthavivarna – discoloration of the tongue

• Dvijaharsha – tingling sensation in the teeth

• Hanustambha – stiffness of the jaw bones (mandibular joints)

• Aasyadaha – burning sensation in the face

• Lala – salivation and

• Gala vikara- morbidity in the throat

If the poisoned food and drinks have entered into the stomach, then the patient suffers from:

• Vaivarnya – discoloration

• Sweda – sweating

• Sadana – Asthenia

• Utkleda – Nausea

• Drshtiuparodha – impairment of the vision

• Hrdayauparodha – arrest of cardiac functions and

• Bindu shatachiyateangam – appearance of drop like impels all over the limbs

If the poisoned food and drinks enter into the colon, then the patient suffers from

• Murccha -fainting

• Mada – intoxication

• Moha – unconsciousness

• Daha – burning sensation

• Balanasha – weakness

• Tandra – drowsiness and

• Karshya – emaciation

The patient suffers from Pandu (anaemia) when the poisoned food and drinks get localized in the abdomen. If the tooth brushing twig is poisoned, when the brush–like tip of it gets withered, and the patient suffers from oedema of the teeth, lips and muscles of the mouth.

If the oil for application over the head is poisoned, then the patient suffers from hair fall, headache and tumours in the head.

If the collyrium is poisoned, then the patient suffers from burning sensation, excess lacrimation and excess production of sticky material, oedema and redness of the eyes.

Intake of poisoned food vitiates the Kostha (gastrointestinal tract) and external application of poisoned material afflicts the skin in the beginning.

If the materials for the bath, massage, unction, clothing, ornaments and Varnaka (cosmetics) are poisoned, then the patient suffers from pruritis, pain, urticaria, pimples, horripilation, tingling sensation and oedema.

Burning sensation and pricking pain in the hands and feet, fatigue and indigestion are caused by the poisoning of the earth (where one moves), shoes, horse, elephant, weapons, flags, bed and seat.

A poisoned garland loses its aroma and gets withered soon. It causes headache and horrification. The poisoned fume causes stiffness in the channels of circulation and impairment of the functioning of the nose and eyes.

If the water of wells and ponds are poisoned, then the water becomes foul-smelling, dirty and discoloured. Intake of this poisoned water causes:

• Shotha – oedema

• Urticaria and

• Pimples and

• Even death

If the poison has reached the stomach, then the physician in the beginning should be administered with emetic therapy. If the poisonous material is located in the skin, then ointments and fomentation therapy, etc is administered. These therapeutic measures are administered, keeping in view the nature of the Doshas and the strength of the patient. Thus, the specific nature of the root poisons is explained. [112- 123½]

Jangama Visha – Animal Poisons:

... शृणु जङ्गमस्यातः|

सविशेष चिकित्सितमेवादौ तत्रोच्यते तु सर्पाणाम्||१२३||

इह दर्वीकरः सर्पा मण्डली राजिमानिति| त्रयो यथाक्रमं वात पित्त श्लेष्म प्रकोपणाः||१२४||

दर्वीकरः फणी ज्ञेयो मण्डली मण्डलाफणः| बिन्दुलेख विचित्राङ्गः पन्नगः स्यातु राजिमान्||१२५||

विशेषादूक्ष कटुकमम्लोष्णं स्वादु शीतलम्| विषं यथाक्रमं तेषां तस्माद्वातादिकोपनम्||१२६||

दर्वीकरकृतो दंशः सूक्ष्मदंष्ट्रापदोऽसितः| निरुद्धरक्तः कूर्माभो वातव्याधिकरो मतः||१२७||

पृथ्वर्पितः सशोथश्च दंशो मण्डलिना कृतः| पीताभः पीतरक्तश्च सर्वपित्त विकारकृत्||१२८||

कृतो राजिमता दंशः पिच्छिलः स्थिर शोफकृत्| स्निग्धः पाण्डुश्च सान्द्रासृक् श्लेष्मव्याधि समीरणः||१२९||

JangamaVisha – Animal Poisons:

Snake poisoning:

Now hear about the exposition of animal poisons. In the beginning, the snakes and the special treatment for snakebite will be explained.

Snakes are classified into 3 categories, viz.,

• Darvikara has a spoon like hood and its poison is dry and pungent because of which it causes Vayu aggravation

• Mandali has a rounded hood and its poison is sour and hot because of which it causes Pitta aggravation

• Rajiman has its body of varieties of colour with drop like spots on it and its poison is sweet and cold because of which it causes Kapha aggravation

The bite by the Darvikara snake is characterized by subtle black marks of the teeth (fangs), absence of bleeding, swelling, having the shape of a tortoise and manifestation of diseases caused by Vata.

Bite by Mandali snake is characterized by gross and deep marks of teeth (fangs), oedema, yellowishness of the place of bite, yellow coloration of the exuding blood and manifestation of diseases caused by pitta.

Bite by Rajiman snake is characterized by sliminess, stable oedema, unctuousness, Paleness, thickness of the exuding blood and manifestation of diseases caused by Kapha [123 ¾ – 129]

Identification of sex and Breed of biting Snake:

वृत्तभोगो महाकायः श्वसन्नूर्ध्वेक्षणः पुमान्| स्थूलमूर्धा समाङ्गश्च स्त्री त्वतः स्यादिवपर्ययात्||१३०||

क्लीबस्त्रसत्यधोदृष्टिः स्वरहीनः प्रकम्पते| स्त्रिया दष्टो विपर्यस्तैरेतैः पुंसा नरो मतः||१३१||

व्यामिश्रलिङ्गैरेतैस्तु क्लीबदष्टं नरं वदेत्| इत्येतदुक्तं सर्पाणां स्त्रीपुङ्क्लीब निदर्शनम्||१३२||

पाण्डु वक्त्रस्तु गर्भिण्या शूनौष्ठोऽप्यसितेक्षणः| जृम्भा क्रोधोपजिह्वार्तः सूतया रक्तमूत्रवान्||१३३||

सर्पो गौधेर(य)को नाम गोधायां स्याच्चतुष्पदः| कृष्णसर्पेण तुल्यः स्यान्नाना स्युर्मिश्रजातयः||१३४||

गूढसम्पादितं वृत्तं पीडितं लम्बितार्पितम्| सर्पितं च भृशाबाधं, दंशा येऽन्ये न ते भृशाः||१३५||

The male snake is characterized by a round hood, big body, hissing sound, and upward look, grossness of the head and evenness of the body.

The female snake has opposite characteristic features.

The Napumsaka (impotent) snake is timid in nature.

Patient bitten by a female snake looks downwards, he becomes voiceless and he trebles. Bite by a male snake produces opposite symptoms. If a person is bitten by a Napumsaka (impotent) snake, then the symptoms of both of these (bite by male and female snakes) in a combined form are manifested.

In a person bitten by a pregnant snake, the face becomes pale; the lips get swollen and the eyes become black. A person suffers from yawning, anger, inflammation of the epiglottis (Upajihva) and hematuria

Godheryaka is a hybrid offspring of male snake and female Godha (Iguana), and is quadrupled. Its bite produces signs and symptoms like those of a black snake (Krishna Sarpa). There are several other types of hybrid snakes.

If the mark of bite is very deep, if the lace of bite is circularly elevated, if it is painful, if it is elongated and if it is with all the teeth marks, and if it is of spreading nature, then the condition is serious. Other types of bite are not so serious. [130 -135]

Virulence of poison on the Basis of Age of Snakes:

तरुणाः कृष्णसर्पास्तु गोनसाः स्थविरास्तथा| राजिमन्तो वयोमध्ये भवन्त्याशीविषोपमाः||१३६||

The poison of black snakes when they are young, of the Gonasas when they are old, and of the rajiman types of snakes when they are of middle age, is highly virulent like that of Asivisha (snakes whose poison is transmitted through their very sight and breath resulting in instant (death).

Color of Fangs and Quantity of Poison:

सर्पदंष्ट्राश्चतस्रस्तु तासां वामाधरा सिता| पीता वामोत्तरा दंष्ट्रा रक्तश्यावाऽधरोत्तरा ||१३७||

यन्मात्रः पतते बिन्दुर्गोबालात् सलिलोद्धृतात्| वामाधरायां दंष्ट्रायां तन्मात्रं स्यादहेर्विषम्||१३८||

एकद्वित्रिचतुर्वृद्धविषभागोत्तरोत्तराः| सवर्णास्तत्कृता दंशा बहुतरविषा भृशाः||१३९||

Snakes have 4 fangs. Of these the lower left one is white in colour, the upper left one is yellow in colour, the lower right one is red in colour, and the upper right one is brownish in colour.

The quantity of poison contained in the lower left fang is equal to the number of drops which fall from the hair of the tail of a cow when it is dipped in water and then flirted up. The poison contained in the upper left, lower right and upper right fangs is respectively double, 3 times and 4 times of the poison contained in the power left fang. The colours of the sites of the bite are the same as the colour of the fang through which the person is bitten.

The poisons coming out of these fangs viz, lower left, upper left and upper right are progressively more and more virulent, and more and more incurable. [137- 139]

Insect Poison:

सर्पाणामेव विण्मूत्रात् कीटाः स्युः कीट सम्मताः| दूषी विषाः प्राणहरा इति सङ्क्षेपतो मताः||१४०||

गात्रं रक्तं सितं कृष्णं श्यावं वा पिडकान्वितम्| सकण्डू दाह वीसर्पपाकि स्यात् कुथितं तथा||१४१||

कीटे दूषी विषैर्दष्टं लिङ्गं प्राणहरं शृणु| सर्पदष्टे यथा शोथो वर्धते सोग्रगन्ध्यसृक्||१४२||

दंशोऽक्षि गौरवं मूर्च्छा स रुगार्तः श्वसित्यपि| तृष्णारुचि परीतश्च भवेद्दूषी विषार्दितः||१४३||

Keeta (insects) are so called because they are procreated from the Kit or waste products like stool and urine of the snakes.

In brief, these are of 2 types viz,

• Dushivisha (those causing chronic poisoning) and

• Prana Hara (those causing death).

The insects belonging to Dushivisha (causing chronic poisoning) category cause red, white, black or brownish black coloration over the body part which is bitten, and the area becomes covered with pimples / boils. The patient suffer from

• Kandu – itching
• Daha – burning sensation
• Visarpa – erysipelas
• Apaki – suppuration and
• Kuthitam – sloughing

The insect bite of pranahara (causing death) category produces expanding oedema, as it happens in snake bite, associated with strong smell and bleeding. The patient suffers from heaviness of the eyes, fainting, pain and dyspnoea.

The patient afflicted with Dushivisha (bite of insects causing chronic poisoning) suffers from morbid thirst and anorexia in excess [140-143]

Spider poison – LuthaVisha:

दंशस्य मध्ये यत् कृष्णं श्यावं वा जालकावृतम्| दग्धाकृति भृशं पाकि क्लेद शोथ ज्वरान्वितम्||१४४||

दूषीविषाभिर्लूताभिस्तं दष्टमिति निर्दिशेत्| सर्वासामेव तासां च दंशे लक्षणमुच्यते||१४५||

शोफः श्वेतासिता रक्ताः पीता वा पिडका ज्वरः| प्राणान्तिको भवेच्छवासो दाह हिक्का शिरोग्रहाः||१४६||

Spider poison – LuthaVisha:

If the center of the bite-place is blackish brown, surrounded by a network, if the area appears as if burnt, if it gets suppurated quickly, if it is associated with slough and oedema and if the patient has fever, then it is to be diagnosed as spider bite of Dushi- visha (slow poisoning) type.

General symptoms of spider bite:

• Shopha – oedema,
• Sveta asitarakta pita pidaka – pimples / eruptions of white, black, red or yellow colour,
• Shvasa – terminal dyspnoea,
• Daha – burning sensation,
• Hikka – hiccup and
• Shiro graha – stiffness of the head [144- 146]

Rat Poison – AkhuVisha:

आदंशाच्छोणितं पाण्डु मण्डलानि ज्वरोऽरुचिः| लोमहर्षश्च दाहश्चाप्याखु दूषी विषार्दिते||१४७||

मूर्च्छाङ्ग शोथ वैवर्ण्य क्लेद शब्दाश्रुति ज्वराः| शिरोगुरुत्वं लालासृक्छर्दिश्चासाध्य मूषिकैः||१४८||

The bite by the rat of Dushivisha (slow poisoning) type produces signs and symptoms like

• Adamshat shonitapandu – exudation of blood having pale yellow colour from the site of the bite,
• Mandalani – circular patches,
• Jwara – fever
• Aruchi – anorexia
• Loma harsha – horripilation and
• Daha – burning sensation.

If person is bitten by a rat of Asadhya (incurable) or Pranahara (causing death) type, then he suffers from

• Murchha – fainting
• Angashotha – oedema of limbs,
• Vaivarnya – discoloration of the skin
• Kleda – sloughing
• Shabdaashruti – deafness
• Jwara – fever

- Shiro gurutvam – heaviness of the head
- Lala praseka – excessive salivation and
- Asrkchardi – haematemesis [147- 148]

Chameleon Poison:

श्यावत्वमथ काष्ण्र्य वा नानावर्णत्वमेव वा| मोहः पुरीषभेदश्च दष्टे स्यात् कृकलासकैः||१४९||

Bite by a Krukalasaka (Chameleon) causes brownish black or black or variegated coloration, unconsciousness and diarrhoea [149]

Scorpion Poison – Vruschika Visha:

दहत्यग्निरिवादौ तु भिनत्तीवोर्ध्वमाशु च| वृश्चिकस्य विषं याति दंशे पश्चात् तिष्ठति||१५०||

दष्टोऽसाध्यस्तु दृग्घ्राणरसनोपहतो नरः| मांसैः पतद्भिरत्यर्थं वेदनार्तो जहात्यसून्||१५१||

Scorpion Poison – Vruschika Visha:

Sting of a scorpion (of Dushi- visha or slow poisoning type) causes burning sensation like in the beginning, and thereafter, pinching pain which spreads upwards instantaneously. At the end, the burning sensation and pain is localized at the site of the sting.

If stung by a scorpion of Asadhya (incurable) type, the patient loses his power of vision, smell and taste his muscle tissue gets sloughened and falls out; he suffers from excessive pain and he succumbs to death. [150-151]

Kanabha (Hornet) Poison:

विसर्पः श्वयथुः शूलं ज्वरश्छर्दिरथापि च| लक्षणं कणभैर्दष्टे दंशश्चैव विशीर्यते||१५२||

The sting of a Kanabha (hornet) causes

- Visarpa – erysipelas
- Shvayathu – oedema
- Shula – colic pain
- Jvara – fever
- Chardi – vomiting and withering out of the site of the bite. [152]

Ucchitinga (Crab) Poison:

हृष्टरोमोच्चिटिङ्गेन स्तब्ध लिङ्गो भृशार्तिमान्| दष्टः शीतोदकेनेव सिक्तान्यङ्गानि मन्यते||१५३||

Sting of an Uccitinga (poisonous crab) causes

- Hrstaroma – horrification
- Stabdhalinga – stiffness of the phallus
- Bhrsha aarti – excessive pain and
- Shitaudakanevasikta – a feeling as if the whole body is effused with cold water [153]

Manduka (Toad) Poison:

एकदंष्ट्रादितः शूनः सरुक् स्यात् पीतकः सतृट्| छर्दि निद्रा च मण्डूकैः सविषैर्दष्ट लक्षणम्||१५४||

If bitten by a poisonous toad, then there will be the mark of only 1 fang.

There will be

- Shunahsaruk – oedema with pain
- Pitaka satrt – yellow colouration with morbid thirst
- Chardi – vomiting and
- Nidra – excessive sleep [154]

Poison of Fish and Leech:

मत्स्यास्तु सविषाः कुर्युर्दाह शोफ रुजस्तथा| कण्डूं शोथं ज्वरं मूर्च्छां सविषास्तु जलौकसः||१५५||

Bite or sting by poisonous fish causes
• Daha – burning sensation
• Shopha – oedema and
• Ruja – pain
Bite by poisonous leeches causes
• Kandu – itching,
• Shotha – oedema,
• Jwara – fever and
• Murchha – fainting. [155]

Poison of House- Lizard and Centipede:

दाह तोद स्वेद शोथकरी तु गृहगोधिका | दंशे स्वेदं रुजं दाहं कुर्याच्छतपदी विषम्||१५६||

The poison of Grha- Godhika (house lizard) causes
• Daha – burning sensation
• Toda – pricking pain
• Sveda – sweating and
• Shotha – oedema
The poison of Sata- Padi (centipede) causes
• Sweda – sweating
• Rujam – pain and
• Daha – burning sensation at the site of the bite. [156]

Mosquito poison:

कण्डूमान्मशकैरीषच्छोथः स्यान्मन्द वेदनः| असाध्य कीट सदृशमसाध्यमशकक्षतम्||१५७||

Mosquito bite (sting) causes
• Kandu – itching,
• Shotha – oedema and
• Manda vedana – mild pain
The symptoms of bite of the mosquito of Asadhya (incurable) variety would resemble the symptoms of bite of incurable variety of Keetas (insects) [157]

Makshika (Bee or fly) poison:

सद्यःप्रस्राविणी श्यावा दाह मूर्च्छा ज्वरान्विता| पीडका मक्षिकादंशे तासां तु स्थगिकाऽसुहृत्||१५८||

Bite by Makshika (Bee or fly) causes pimples of Blackish brown colour with instant exudation. The patient suffers from
• Daha – burning sensation,
• Murchha – fainting and
• Jwara – fever
The poison of the sthagika type of bee (fly) causes death. [158]

Features of incurable poisonous bites:

श्मशान चैत्य वल्मीक यज्ञाश्रमसुरालये| पक्ष सन्धिषु मध्याह्ने सार्धरात्रेऽष्टमीषु च||१५९||
न सिद्ध्यन्ति नरा दष्टाः पाषण्डायतनेषु च| दृष्टिश्वास मल स्पर्श विषैराशी विषैस्तथा||१६०||
विनश्यन्त्याशु सम्प्राप्ता दष्टाः सर्वेषु मर्मसु|१६१|

Features of incurable poisonous bites:

Persons bitten by snakes in a cremation ground, under a sacred tree, near an ant- hill, in the place of Yajna (vedic sacrifice), Ashrama (hermitage) or temple, during the time of conjunction of 2 fort-nights (viz, full moon day and new-moon day), mid day, mid night or eight- day of the lunar fortnight, and in the abodes of Pakhandas (hermits of Kapalika sect) and others do not get cured.

Persons afflicted with the bite by Asivisha transmitting poison through vision, breath, waste- products and simple touch and persons bitten over the vital organs succumb to death instantaneously.

The description given above (regarding the place, time and nature) of transmission is applicable to any type of snake. [156- 161]

Augmentation and Diminution of poisoning Effects:

विषं प्रकृतिकालौ च तुल्यौ प्राप्याल्पमन्यथा |१६२||

वारिविप्रहताः क्षीणा भीता नकुलनिर्जिताः|

वृद्धा बालास्त्वचो मुक्ताः सर्पा मन्दविषाः स्मृताः||१६३||

सर्वदेहाश्रितं क्रोधादि्विषं सर्पो विमुञ्चति|

तदेवाहारहेतोर्वा भयाद्वा न प्रमुञ्चति||१६४|

The effects of poisoning get aggravated by fear, intoxication, weakness, heat, hunger and thirst of the patient similarly, if the physical constitution and time of bite are similar to the poison, then the effects get augmented.

If the snakes, etc., are afflicted by fast moving water, if they are emaciated, if they are fearful, if they are afflicted by the attacks of mongoose, if they are old or too young or if they have shed their scales, then the poison transmitted by them has mild effects.

The poison pervades the entire body of the snake, and it comes out through the fangs because of their anger. But when they bite for food or when they are fearful, then the poison does not come out of their fangs. [162-164]

Nature (Vatika, etc) of Poisons and Their Characteristic Signs:

वातोल्बण विषाः प्राय उच्चिटिङ्गाः सवृश्चिकाः| वातपित्तोल्बणाः कीटाः श्लैष्मिकाः कणभादयः||१६५||

यस्य यस्य हि दोषस्य लिङ्गाधिक्यानि लक्षयेत्| तस्य तस्यौषधैः कुर्यादि्वपरीतगुणैः क्रियाम्||१६६||

हृत्पीडोर्ध्वानिलः स्तम्भः सिरायामोऽस्थिपर्वरुक्| घूर्णनोद्वेष्टनं गात्रश्यावता वातिके विषे||१६७||

सञ्ज्ञानाशोष्णनिश्वासौ हृद्दाहः कटुकास्यता| दंशावदरणं शोथो रक्तपीतश्च पैत्तिके||१६८||

वम्यरोचक हृल्लास प्रसेकोत्क्लेश गौरवैः|

सशैत्य मुखमाधुर्यैर्विद्याच्छ्लेष्माधिकं विषम्||१६९||

Nature (Vatika, etc) of Poisons and Their Characteristic Signs:

The poison of ucchitinga (poisoning crabs) and scorpion is dominated by Vayu, that of Keeta (insect) is dominated by Vayu and pitta, and the poison of Kanabha (hornet), etc, is dominated by Kapha.

To treat the patient afflicted with poison, the physician should employ therapeutic measures having attributes opposite to the aggravated Doshas which can be ascertained from the manifested signs and symptoms.

Vayu- aggravating poison results in

• Hrtpida – pain in the cardiac region

• Urdhvaanila – upward movement of the Vayu

• Stambha – stiffness

• Sira aayama – dilatation of the veins,

• Asthi parva ruk – pain in the bones and joints,

• Giddiness

• Cramps and

• Blackish brown colouration of the body

Pitta- aggravating poison exhibits –

• Sanjnanasha – Unconsciousness

• Ushnasvasa – Hot breath

• Hrtdaha – Burning sensation in the cardiac region

• Katukaaasya – pungent taste in the mouth

• Damshavataavarana – Cracking of the tissue in the lace of the bite
• Shotha – Oedema and
• Rakta pita shotha – Red as well as yellow coloration of the skin at the site of the bite
Kapha- aggravating poison exhibits:
• Chardi – vomiting
• Arochaka – anorexia
• Hrllasa – Nausea
• Utklesha – Salivation
• Stretching
• Gaurava – heaviness
• Sa shaityaMukhamadhurya – feeling of cold and sweet taste in the mouth. [165- 169]

Visha Chikitsa Suthra – Line of Treatment:
खण्डेन च व्रणालेपस्तैलाभ्यङ्गश्च वातिके| स्वेदो नाडीपुलाकाद्यैर्बृंहणश्च विधिर्हितः||१७०||
सुशीतैः स्तम्भयेत् सेकैः प्रदेहैश्चापि पैतिकम्| लेखन च्छेदन स्वेद वमनैः श्लैष्मिकं जयेत्||१७१||
विषेष्वपि च सर्वेषु सर्व स्थानगतेषु च| अवृश्चिकोच्चिटिङ्गेषु प्रायः शीतो विधिर्हितः||१७२||
वृश्चिके स्वेदमभ्यङ्गं घृतेन लवणेन च| सेकांश्चोष्णान् प्रयुञ्जीत भोज्यं पानं च सर्पिषः||१७३||
एतदेवोच्चिटिङ्गेऽपि प्रतिलोमं च पांशुभिः| उद्वर्तनं सुखाम्बूष्णैस्तथाऽवच्छादनं घनैः||१७४||
VishaChikitsaSuthra – Line of Treatment:
Vataja Visha Chikitsa:

In case of affliction by the Vata- aggravating poison, the patient is treated by the application of Khanda (Paste of sugar or the sesame) over the wound, massage with sesame oil, Nadi and Pulaka types of fomentation therapies and nourishing diet.

Pitta Dosha VishaChikitsa:

In case of affliction by the Pitta- aggravated poison, the patient is treated with affusion which is very cold and which is Stambhana (arresting the movement of fluids in the body) and the application of cold ointments.

Kapha Dosha VishaChikitsa:

Affliction by Kapha- aggravating poison is treated with Lekhana (which scrapes out the tissues), Chedana (which causes incision in the tissues), fomentation and emetic therapies.

For all the types of poison evading the various parts of the body, excepting the poison of crabs and scorpions, generally cooling therapy is useful.

In case of scorpion poison, the patient is given fomentation and massage and affusions with warm ghee mixed with salt. He is given ghee for food and drinks.

For the poison of crabs, the above mentioned therapies (described for scorpion- bite) is administered. In addition, the patient is rubbed downwards (from the proximal side to the distal side) with sand mixed luke- warm water. The site of the bite is then covered with a thick layer of this sand mixed with luke- warm water. [170- 174]

Poison of Rabid Dog and other wild Animals:
श्वा त्रिदोष प्रकोपान्तु तथा धातु विपर्ययात्| शिरोऽभितापी लालास्राव्यधो वक्त्रस्तथा भवेत्||१७५||
अन्येऽप्येवंविधा व्यालाः कफवातप्रकोपणाः| हृच्छिरोरुग्ज्वर स्तम्भ तृषा मूर्च्छाकरा मताः||१७६||
Because of aggravation of all the 3 Doshas and impairment of tissue elements, the rabid dog suffers from
• Shiro abhitapa – burning sensation in the head
• Lala srava – excessive salivation and
• Adhovaktra – dropping of the head
The same symptoms are also manifested in a person bitten by the rabid dog.
There are other wild animals whose poison causes aggravation of Kapha and Vayu. Bite by these animals causes pain in the cardiac region, headache, fever, stiffness, morbid thirst and fainting. [175-176]

Signs and Symptoms of Poisonus and Non-poisoning bites:

कण्डू निस्तोद वैवर्ण्य सुप्ति क्लेदोपशोषणम्| विदाह राग रुक्पाकाः शोफो ग्रन्थि निकुञ्चनम्||१७७||

दंशावदरणं स्फोटाः कर्णिका मण्डलानि च| ज्वरश्च सविषे लिङ्गं विपरीतं तु निर्विषे||१७८||

The symptoms of poisonous bites are - Kandu – Itching, Nistoda – pain, Vaivarnya – discoloration of the skin, Supti – numbness, Kleda – sloughing. Ruksha – dryness, Vidahashopho – oedema associated with burning sensation, Raga – redness, Ruk – pain and Paka – suppuration, Sphota – adenitis, ContractionCracks in the site of the bite, Pustular eruptions, Karnika (polyp), circular and elevated patches and Jwara – fever.

The opposite symptoms pertain to non- poisonous bites. [177-178]

Visha Chikitsa – Treatment of Poisoning:

तत्र सर्वे यथावस्थं प्रयोज्याः स्युरुपक्रमाः| पूर्वोक्ता विधिमन्यं च यथावद्ब्रुवतः शृणु||१७९||

हृद्दि दाहे प्रसेके वा विरेक वमनं भृशम्| यथावस्थं प्रयोक्तव्यं शुद्धे संसर्जनक्रमः||१८०||

शिरोगते विषे नस्तः कुर्यान्मूलानि बुद्धिमान्| बन्धुजीवस्य भार्ग्याश्च सुरसस्यासितस्य च||१८१||

दक्ष काक मयूराणां मांसासृङ्मस्तके क्षते| उपधेयमधोदष्टस्योर्ध्वदष्टस्य पादयोः||१८२||

पिप्पली मरिच क्षार वचा सैन्धव शिग्रुकाः| पिष्टा रोहित पितेन घ्नन्त्यक्षिगतमञ्जनात्||१८३||

कपित्थमामं ससिताक्षौद्रं कण्ठगते विष| लिह्यादामाशयगते ताभ्यां चूर्णपलं नतात्||१८४||

विषे पक्वाशयगते पिप्पलीं रजनीद्वयम्| मञ्जिष्ठां च समं पिष्ट्वा गोपितेन नरः पिबेत्||१८५||

रक्तं मांसं च गोधायाः शुष्कं चूर्णीकृतं हितम्| विषे रसगते पानं कपित्थ रस संयुतम्||१८६||

शेलोर्मूलत्वग्ग्राणि बादरौदुम्बराणि च| कटभ्याश्च पिबेद्रक्तगते, मांसगते पिबेत्||१८७||

सक्षौद्रं खदिरारिष्टं कौटजं मूलमम्भसा| सर्वेषु च बले द्वे तु मधूकं मधुकं नतम्||१८८||

VishaChikitsa – Treatment of Poisoning:

For the treatment of poisoning, all the 24 therapeutic measures described earlier (vide verse nos. 35-37) are employed in appropriate stages. Now hear about the other treatment measures to be employed in appropriate stages. HrudgataVisha – If there is burning sensation in the cardiac region, and salivation, then purgation and emetic therapies are to be employed frequently at appropriate stages. After Shodhana, the patient is given Samsarjana-Krama (rehabilitating diet).

ShirogataVisha – If the patient is bitten by the poisonous creature at the head / scalp, then the scalp is scarified (scrapped) and the meat as well as blood of cock, crow and pea-cock is applied over it. If the bite is in the upper art of the body, then the feet is scarified and the meat as well as blood of the above mentioned birds is applied over it.

Chakshugata Visha – The poison afflicting the eyes gets cured by the application of the collyrium (Anjana) prepared of Pippali – Long pepper fruit – Piper longum, maricha – Piper nigrum, Kshara, Vacha (Acorus calamus Linn.), Saindhava and Shigru – Moringa oliefera which are made to a paste by triturating with the bile of Rohita type of fish.

Kantha gata Visha If the poison has reached the throat, then the patient is given green Kapittha (Feronia limonia) along with sugar and honey. If it has reached the stomach, then the patient is given one Pala of the powder of Nata (Valeriana wallicii) along with sugar and honey.

Koshtagata Visha – If the poison has reached colon, then the patient should take Pippali – Long pepper fruit – Piper longum, Haridra (turmeric), Daru Haridra (turmeric – Curcuma longa) and Manjistha – Rubia cordifolia, taken in equal quantities and made to a paste by triturating with cow's bile.

Raktagata Visha – If the poison has reached blood, then the patient should take root, bark and tender branches of Selu (Slesmataka), Badara – Zizyphus jujuba and Udumbara – Ficus racemosa along with Katabhi.

Mamsagata Visha – If the poison has reached muscle tissue, then the patient the patient should take the potion containing Bala – Country mallow (root) – Sida cordifolia, Maha-Bala – Country mallow (root) – Sida cordifolia, Madhuka– Licorice – Glycyrrhiza glabra, Madhuka– Licorice – Glycyrrhiza glabra and Nata (Valeriana wallicii). [179- 188]

Sarpavisha Aushadha –

पिप्पलीं नागरं क्षारं नवनीतेन मूर्च्छितम्| कफे भिषगुदीर्णं तु विदध्यात्प्रतिसारणम्||१८९||
मांसी कुङ्कुम पत्रत्वग्रजनी नत चन्दनैः| मनःशिला व्याघ्रनख सुरसैरम्बु पेषितैः||१९०||
पाननस्याञ्जनालेपाः सर्वशोथ विषापहाः| चन्दनं तगरं कुष्ठं हरिद्रे द्वे त्वगेव च||१९१||
मनःशिला तमालश्च रसः कैशर एव च| शार्दूलस्य नखश्चैव सुपिष्टं तण्डुलाम्बुना||१९२||
हन्ति सर्वविषाण्येव वज्रिवज्रमिवासुरान्| रसे शिरीष पुष्पस्य सप्ताहं मरिचं सितम्||१९३||
भावितं सर्पदष्टानां नस्यपानाञ्जने हितम्| द्विपलं नत कुष्ठाभ्यां घृतक्षौद्र चतुष्पलम्||१९४||
अपि तक्षकदष्टानां पानमेतत् सुखप्रदम्| सिन्धुवारस्य मूलं च श्वेता च गिरिकर्णिका||१९५||
पानं दर्वीकरैर्दष्टे नस्यं समधु पाकलम्| मञ्जिष्ठा मधुयष्टी च जीवकर्षभकौ सिता||१९६||
काश्मर्य वटशुङ्गानि पानं मण्डलिनां विषे| व्योषं सातिविष कुष्ठं गृहधूमो हरेणुका||१९७||
तगरं कटुका क्षौद्रं हन्ति राजीमतां विषम्| गृहधूमं हरिद्रे द्वे समूलं तण्डुलीयकम्||१९८||
अपि वासुकिना दष्टः पिबेन्मधु घृताप्लुतम् |१९९|

Medicnes for snake poisoning:

If Kapha is aggravated because of poisoning, then the paste of pippali – piper longum, Nagara – Zingiber officinale and Ksara (Alkali preparation) triturated with butter is applied over the site of bite for Pratisarana (exudation of liquid).

Administration of Jatamamsi, Kunkuma, Patra – Cinnamomum tamala Nees and Eberum., Tvak, Rajani (Turmeric), Nata , Chandana (Sandalwood – Santalum album), Manahshila, VyaghraNakha and surasa (made into paste by triturating with water, or administered orally or through Nasya, Anjana or Lepa (external application in the form of paste) cures all types of oedema and poisons.

Chandana (Sandalwood – Santalum album), Tagara, Kushta – Saussurealappa, Haridra (turmeric – Curcuma longa), Daruharidra (Berberis aristata), Tvak, Manah-Sila, Tamala, Juice of Kesara, Sardula- Nakha or Vyaghra-Nakha (Nakhi) is made to a paste by triturating with Tandulambu (rice wash). Administration of this recipe cures all the types of poisons as the thunder- bolt of Indra destroyed all the Demons.

White variety of Maricha – Black pepper fruit – piper nigrum is impregnated with the juice of the flower of Sirisha (Albizia lebbeck) for 7 days. Administration of this potion in the forms of Nasya (inhalation therapy), pana (taking internally) and Anjana (collyrium) is useful in snakebite.

Intake of the potion containing 2 Palas of ghee and honey is useful even for a patient bitten by Taksaka (celestial snake).

To a patient bitten by a Darvikara type of snake, the root of Sindhuvara (Vitex negundo) and white variety of GiriKarnika (Kutaja) is administered internally. He is given Pakala (Kushta – Saussurea lappa) along with honey for inhalation.

A person afflicted with the poison of a Mandali Snake should take the potion comprising Manjistha – Rubia cordifolia, Madhuyasti – Glycrrhrizza glabra, Jivaka – Malaxis acuminata, Rishabhaka – Manilkara hexandra, Suar, Kasmarya and the still root of Vata – Ficus bengalensis.

The potion comprising Sunthi – Zingiber officinale, Pippali – Piper longum, Maricha – Black pepper fruit – piper nigrum, ativisha – Aconitum heterophyllum, Kushta – Saussurea lappa, Grha- Dhuma (Kitchen- soot), Harenu, Tagara, Katuka and Honey cures the poison of a Rajiman type of Snakes.

The potion comprising Griha-Dhuma (Kitchen-soot), Haridra (turmeric – Curcuma longa), Daruharidra – Berberis aristata and Tanduliyaka along with its root is a mixed liberal quantity of honey and ghee. Intake of this cures a patient even if he is bitten by Vasuki (a celestial snake). [189 –199½]

Medicines for Poisons of Insects, Etc:

क्षीरिवृक्षत्वगालेपः शुद्धे कीट विषापहः||१९९||
मुक्तालेपो वरः शोथ दाह तोद ज्वरापहः| चन्दनं पद्मकोशीरं शिरीषः सिन्धुवारिका||२००||
क्षीर शुक्ला नतं कुष्ठं पाटलोदीच्यसारिवाः| शेलुस्वरसपिष्टोऽयं लूतानां सार्वकार्मिकः||२०१||
(यथायोगं प्रयोक्तव्यः समीक्ष्यालेपनादिषु)|

मधूकं मधुकं कुष्ठं शिरीषोदीच्य पाटलाः| सनिम्ब सारिवा क्षौद्राः पानं लूता विषापहम्||२०२||
कुसुम्भपुष्पं गोदन्तः स्वर्णक्षीरी कपोत विट्| दन्ती त्रिवृत्सैन्धवं च कर्णिकापातनं तयोः||२०३||
कटभ्यर्जुनशैरीषशेलुक्षीरिद्रुमत्वचः| कषाय कल्क चूर्णाः स्युः कीट लूता व्रणापहाः||२०४||
त्वचं च नागरं चैव समांशं श्लक्ष्ण पेषितम्| पेयमुष्णाम्बुना सर्व मूषिकाणां विषापहम्||२०५||
कुटजस्य फलं पिष्टं तगरं जालमालिनी| तिक्तेक्ष्वाकुश्च योगोऽयं पान प्रधमनादिभिः||२०६||
वृश्चिकोन्दुरुलूतानां सर्पाणां च विषं हरेत्| समानो ह्यमृतेनायं गराजीर्णं च नाशयेत्||२०७||
सर्वेऽगदा यथादोषं प्रयोज्याः स्युः कृकण्टके| कपोत विण्मातुलुङ्गं शिरीष कुसुमाद्रसः||२०८||
शङ्खिखिन्यार्क पयः शुण्ठी करञ्जो मधु वार्श्चिके| शिरीषस्य फलं पिष्टं स्नुहीक्षीरेण दार्दुरे||२०९||
मूलानि श्वेतभण्डीनां व्योषं सर्पिश्च मत्स्यजे| कीटदष्ट क्रियाः सर्वाः समानाः स्युर्जलौकसाम्||२१०||
वातपित्तहरी चापि क्रिया प्रायः प्रशस्यते| वार्श्चिको ह्युच्चिटिङ्गस्य कणभस्यौन्दुरोऽगदः ||२११||

Medicines for Poisons of Insects, Etc:

Application of the paste of the bark of Ksheeri- Vrukshas (trees having Milky –Latex, viz, Nyagrodha, Udumbara, Asvattha, Vetasa and Plaksa) after purification (administration of 5 elimination therapies) cures insect poison application of the paste of pearl prepared by triturating with water is excellent for curing oedema, burning sensation, pain and fever.

Chandana – Santalum album, padmaka, Ushira – Vetiver – Vetiveria zizanioides, Sirisha Albizia lebbeck Benth.), Sindhuvarika, Ksirasukla, Nata (Valeriana wallicii), Kushta – Saussurea lappa, Patala – Stereospermum suaveolens, Udichya and Sariva – Indian Sarsaparilla is made to a paste by triturating with the juice of Selu.

This recipe is useful in the form of all therapeutic measures for the treatment of the poison of the spider. After proper examination, this recipe is used appropriately in Lepana (external application), etc.

Intake of Madhuka– Licorice, Kushta – Saussurea lappa, Sirisha (Albizia lebbeck), Udichya and Patala – Sterospermumsuaveolens, along with Nimba – Neem, Sariva – Indian Sarsaparilla – Hemidesmus indicus and honey cures the poison of spiders.

Flower of Kusumbha – Carthamus tinctorius, Godanta (tooth of a cow), Svarna- Ksiri, stool of Kapota, Danti – Baliospermum montanum, Trivrt – Operculina turpethum and Saindhava cures the Karnika (granulomatus growth) in the wound caused by the bite of insects and spiders.

The decoction, paste and powder of Katabhi, Arjuna (Terminalia arjuna), bark of Sirisha Albizia lebbeck Benth.), Selu and the barks of late bearing trees(Nyagrodha, Udumbara, Asvattha, Vetasa and Plaksa) cure ulcers caused by the bite of insects and spiders.

Tvak (cinnamon) and Nagara – Zingiber officinale taken in equal quantities is made to a fine paste, and taken along with hot water, cures poison of all types of rats. The recipe comprising the paste of the fruit of Kutaja – Connessi Albizia lebbeck Wall.), Tagara, Jala- Malini (Devadataka or Devadali) and bitter variety of Iksvaku is administered in the form of pana (taking internally), pradhamana (a type of Inhalation therapy), etc. cures the poisons of scorpions, rats, spiders and snakes? This recipe is like Ambrosia, and it also cures indigestion of Gara (artificial poisoning).

All the above mentioned recipes are useful for the ailments caused by the poison of Krkantaka or Krkalasa (Chamelion) and are used according to the Doshas provoked by such poison.

The recipe comprising the stool of Kapota, Matulunga – Lemon variety – Citrus decumana / Citrus limon, the juice of the flowers of Shirisha (Albizia lebbeck Benth.), Shankini – Canscora decussata and the milky latex of Arka – Calotropis gigantea, Sunthi –ginger, karanja – Pongamia pinnata and honey cures scorpion poison.

The paste of the fruit of Sirisha – Albizia lebbeck prepared by triturating with the milky latex of Sunthi – Zingiber officinale is useful in curing the ailments caused by frog- bite.

The paste of the root of the white variety of Bh(m)andi (Aparajita), Sunthi, Pippali – Long pepper fruit – Piper longum, Maricha – Black pepper fruit – piper nigrum, and honey is useful in curing fish- poison.

All the therapeutic measures prescribed for the treatment of insect- bite are equally good for the treatment of leech- poison. In such cases, generally, therapeutic measures for the alleviation of Vayu and Pitta are useful.

The therapies prescribed for scorpion- bite are useful for Crab- bite. Therapeutic measures prescribed for rat bite are useful for hornet- bite. [199 ½- 211]

Paramo Agada – Remedy Par Excellence: Best antidote:

वचां वंशत्वचं पाठां नतं सुरसमञ्जरीम्| द्वे बले नाकुली कुष्ठं शिरीषं रजनीद्वयम्||२१२||

गुहामतिगुहां श्वेतामजगन्धां शिलाजतु| कत्तृणं कटभीं क्षारं गृहधूमं मनःशिलाम्||२१३||

रोहीतकस्य पित्तेन पिष्ट्वा तु परमोऽगदः| नस्याञ्जनादिलेपेषु हितो विश्वम्भरादिषु||२१४||

Paramo Agada – Remedy Par Excellence: Best antidote:

Vacha (Acorus calamus Linn.), Bark of Vamsa, Patha – Cissampelos parriera, Nata (Valeriana wallicii), inflorescence of Surasa, Bala – Country mallow (root) – Sida cordifolia, Maha-Bala – Country mallow (root) – Sida cordifolia, Nakuli, Kushta – Saussurea lappa, Sirisha Albizia lebbeck Benth.), Haridra (turmeric – Curcuma longa), Daru-Haridra (turmeric – Curcuma longa), Guha, Atiguha, Sveta, Ajagandha, Silajatu, Kattrna, Katabhi, Ksara, (alkali reparation), Grha- Dhuma(Kitchen- Soot) and Manah-Sila is made to a paste by attributing with the bile of Rohita (a type of fish). This is called "Paramo Agada' remedy par excellence. Administration of this recipe in the form of Nasya (inhalation therapy) Anjana (collyrium), Leech (external application). Etc., is useful in the poisonous insect bites like Visvambharas. [212- 214]

Recipe for Centipede Poison:

स्वर्जिकाऽजशकृत्क्षारः सुरसाऽथाक्षिपीडकः | मदिरामण्डसंयुक्तो हितः शतपदी विषे||२१५||

Use of Svarjika Ksara of the goat's droppings, Surasa and Aksi- Pidaka (a type of Simbi having white and yellow colour) triturated with the supernatant part of madira (a type of alcohol) is useful in centipede- poison. [215]

Recipe for house – lizard poison:

कपित्थमक्षिपीडोऽर्कबीजं त्रिकटुकं तथा| करञ्जो द्वे हरिद्रे च गृहगोधा विषं जयेत्||२१६||

The recipe comprising Kapittha (Feronia limonia), Aksi-Pida(a type of Simbi having white and yellow color), seeds of Arka – Calotropis gigantea, Sunthi – Zingiber officinale, Pippali – Long pepper fruit – Piper longum, Maricha – Black pepper fruit – piper nigrum, Karanja (Pongamia pinnata), Lata Karanja, Haridra (turmeric – Curcuma longa) and Daru Haridra (turmeric – Curcuma longa) cures the poison of House- lizard. [216]

Recipes for all Poisons

काकाण्ड रससंयुक्तो विषाणां तण्डुलीयकः| प्रधानो बर्हिपित्तेन तद्वद्वायस पीलुकः||२१७||

Tanduliyaka triturated with the juice of Kakanda (Kakatinduka) is useful in all types of poison. Similarly, Vayasa-Piluka (Kakamachi) triturated with peacock- bile is useful in all types of poison. [217]

PanchaShireesha Agada

शिरीषफलमूलत्वक्पुष्पपत्रैः समैर्धृतैः|

श्रेष्ठः पञ्च शिरीषोऽयं विषाणां प्रवरो वधे||२१८||

इति पञ्चशिरीषोऽगदः|

The excellent recipe containing [the 5 parts, viz.,] fruits, roots, barks, flowers and leaves of Sirisha Albizia lebbeck Benth.), all taken in equal quantities is added with ghee this is called Pancha- Sirisha (Albizia lebbeck .) It is the most effective remedy for all types of poison.

Thus, ends the description of PanchShirisha Agada [218]

Recipe for poisons of Nails and teeth:

चतुष्पद्भिर्द्विपद्भिर्वा नखदन्तक्षतं तु यत्| शूयते पच्यते चापि स्रवति ज्वरयत्यपि||२१९||

सोमवल्कोऽश्वकर्णश्च गोजिह्वा हंसपद्यपि| रजन्यौ गैरिकं लेपो नखदन्तविषापहः||२२०||

A person injured by the nails (claws) and the teeth of quadrupeds and bipeds suffers from oedema, suppuration, exudation of liquid material from the place of bite and fever. Application of the paste of soma-valka, Asva- Karma, Gojihva, Hamsa-Padi, Haridra (turmeric – Curcuma longa), Daru- Haridra (turmeric – Curcuma longa) and Gairika cures these poisons of nails and teeth. [219- 220]

Shanka-visha (Fear of Poison) and its Management:

दुरन्धकारे विद्धस्य केनचिद्विषशङ्कया| विषोद्वेगाज्ज्वरशछर्दि मूर्च्छा दाहोऽपि वा भवेत्||२२१||

ग्लानि र्मोहोऽतिसारश्चाप्येतच्छङ्काविषं मतम्| चिकित्सितमिदं तस्य कुर्यादाश्वासयन् बुधः||२२२||

सिता वैगन्धिको द्राक्षा पयस्या मधुकं मधु| पानं समन्त्रपूताम्बु प्रोक्षणं सान्त्वहर्षणम्||२२३||

Shanka-visha (Fear of Poison) and its Management:

When a person is bitten by something (non- poisonous creature) in pitch darkness, the fear or suspicion (Sanka) of being bitten by a poisonous creature causes manifestation of symptoms of pseudo- poison in the form of fever, vomiting, fainting, burning sensation, prostration, unconsciousness and diarrhoea. This condition is called Sanka-visha (fear- poison).

For the treatment of this ailment, the wise physician should console the patient. He is given sugar, purified sulphur, Draksha – Raisin – Vitis vinifera, ayasya, Madhuka– Licorice – Glycyrrhiza glabra to drink honey along with water impregnated with Mantra to drink. This sanctified water is sprinkled over his body, he is consoled and made cheerful. [221- 223]

Diet and Regimes:

शालयः षष्टिकाश्चैव कोरदूषाः प्रियङ्गवः| भोजनार्थे प्रशस्यन्ते लवणार्थे च सैन्धवम्||२२४||

तण्डुलीयकजीवन्तीवार्ताकसुनिषण्णकाः| चुच्चूर्मण्डूकपर्णी च शाकं च कुलकं हितम्||२२५||

धात्री दाडिममम्लार्थे यूषा मुद्गहरेणुभिः| रसाश्चैणशिखिश्वाविल्लावतैतिरपार्षताः||२२६||

विषघ्नौषधसंयुक्ता रसा यूषाश्च संस्कृताः| अविदाहीनि चान्नानि विषार्तानां भिषग्जितम्||२२७||

विरुद्धाध्यशनक्रोधक्षुद्भयायासमैथुनम्| वर्जयेद्विषमुक्तोऽपि दिवास्वप्नं विशेषतः||२२८||

Diet and regimen in poisoning care:

For a person suffering from ailments caused by poisoning, Sali rice, Sastika rice, kora- dusa and Priyangu (Callicara macrophylla) are useful as food, and Saindhava (rock salt) is given as salt. As vegetables, Tanduliyaka, Jivanti – Leptadenia reticulata, Vartaka, Sunisannaka, Cuccu, Manduka- parni and Kuaka (Karavellaka or Patola) are useful. To cause sourness in food, Amalaki – Phyllanthus emblica and Dadima – Pomegranate – Punica granatum are useful. Mudga and Harenu are used for preparing vegetable- soup for him the meat of Ena, Sikhi, Svavit lava, Tittiri and Prsat is used for preparing meat soup.

These meat- soups and vegetable- soups are sizzled by adding ingredients which are antidotes of poisons. Food ingredients which do not cause burning sensation (Avidahi) are useful in the treatment of a person suffering from ailments caused by poisons.

The patient should avoid such diets, ingredients of which are mutually contradictory (Viruddha), and intake of food before the previous meal is digested he should also refrain from anger, hunger, fear, exhaustion and sexual intercourse he should, specially, avoid sleep during the day time, even if he is cured of the poison. [224- 228]

Signs and Symptoms of poison in Quadrupeds:

मुहुर्मुहुः शिरोन्यासः शोथः स्रस्तौष्ठकर्णता | ज्वरः स्तब्धाक्षिगात्रत्वं हनुकम्पोऽङ्गमर्दनम्||२२९||

रोमापगमनं ग्लानिररति वेपथु भ्रमः| चतुष्पदां भवत्येतद्दष्टानामिह लक्षणम्||२३०||

If quadrupeds are afflicted by poisonous bites, then symptoms like

• Muhurmuhshironyasa – repeated jerks of the head,

• Shotha – oedema,

• Srastaosthakarnata – dropping of the lips and ears,

• Malaise,

• Roma upagamana – hair fall,

• Glani – exhaustion,

• Arati – Disliking for everything,

• Vepathu – trembling and
• Bhrama – giddiness appear [229-230]

Treatment of Poisoned Quadrupeds:
देवदारु हरिद्रे द्वे सरलं चन्दनागुरु| रास्ना गोरोचनाऽजाजी गुग्गुल्विक्षुरसो नतम्||२३१||
चूर्णं ससैन्धवानन्तं गोपित्तं मधु संयुतम्| चतुष्पदानां दष्टानामगदः सार्वकार्मिकः||२३२||
The recipe comprising
Devadaru (Cedrus deodara),
Haridra – Curcuma longa
Daru- Haridra (Berberis aristata),
Sharaa,
Chandana (Sandalwood – Santalum album),
Rasna (Pluchea lanceolata),
Goracana,
Ajaji – Nigella sativa
Guggulu (commiphora mukul Engl.),
Sugarcane juice,
Tagara – Valerianawalichii
Saindhava and
Ananta is made to a powder and mixed with cow's bile and honey.
This recipe is used in all the different forms of therapeutic measures for the treatment of the poisoned quadrupeds.
[231- 232]

GaravishaLakshana – Signs Symptoms and treatment of Gara Type of Poison:
सौभाग्यार्थं स्त्रियः स्वेदरजोनानाङ्गजान्मलान्| शत्रुप्रयुक्तांश्च गरान् प्रयच्छन्त्यन्नमिश्रितान्||२३३||
तैः स्यात् पाण्डुः कृशोऽल्पाग्निर्गरश्चास्योपजायते| मर्म प्रधमनाध्मानं श्वयथुं हस्त पादयोः||२३४||
जठरं ग्रहणीदोषो यक्ष्मा गुल्मः क्षयो ज्वरः | एवंविधस्य चान्यस्य व्याधिलिङ्गानि दर्शयेत्||२३५||
स्वप्ने मार्जार गोमायुव्यालान् सनकुलान् कपीन्| प्रायः पश्यति नद्यादीञ्छुष्कांश्च सवनस्पतीन्||२३६||
कालश्च गौरमात्मानं स्वप्ने गौरश्च कालकम्| विकर्ण नासिकं वाऽपि प्रपश्येदिवहतेन्द्रियः||२३७||
तमवेक्ष्य भिषक् प्राज्ञः पृच्छेत् किं कैः कदा सह| जग्धमित्यवगम्याशु प्रदद्यादवमनं भिषक्||२३८||
सूक्ष्मं ताम्र रजस्तस्मै सक्षौद्रं हृदिविशोधनम्| शुद्धे हृदि ततः शाणं हेमचूर्णस्य दापयेत्||२३९||
हेम सर्वविषाण्याशु गरांश्च विनियच्छति| न सज्जते हेमपाङ्गे विषं पद्मदलेऽम्बुवत्||२४०||
नागदन्ती त्रिवृद्दन्ती द्रवन्ती स्नुक्पयःफलैः| साधितं माहिष सर्पिः सगोमूत्राढकं हितम्||२४१||
सर्प कीट विषार्तानां गरार्तानां च शान्तये|२४२|
GaravishaLakshana – Signs Symptoms and treatment of Gara Type of Poison:
Women, in order to gain favour from their husbands, at times, administer their sweat, menstrual blood and different types of waste products of their body along with food. Even (as spies) lying in the hands of enemies, sometimes, administer various types of Gara (artificial poison) along with food preparations.
Because of these poisons, a person suffers from
• Pandu – anemia,
• Karshya – emaciation,
• suppression of the power of digestion,
• Visha – poisoning,
• Palpitation of vital organs (like heart),
• flatulence,
• oedema in the hands and feet,
• Jathara (obstinate Syndrome),

- Tuberculosis,
- Gulma (phantom tumour),
- Consumption,
- Jwara – fever

Amruta Ghrita:

शिरीष त्वक् त्रिकटुकं त्रिफलां चन्दनोत्पले||२४२||

द्वे बले सारिवा स्फोता सुरभी निम्ब पाटलाः| बन्धु जीवाढकी मूर्वा वासा सुरस वत्सकान्||२४३||

पाठाङ्कोलाश्वगन्धार्कमूलयष्ट्याह्व पद्मकान्| विशालां बृहतीं लाक्षां कोविदारं शतावरीम्||२४४||

कटभी दन्त्यपामार्गान् पृश्निपर्णी रसाञ्जनम्| श्वेतभण्डाश्वखुरकौ कुष्ठदारु प्रियङ्गुकान्||२४५||

विदारीं मधुकात् सारं करञ्जस्य फलत्वचौ| रजन्यौ लोध्रमक्षांशं पिष्ट्वा साध्यं घृताढकम्||२४६||

तुल्याम्बुच्छाग गोमूत्रत्र्याढके तद्विषापहम्| अपस्मार क्षयोन्माद भूतग्रहगरोदरम्||२४७||

पाण्डुरोग क्रिमी गुल्म प्लीहोरुस्तम्भ कामलाः| हनुस्कन्ध ग्रहादींश्च पानाभ्यञ्जन नावनैः||२४८||

हन्यात् सञ्जीवयेच्चापि विबोद्बन्धमृतान्नरान्| नाम्नेदममृतं सर्वविषाणां स्याद्घृतोत्तमम्||२४९||

इत्यमृतघृतम्|

1 Adhaka of Ghee (according to Mana- Paribhasa the quantity of ghee is 2 Adhakas) is cooked by adding the paste of
1 Aksa each of the
Bark of Sirisha, Sunthi, Pippali, Maricha, Haritaki, Bibhitaka, Amalaki, Chandana, Utpala, Bala, MahaBala, Sariva, Ashpota, Surabhi, Nimba, Patala, Bandhu-jiva, Adhaki, Murva, Vasa, Surasa, Vatsaka, Patha, Ankola, Asvagandha, Root of Arka, Yasti-madhu, Padmaka, Visala,Brihati, Laksa, Kovidara, Satavari, Katabhi, Danti, Apamarga, Prisniparni,Rasanjana, Sveta- Bhanda, Asvakhuraka, Khuraka, Kustha, Daru, Priyangu, Vidari, Exudate of madhuka, Fruits and bark of karanja, Haridra,Daru- Haridra and Lodhra,
2 Adhakas of water,
3 Adhakas of goat's urine and
3 Adhakas of cow's urine
Indications:
When used in the form of pana (drink), Abhyanga (massage) and Navana (inhalation therapy) it helps cure of:
Visha – poisons, Apasmara – epilepsy, Kshaya – consumption, Unmada – insanity, Seizures of evil spirits, Garavisha – Artificial poisons, Udara (obstinate abdominal disorders including ascites), Pandu – anemia,
Krimi – parasitic infestation, Gulma (phantom tumour), Pliha – splenic disorders, Urustambha (stiffness of the thighs), Kamala – Jaundice, Stiffness of Jaws and shoulders etc.,
It helps in the revival of persons who appear to be dead because of poison and hanging. This excellent recipe of medicated ghee is called Amrta-ghrta and it is like Ambrosia for curing all type of Poisons.
Thus, ends the description of Amrita Ghruta [242 ½ – 249]
Preventive measures against snake bite:

भवन्ति चात्र-

छत्री झर्झरपाणिश्च चरेद्रात्रौ तथा दिवा| तच्छायाशब्द वित्रस्ताः प्रणश्यन्त्याशु पन्नगाः||२५०||

दष्टमात्रो दशेदाशु तं सर्पं लोष्टमेव वा| उपर्यरिष्टां बध्नीयाद्दंशं छिन्द्याद्दहेत्तथा||२५१||

वज्रं मरकतः सारः पिचुको विष मूषिका| कर्कतनः सर्प मणि वैंदूर्यं गज मौक्तिकम्||२५२||

धार्यं गरमणिर्याश्च वरौषध्यो विषापहाः| खगाश्च शारिका क्रौञ्च शिखि हंस शुकादयः||२५३||

Preventive measures against snake bite:
Thus it is said that one should move about with an umbrella during the day time and with a ratting stick in hand at night so that with their shade and sound respectively, the snakes get frightened and go away [without biting the person].
Immediately after the snake- bite, the person should bite the snake itself (if possible) or otherwise bite a clod of earth. Thereafter, a tourniquet is tied above (at the proximal end of) the site of bite and the place of the bite is incised

as well as cauterized.

Wearing of diamond, Marakata (emerald), Sara, icuka, visha- Musika, (visha-Mani), Karketana (Padma – Lotus (Nelumbo nucifera)- Raga, Sara-Mani (A type of pearl or gem collected from the head of the snake), Vaidurya (LaisLauli), Gaja Mani (different types of gems which are antidotes of poisons) and Varasadha (Talisman or amulet containing herbs which are antidotes of poisons) gives immunity against poisons.

Keeping (domesticating) birds like Sarika (Myna), Krauncha (crane), Peacock, Swan and parrots is also useful to overcome poisons. [250- 253]

तत्र श्लोकः-

इतीदमुक्तं द्विविधस्य विस्तरैर्बहुप्रकारं विषरोगभेषजम्| अधीत्य विज्ञाय तथा प्रयोजयन् व्रजेद्विषाणामविषह्यतां बुधः||२५४||

Thus, details of 2 categories of poisons along with several types of medicines to cure the ailments caused by these poisons are described. If the wise physician has a thorough knowledge of these poisons and skilfully administers treatments to get rid of them, he can definitely overcome these poisons by the application of his knowledge and experience. [254]

इत्यग्निवेशकृते तन्त्रे चरक प्रतिसंस्कृते चिकित्सा स्थाने विष चिकित्सितं नाम त्रयोविंशोऽध्यायः||२३||

Thus, ends the 23rd chapter of the ChikitsaSthana dealing with the treatment of poisons of Agnivesha's work as redacted by Master Charaka.

7

Chikitsasthana Chapter 24
Madatyaya Chikitsitam

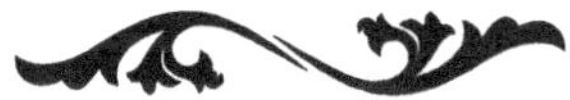

The 24th chapter of Charaka Samhita Chikitsa Sthana deals with symptoms and treatment for alcoholism. It is called Madatyaya Chikitsa Adhyaya.

अथातो मदात्यय चिकित्सितं व्याख्यास्यामः||१||
इति ह स्माह भगवानात्रेयः||२||
We shall now explain the Treatment of Alcoholism. Thus, said Lord Atreya. [1-2]

Appreciation of Sura – alcohol:
सुरैः सुरेश सहितैर्या पुरा परिपूजिता| सौत्रामण्यां हूयते या कर्मिभिर्या प्रतिष्ठिता||३||
यज्ञौही या यया शक्रः सोमातिपतितो भृशम्| निरोजस्तमसाऽऽविष्टस्तस्माद्दुर्गात् समुद्धृतः||४||
विधिभिर्वेदविहितैर्वा यजद्भिर्महात्मभिः| दृश्या स्पृश्या प्रकल्प्या च यज्ञीया यज्ञसिद्धये||५||
योनि संस्कार नामाद्यैर्विशेषैर्बहुधा च या| भूत्वा भवत्येक विधा सामान्यान्मद लक्षणात्||६||
या देवानमृतं भूत्वा स्वधा भूत्वा पितृंश्च या| सोमो भूत्वा द्विजातीन् या युङ्क्ते श्रेयोभिरुत्तमैः||७||
आश्विनं या महतेजो बलं सारस्वतं च या| वीर्यमैन्द्रं च या सिद्धा सोमः सौत्रामणौ च या||८||
शोकारतिभयोद्वेगनाशिनी या महाबला| या प्रीतिर्या रतिर्या वाग्या पुष्टिर्या च निर्वृतिः||९||
या सुरा सुरगन्धर्वयक्ष राक्षस मानुषैः| रतिः सुरेत्यभिहिता तां सुरां विधिना पिबेत्||१०||

The Drink, which, in the time of Yore, was adored by the gods along with their master Indra, which is offered as oblation to fire during Satramani sacrifice (for details of this type of Vedic ritual, Vide Suka- Yajurveda: Kanvasakha Chapters 21- 23 – reference from CS by Bhagwan Dash and Sharma PK); which is respected by the priests, which sustains the Vedic rituals: which when taken appropriately eliminated the miseries of Indra who had fallen down, lost his energies (ojas), and was afflicted with diseases because of excessive alcoholic intake; which is a visible, touchable and applicable instrument of sacrifice conducive to its successful completion as enjoyed by the great sages performing sacrifices according to the methods prescribed by the Vedas; which has different types depending upon its specific source material, Samskara (method of reparation), nomenclature, etc, which is at the same time unitary in character on account of the common feature of intoxication which bestows auspiciousness par excellence by providing nourishment to the gods in the form of ambrosia, to the pitrus (Manes) in the form of Svadha (the term used for offering oratory offerings to the manes), to Dvijas (the twice born, viz, Brahmanas, Kshatriyas and Vaisyas) in the form of Soma; which represents the great Lustre of the Ashvini Kumaras, the prowess of the mantras, and the supremacy of Indra; which is perfected Soma in the Sautramani sacrifice; which eradicates grief, depression, fear and bewilderness; which in itself represents the invincible strength, love, voice, nourishment and peace; and which is called Sura by the Gods, Gandharvas (celestial musicians), Yakshas, Raksas and human beings, is taken appropriately (according to the prescription of the Shastra).[3-10]

The right method of Alcohol consumption:

शरीरकृत संस्कारः शुचिरुत्तम गन्धवान्| प्रावृतो निर्मलैर्वस्त्रैर्यथर्तूद्दामगन्धिभिः||११||

विचित्र विविध स्रग्वी रत्नाभरण भूषितः| देवद्विजातीन् सम्पूज्य स्पृष्ट्वा मङ्गलमुत्तमम्||१२||

देशे यथर्तुके शस्ते कुसुमप्रकरीकृते| सरसासम्मते मुख्ये धूप सम्मोदबोधिते||१३||

सोपधाने सुसंस्तीर्णे विहिते शयनासने| उपविष्टोऽथवा तिर्यक् स्व शरीर सुखे स्थितः||१४||

सौवर्णे राजतैश्चापि तथा मणिमयैरपि| भाजनैर्विमलैश्चान्यैः सुकृतैश्च पिबेत् सदा||१५||

रूप यौवनमत्ताभिः शिक्षिताभिर्विशेषतः| वस्त्राभरणमाल्यैश्च भूषिताभिर्यथर्तुकैः||१६||

शौचानुरागयुक्ताभिः प्रमदाभिरितस्ततः| संवाह्यमान इष्टाभिः पिबेन्मद्यमनुत्तमम्||१७||

मद्यानुकूलैर्विविधैः फलैर्हरितकैः शुभैः| लवणैर्गन्धपिशुनैरवदंशैर्यथर्तुकैः||१८||

भृष्टैर्मांसैर्बहुविधैर्भूजलाम्बरचारिणाम्| पौरोगवर्ग विहितैर्भक्ष्यैश्च विविधात्मकैः||१९||

पूजयित्वा सुरान् पूर्वमाशिषः प्राक् प्रयुज्य च| प्रदाय सजलं मद्यमर्थिभ्यो वसुधातले||२०||

The following rules are observed for taking alcohol:

1. Before taking alcohol, the person should follow proper rituals (Samskara), hygiene (Shuchi).

2. He should wear the most pleasing perfumes and have pleasant disposition

3. He should wear clean clothes and follow rituals as per the requirement of the season,

4. He should wear different types of garlands of different colours, jewels and ornaments.

5. He should offer prayer to the Gods and Dvijas or the Twice born (Brahmanas, Kshatriyas and Vaisyas)

6. He should touch auspicious objects

7. Alcohol is taken in an air-conditioned (Yathartuka) place which is surrounded with trees having falling flowers, which is exceedingly liked by the beloved ones, which is perfumed with the aroma of incense and which is provided with well spread beds and seats along with pillows;

8. The person comfortably sitting or lying in an incumbent posture over the above-mentioned seats or bed should drink alcohol served to him in a beaker of gold, silver or costly stone or in other clean and well-prepared vessels.

9. While taking alcohol, he should sit or lie down in an incumbent posture over the above-mentioned seats or bed should drink alcohol served to him in a beaker of gold, silver or costly stone or in other clean and well-prepared vessels.

10. While drinking alcohol, he should eat delicious refreshments like fruits, Haritaka (green salads) which are sauted and made aromatic, and which go well with types of alcohol and seasonal needs

11. Along with alcohol, he should take different types of roasted meat- preparations of animals and birds inhabiting land and, water and sky, and other various types of eatables prepared by expert cooks

12. Before drinking, he should offer prayer to the gods and solicit their blessings and.

13. He should pour of the alcohol along with water on the ground for the needy (celestial beings like Baladeva, chandi and Yaksa) before starting to consume the drink [11-20]

Regimes to be followed by Persons of Different Body Types

अभ्यङ्गोत्सादन स्नान वासोधूपानुलेपनैः| स्निग्धोष्णैर्भावितश्चान्नैर्वातिको मद्यमाचरेत्||२१||

शीतोपचारै र्विविधै मधुर स्निग्ध शीतलैः| पैत्तिको भावितश्चान्नैः पिबन्मद्यं न सीदति||२२||

उपचारैरशिशिरैर्यैव गोधूम भुक् पिबेत्| श्लैष्मिको धन्वजैर्मांसैर्मद्यं मारिचकैः सह||२३||

विधिर्वसुमतामेष भविष्यदिवभवाश्च ये| यथोपपत्ति तैर्मद्यं पातव्यं मात्रया हितम्||२४||

वातिकेभ्यो हितं मद्यं प्रायो गौडिक पैष्टिकम्| कफपित्ताधिकेभ्यस्तु माद्वीकं माधवं च यत्||२५||

A person having Vatika type of constitution should drink alcohol after

• Abhyanga – massage

• Utsadana – Unction

• Snana – Bath

• Dhupana – Fumigation and

• Snigdha Anu lepana – Application of unguent and

• After having taken food which is unctuous and hot

A person having Pitta body type does not get adversely afflicted if he drinks alcohol after restoring to different types of cooling regimens, and take food- preparations which are sweet, unctuous and cooling regimens, and take food- preparations which are sweet, unctuous and cooling.

The person having kapha type of constitution should drink alcohol after resorting to heating regimens, and along with food prepared of Barley, wheat and meat of animals inhabiting arid zone mixed black pepper.

The rules of drinking alcohol described above are meant for wealthy persons or for those who are going to attain wealth (in near future). However, drinking alcohol is useful for them only when appropriate procedure is followed and the drink is taken in proper quantity.

For persons of Vatika constitution, alcohol prepared of Jaggery and Pishta (paste of the flour of wheat, etc) is generally useful. For persons dominated by Kapha (having Kaphaja constitution) alcohol prepared with honey is useful. Similarly, for persons having Paittika type of constitution, alcohol prepared with grapes is useful. [21-25]

Good and ill Effects of Alcohol

बहुद्रव्यं बहुगुणं बहुकर्म मदात्मकम्| गुणैर्दोषैश्च तन्मद्यमुभयं चोपलक्ष्यते||२६||

विधिना मात्रया काले हितैरन्नैर्यथाबलम्| प्रहृष्टो यः पिबेन्मद्यं तस्य स्यादमृतं यथा||२७||

यथोपेतं पुनर्मद्यं प्रसङ्गाद्येन पीयते| रूक्षव्यायामनित्येन विषवद्याति तस्य तत्||२८||

Alcoholic drinks are prepared with different types of ingredients; they have different qualities and actions, and they are intoxicating in nature. Therefore, they have both useful and harmful effects.

If taken in an appropriate manner, in the right dose, at an appropriate time, along with a cheerful mind, alcohol works like ambrosia.

If, however, a person drinks whichever type of alcohol is available (without considering its appropriateness), and that too in excess quantity, and if his body is regularly un-unctuous / dry and exhausted because of physical exercise (Vyayama), then it works as a poison. [26- 28]

Attributes of alcohol vis a vis Ojas:

मद्यं हृदयमाविश्य स्वगुणैरोजसो गुणान्| दशभिर्दश सङ्क्षोभ्य चेतो नयति विक्रियाम्||२९||

लघूष्ण तीक्ष्ण सूक्ष्माम्ल व्यवाय्याशुगमेव च| रूक्षं विकाशि विशदं मद्यं दशगुणं स्मृतम्||३०||

गुरु शीतं मृदु श्लक्ष्णं बहलं मधुरं स्थिरम्| प्रसन्नं पिच्छिलं स्निग्धमोजो दशगुणं स्मृतम्||३१||

गुरुत्वं लाघवाच्छैत्यमौष्णादम्ल स्वभावतः| माधुर्यं मार्दवं तैक्ष्ण्यात्प्रसादं चाशुभावनात्||३२||

रौक्ष्यात् स्नेहं व्यवायित्वात् स्थिरत्वं श्लक्ष्णतामपि| विकासिभावात्पैच्छिल्यं वैशद्यात्सान्द्रतां तथा||३३||

सौक्ष्म्यान्मद्यं निहन्त्येवमोजसः स्वगुणैर्गुणान्| सत्त्वं तदाश्रयं चाशु सङ्क्षोभ्य जनयेन्मदम्||३४||

रसवातादिमार्गाणां सत्त्वबुद्धीन्द्रियात्मनाम्| प्रधानस्यौजसश्चैव हृदयं स्थानमुच्यते||३५||

अतिपीतेन मद्येन विहतेनौजसा च तत्| हृदयं याति विकृतिं तत्रस्था ये च धातवः||३६||

Alcohol, while reaching the Hrdaya (heart), afflicts the 10 qualities of Ojas (located in the heart), by virtue of its 10 qualities, giving rise to mental distortions.

Madya Dasha Guna – The 10 qualities of alcohol are

Laghu – light to digest – lightness, Ushna – hot, Tikshna – Sharpness, Sukshma – subtleness, Amla – sourness, Vyavayi – pervasiveness or the quality of a substance which first of all pervades the entire body and thereafter gets digested, Ashuga – Swiftness, Rooksha – Dryness, Vikasi – expansiveness and Vishada (non- sliminess)

The 10 qualities of Ojas are

Guru – heaviness, Sita – cold, Mrudu – softness, Slaksna – smoothness, Bahala – density, Madhura – sweetness, Sthira – Stability, Passanna - clearness or leisureliness, Picchila – Sliminess and Snigdha – unctuousness

The counteraction of Ojas –

Heaviness of Ojas is counteracted by the lightness of alcohol;

The cold attribute of Ojas is counteracted by the heating attribute of alcohol;

The sweet attribute of Ojas is conteracted by sourness of alcohol;

The softness of Ojas is counteracted b the sharpness of alcohol;

The leisureliness or clarity of Ojas is counteracted by the swiftness of alcohol;

The unctuousness of ojas is counteracted by the dryness of alcohol

The stability of Ojas is counteracted by the pervasiveness of alcohol

The smoothness of Ojas is counteracted b the expansiveness of alcohol

The sliminess of Ojas is counteracted by the non sliminess of alcohol and

The density of Ojas is counteracted by the subtleness of alcohol.

Thus, alcohol destroys all the attributes of Ojas which is the abode of Sattva (mind) by Virtue of its 10 attributes, and as result of this affliction, the mind gets agitated, and so causes intoxication.

Heart is the abode (controlling organ) of the channels of circulation of Rasa (plasma), Vata, etc, the Sattva (mind), the Buddhi (wisdom), indriyas (senses), Atman (soul) and Ojas (vital essence) gets destroyed by the excess intake of alcohol, and morbidities appear in the heart and in the Dhatus (Sattva, Etc) Located in it. [29-36]

Affliction of Ojas in Different Stages of Intoxication:

ओजस्यविहते पूर्वो हृदि च प्रतिबोधिते| मध्यमो विहतेऽल्पे च विहते तूत्तमो मदः||३७||

There are 3 stages of intoxication caused by the intake of alcohol during the

First stage, the Ojas (Vital essence) is not afflicted but the heart gets stimulated

Middle stage, Ojas is mildly afflicted, and

Third stage, Ojas is entirely afflicted and produces Mada – intoxication. [37]

Specific Nature of Alcohol Prepared of Cereals (Paishtika)

नैवं विघातं जनयेन्मद्यं पैष्टिकमोजसः| विकाशि रूक्ष विशदा गुणास्तत्र हि नोल्बणाः||३८||

The Paistika type of alcohol (prepared from the paste of cereals) does not cause extreme affliction of the Ojas (Vital Essence), because it is not dominated by attributes like Vikasi (expansiveness), dryness and Vishada (non-sliminess). [38]

Effects of Excessive Intake of Alcohol:

हृदि मद्यगुणाविष्टे हर्षस्तर्षो रतिः सुखम्| विकाराश्च यथासत्त्वं चित्रा राजस तामसाः||३९||

जायन्ते मोह निद्रान्ता मद्यस्यातिनिषेवणात्| स मद्यविभ्रमो नाम्ना 'मद' इत्यभिधीयते||४०||

The heart gets afflicted by the excessive intake of alcohol on account of the attributes of alcohols resulting in

Exhilaration

Passionate desire

Erotic stimulation

Sense of pleasure and

Varieties of psychic morbidities of Rajasika (dynamic) and Tamasika (sluggish) nature depending upon the mental attitude of the person culminating in Moha- Nidra (Coma)

This mental perversion caused by alcohol (Madya-Vidhrama) is called Mada or Intoxication.

Prathama Mada – First Stage of Alcoholic Intoxication:

पीयमानस्य मद्यस्य विज्ञातव्यास्त्रयो मदाः| प्रथमो मध्यमोऽन्त्यश्च लक्षणैस्तान् प्रचक्ष्महे||४१||

प्रहर्षणः प्रीतिकरः पानान्नगुणदर्शकः| वाद्यगीत प्रहासानां कथानां च प्रवर्तकः||४२||

न च बुद्धि स्मृतिहरो विषयेषु न चाक्षमः| सुखनिद्रा प्रबोधश्च प्रथमः सुखदो मदः||४३||

Intake of alcohol results in 3 stages of intoxication, viz, the beginning (first), the middle (second), and the last (third) stages;their characteristic features will be described hereafter.

The first stage is characterised by

Praharshana – Exhilaration

Priti karah – Passion

Pana anna guna darshakah – Proper manifestation of the attributes of food and drinks, and

Vadya gita praharshanam kathanam cha pravartaka – Creativity of music, song, humour and stories

Na cha buddhi smrti haro viṣayeṣu na cākṣamaḥ – It does not impair wisdom and memory and does not cause inability for the senses to perceive their objects.

This first stage of intoxication results in Sukha nidra (sound sleep) and post –waking feeling of freshness. Thus, this stage of intoxication brings happiness [41- 43]

Dwiteeya Mada – Second Stage of Alcoholic intoxication:

मुहुः स्मृति मुहुर्मोहो(s)व्यक्ता सज्जति वाइमुहुः| युक्तायुक्त प्रलापश्च प्रचलायनमेव च||४४||

स्थानपानान्नसाइकथ्ययोजना सविपर्यया| लिङ्गान्येतानि जानीयादाविष्टे मध्यमे मदे||४५||

During the second stage of intoxication, the person often remembers things and often forgets them. His voice becomes inarticulate and confused, and speaks sense and nonsense simultaneously.

His movement, posture, drinking, eating and talking are all appropriately funny these are the signs and symptoms of the second stage of intoxication. [44- 45]

Truteeya madatyaya Lakshana – Third Stage of Alcoholic Intoxication:

मध्यमं मदमुत्क्रम्य मदमाप्राप्य चोत्तमम्| न किञ्चिन्नाशुभं कुर्युर्नरा राजस तामसाः||४६||

को मदं ताद‌शं विद्वानुन्मादमिव दारुणम्| गच्छेदध्वानमस्वन्तं बहुदोषमिवाध्वगः||४७||

तृतीयं तु मदं प्राप्य भग्नदार्विव निष्क्रियः| मद मोहावृतमना जीवन्नपि मृतैः समः||४८||

रमणीयान् स विषयान्न वेत्ति न सुहृज्जनम्| यदर्थं पीयते मद्यं रतिं तां च न विन्दति||४९||

कार्याकार्य सुखं दुःखं लोके यच्च हिताहितम्| यदवस्थो न जानाति कोऽवस्थां तां व्रजेद्बुधः||५०||

स दूष्यः सर्वभूतानां निन्द्यश्चाग्राह्य एव च| व्यसनित्वादुदर्के च स दुःखं व्याधिमश्नुते||५१||

Truteeya mada Lakshana – Third Stage of Alcoholic Intoxication:

After crossing the second stage and in the beginning of the third stage, there comes a stage when the person is afflicted with Rajas and Tamas. This stage predisposes the person to serious complications like insanity. This can be compared to a person walking to an unhappy destination with a lot of dangers. So, a wise person would not subject himself as a victim of that stage.

At the third stage of Madatyaya, a person becomes inactive like a broken tree with his mind afflicted with intoxicating morbid deities and unconsciousness though alive, he resembles a dead person.

He becomes incapable of recognizing pleasing things and friends. He is soon deprived of all happiness for which he had taken alcohol in this stage of intoxication. He loses the very sense of distinction of rightful, happy and useful items from the wrong, miserable and harmful ones respectively.

No wise person will ever like to place himself in such a stage of intoxication. He is condemned and censured by all persons, and disliked by them. As the natural outcome of this indulgence, he suffers from miseries and diseases of alcoholism all the time [46- 51]

Adverse effects of Alcohol:

प्रेत्य चेह च यच्छ्रेयः श्रेयो मोक्षे च यत् परम्| मनःसमाधौ तत् सर्वमायत्तं सर्व देहिनाम्||५२||

मद्येन मनसश्चास्य सङ्क्षोभः क्रियते महान्| महामारुत वेगेन तटस्थस्येव शाखिनः||५३||

मद्य प्रसङ्गं तं चाज्ञा महादोषं महागदम्| सुखमित्यधिगच्छन्ति रजो मोहपराजिताः||५४||

मद्योपहतविज्ञाना वियुक्ताः सात्विकैर्गुणैः| श्रेयोभिर्विप्रयुज्यन्ते मदान्धा मदलालसाः||५५||

मद्ये मोहो भयं शोकः क्रोधो मृत्युश्च संश्रितः| सोन्मादमदमूर्च्छायाः सापस्मारापतानकाः||५६||

यत्रैकः स्मृतिविभ्रंशस्तत्र सर्वमसाधुवत्| इत्येवं मद्यदोषज्ञा मद्यं गर्हन्ति यत्नतः||५७||

Whatever is useful after death, whatsoever is good for the present life, and whatsoever is supreme for attaining salvation are based on the tranquillity of the mind of an individual. Alcohol considerably agitates this mind as a strong wind shakes the tree located on the bank of a river.

Unwise people, ignorant of the serious adverse effects of alcohol and serious nature of intoxication (mahagada), being impelled by Rajas and Moha (illusion), consider indulgence in drinking alcohol as a source of happiness

Their minds get afflicted by the adverse effects of alcohol and become derived from the Sattvika qualities. These people, with a craving for intoxication, become blinded by alcohol, and lose all happiness of life.

Illusion, fear, grief, anger and death and diseases like insanity, intoxication, fainting, epilepsy and apatanaka (convulsion) are caused by alcohol.

Wherever there is impairment of memory, all the evil deeds are manifested there. Because of this; people acquainted with the adverse effects of alcohol vehemently condemn its drinking. [52-57]

Food Value of Alcohol:

सत्यमेते महादोषा मद्यस्योक्ता न संशयः| अहितस्यातिमात्रस्य पीतस्य विधि वर्जितम्||५८||

किन्तु मद्यं स्वभावेन यथैवान्नं तथा स्मृतम्| अयुक्तियुक्तं रोगाय युक्तियुक्तं यथाऽमृतम्||५९||

प्राणाः प्राणभृतामन्नं तदयुक्त्या निहन्त्यसून्| विषं प्राणहरं तच्च युक्तियुक्तं रसायनम्||६०||

Food Value of Alcohol:

The serious adverse effects of alcohol described above are undoubtedly true. Such adverse effects are produced when an unwholesome type of alcohol is taken in excess quantity without observing the appropriate procedure.

But alcohol is like food which when taken in excess quantity without observing the appropriate procedure can result in diseases. Alcohol, like food, when taken appropriately, is like ambrosia (Amruta).

For all living beings, food is the sustainer of life, but when taken inappropriately, it causes death. Similarly, poison which causes death works like Rasayana (rejuvenating agent) when used appropriately [58- 60]

Good effects of Alcohol Taken in appropriate manner:

हर्षमूर्जं मुदं पुष्टिमारोग्यं पौरुषं परम् | युक्त्या पीतं करोत्याशु मद्यं सुखमदप्रदम्||६१||

Alcohol taken in appropriate manner produces

• Harsha – Exhilaration

• Urja – energy

• Mudam – happiness (mental satisfaction),

• Pushti – nourishment,

• Aarogyam – good health,

• Paurushyam – excellent virility and

• Sukha madya – pleasant intoxication instantaneously. [61]

In Praise of Alcohol Taken Appropriately

रोचनं दीपनं हृद्यं स्वर वर्णं प्रसादनम्| प्रीणनं बृंहणं बल्यं भय शोक श्रमापहम्||६२||

स्वापनं नष्ट निद्राणां मूकानां वाग्विबोधनम्| बोधनं चातिनिद्राणां विबद्धानां विबन्धनुत्||६३||

वध बन्ध परिक्लेश दुःखानां चाप्यबोधनम्| मद्योत्थानां च रोगाणां मद्यमेव प्रबाधकम्||६४||

रतिर्विषयसंयोगे प्रीतिसंयोगवर्धनम्| अपि प्रवयसां मद्यमुत्सवामोदकारकम्||६५||

पञ्चस्वर्थेषु कान्तेषु या रतिः प्रथमे मदे| यूनां वा स्थविराणां वा तस्य नास्त्युपमा भुवि||६६||

बहुदुःखहतस्यास्य शोकेनोपहतस्य च| विश्रामो जीव लोकस्य मद्यं युक्त्या निषेवितम्||६७||

Alcohol taken appropriately produces invigorating effects as follows:

It promotes Rochana (appetite), Dipanam (stimulates the power of digestion), Hrdyam (tones up the heart), promotes Svara (voice) and Varna (complexion), Prasadanam (produces the feeling of refreshment) and Prinanam (corpulence), balyam (increases strength), and removes Bhaya (fear), Shoka (grief) and Shrama (fatigue).

Patients suffering from insomnia enjoy sound sleep by taking alcohol and it stimulates speech in dumb persons (Mooka = lit dumb);

It helps persons having excessive sleep to remain awake and causes bowel movement in constipated patients

It renders the mind insensitive to the miseries of injury, imprisonment and fatigue.

Alcohol itself cures the diseases caused by its excessive and inappropriate intake.

It represents erotic passion, and when associated with an object, it promotes the association of pleasure in it.

It stimulates passion and hilarity even in persons of old age

The enjoyment derived from the 5 enjoyable objects of senses by the young or old during the first stage of alcoholic intoxication has no parallel in this world and

it provides respite to persons afflicted with multitudinous suffering and grief. [62-67]

Appropriateness of Alcohol Intake

अन्नपान वयो व्याधि बलकाल त्रिकाणि षट्| त्रीन्दोषांस्त्रिविधं सत्त्वं ज्ञात्वा मद्यं पिबेत्सदा||६८||

तेषां त्रिकाणामष्टानां योजना युक्तिरुच्यते| यया युक्त्या पिबन्मद्यं मद्यदोषैर्न युज्यते||६९||

मद्यस्य च गुणान् सर्वान् यथोक्तान् स समश्नुते| धर्मार्थयोरपीडायै नरः सत्वगुणोच्छ्रितः||७०||

सत्वानि तु प्रबुध्यन्ते प्रायशः प्रथमे मदे| द्वितीयेऽव्यक्ततां यान्ति मध्ये चोत्तम मध्ययोः||७१||

सस्य सम्बोधकं वर्ष, हेम प्रकृति दर्शकः| हुताशः, सर्वसत्वानां मद्यं तूभयकारकम्||७२||

प्रधानावरमध्यानां रूपाणां व्यक्ति दर्शकः| यथाऽग्निरेवं सत्वानां मद्यं प्रकृति दर्शकम्||७३||

One should always drink alcohol with due regard to the 3 varieties of each of the 6 factors, viz food, drinks, age, diseases, strength and season and of the Doshas and mental faculties.

Proper application of the triads of these 8 factors is called Yukti or appropriateness in view, and then a person does not suffer from the evil effects of drinking. On the other hand, he with his exalted state of mind enjoys all the good effects of alcohol as stated before without endangering Dharma (religious virtues) and Artha (satisfaction of senses). During the first stage of intoxication, the mental facilities generally get stimulated.

During the second stage and in between the second and third stages of intoxication, these faculties get suppressed or become un-manifested.

Simile – As the rain stimulates the growth of crops, and fire demonstrates the real nature (Purity) of gold, similarly, alcohol both stimulates and demonstrates the minds of all creatures.

As fire demonstrates the nature of superior, medium and inferior qualities of gold, similarly alcohol demonstrates the characteristic features of the (different types of) mind. [68- 73]

Effects of Alcohol on Sattvika, Rajasika and Tamasika Faculties:

सुगन्धिमाल्य गन्धर्व सुप्रणीतममाकुलम्| मिष्टान्नपान विशदं सदा मधुर सङ्कथम्||७४||

सुख प्रपानं सुमदं हर्ष प्रीति विवर्धनम्| स्वन्तं सात्विकमापानं न चोत्तममदप्रदम्||७५||

वैगुण्यं सहसा यान्ति मद्य दोषैर्न सात्विकाः| मद्यं हि बलवत्सत्वं गृह्णाति सहसा न तु ||७६||

सौम्यासौम्य कथाप्रायं विशदाविशदं क्षणात्| चित्रं राजसमापन्नं प्रायेणास्वन्तकाकुलम्||७७||

हर्ष प्रीति कथापेतमतुष्टं पानभोजने| सम्मोह क्रोध निद्रान्तमापानं तामसं स्मृतम्||७८||

A person having Sattvika type of mental faculty drinks alcohol while wearing aromatic garlands and while hearing songs. The alcohol he takes is well prepared and not polluted. While taking alcohol, he takes wholesome and delicious food as well as drinks, while drinking alcohol, he always engages himself in delightful conversations. He takes alcohol in a happy mood leading to a pleasing type of intoxication which promotes cheerfulness and poison. It terminates as a pleasing event, and it does not lead to the third stage of intoxication. Sattvika type of persons do not exhibit perverted activities immediately after taking alcohol because alcohol is incapable of adversely afflicting the powerful minds of Sattvika persons instantaneously.

A person having Rajasik type of mental faculty generally talks some time gently and at times rudely, some time distinctly and at times indistinctly, and so demonstrates his irregular varieties of behaviours after taking alcohol. It terminates as a tragic event.

A person having Tamasika type of mental faculty, after taking alcohol, becomes excited and passionate in his talks, he never gets satisfaction in eating and drinking, and his alcoholic intoxication terminates in unconsciousness, anger and sleep. [74- 78]

Friends to be associated while Drinking Alcohol:

आपाने सात्विकान् बुद्ध्वा तथा राजस तामसान्| जह्यात्सहायान् यैः पीत्वा मद्य दोषानुपाश्नुते||७९||

While drinking alcohol, one should ascertain the Satvika, Rajasika and Tamasika nature of the friends (keeping company in drinking) and should avoid the company of the Rajasika and Tamasika types of friends, because drinking along with them may lead to the transgression of alcohol quantity which may result in the adverse effects of alcohol. [79]

Characteristics of Good Friends for Company during Drinking Alcohol:

सुखशीलाः सुसम्भाषाः सुमुखाः सम्मताः सताम्| कलास्वबाह्या विशदा विषय प्रवणाश्च ये||८०||

परस्पर विधेया ये येषामैक्यं सुहृत्तया| प्रहर्ष प्रीति माधुर्यैरापानं वर्धयन्ति ये||८१||

उत्सवादुत्सवतरं येषामन्योन्यदर्शनम्| ते सहायाः सुखाः पाने तैः पिबन्सह मोदते||८२||

Persons who are pleasure-loving, who talk pleasantly, who are amiable in disposition, who are admired by the wise, who have artistic talent, who are friendly, who are experts in different fields of knowledge, who are sympathetic to each other, who are united because of sincere friendship, who promote the good effects of alcohol by their joyful attitude, affection and sweetness, and whose company provide more and more of delightfulness among each other are the best friends to (Keep company with). One derives maximum delight in drinking alcohol in their company. [80-82]

Good environment for Drinking Alcohol:

रूप गन्ध रस स्पर्शैः शब्दैश्चापि मनोरमैः| पिबन्ति सुसहाया ये ते वै सुकृतिभिः समाः||८३||

पञ्चभिर्विषयैरिष्टैरुपेतैर्मनसः प्रियैः| देशे काले पिबेन्मद्यं प्रहृष्टेनान्तरात्मना||८४||

Persons who drink alcohol in the company of good friends while enjoying the easing objects of senses like sight, smell, taste, touch and sound are [really fortune] like the most virtuous ones.

One should drink alcohol with happiness of the mind (soul), at an appropriate time with the pleasing environment represented by the most enjoyable objects of the 5 senses organs. [83- 84]

Persons who do not get Intoxicated Easily:

स्थिर सत्व शरीरा ये पूर्वान्ना मद्यपान्वयाः| बहुमद्योचिता ये च माद्यन्ति सहसा न ते||८५||

Persons having strong mind and stable body, who have taken food before drinking alcohol, the person born in a family accustomed to drink alcohol, and those who are accustomed to take large quantities of alcohol regularly (addict) do not get intoxicated by alcohol immediately [85]

People who get intoxicated very quickly:

क्षुत्पिपासा परीताश्च दुर्बला वात पैत्तिकाः| रूक्षाल्प प्रमिताहारा विष्टब्धाः सत्व दुर्बलाः||८६||

क्रोधिनोऽनुचिताः क्षीणाः परिश्रान्ता मद क्षताः| स्वल्पेनापि मदं शीघ्रं यान्ति मद्येन मानवाः||८७||

Persons who are afflicted with hunger and thirst, who are weak, who are of Vatika and Paittika types of constitution, who are given to dry food, less of food and limited quantity of food, who are constipated, who are weak mind, who are wrathful in nature, who are not accustomed to taking alcohol, who are weak and fatigued, and who are afflicted by alcoholism, get intoxicated quickly after drinking alcohol even in small quantity. [86-87].

Etiology, signs and symptoms of Vatika Madatyaya:

ऊर्ध्वं मदात्ययस्यातः सम्भवं स्वस्वलक्षणम्| अग्निवेश! चिकित्सां च प्रवक्ष्यामि यथाक्रमम्||८८||

स्त्री शोक भय भाराध्व कर्मभिर्योऽतिकर्शितः| रूक्षाल्प प्रमिताशी च यः पिबत्यतिमात्रया||८९||

रूक्षं परिणतं मद्यं निशि निद्रां विहत्य च| करोति तस्य तच्छीघ्रं वात प्रायं मदात्ययम्||९०||

हिक्का श्वास शिरःकम्प पार्श्वशूल प्रजागरैः| विद्याद्बहु प्रलापस्य वात प्रायं मदात्ययम्||९१||

O! Agnivesha, I shall explain seriatim the aetiology, signs and symptoms and treatment of (the various types of) Madataya (alcoholic intoxication).

If a person excessively emaciated because of indulgence in women, grief, fear, carrying heavy load, walking long distance and other strenuous activities, while eating dry food, less quantity of food or limited quantity of food, drinks alcohol which is dry in nature and which is excessively fomented, at night, then this leads to the impairment of his sleep, and Vatika type of Madatyaya instantaneously.

This Vatika type of Madataya is characterized by signs and symptoms like

Hikka – hiccup, Shvasa – Asthma

Shira kampa – Tremors in the head

Parshva shoola – pain in the sides of the chest

Nidra nasha – insomnia and

Pralapa – Delirium in excess [88- 91]

Pittaja Madatyaya Nidana Lakshana:

तीक्ष्णोष्णं मद्यमम्लं च योऽतिमात्रं निषेवते| अम्लोष्णतीक्ष्णभोजी च क्रोधनोऽग्न्यातपप्रियः||९२||

तस्योपजायते पित्तादिविशेषेण मदात्ययः| स तु वातोल्बणस्याशु प्रशमं याति हन्ति वा||९३||

तृष्णा दाह ज्वर स्वेद मूर्च्छातीसार विभ्रमैः| विद्याद्धरित वर्णस्य पित्तप्रायं मदात्ययम्||९४||

Etiology, signs and symptoms of Paittika Madatyaya:

If a person, indulging in food which is sour, hot and Tikshna (sharp), having wrathful disposition, and having liking for excessive expose to the fire and sun, drinks excess quantity of alcohol which is Tikshna (sharp), heat- producing and sour, then he suffers from Paittika type of Madatyaya.

If this Paittika type of Madatyaya is also dominated by aggravated Vata, then the ailment may either get cured immediately or may cause instantaneous death.

This Paittika type of Madataya is characterised by signs and symptoms like

Trshna – Morbid thirst

Daha – burning sensation

Jvara – fever

Sweda – sweating

Murchha – fainting

Atisara – diarrhoea

Vibhrama – giddiness and

Harita varna – green coloration of the body [92-94]

Kaphaja Madatyaya Nidana, Lakshana:

तरुणं मधुर प्रायं गौडं पैष्टिकमेव वा| मधुर स्निग्ध गुर्वाशी यः पिबत्यतिमात्रगा||९५||

अव्यायाम दिवास्वप्न शय्यासनसुखे रतः| मदात्ययं कफप्रायं स शीघ्रमधिगच्छति||९६||

छर्द्यरोचक हृल्लास तन्द्रा स्तैमित्य गौरवैः| विद्याच्छीतपरीतस्य कफप्रायं मदात्ययम्||९७||

Aetiology, Signs and Symptoms of Kaphaja Madatyaya:

If a person who is habituated to sweet, unctuous and heavy food, who does not undertake exercise, who sleeps during the day- time, and indulges in the comforts of beds and seats, excessively drinks alcohol which is not fermented well or which in generally sweet in taste like Gauda (alcohol prepared of Guda or Jaggery) and Paistika (alcohol prepared of the assets of cereals), then he immediately develops Madatyaya dominated by Kapha.

Kaphaja type of Madatyaya is characterised by the signs and symptoms like

Chardi – vomiting

Arochaka – anorexia

Hrllasa – Nausea

Tandra – drowsiness

Staimitya – timidity

Gaurava – heaviness and chilliness [95- 97]

Sannipatika Nature of all the Madatyaya (Alcoholism):

विषस्य ये गुणा दृष्टाः सन्निपात प्रकोपणाः| त एव मद्ये दृश्यन्ते विषे तु बलवत्तराः||९८||

हन्त्याशु हि विषं किञ्चित् किञ्चिद्रोगाय कल्पते| यथा विषं तथैवान्त्यो ज्ञेयो मद्यकृतो मदः||९९||

तस्मात् त्रिदोषजं लिङ्गं सर्वत्रापि मदात्यये| दृश्यते रूप वैशेष्यात् पृथक्त्वं चास्य लक्ष्यते||१००||

Qualities of Visha (poison) which cause aggravation of all the 3 Doshas (Sannipata) are also found in the alcohol, the only difference being in poison, these attributes are more powerful.

Poison at times, causes death, and at times, causes diseases in the afflicted person. Like poison, the intoxicating effect of alcohol, at times, leads to death and, at times, causes diseases as the ultimate effect. Therefore, in all types of Madatyaya, the signs and symptoms of all the 3 Doshas are manifested. But on the basis of the specific nature or predominance of the signs and symptoms of a Dosha, these ailments are classified into different types [namely Vatika, Paittika and Kaphaja Madatyaya] [98- 100]

Signs and Symptoms of Madatyaya (Alcoholism) in General:

शरीर दुःखं बलवत् सम्मोहो हृदयव्यथा| अरुचिः प्रतता तृष्णा ज्वरः शीतोष्ण लक्षणः||१०१||

शिरःपार्श्वास्थि सन्धीनां विद्युत्तुल्या च वेदना| जायतेऽतिबला जृम्भा स्फुरणं वेपनं श्रमः||१०२||

उरो विबन्धः कासश्च हिक्का श्वासः प्रजागरः| शरीर कम्पः कर्णाक्षि मुखरोगस्त्रिकग्रहः||१०३||

छर्द्यतीसार हृल्लासा वात पित्त कफात्मकाः| भ्रमः प्रलापो रूपाणामसतां चैव दर्शनम्||१०४||

तृण भस्म लता पर्ण पांशुभिश्चावपूरणम्| प्रधर्षणं विहङ्गैश्च भ्रान्तचेताः स मन्यते||१०५||

व्याकुलानाम शस्तानां स्वप्नानां दर्शनानि च| मदात्ययस्य रूपाणि सर्वाण्येतानि लक्षयेत्||१०६||

All the signs and symptoms manifested in Madatyaya are as follows:

Sharira dukha – Excruciating pain in the body

Sammoha – Unconsciousness

Hrdi vyatha – pain in the cardiac region

Aruchi – anorexia and

Pratata trshna – incessant thirst

Shita ushna jvara – Fever having the characteristics of cold and heat

Shirah, pārśvāsthi sandhīnām vidyuttulyā ca vedanā – Lightening pain in the head, sides of the chest, bones and joints

Ati jrmbha – severe yawning, Sphuranam – throbbing, Vepanam – twitching, Shrama – Fatigue

Uro vibandha – obstruction in the chest

Kasa – coughing, Hikka – hiccup, Shvasa – Asthma

Prajagaran – insomnia and Sharira kampa – trembling of the body

Karna akshi mukha roga – Diseases of the ears, eyes and mouth

Trika graha – Stiffness of the Trika (sacro- iliac joint)

Chardi – Vomiting,

Atisara – diarrhoea and

Vata, pitta , kapha hrllasa – Nausea caused by Vata, Pitta and Kapha

Bhrama – Giddiness, Pralapa – delirium and

Rupanam cha mastanam cha darshana – Visualisation of non- existing objects

tṛṇa bhasma latā parṇa pāṃśubhiścāvapūraṇam – Feeling as if the body is covered with grass, ash, creepers, leaves and dust and dashing of birds over the body because of bewilderment and

pradharṣaṇaṃ vihaṅgaiśca bhrāntacetāḥ sa manyate – Dreaming of terrifying and inauspicious objects [101- 106]

Madatyaya Chikitsa Sutra:

सर्व मदात्ययं विद्यात् त्रिदोषमधिकं तु यम्| दोष मदात्यये पश्येत् तस्यादौ प्रतिकारयेत्||१०७||

कफस्थानानुपूर्व्या च क्रिया कार्या मदात्यये| पित्त मारुत पर्यन्तः प्रायेण हि मदात्ययः||१०८||

मिथ्यातिहीनपीतेन यो व्याधिरुपजायते| समपीतेन तेनैव स मद्येनोपशाम्यति||१०९||

जीर्णममद्यदोषाय मद्यमेव प्रदापयेत्| प्रकाङ्क्षालाघवे जाते यद्यदस्मै हितं भवेत्||११०||

सौवर्चलानुसंविद्धं शीतं सबिड सैन्धवम्| मातुलुङ्गार्द्रकोपेतं जलयुक्तं प्रमाणवित् ||१११||

Line of treatment

All the types of Madatyaya are caused by the vitiation of all the 3 Doshas. In the beginning, treatment is given for the most predominant Dosha. If all the Doshas are equally aggravated, the treatment is started from the location of Kapha, followed by that of Pitta, and lastly that of Vata.

The ailments caused by the drinking of alcohol in wrongful manner or in excess quantity or in less quantity can be cured by taking the same alcohol in appropriate manner and quantity.

After the morbidity caused by the immaturity of the digestion and metabolism of alcohol is overcome by its proper digestion and metabolism, when the patient desires to have food and drinks, and when there is a feeling of lightness of the body, he is given alcohol which is cooling in effect, which is added with Bida and Saindhava types of salt, and which is diluted with the juice of Matulunga – Lemon variety – Citrus decumana / Citrus lemon and water by a physician well versed with posology i.e. appropriate quantity. [107- 111]

Justification of Giving Alcohol in Alcoholism

तीक्ष्णोष्णेनातिमात्रेण पीतेनाम्ल विदाहिना| मद्येनान्नरसोत्क्लेदो विदग्धः क्षारतां गतः||११२||

अन्तर्दाहं ज्वरं तृष्णां प्रमोहं विभ्रमं मदम्| जनयत्याशु तच्छान्त्यै मद्यमेव प्रदापयेत्||११३||

क्षारो हि याति माधुर्यं शीघ्रमम्लोपसंहितः| श्रेष्ठमम्लेषु मद्यं च यैर्गुणैस्तान् परं शृणु||११४||

मद्यस्याम्लस्वभावस्य चत्वारोऽनुरसाः स्मृताः| मधुरश्च कषायश्च तिक्तः कटुक एव च||११५||

गुणाश्च दश पूर्वोक्तास्तैश्चतुर्दशभिर्गुणैः| सर्वेषां मद्यमम्लानामुपर्युपरि तिष्ठति||११६||

Intake of excessive alcohol which is Teekshna (sharp), hot , sour and Vidahi (causing burning sensation) makes the Anna Rasa (juice of the food after digestion) sticky and improperly digested (Vidagdha) which ultimately turns alkaline (Ksara), and causes Antardaha (Burning sensation in the interior of the body), Jwara (fever), Trishna (thirst), Pramoha (unconsciousness), Vibhrama (giddiness) and Madam (intoxication) instantaneously.

To correct these ailments, alcohol is administered because when an alkaline substance (Ksara) gets mixed with a sour substance, the outcome becomes sweet in taste, and alcohol is the best among the articles having sour taste.

Now, hear about the attributes of alcohol which make it best among the sour articles. Alcohol by nature is sour and it has 4 subsidiary tastes like sweet, astringent, bitter and pungent. Thus, along with the ten attributes described before (in verse no 31), alcohol has 14 qualities in total. It is because of these 14 attributes; alcohol stands supreme among all the sour articles. [112- 116]

Pathogenesis and Treatment of Vatika Madatyaya:

मद्योत्क्लिष्टेन दोषेण रुद्धः स्रोतःसु मारुतः| करोति वेदनां तीव्रां शिरस्य स्थिषु सन्धिषु||११७||

दोष विष्यन्दनार्थं हि तस्मै मद्यं विशेषतः| व्यवायि तीक्ष्णोष्णतया देयमम्ले(न्ये)षु सत्स्वपि||११८||

स्रोतो विबन्धनुन्मद्यं मारुतस्यानुलोमनम्| रोचनं दीपनं चाग्नेरभ्यासात् सात्म्यमेव च||११९||

रुजः स्रोतःस्वरुद्धेषु मारुते चानुलोमिते| निवर्तन्ते विकाराश्च शाम्यन्त्यस्य मदोदयाः||१२०||

Pathogenesis and Treatment of Vatika Madatyaya:

The Dosha incited by alcohol causes obstruction of the movement of Vata in the channels of circulation as a result of which the patient suffers from tivra shira asthi, sandhi shoola – excruciating pain in the head, bones and joints.

In spite of the availability of other sour ingredients, alcohol should specifically be administered to such a patient for causing melting and elimination of the Doshas because of its Vyavayi (diffusive), Tikshna (sharp) and hot attributes.

Alcohol removes:

Sroto vibandha (obstruction in the channels of circulation)

Marutasya anuloman – helps in the downward movement of Vata,

Rochana – acts as an appetiser,

Dipanam – stimulates the power of digestion, and

Satmya – becomes wholesome when consumed habitually.

When the obstruction in the channels is removed, and Vata moves downwards, the pain subsides and the ailments caused by alcoholism get cured. [117- 120]

Recipe for Vatika Madatyay:

बीजपूरक वृक्षाम्ल कोल दाडिम संयुतम्‌| यवानी हपुषाजाजी शृङ्गवेरावचूर्णितम्‌||१२१||

सस्नेहैः शक्तुभिर्युक्तमवदंशैर्विरोचितम्‌ | दद्यात्‌ स लवणं मद्यं पैष्टिकं वात शान्तये||१२२||

For the alleviation of Vayu, alcohol prepared of the

Paistika- Madya – paste of cereals mixed with

Bija- Puraka – Citrus medica

Vrksamla – Garcinia gummigatta

Kola – Zizyphus jujuba and

Dadima – pomegranate and

Sprinkled with the powder of

Yavani – Trachyspermum ammi

Hapusa – Juniperus communis

Ajaji – Cuminum cyminum and

Sringavera – ginger is taken along with salt.

While taking this alcohol, the patient should take delicious snacks prepared of Saktu (roasted flour of cereals) by adding ghee. [121- 122]

Meat soup for Vatika Madatyaya

दृष्ट्वा वातोल्बणं लिङ्गं रसैश्चैनमुपाचरेत्‌| लाव तित्तिर दक्षाणां स्निग्धाम्लैः शिखिनामपि||१२३||

पक्षिणां मृग मत्स्यानामानूपानां च संस्कृतैः| भूशय प्रसहानां च रसैः शाल्योदनेन च||१२४||

After observing the signs and symptoms of aggravated Vata Dosha in the patient suffering from alcoholism, he is given the soup of the meat of Lava, Tittiri – Patridge, chicken and peacock, or birds, animals and fish inhabiting marshy land and burrows (Bhusaya) and of the meat of Prasaha (those who eat their food by hunting / beast or bird of prey) type of animals with Shali types of rice. [123- 124]

Vesavara and Pan-Cakes for Vatika Alcoholism:

स्निग्धोष्ण लवणाम्लैश्च वेशवारैर्मुखप्रियैः| चित्रै गौधूमिकैश्चान्नै वारुणी मण्ड संयुतैः ||१२५||

पिशितार्द्रक गर्भाभिः स्निग्धाभिः पूपवर्तिभिः| माष पूपलिकाभिश्च वातिकं समुपाचरेत्‌||१२६||

The person suffering from Vatika type of alcoholism is given delicious Vesara (a type of appetiser) added with ghee, hot (pungent) ingredients, salt and sour articles.

He is given different food articles prepared of wheat by adding Varuni (a type of alcohol), Pupa- Vartis (Scrolls) stuffed with meat and ginger, and made unctuous by adding ghee are useful for him. Pupalikas (pan- cakes) prepared of Masha are also useful for Vatika type of alcoholism. [125- 126]

Meat and pastries for Vatika Alcoholism:

नाति स्निग्धं न चाम्लेन युक्तं समरिचार्द्रकम्‌| मेद्यं प्रागुदितं मांसं दाडिम स्वरसेन वा||१२७||

पृथ्विक्रजातकोपेतं स धान्य मरिचार्द्रकम्‌| रस प्रलेपि सम्पूपैः सुखोष्णैः सम्प्रदापयेत्‌||१२८||

Meat of the fatty animals described before (in verse nos 123- 124) which is neither too unctuous nor sour is added with black pepper and ginger, and given to the patient along with the juice of Dadima – Pomegranate.

Pastries smeared with sugar syrup (Rasa- pralepi) which are luke- warm, and which are added with Trijataka (Cinnamon, cardamom and cinnamon leaves), Dhanya, and Maricha – Black pepper fruit and is given to such a patient. [127- 128]

Post- Prandial Drinks for Vatika Madatyaya

भुक्ते तु वारुणी मण्डं दद्यात्‌ पातुं पिपासवे| दाडिमस्य रसं वाऽपि जलं वा पाञ्चमूलिकम्‌||१२९||

धान्य नागर तोयं च दधिमण्डमथापि वा| अम्ल काञ्जिक मण्डं वा शुक्तोदकमथापि वा||१३०||

After taking food if the patient feels thirsty, he is given supernatant part of the Varuni type of wine or the juice of Dadima – Pomegranate or the decoction of panchamoola (the roots of Bilva – bael, Syonaka – Oroxylum indicum, Gambhari – Gmelina arborea, patala – Stereospermum suaveolens and Ganikarika –Premna integrifolia) or the decoction of Dhanya and Nagara or the supernatant part of curd or the supernatant part of sour Kanji (a sour drink) or vinegar to drink [129- 130]

Effects of Therapies:

कर्मणाऽनेन सिद्धेन विकार उपशाम्यति| मात्राकालप्रयुक्तेन बलं वर्णश्च वर्धते||१३१||

The above mentioned effective therapeutic measures administered in appropriate dose and time, the ailment gets cured. These measures also help in the promotion of strength and complexion of the patient. [131]

Other Regimes for Vatika Madatyaya:

राग षाडव संयोगै र्विविधै भंक्त रोचनैः| पिशितैः शाक पिष्टान्नैर्यव गोधूम शालिभिः||१३२||

अभ्यङ्गोत्सादनैः स्नानैरुष्णैः प्रावरणैर्घनैः| घनेरगुरुपङ्कैश्च धूपैश्चागुरुजैर्घनैः||१३३||

नारीणां यौवनोष्णानां निर्देयैरुपगूहनैः| श्रोण्यूरुकुचभारैश्च संरोधोष्णसुखावहैः||१३४||

शयनाच्छादनैरुष्णैरुष्णैश्चान्तर्गृहैः सुखैः| मारुतप्रबलः शीघ्रं प्रशाम्यति मदात्ययः||१३५||

Madatayaya caused by the predominantly aggravated vata gets immediately cured by the following regimens:
1. Intake of meat, vegetable preparations, Pastries, Barley, wheat and Shali- rice mixed with different types of appetising Ragas and Shadava (pungent, sour and Saline reparations)
2. Massage, unction and bath with hot ingredients
3. Wearing of thick blankets
4. Application of thick paste of Aguru – Aquilaria agallocha, and thick fumigation with smoke of Aguru
5. Strong embracement of ladies having the warmth of youth, and enjoying of the warmth
6. Use of warm beds and bed-sheets and
7. Enjoyment of the happiness of the interior apartments which are warm [132- 135]

Treatment for Paittkia Madatyaya:

Drinks for Paittika Madatyaya:

भव्य खर्जूर मृद्वीका परूषक रसैर्युतम्| स दाडिम रसं शीतं सक्तुभिश्चावचूर्णितम्||१३६||

सशर्करं शार्करं वा माद्वीकमथवाऽपरम्| दद्याद्बहूदकं काले पातुं पित्त मदात्यये||१३७||

In the alcoholism caused by Pitta, the patient is given in appropriate time, Sarkara (made of sugar) or Mrdvika (made of grapes) types of alcohol added with sugar along with the juice of Bhavya Kharjura, Mrdvika and parusaka, or along with the Juice of Dadima – Pomegranate, after making them cool, after sprinkling Saktu (roasted flour of cereals) over them and after diluting with large quantity of water. [136- 137]

Food for Patitika Alcoholism:

शशान् कपिञ्जलानेणाँल्लावानसितपुच्छकान्| मधुराम्लान् प्रयुञ्जीत भोजने शालि षष्टिकान्||१३८||

The patient suffering from paittika alcoholism should take the meat of Shasha, Kapinjala, Ena, Lava and Asita Puccha, Sweet and sour ingredients and Shali and Sastika types of rice as food. [138]

Soups for Paittika Alcoholism:

पटोल यूषमिश्रं वा छागलं कल्पयेद्रसम्| सतीन मुद्गमिश्रं वा दाडिमामलकान्वितम्||१३९||

द्राक्षामलक खर्जूर परूषक रसेन वा| कल्पयेत्तर्पणान् यूषान् रसांश्च विविधात्मकान्||१४०||

The soup of the meat of goat is prepared by adding the soup of Patola or the soup of Satina and Mudga, and mixed with Dadima – Pomegranate and Amalaka – Phyllanthus emblica. Similarly, different types of Tarpanas (refreshing drinks), Yusha (soup) and Rasa (meat soup) is reared by adding the juice of Draksha – Raisin – Vitis vinifera,

Amalaka – Phyllanthus emblica, Kharjura – Phoenix sylvestris and Parusaka – Grewia asiatica which are useful for the patient suffering from Paittika type of Alcoholism. [139 – 140]

Vamana for Paittika Alcoholism:

आमाशयस्थमुत्क्लिष्टं कफपित्तं मदात्यये| विज्ञाय बहुदोषस्य दह्यमानस्य तृष्यतः||१४१||

मद्यं द्राक्षारसं तोयं दत्त्वा तर्पणमेव वा| निःशेषं वामयेच्छीघ्रमेवं रोगादि्वमुच्यते||१४२||

If in the patient of alcoholism, Kapha and Pitta located in the Amashaya (stomach including small intestine) are incited, if there is excess of morbidity, and if he is suffering from Daha (burning sensation) and Trshna (morbid thirst), then they are given alcohol, grapes juice, water or Tarpana (refreshing drink), and thereafter, administered emetic therapy to eliminate the morbid matter completely. This makes the patient free from Paittika alcoholism instantaneously. [141-142]

Samsarjana Krama:

काले पुनस्तर्पणाद्यं क्रमं कुर्यात् प्रकाङ्क्षिते| तेनाग्निर्दीप्यते तस्य दोष शेषान्नपाचकः||१४३||

In appropriate time, when the patient is hungry, Tarpana (refreshing drinks), etc., is given as Krama (post therapeutic dietary regimen), by which the power of digestion gets stimulated, and the residual Doshas (morbid matter adhered to the wall of the Intestines) and food get digested. [143]

Treatment of Complications:

कासे सरक्तनिष्ठीवे पार्श्वस्तनरुजासु च| तृष्यते सविदाहे च सोत्क्लेशे हृदयोरसि||१४४||

गुडूची भद्र मुस्तानां पटोलस्याथवा भिषक्| रसं सनागरं दद्यात् तित्तिरि प्रतिभोजनम्||१४५||

If the patient of Paittika alcoholism suffers from

Kasa (cough),

Rakta sthivana – spitting of blood,

Parshva stana ruja – pain in the sides of the chest and breasts,

Trishna – morbid thirst,

Daha – burning sensation,

Hrudaya ura utklesha – agitation in the heart and chest then he is given the decoction of

Guduchi –Tinospora cordifolia and

Bhadra-Musta (Cyperus rotundus) or

Patola along with Nagara – Zingiber officinale After its digestion, the soup of the meat of Tittiri- bird is given to him along with food [144-145]

Treatment of excess Thirst:

तृष्यते चातिबलवद्वातपित्ते समुद्धते| दद्याद्द्राक्षारसं पातुं शीतं दोषानुलोमनम्||१४६||

जीर्णे समधुराम्लेन छागमांसरसेन तम्| भोजनं भोजयेन्मद्यमनुतर्षं च पाययेत्||१४७||

अनुतर्षस्य मात्रा सा यया नो दूष्यते मनः|

If along with morbid thirst, there is excessive aggravation of Vayu and Pitta, then the patient is given cold grape-juice to drink which causes downward movement of the Doshas (morbid matter).

After its digestion, he is given food along with the sweet and sour soup of the meat of the goat.

If there is thirst, then the patient is given alcohol as anurasa or Anupana (post- prandial drink) in such quantity as would not adversely affect the mind. [146 -½ 148]

Method of Giving Alcohol:

तृष्यते मद्यमल्पाल्पं प्रदेयं स्याद्बहूदकम्||१४८||

तृष्णा येनोपशाम्येत मदं येन च नाप्नुयात्|

To the patient having morbid thirst, alcohol diluted with water in large quantity is given in small quantities by which the thirst is alleviated with any intoxicating effect [148 ½ – ½ 149]

Recipes of excess Thirst:

परूषकाणां पीलूनां रसं शीतमथापि वा||१४९||

पर्णिनीनां चतसृणां पिबेद्वा शिशिरं जलम्| मुस्त दाडिम लाजानां तृष्णाघ्नं वा पिबेद्रसम्||१५०||

The following recipes alleviate thirst

1. Cold infusion of Parusaka – Grewia asiatica and Pilu – Salvadora oleoides.
2. Cold infusion of 4 types of Parni (Shala- Parni , Prsni- Parni, Masa- parni – Phaseolus mungo and Mudga- Parni – Phaseolus trilobus) and
3. The decoction (cold) of musta (Cyperus rotundus), Dadima – Pomegranate and laja (roasted Paddy). [149 ½- 150]

Panchamalaka Yoga:

कोल दाडिम वृक्षाम्ल चुक्रीकाचुक्रिकारसः| पञ्चाम्लको मुखालेपः सद्यस्तृष्णां नियच्छति||१५१||

Application of the juice of Panchamlaka (5 sour- drugs), viz,

• Kola – Zizyphus jujuba,
• Dadima – Pomegranate
• Vrikshamla – Garcinia morella,
• Cukrika (Cangeri) – Oxalis corniculata and
• Cukrika – Tamarindus indica as mouth –paint instantaneously cures morbid thirst. [151]

External Therapy for Paittika Alcoholism:

शीतलान्यन्नपानानि शीत शय्यासनानि च| शीत वात जल स्पर्शाः शीतान्युपवनानि च||१५२||

क्षौम पद्मोत्पलानां च मणीनां मौक्तिकस्य च| चन्दनोदक शीतानां स्पर्शाश्चन्द्रांशु शीतलाः||१५३||

हेमराजतकांस्यानां पात्राणां शीतवारिभिः| पूर्णानां हिमपूर्णानां दृतीनां पवनाहताः||१५४||

संस्पर्शाश्चन्दनार्द्राणां नारीणां च समारुताः| चन्दनानां च मुख्यानां शस्ताः पित्तमदात्यये ||१५५||

शीतवीर्यं यदन्यच्च तत् सर्वं विनियोजयेत्| कुमुदोत्पलपत्राणां सिक्तानां चन्दनाम्बुना||१५६||

हिताः स्पर्शा मनोज्ञानां दाहे मद्यसमुत्थिते| कथाश्च विविधाः शस्ताः शब्दाश्च शिखिनां शिवाः||१५७||

तोयदानां च शब्दा हि शमयन्ति मदात्ययम्| जलयन्त्राभिवर्षाणि वात यन्त्रवहानि च||१५८||

कल्पनीयानि भिषजा दाहे धारागृहाणि च| फलिनीसेव्यलोध्राम्बुहेमपत्रं कुटन्नटम्||१५९||

कालीयक रसोपेतं दाहे शस्तं प्रलेपनम्| बदरीपल्लवोत्थश्च तथैवारिष्टकोद्भवः||१६०||

फेनिलायाश्च यः फेनस्तैर्दाहे लेपनं शुभम्| सुरा समण्डा दध्यम्लं मातुलुङ्गरसो मधु||१६१||

सेके प्रदेहे शस्यन्ते दाहघ्नाः साम्लकाञ्जिकाः| परिषेकावगाहेषु व्यञ्जनानां च सेवने||१६२||

शस्यते शिशिरं तोयं दाह तृष्णा प्रशान्तये| मात्रा काल प्रयुक्तेन कर्मणाऽनेन शाम्यति ||१६३||

धीमतो वैद्यवश्यस्य शीघ्रं पित्तमदात्ययः|१६४|

External therapies for Paittik Madatyaya:

For Paitika types of Alcoholism, the following cooling regimes are useful

1. Intake of cooling food and drinks
2. Use of cooling beds and seats
3. Contact of cold air and water
4. Movement in cooling parks
5. Wearing of silken garments, lotus, water-lily, gems and pearls and pearl and application of sandal paste added with water which is cooling like the cooling rays of the moon.
6. Touch of the vessels of gold, silver and bronze filled with cold water, and of leather bags filled with ice which is exposed to wind.
7. Contact of woman smeared with sandal paste, and of breeze perfumed with the best type of sandal scent
8. Application of all such regimens which are cold in potency.

9. If there is burning sensation in alcoholism, then the contact of beautiful leaves of Kumuda – Nymphaea alba and Utpala sprinkled with sandal water is useful.

10. Hearing different pleasing stories, the sound of peacock and the roaring of the cloud cure alcoholism.

11. To cure burning sensation the physician should ask the patient to use Jala- Yantra (instrument for the shower of water) for sprinkling water, Vata- Yantra (instrument for movement of air) for blowing air in the room, and Dhara-Grha (a room where water sprinkles from the roof) for the stay;

12. For curing Daha (burning sensation), application of the paste of phalini, Sevya, Lodhra – Symplocos racemosa, Hema (Mesua ferrea), Patra and Kutannata reared by triturating with the juice of kaliyaka is useful

13. Application of the lather prepared of the pieces of Baari, Aristaka (Nimba – Neem (Azadirachta indica)) and Phenila is useful in curing the burning sensation

14. Sura (alcohol), Sura- Manda (Supernatant art of alcohol), sour yoghurt (curd), juice of Matulunga – Lemon variety – Citrus decumana / Citrus limon, honey and sour Kanji (a fermented liquid) are useful as seka (sprinkling) and Pradeha (application in the form of a paste by adding to other drugs) for curing burning sensation and

15. Use of cold water for affusion and bath, and for making the fan wet is useful in curing burning sensation and morbid thirst

Use of the above-mentioned therapies in appropriate dose and time person would get cured of the Paittika type of alcoholism. [152- ½ 164]

Treatment of Kaphaja Madatyaya:

उल्लेखनोपवासाभ्यां जयेत् कफ मदात्ययम्||१६४||

तृष्यते सलिलं चास्मै दद्याद्ध्रीबेरसाधितम्| बलया पृश्निपर्ण्या वा कण्टकार्याऽथवा शृतम्||१६५||

सनागराभिः सर्वाभिर्जलं वा शृतशीतलम्| दुःस्पर्शन समुस्तेन मुस्तपर्पटकेन वा||१६६||

जलं मुस्तैः शृतं वाऽपि दद्याद्दोषविपाचनम्| एतदेव च पानीयं सर्वत्रापि मदात्यये||१६७||

निरत्ययं पीयमानं पिपासा ज्वर नाशनम्| निरामं काङ्क्षितं काले सक्षौद्रं पाययेतु तम्||१६८||

शार्करं मधु वा जीर्णमरिष्टं सीधुमेव वा| रूक्ष तर्पण संयुक्तं यवानी नागरान्वितम्||१६९||

The physician should overcome the Kaphaja type of Madatyaya by emetic therapy and fasting therapy (Upavasa).

If the patient suffers from morbid thirst, then he is given the decoction of

Hribera – Coleus vettiveroides

Bala – Sida cordifolia

Prsni-Parni or

Kantakari – Solanum xanthocarpum

He may also be given the boiled and cooled decoction of all the above mentioned drugs along with Nagara – Zingiber officinale

The patient is given water boiled with either Dusparsa and Musta (Cyperus rotundus) or

Musta (Cyperus rotundus) and parpataka or

Musta (Cyperus rotundus) alone for the pachana (metabolic transformation) of Doshas.

The above-mentioned drinks (decoctions) can be safely administered in all types of Madatyaya for curing morbid thirst and fever.

When the patient is free from Ama – A product of indigestion and altered metabolism (Product of improper digestion and metabolism), and if he so desires, he may be given Sarkara (alcohol prepared of sugar), Madhu (Alcohol prepared of honey), old Arista (a type of wine) and Sidhu (another type of wine) along with honey, by adding dry type of Tarpana (refreshing drink), Yavani and Nagara. [164 ½- 169]

Food and drinks for Kaphaja Alcoholism:

यावगौधूमिकं चान्नं रूक्ष यूषेण भोजयेत्| कुलत्थानां सुशुष्काणां मूलकानां रसेन वा||१७०||

तनुनाऽल्पेन लघुना कट्वम्लेनाल्पसर्पिषा| पटोल यूषमम्लं वा यूषमामलकस्य वा||१७१||

प्रभूत कटु संयुक्तं सयवान्नं प्रदापयेत्| व्योष यूषमथाम्लं वा यूष वा साम्लवेतसम्||१७२||

छागमांसरसं रूक्षमम्लं वा जाङ्गलं रसम्| स्थाल्यां वाऽथ कपाले वा भृष्टं निर्द्रववर्तितम्||१७३||

कट्वम्ल लवणं मांसं भक्षयन् वृणयान्मधु| व्यक्त मारीचकं मांसं मातुलुङ्ग रसान्वितम्||१७४||

प्रभूत कटु संयुक्तं यवानी नागरान्वितम्| भृष्टं दाडिम साराम्लमुष्णपूपोपवेष्टितम्||१७५||

यथाग्नि भक्षयेत् काले प्रभूतार्द्रक पेशिकम्| पिबेच्च निगदं मद्यं कफप्राये मदात्यये||१७६||

The patient suffering from Kaphaja alcoholism is given food prepared of barley and wheat along with the dry soup of Kulattha or dried radish. This vegetable - soup is thin, small in quantity and light for digestion. It is added with pungent and sour ingredients, and ghee in small quantities.

He may be given food prepared of barley along with the soup of Patola – Trichosanthes dioica prepared by adding sour ingredients or the soup of Amalaki added with pungent ingredients profusely or the sour soup of Vyosa (sunthi – Zingiber officinale, Pippali – Piper longum and Maricha – Piper nigrum) or the soup of Amla-Vetasa – Garcinia pedunculata or the soup of the meat of goat and animals inhabiting arid zone (Jangala) prepared by adding ingredients, and without adding ghee.

Meat is roasted in a metal pan or earthen pan till it becomes completely dry. This is added with pungent, sour and saline ingredients. After taking this meat preparation, the patient of Kaphaja alcoholism should drink Madhu (alcohol prepared with honey).

Meat mixed with profuse quantities of Maricha – Piper nigrum, and added with the juice of matulunga – Citrus medica, pungent ingredients in large quantities, Yavani – Carum copticum and Nagara – Zingiber officinale is roasted. This is then made sour by adding the juice of Dadima – pomegranate and stuffed into a roll of pancake. Depending upon the power of digestion, the patient suffering from Kaphaja type of alcoholism should eat it along with pieces of ginger mixed copiously. Thereafter, he should drink wholesome alcohol. [170- 176]

Asthanga Lavana:

सौवर्चलमजाजी च वृक्षाम्लं साम्लवेतसम्| त्वगेला मरिचार्धांशं शर्कराभागयोजितम्||१७७||

एतल्लवणमष्टाङ्गमग्नि सन्दीपनं परम्| मदात्यये कफप्राये दद्यात् स्रोतोविशोधनम्||१७८||

एतदेव पुनर्युक्त्या मधुराम्लैर्द्रवीकृतम्| गोधूमान्नयवान्नानां मांसानां चातिरोचनम्||१७९||

One part of each of Sauvarcala,

Ajaji – Cuminum cyminum,

Vriksamla – Garcinia gummigutta and

Amlavetasa – Garcinia pedunculata,

half part of each of Tvak – Cinnamonum zeylanica, Ela – Elettaria cardamomum and marica – Piper nigrum, and one part of sugar is mixed together. This is called Astanga- Lavana.

It is an excellent promoter of the power of digestion, and is given to the patient suffering from alcoholism caused by the predominance of Kapha for cleansing the channels of circulation.

Being diluted appropriately with sweet and sour ingredients, the above-mentioned recipe may be added to the preparation of wheat and barley or to different types of meat- preparations to make them exceedingly delicious. [177- 179]

Recipes of digestive Stimulants:

पेषयेत् कटुकैर्युक्तां श्वेतां बीजविवर्जिताम्| मृद्वीकां मातुलुङ्गस्य दाडिमस्य रसेन वा||१८०||

सौवर्चलैला मरिचैरजाजी भृङ्ग दीप्यकैः| स रागः क्षौद्रसंयुक्तः श्रेष्ठो रोचन दीपनः ||१८१||

मृद्वीकाया विधानेन कारयेत् कारवीमपि| शुक्त मत्स्यण्डिकोपेतं रागं दीपन पाचनम्||१८२||

आम्रामलकपेशीनां रागान् कुर्यात् पृथक् पृथक्| धान्य सौवर्चलाजाजी कारवी मरिचान्वितान्||१८३||

गुडेन मधुयुक्तेन व्यक्ताम्ल लवणीकृतान्| तैरन्नं रोचते दिग्धं सम्यग्भुक्तं च जीर्यति||१८४||

Recipes of digestive Stimulants:

White variety of Mrudveeka – raisins free from seeds is made to a paste by adding pungent ingredients, and the juice of Matulunga – Citrus medica or Dadima – pomegranate. To this paste, sauvarcala, Ela – Elattaria cardamum, Maricha – Piper nigrum, Ajaji – Cuminum cyminum, Bhrnga (Tvak) and Dipyaka are added. This Raga (sweet, sour, Saline and pungent appetizer), taken along with honey is an excellent appetiser and digestive stimulant.

Following the above procedure, the Raga of Karavi (small variety of grape) is prepared. Intake of this along with Sukta (Vinegar) and Matsyandika (a preparation of jaggery) stimulates the power of digestion, and it is carminative (Panaca).

Similarly, separate Ragas are prepared of the plup of Amra – Mangifera indica and Amalaka – Phyllanthus emblica by adding Dhanya, Sauvarcala, Ajaji – Cuminum cyminum, Karavi – Carum carvi and Marica – Piper nigrum. These recipes along with jaggery, honey and a profuse quantity of sour and saline ingredients are taken. Food along with these recipes becomes very delicious, and gets digested properly. [180- 184]

Other Regimens for Kaphaja Alcoholism

रूक्षोष्णेनान्नपानेन स्नानेनाशिशिरेण च| व्यायाम लङ्घनाभ्यां च युक्त्या जागरणेन च||१८५||

कालयुक्तेन रूक्षेण स्नानेनोद्वर्तनेन च| प्राण वर्णकराणां च प्रघर्षाणां च सेवया||१८६||

सेवया वसनानां च गुरूणामगुरोरपि| सङ्कोचोष्णसुखाङ्गीनामङ्गनानां च सेवया||१८७||

सुख शिक्षित हस्तानां स्त्रीणां संवाहनेन च| मदात्ययः कफप्रायः शीघ्रमेवोपशाम्यति||१८८||

Alcoholism caused by the predominance of Kapha gets cured quickly by the following regimes:

1. Intake of food and drinks which are dry and hot in potency

2. Hot water bath

3. Physical exercise and fasting therapy

4. Remaining awake at night appropriately

5. Bath and unction with dry articles at appropriate time.

6. Rubbing the body with ingredients which are promoters of life and complexion

7. Wearing of heavy clothing

8. Application of the past of Aguru – Aquillaria agallocha all over the body

9. Embracing women whose pleasant limbs are smeared with Sankoca (Kunkuma or saffron) and

10. Pleasant massages by women whose hands are warm and who is well trained. [158- 188]

Treatment of Sannipatika Alcoholism:

यदिदं कर्म निर्दिष्टं पृथग्दोषबलं प्रति| सन्निपाते दश विधे तद्विकल्प्यं भिषग्विदा||१८९||

यस्तु दोष विकल्पज्ञो यश्चौषधि विकल्पवित्| स साध्यान्साधयेद्व्याधीन् साध्यासाध्यविभागवित्||१९०||

The therapeutic measures described above for the treatment of 3 different types of alcoholism separately for each Dosha is carefully combined by the wise physician for the treatment of the (remaining) ten types of alcoholism caused by Sannipata (or simultaneous aggravation of all the 3 Doshas).

The physician who is well versed with the knowledge of proportionate increase or decrease of different aggravated Doshas (Dosha- Vikalpana), who is well versed with the knowledge of preparing medicines to carter to the requirement of these differently aggravated Doshas (Ausadhi- Vikalpavit), and who is well versed with the knowledge of curability and incurability of diseases (Sadhyasadhya- Vidhagavit) is capable of curing all the curable diseases. [189- 190]

Regimens for Alcoholism:

वनानि रमणीयानि सपद्माः सलिलाशयाः| विशदान्यन्नपानानि सहायाश्च प्रहर्षणाः||१९१||

माल्यानि गन्धयोगाश्च वासांसि विमलानि च| गान्धर्व शब्दाः कान्ताश्च गोष्ठ्यश्च हृदयप्रियाः||१९२||

सङ्कथाहास्यगीतानां विशदाश्चैव योजनाः| प्रियाश्चानुगता नार्यो नाशयन्ति मदात्ययम्||१९३||

The following factors help a person to overcome alcoholism

1. Beautiful forests

2. Ponds and lakes with lotus- flowers

3. Clean food and drinks

4. Exciting companions

5. Use of garlands and perfumes

6. Clean garments

7. Musical performances

8. Pleasing and delightful companions

9. Exposition of refreshing stories, jokes and songs and

10. Companionship of lovely and devoted women. [191- 193]

Psychotherapy for Alcoholism:

नाक्षोभ्य हि मनो मद्यं शरीरमविहत्य च| कुर्यान्मदात्ययं तस्मादेष्टव्या हर्षणी क्रिया||१९४||

Alcoholism does not cause alcoholism without causing agitation of the mind without causing morbidity in the body. Therefore,

a patient suffering from alcoholism, therapeutic measures (psyho- therapy) for the cheerfulness of the mind are administered. [194]

Milk for Alcoholism:

आभिः क्रियाभिः सिद्धाभिः शमं याति मदात्ययः| न चेन्मद्यविधिं मुक्त्वा क्षीरमस्य प्रयोजयेत्||१९५||

लङ्घनैः पाचनै दोष शोधनैः शमनैरपि| विमद्यस्य कफे क्षीणे जाते दौर्बल्य लाघवे||१९६||

तस्य मद्य विदग्धस्य वात पित्ताधिकस्य च| ग्रीष्मोप तप्तस्य तरोर्यथा वर्षा तथा पयः||१९७||

पयसाऽभिहृते रोगे बले जाते निवर्तयेत्| क्षीर प्रयोगं मद्यं च क्रमेणाल्पाल्पमाचरेत्||१९८||

The above mentioned effective therapeutic measures cure alcoholism. If not, then the physician should give up therapies comprising alcohol, and administer milk for its treatment. With withdrawal of liquor, due to administration of langhana (Lightening therapies) Pachana (Ama removing measures) , Dosha sodhana (Cleansing the doshas / Purification therapies and Samahna (Paliative treatments), when kapha is diminished and debility and agility occurs due to fasting, and purifying metabolism of toxins, alleviating measures and vata pitta get dominant in the person wreaked with liquor, the milk acts as a boon like the rains for the tree in intense summer.

After the diseases are cured by the administration of milk, and after the patient has gained strength, the milk is gradually withdrawn, and alcohol is substituted in its place little by little. [195- 198]

Dhvamsaka and Vikshaya:

विच्छिन्न मद्यः सहसा योऽतिमद्यं निषेवते| ध्वंसको विक्षयश्चैव रोगस्तस्योपजायते||१९९||

व्याध्युप क्षीण देहस्य दुश्चिकित्स्यतमौ हि तौ| तयोलिङ्गं चिकित्सा च यथावदुपदेक्ष्यते||२००||

श्लेष्मप्रसेकः कण्ठास्य शोषः शब्दासहिष्णुता| तन्द्रा निद्रातियोगश्च ज्ञेयं ध्वंसक लक्षणम्||२०१||

हृत्कण्ठरोगः सम्मोह श्छर्दिरङ्गरुजा ज्वरः| तृष्णा कासः शिरःशूलमेतद्विक्षयलक्षणम्||२०२||

तयोः कर्म तदेवेष्टं वातिके यन्मदात्यये| तौ हि प्रक्षीण देहस्य जायेते दुर्बलस्य वै||२०३||

बस्तयः सर्पिषः पानं प्रयोगः क्षीर सर्पिषोः| अभ्यङ्गोद्वर्तनस्नानान्यन्नपानं च वातनुत्||२०४||

ध्वंसको विक्षयश्चैव कर्मणाऽनेन शाम्यति| युक्त मद्यस्य मद्योत्थो न व्याधिरुपजायते||२०५||

Dhvamsaka and Vikshaya:

If a person who has stopped drinking alcohol suddenly takes recourse to drinking alcohol in excess, he suffers from 2 diseases, viz, Dhvamsaka and Viksaya. Since such a person is already emaciated because of his earlier drinking habit, these 2 diseases appearing in him are very difficult to cure. Their signs, symptoms and treatment will not be described appropriately.

The signs and symptoms of Dhvamsaka:

• Sleshma praseka – Excessive salivation

• Kantha aasya shosha – dryness of the throat and mouth

• Shabda asahisnuta – intolerance to noise and

• Tandra – excessive drowsiness and

• Nidra ati yoga – sleep

The signs and symptoms of Viksaya:
• Hrt roga – Cardiac disorder
• Kantha roga – throat- disorder
• Sammoha – unconsciousness
• Chardi – vomiting
• Anga ruja – pain in the limbs,
• Jvara – fever,
• Trshna – morbid thirst,
• Kasa – cough
• Shiro ruja – headache

Since both these ailments appear in an emaciated and weak person, their treatment is done on the line suggested for the treatment of Vatika type of Madatyaya.

Treatment: Basti (medicated enema), Sarpis (medicated ghee), milk, ghee, massage, unction, bath, food and drinks which cause alleviation of Vata Dosha. By the above-mentioned therapeutic measures, Dhvamsaka and Viksaya get alleviated.

Intake of alcohol in an appropriate manner will not give rise to disease caused by [excessive intake of] alcohol. [190-205]

Virtues of Abstinence from Alcohol:

निवृत्तः सर्वमद्येभ्यो नरो यश्च जितेन्द्रियः| शारीर मानसै र्धीमान् विकारैर्न स युज्यते||२०६||

A wise person who has self- control over the senses and who abstains from drinking all types of alcohol preparations never gets afflicted with physical and mental disorders. [206]

Summary:

तत्र श्लोकाः:-

यत्प्रभावा भगवती सुरा पेया यथा च सा| यद्द्रव्या यस्य या चेष्टा योगं चापेक्षते यथा||२०७||

यथा मद्यते यैश्च गुणैर्युक्ता महागुणा| यो मदो मदभेदाश्च ये त्रयः स्वस्वलक्षणाः||२०८||

ये च मद्यकृता दोषा गुणा ये च मदात्मकाः| यच्च त्रिविधमापानं यथासत्त्वं च लक्षणम्||२०९||

ये सहायाः सुखाः पाने चिरक्षिप्रमदा नराः| मदात्ययस्य यो हेतु र्लक्षणं यद् यथा च यत्||२१०||

मद्यं मद्योत्थितान् रोगान् हन्ति यश्च क्रियाक्रमः| सर्वं तदुक्तमखिलं मदात्यय चिकित्सिते||२११||

In this chapter on the "Treatment of Alcoholism", the following topics are described in their entirety:

The powers of the goddess Sura (alcohol)

The method of drinking alcohol

The ingredients with which alcohol is to be taken

Wholesomeness of different varieties of alcohol for different types of persons

The methods of its appropriate use

The process by which intoxication is caused

The properties of alcohol which is endowed with great attributes

Signs and symptoms of alcoholic intoxication

Different stages of alcoholic intoxication

Signs and symptoms of each of the three stages of alcoholic intoxication

Adverse effects of alcohol

Good effects of alcohol

Use of alcohol keeping in view the three varieties [of eight factors]

Signs and symptoms manifested in persons having 3 types of mental faculties.

Characteristics of good companions in drinking parties

Characteristics of persons who get drunk slowly and who get drunk quickly

causes, signs and symptoms of Madatyaya
The type of alcohol and the manner in which alcohol cures Madatyaya and
Line of treatment of Madatyaya; [207- 211]

Colophon:
इत्यग्निवेशकृते तन्त्रे चरकप्रतिसंस्कृते चिकित्सास्थाने मदात्ययचिकित्सितं नाम चतुर्विंशोऽध्यायः||२४||
Thus, ends the 24th chapter of Cikitsa –sthana (section on the treatment of diseases) dealing with the treatment of Madatyaya in the Agnivesha's work as redacted by Charaka

8

Chikitsasthana Chapter 25 Vrana Chikitsitam

25th chapter of Charaka Samhita, Chikitsa Sthana deals with symptoms and treatment of internal and external wounds and ulcers. It is called Vrana Chikitsa Adhyaya.

अथातो द्विव्रणीय चिकित्सितं व्याख्यास्यामः||१||

इति ह स्माह भगवानात्रेयः||२||

We shall now explore the treatment of 2 types of Ulcers. Thus, said Lord Atreya. [1-2]

Prologue:

परावरज्ञमात्रेयं गतमान मद व्यथम्| अग्निवेशो गुरुं काले विनयादिदमब्रवीत्||३||

भगवन्! पूर्वमुद्दिष्टौ द्वौ व्रणौ रोग सङ्ग्रहे| तयोर्लिङ्गं चिकित्सां च वक्तुमर्हसिशर्मद!||४||

Finding an opportune moment, Agnivesha respectfully requested his preceptor, Lord Atreya who was well versed in the spiritual and physical sciences, and as free from the afflictions of self- pride as well as vanity, as follows:

"O! Lord. 2 types of Ulcers are enumerated in the chapter dealing with the complications of diseases (vide Sutra 19:4:7) O! Bestower of happiness, you may kindly expound the signs and symptoms as well as treatment of these two types of ulcers. [3-4]

Guru's reply:

इत्यग्निवेशस्य वचो निशम्य गुरुरब्रवीत्| यौ व्रणौ पूर्वमुद्दिष्टौ निजश्चागन्तुरेव च||५||

श्रूयतां विधिवत् सौम्य! तयोर्लिङ्गं च भेषजम्|

Having heard this query, the Preceptor replied, as follows:

O! disciple, now listen about the Linga (signs and symptoms including aetiology) and Bheshaja (therapeutic measures) of both the types of ulcers, viz, nija (endogenous) and Agantuja (Exogenous) which were enumerated, in brief, earlier (in Sutra 19;4: 7) [5- ½ 6]

Nija and Agantuja Vrana – Endogenous and exogenous ulcers:

निजः शरीरदोषोत्थ आगन्तुर्बाह्यहेतुजः||६||

वध बन्ध प्रपतनाद्दंष्ट्रा दन्त नख क्षतात्| आगन्तवो व्रणास्तद्वद्विषस्पर्शाग्निशस्त्रजाः||७||

मन्त्रागद प्रलेपाद्यैर्भेषजैर्हेतुभिश्च ते| लिङ्गैकदेशैर्निर्दिष्टा विपरीता निजैर्व्रणैः ||८||

The Nija or endogenous type of Vrana (ulcer) are caused by the vitiation of Doshas of the body, and

The Agantuja type of ulcer is caused by external factors like Vadha (wound caused by stabbing, etc,), Bandha (wound caused by tying with a rope etc), fall and injury by fangs, teeth and nails. This type of exogenous ulcer is also caused by exposure to (contact with) poison, fire and sharp- edged weapons.

The exogenous ulcer bears special characteristic features in as much as these can be cured by

- Mantra (Incantation)
- Agada (Talisman) and
- External application of drugs in the form of paste

They have specific causative factors, and they have specific signs and symptoms (which are localised). The Nija or endogenous and types of ulcers, however, bears opposite characteristic features. [6 ½- 8]

व्रणानां निज हेतूनामागन्तूनामशाम्यताम्| कुर्याद्दोषबलापेक्षी निजानामौषधं यथा||९||

If the endogenous type of ulcer does not yield to the treatment (specified above) because of its association with the Doshas of the body, then even such exogenous ulcer is treated with medicines (to be) prescribed for endogenous ulcer, depending upon the strength of the aggravated Doshas. [9]

Pathogenesis of Endogenous Ulcers:

यथास्वैर्हेतुभिर्दुष्टा वात पित्त कफा नृणाम्| बहिर्मार्गं समाश्रित्य जनयन्ति निजान् व्रणान्||१०||

Vata, Pitta and Kapha being aggravated by their respective causative factors get lodged in the exterior (eternal pathway) of the body to give rise to endogenous type of ulcer in the human beings [10]

Vataja Vrana Lakshana:

स्तब्धः कठिन संस्पर्शो मन्द स्रावोऽति तीव्र रुक् | तुद्यते स्फुरति श्यावो व्रणो मारुत सम्भवः||११||

Vatika type of ulcer is characterised by

- Stabdha – stiffness
- Kathina samsparsha – hardness in touch
- Manda srava – scant discharge
- Ati tivra ruk – excruciating pain
- Tudyate – pricking sensation
- Sphurana – throbbing and
- Shyava aruna maruta sambhava – bluish black coloration [11]

Treatment of Vatika Ulcer:

सम्पूरणैः स्नेहपानैः स्निग्धैः स्वेदोपनाहनैः| प्रदेहैः परिषेकैश्च वात व्रणमुपाचरेत्||१२||

The patient suffering from Vatika type of ulcer is treated with

- Sampurna – filling buccal cavity of the ulcer
- Snehapana – oleation therapy and
- Snigdha – fomentation
- Upanaha – application of hot paste of drugs
- Pradeha – application of ointment and
- Pariseka - (affusion) which are of unctuous nature [12]

Signs and Symptoms of Paittika Vrana:

तृष्णा मोह ज्वर स्वे(क्ले)द दाह दुष्ट्यवदारणैः| व्रणं पित्तकृतं विद्यादगन्धैः स्रावैश्च पूतिकैः||१३||

The patient suffering from Paittika type of ulcer gets

- Trishna – thirst
- Moha – unconsciousness
- Jwara – fever
- Sweda – sweating
- Daha – burning sensation
- Dushti – putrification and
- Avadarana – sloughing out of tissues and

• Vidyat gandhaih putika srava – elucidation of foul-smelling material (pus) from the ulcer [13]

Treatment of Paittika Ulcer:

शीतलै मधुरैस्तिक्तैः प्रदेह परिषेचनैः| सर्पिष्पाने विरेकैश्च पैतिकं शमयेद्व्रणम्||१४||

Paittika type of ulcer is treated with

• Pradeha – application of hot paste of drugs and

• Parisechana (affusion)

• Sarpi pana – intake of medicated ghee and

• Virechana – purgation therapy prepared of cooling, sweet and bitter drugs. [14]

Signs and Symptoms of Kaphaja Vrana:

बहु पिच्छो गुरुः स्निग्धः स्तिमितो मन्द वेदनः| पाण्डुवर्णोऽल्प सङ्क्लेदश्चिरकारी कफव्रणः||१५||

The Kaphaja type of ulcer is characterised by

• Bahu piccha – excessively slime exudation

• Guru – heaviness

• Snigdha – unctuousness

• Stimita – still / motionless / steady / moist

• Manda vedana – mild pain

• Pandu varna – pallor

• Alpa sanklesha – less of sloughing and

• Chira kari — long duration (chronic nature). [15]

Treatment of Kaphaja Vrana:

कषाय कटु रूक्षोष्णैः प्रदेह परिषेचनैः| कफव्रणं प्रशमयेत्तथा लङ्घन पाचनैः ||१६||

Kaphaja type of ulcer is treated with

• Pradeha (application of hot paste of drugs) and

• Parisechana (affusion) prepared drugs which are Kashaya (astringent), Katu (pungent), Ruksha (dry) and Ushna (hot).

The patient suffering from this type of ulcer is given

• Langhana (Fasting) and

• Pachana (which helps in the metabolic transformation of uncooked material of the body) therapies [16]

Characteristic Features:

तौ द्वौ नानात्वभेदेन निरुक्ता विंशति द्रणाः| तेषां परीक्षा त्रिविधा, प्रदुष्टा द्वादश स्मृताः||१७||

स्थानान्यष्टौ तथा गन्धाः, परिस्रावाश्चतुर्दश| षोडशोपद्रवा दोषाश्चत्वारो विंशतिस्तथा||१८||

तथा चोपक्रमाः सिद्धाः षट्त्रिंशत् समुदाहृताः| विभज्यमानाञ्छृणु मे सर्वानेतान् यथेरितान्||१९||

These types of ulcers have the following characteristic features:

1. These are further classified into 20 varieties, depending upon the differences in their nature

2. These are to be examined in 3 different ways

3. In the advanced stage of their manifestation, they exhibit 12 characteristic features

4. Their locations are 8 in number

5. They are associated with 8 types of foul odours

6. They have 14 types of discharges

7. They have 16 types of complications

8. There are 24 factors which cause impediments in the healing of these ulcers and

9. There are 36 effective therapeutic measures for the treatment of these ulcers.

All the above-mentioned factors will be described hereafter individually. Listen to me! [17-19]

Vrana Bheda – Twenty varieties of Ulcers:

कृत्योत्कृत्यस्तथा दुष्टोऽदुष्टो मर्मस्थितो न च| संवृतो दारुणः स्रावी सविषो विषमस्थितः||२०||

उत्सङ्ग्युत्सन्न एषां च व्रणान् विद्यादिवपर्ययात्| इति नानात्वभेदेन निरुक्ता विंशति व्रणाः||२१||

Depending upon their various characteristic features, ulcers are of 20 varieties as follows

1. Krtya or those requiring intervention, viz, incision, etc, [this term is also interpreted as "curable"].

2. Akrtya or those not requiring surgical intervention. These are just to be healed [this term is also interpreted as" incurable]

3. Dusta or putrified ulcer

4. Adusta or ulcers which are not putrified

5. Marmasthita or ulcers located in the Marma (vital organs)

6. Amarmasthita or ulcers not located in the vital organs

7. Samvrta or closed ulcers

8. Vivrata or open (exposed) ulcers

9. Daruna or hard ulcers

10. Adaruna or soft ulcer

11. Sravin or ulcers with profuse discharge

12. Asravin or ulcers with no discharge or scanty discharge

13. Savisa or ulcers having poisonous effects or those caused by poisons

14. Avisa or ulcers which are not poisonous or which are not caused by poisons

15. Visamasthita or ulcers having regular borders or which are located in the uneven parts of the body.

16. Samasthita or ulcers having regular borders or which are located in the uneven parts of the body

17. Utsangi or ulcers which are elevated / having raised borders

18. Anutsangi or ulcers which are not elevated / not having raised borders

19. Utsanna or ulcers having elevated surface and

20. Anutsanna or ulcers having a depressed surface. [20-21]

Methods of Examination:

दर्शन प्रश्न संस्पर्शैः परीक्षा त्रिविधा स्मृता| वयो वर्ण शरीराणामिन्द्रियाणां च दर्शनात्||२२||

हेत्वर्ति सात्म्याग्निबलं परीक्ष्यं वचनाद्बुधैः| स्पर्शान्मार्दवशैत्ये च परीक्ष्ये सविपर्यये||२३||

Examination of the ulcer and the patient suffering from this ailment is to be carried out in 3 different ways, viz,

• Darshana – inspection

• Prashna – interrogation and

• Samsparsha – palpation

To be examined by Darshana (inspection):

• Vaya – age

• Varna – color

• Sharira – nature of the physique and

• Indriya – sense organs

To be examined by Prashna (interrogation):

• Hetu – etiology

• Arti – nature of the pain

• Satmya (wholesomeness of food, drugs, etc.) and

• Agni Bala (power of digestion and metabolism)

To be examined by Samsparsha (palpation):

• Mardava – Stiffness or hardness and

• Shaitya – coldness or heat in the ulcerated part of the body are [22-23]

Characteristic Features of Ulcer in Advanced Stage:

श्वेतोऽवसन्नवर्मांऽतिस्थूलवर्मांऽतिपिञ्जरः| नीलःश्यावोऽतिपिडको रक्तः कृष्णोऽतिपूतिकः||२४||

रोप्यः कुम्भीमुखश्चेति प्रदुष्टा द्वादश व्रणाः| चतुर्विंशतिरुद्दिष्टा दोषाः कल्पान्तरेण वै||२५||

12 characteristic features indicating the advanced stage of morbidity of an ulcer are as follows

1. Svetatva – Paleness of the ulcer

2. Avasanna Vartmatva – depression of the margin of the ulcer

3. Ati SthulaVartmatva – excessive thickness of the margin of the ulcer

4. ati Pinjaratva – excessively red and yellow mixed coloration of the ulcer

5. Neelatva – blue coloration of the ulcer

6. Shyavatva – blackish brown coloration of the ulcer

7. Ati pidakatva – appearance of eruptions in excess around the ulcer

8 – 9 Rakta-Krsnatva – red or black coloration of the ulcer

10. Ati putitva – excessive putrefaction of the ulcer

11. ropyatva – recurrence of the ulcer, after it is healed and

12. Kumbhi mukhatva – the ulcer having a narrow opening with an expanded base like a jar

These morbid conditions are also classified into 24 categories depending upon their association with causative factors like Snayu-kleda (sloughing of ligament). [24-25]

Vrana Sthana – Seats of Manifestation of Ulcers:

त्वक्सिरा मांस मेदोऽस्थि स्नायु मर्मान्तराश्रयाः| व्रणस्थानानि निर्दिष्टान्यष्टावेतानि सङ्ग्रहे||२६||

Ulcers, in brief, are manifested in the following 8 locations:

1. Tvag Ashraya – located in the skin

2. Sira ashraya – located in the vessels

3. Mamsa ashraya – located in the muscle tissue

4. Medas-Ashraya – located in the fat tissue

5. Asthi Ashraya – located in the bones

6. Snayu- Ashraya – located in the ligaments

7. Marma-Ashraya – located in the vital organs and

8. Antarashraya or Kosthashraya – located in the visceras of the chest and abdomen [26]

Vrana Gandha – Different Odours of Ulcer:

सर्पिस्तैल वसा पूय रक्त श्यावाम्ल पूतिकाः| व्रणानां व्रण गन्धज्ञैरष्टौ गन्धाः प्रकीर्तिताः||२७||

According to the physicians specialised in determining different types of odours, the smell emanating from the ulcers are of 8 types, as follows:

1. Sarpis – smell of the ghee

2. Taila – smell of oil

3. Vasa – smell of fat

4. Puya – smell of pus

5. Rakta – smell of blood

6. Syava – smell which emanates when curd is rubbed over copper

7. Amla -smell associated with a sour substance and

8. Puti – putrid smell [27]

Vrana Srava – Nature of discharge from ulcers:

लसीका जल पूयासृग्घारिद्रारुण पिञ्जराः| कषाय नील हरित स्निग्ध रूक्ष सितासिताः||२८||

इति रूपैः समुद्दिष्टा व्रणस्रावाश्चतुर्दश|

Discharges from ulcers are, in brief, of 14 types, as follows

1. Lasika-Srava – discharge of lymph –like fluid

2. Jala Srava – watery discharge

3. Puya-Srava – Discharge of Pus

4. Asrk- Srava – blood discharge

5. Haridra Srava – discharge which is yellow like turmeric

6. Aruna- Srava – discharge which is reddish in colour

7. Pinjara-Srava – discharge which is mixed red and yellow in colour

8. Kasaya- Srava – discharge of brownish black colour

9. Neela Srava – discharge of blue colour

10. Harita Srava – discharge of green colour

11. Snigdha Srava – discharge of unctuous nature

12. Rooksha Srava – discharge of Dry nature

13. Sita Srava – discharge of white colour and

14. Asita Srava – discharge of black colour [28 – ½ 29]

Complications of Ulcers:

विसर्पः पक्षघातश्च सिरा स्तम्भोऽपतानकः||२९||

मोहोन्माद व्रण रुजो ज्वरस्तृष्णा हनुग्रहः| कासश्छर्दिरतीसारो हिक्का श्वासः सवेपथुः||३०||

षोडशोपद्रवाः प्रोक्ता व्रणानां व्रण चिन्तकैः|३१|

Complications of ulcers, according to the specialists in this branch are 16 in number as follows

1. Visarpa – erysipelas

2. Paksaghata – hemiplegia

3. Sirastambha – stiffness of vessels

4. Apatanaka – convulsions

5. Moha – unconsciousness

6. Unmada – insanity

7. Vrana ruk – acute pain in ulcers

8. Jvara – fever

9. Trsna – morbid thirst

10. Hanugraha – lock- jaw

11. Kasa – cough

12. Chardi – vomiting

13. Atisara – Diarrhoea

14. Hikka – hiccup

15. Svasa – dyspnoea

16. Vepathu – trembling [29 ½- ½ 31|

Impediments in Healing of Ulcers:

स्नायु क्लेदात्सिराक्लेदाद्गाम्भीर्यात्कृमिभक्षणात् ||३१||

अस्थिभेदात् सशल्यत्वात् सविषत्वाच्च सर्पणात्| नख काष्ठ प्रभेदाच्च चर्मलोमातिघट्टनात् ||३२||

मिथ्याबन्धादति स्नेहादतिभैषज्य कर्षणात्| अजीर्णादतिभुक्ताच्च विरुद्धासात्म्य भोजनात्||३३||

शोकात् क्रोधादिदिवास्वप्नाद्व्यायामान्मैथुनातथा| व्रणा न प्रशमं यान्ति निष्क्रियत्वाच्च देहिनाम्||३४||

Factors which cause impediments in the healing of ulcers are 24 in number, and are as follows:

1. Snayu- Kleda – sloughening of ligaments

2. Sira- Kleda – sloughening of Vessels

3. Gambhirya – when the ulcers are deep seated

4. Krmi- bhaksana – appearance of Maggots, therapy causing denudation of the tissues of the ulcer

5. Asthibheda – fracture of bone near the ulcer

6. Sasalyatva – presence of foreign bodies in the ulcer

7. Savishatva – presence of poison in the ulcer

8. Sarpanatva – spreading of the ulcer

9. Nakha- kastha- prabheda – excessive injury by nails and wood pieces

10. Charma- Atighattana – excessive denudation of the skin

11. Loma- Atighattana – excessive denudation of the small hair near the skin

12. Mitya-Bandha – wrong bandaging

13. Atisneha – excessive oleation

14. Ati- bhaisajya- Karsana – emaciation of the tissues near the ulcer because of application of drugs in excess

15. Ajirna – indigestion

16. Atibhukta – overeating

17. Viruddha-Bhojana – intake of mutually contradictory ingredients of food etc

18. Asatmya- bhojana – intake of unwholesome food

19. Shoka – grief

20. Krodha – anger

21. Diva- svapna – sleep during the day time

22. Vyayama – excessive physical exercise

23. Maithuna- sexual intercourse

24. Niskriyatva – negligence of using proper therapeutic measures [31 ½ – 34]

Reasons of Ulcers becoming difficult of cure:

परिस्रावाच्च गन्धाच्च दोषाच्चोपद्रवैः सह| व्रणानां बहु दोषाणां कृच्छ्त्वं चोपजायते||३५||

If the ulcer is caused by several Doshas (Vayu, pitta and Kapha), and is associated in excess with morbid secretions, odours, Doshas (factors causing impediments in the healing of ulcers) and other complications, then it becomes Kruchra sadhya (difficult of cure). [35]

Vrana Sadha – Asadhyata – Curable, difficult of cure and incurable Ulcers:

त्वङ्मांसजः सुखे देशे तरुणस्यानुपद्रवः| धीमतोऽभिनवः काले सुखसाध्यः स्मृतो व्रणः||३६||

गुणैरन्यतमैर्हीनस्ततः कृच्छ्रो व्रणः स्मृतः| सर्वैर्विहीनो विज्ञेयस्त्वसाध्यो निरुपक्रमः ||३७||

Factors indicating easy curability of ulcers are as follows:

1. Confinements of the ulcer to the skin and muscle tissues alone

2. Location in an easily approachable site

3. Young age of the patient

4. Non-association of the ulcer with complications

5. Enough wisdom of the patient to use appropriate treatment regularly

6. Recent origin of the ulcer and

7. Conduciveness of the season for the treatment of the ulcer

If any of the above-mentioned factors are backing, then the ulcer becomes difficult to cure (Krcchra – Sadhya).

If all the above-mentioned factors are lacking then the ulcer becomes incurable (Asadhya), and its treatment should not be attempted (Nirupakrama). [36- 37]

Shodhana or Elimination Therapy:

व्रणानामादितः कार्यं यथासन्नं विशोधनम्| ऊर्ध्वभागैरधोभागैः शस्त्रैर्बस्तिभिरेव च||३८||

सद्यः शुद्ध शरीराणां प्रशमं यान्ति हि व्रणाः|३९|

In the beginning, the patient suffering from ulcer should appropriately be given elimination therapies for the purification of the body and elimination of the morbid material] through the upward track (Vamana or emesis) and downward track (Virecana or purgation), by venesection with the help of sharp edged instruments, and by medicated enema (basti). When the body becomes cleansed of the morbid matter, the ulcer gets healed up instantaneously. [38-½ 39]

Vrana Chikitsa – Therapeutic Measures:
यथाक्रममतश्चोर्ध्वं शृणु सर्वानुपक्रमान्||३९||
शोफघ्नं षड्विधं चैव शस्त्रकर्मावपीडनम्| निर्वापणं ससन्धानं स्वेदः शमनमेषणम्||४०||
शोधनौ रोपणीयौ च कषायौ सप्रलेपनौ| द्वे तैले तद्गुणे पत्रं छादने द्वे च बन्धने||४१||
भोज्यमुत्सादनं दाहो द्विविधः सावसादनः| काठिन्य मार्दवकरे धूपनालेपने शुभे||४२||
व्रणावचूर्णनं वर्ण्यं रोपणं लोमरोहणम्| इति षट्त्रिंशदुद्दिष्टा व्रणानां समुपक्रमाः||४३||

Now, hear about all the 36 therapeutic measures [for the treatment of ulcers] to be described in the order hereafter. These are, as follows:

1. Shophaghna (therapeutic measures for relieving oedema)
2. 7 Shastra karma (six surgical measures—vide verse no 55)
8. Avapidana (compression by the application of paste of drugs)
9. Nirvana (sprinkling of cooling medicated decoction for alleviating burning sensation and heat of the ulcers)
10. Sandhana (restoration of muscles and fractured bones in the location of the ulcer)
11. Svedana (fomentation)
12. Samana (application of the paste of drugs for the alleviation of pain and burning sensation in the ulcer)
13. Esana (probbing)
14. Sodhana- Kashaya (washing the ulcer with cleansing decoction)
15. Sodhana Pralepa (application of the paste of drugs for cleaning in ulcer)
16. Ropana Kashaya (washing the ulcer with healing decoction)
17. Ropana pralepa – application of the paste of drugs for the healing of ulcer
18. Shodhana Taila ghrta (application of medicated oil and medicated ghee for the cleansing of the ulcer)
19. Ropana Taila ghrta (application of the medicated oil and medicated ghee for the healing of the ulcer)
20. Patra (covering the ulcer with the leaves of the medicinal plants)
21. Chadana (padding the ulcer with gauze)
22. 23 Bandhana (two type of bandaging)
24. Bhojya – diet and regimens
25. Utsadana – elevation of the deep-seated ulcer
26. Avasadana – removal of excessively projected tissues in the ulcer
27. – Daha – cauterization and
28 – Kshara – alkali
29. Kathinyakara Dhupana – fumigation for the hardening of the excessively soft ulcer
30. Mardavakara dhupana – fumigation for softening the excessively hard tissues of the ulcer
31. Kathinyakara alepana – application of ointment for hardening the excessively soft tissues of the ulcer
32. Mardavakara alepana – application of ointment for softening the excessively hard tissues of the ulcer
33. Avachurnana – dusting the powder of drugs over the ulcer
34. Ropana – application of recipes for growth of clear skin over the ulcer
35. Varnya – restoration of the normal colour of the skin over the ulcer
36. Loma- rohana – application of recipes for the restoration of small hair over the skin after the ulcer is healed [39 ½- 43]

Shophaghna Chikitsa (therapeutic measures to relieve oedema):
पूर्वरूपं भिषग्बुद्ध्वा व्रणानां शोफमादितः| रक्तावसेचनं कुर्यादजात व्रण शान्तये||४४||
शोधयेद्बहुदोषांस्तु स्वल्पदोषान् विलङ्घयेत्| पूर्वं कषाय सर्पिर्भिर्जयेद्वा मारुतोत्तरान्||४५||

न्यग्रोधोदुम्बराश्वत्थ प्लक्ष वेतस वल्कलैः| ससर्पिष्कैः प्रलेपः स्याच्छोफ निर्वापणः परम्||४६||

विजया मधुकं वीरा बिसग्रन्थिः शतावरी| नीलोत्पलं नागपुष्पं प्रदेहः स्यात् सचन्दनः||४७||

सक्तवो मधुकं सर्पिः प्रदेहः स्यात् सशर्करः| अविदाहिनि चान्नानि शोफे भेषजमुत्तमम्||४८||

Shophaghna Chikitsa (therapeutic measures to relieve oedema):

In the premonitory stage, when the ulcer(abscess) is not fully manifested, but only oedema is present, the physician, after ascertaining it, should apply blood-letting therapy, to avert its manifestation.

If the Doshas are aggravated in excess, the patient is given- Shodhana (elimination) therapy, and if these Doshas are less aggravated, then Langhana (fasting) therapy is administered. The patient is given decoctions of drugs and medicated ghee for the alleviation of Doshas. In the beginning, however, these therapeutic measures should aim at alleviating the aggravated Vayu followed by other Doshas (Pitta and Kapha).

Application of the paste of bark of Nyagrodha – Ficus benghalensis, Udumbara – Ficus racemosa, Asvattha – Ficus religiosa

a, Plaksa – Ficus lacor and Vetasa along with ghee is, especially effective in order to receive oedema.

Application of the Pradeha (ointment of paste) of

• Vijaya (Bala – Country mallow (root) – Sida cordifolia

• Madhuka– Licorice – Glycyrrhiza glabra

• Vira

• Bisagranthi – Nelumbium speciosum

• Shatavari – Asparagus racemosus

• Nilotpala – Nymphaea stellata and

• Nagapuspa – Messua ferrea along with

• Chandana (Sandalwood – Santalum album) also relieves oedema.

Roasted barley flour and the powder of Madhuka– Licorice – Glycyrrhiza glabra, mixed ghee and sugar is applied for correcting oedema in ulcers.

Food ingredients which do not cause burning sensation (avidahi) are immensely useful for the cure of oedema in ulcers. [44- 48]

Shastrakarma for Vrana – Surgical Interventions:

स चेदेवमुपक्रान्तः शोफो न प्रशमं व्रजेत्| तस्योपनाहैः पक्वस्य पाटनं हितमुच्यते||४९||

तैलेन सर्पिषा वाऽपि ताभ्यां वा सक्तु पिण्डिका| सुखोष्णा शोफपाकार्थमुपनाहः प्रशस्यते||५०||

सतिला सातसीबीजा दध्यम्ला सक्तु पिण्डिका| सकिण्व कुष्ठ लवणा शस्ता स्यादुपनाहने||५१||

रुग्दाह राग तोदैश्च विदग्धं शोफमादिशेत्| जल बस्ति समस्पर्श सम्पक्वं पीडितोन्नतम्||५२||

उमाऽथो गुग्गुलुः सौधं पयो दक्षकपोतयोः| विट् पलाशभवः क्षारो हेमक्षीरी मुकूलकः||५३||

इत्युक्तो भेषजगणः पक्वशोथप्रभेदनः| सुकुमारस्य, कृच्छ्रस्य शस्त्रं तु परमुच्यते||५४||

If oedema does not subside despite the above therapeutic measures, then it is supported by the application of Upanaha (hot paste of drugs). Thereafter opening them (applying opening incisions) are beneficial.

A bolus prepared of Saktu (roasted barley flour) mixed with oil or ghee or both is applied as warm poultice which is useful for causing suppuration of the abscess.

A bolus prepared of Saktu (roasted barly flour) and mixed with Tila – Sesame (Sesamum indicum), Seeds of Atasi – Linum usitatissimum , Sour curd, Kinva (Yeast), Kushta – Saussurea lappa and salt is useful as Upanaha (hot poultice).

If the abscess is characterised by Ruk (pain), Daha (burning sensation), Raga (redness) and Toda (pricking pain), then it is to be diagnosed as Vidagdha or semi matured if it is fully matured (sampakva) or saturated, then it becomes like Jala basti samprasha (after bag to touch), and Pidita unnatam (when pressed it gets elevated of its own again)

These constitute the group of drugs, the external application of which helps in the rupture of the suppurated abscess, these drugs are useful for the patients who are of tender nature (sukumara) who cannot stand surgical intervention:

• Uma – linseed

• Guggulu (Commiphora mukul Engl)

• Sudha-ayas (snuhi- Ksira)

• Stool or Daksa (cock) and Kapota,

• Alkali preparations of Palasa – Butea monosperma, Hema (Mesua ferrea) Ksiri (Kankustha) and Mukulaka (danti)

If the patient is Krcchra (physically and mentally strong), then, incision of the suppurated abscess is an excellent remedial measure. [49- 54]

Shat Vidha Shastrakarma for Vrana – Six surgical Measures:

पाटनं व्यधनं चैव छेदनं लेपनं तथा| प्रच्छनं सीवनं चैव षड्विधं शस्त्रकर्म तत्||५५||

The six types of surgical measures (useful for the treatment of ulcers and abscesses) are as follows:

1. Patana – Incision

2. Vyadhana – Puncturing

3. Chedana – Excision

4. Lepana or Lekhana – Scraping

5. Pracchana – scarification or rubbing and

6. Sivana – Suturing [55]

Patana (incision):

नाडी व्रणाः पक्वशोथास्तथा क्षत गुदोदरम्| अन्तःशल्याश्च ये शोफाः पाट्यास्ते तद्विधाश्च ये||५६||

Incision is useful for the following types of ulcers:

1. Nadi- Vrana – sinus

2. Pakva- Vrana – Suppuratated abscess or ulcer

3. Ksatodara – intestinal perforation

4. Baddha Gudodara – intestine obstruction

5. Antah- Shalya – wounds and ulcers having foreign body inside

6. Similar other ailments [56]

Vyadhana (puncturing):

दकोदराणि सम्पक्वा गुल्मा ये ये च रक्तजाः| व्यध्याः शोणित रोगाश्च विसर्प पिडकादयः||५७||

Puncturing is useful for the following ailments:

1. Dakodara – Ascites

2. Pakva- Gulma – suppurated tumor

3. Rakta- Gulma – uterine tumour and

4. Ailments caused by the vitiation of blood like Visarpa (erysipelas and herpes) and Pidaka (pimple). [57]

Chedana (Excision):

उद्वृत्तान् स्थूल पर्यन्तानुत्सन्नान् कठिणान् व्रणान्| अर्शःप्रभृत्यधीमांसं छेदनेनोपपादयेत्||५८||

Excision is useful in the following types of ulcer:

1. Udvrtta – ulcers having overgrowing granulation tissue

2. Sthula-Paryanta – ulcers having thick margin

3. Utsanna – elevated ulcer

4. Kathina – hard ulcer and

5. Adhi- Mamsa – protruded muscle tissue like Arsas or piles [58]

Lekhana (Scraping):

किलासानि सकुष्ठानि लिखेल्लेख्यानि बुद्धिमान्|

A wise physician should employ the scraping type of surgical measure for the following ailments:

1. Kilasa – leucoderma

2. Kushta – obstinate skin diseases including leprosy and

3. Such other skin diseases requiring scraping therapy [½ 59]

Pracchana (Scarification):

वातासृग्ग्रन्थि पिडकाः सकोठा रक्त मण्डलम्||५९||

कुष्ठान्यभिहतं चाङ्गं शोथांश्च प्रच्छयेदिभिषक्||

A physician should apply scarification therapy for the following:

1. Vatasrk – nodes developed as a result of rheumatoid arthritis and gout

2. Granthi – enlarged lymph glands

3. Pidaka – pimples

4. Kotha – urticarial patches

5. Rakta- Mandala – red and Circular patches in the skin

6. Kushta – lepromatous growths

7. Abhihata- Anga – limbs affected by injury and

8. Sotha – oedematous parts [59 ½ – ½ 60]

Sivana (Suturing):

सीव्यं कुक्ष्युदराद्यं तु गम्भीरं यद्विपाटितम्||६०||

इति षड्विधमुद्दिष्टं शस्त्रकर्म मनीषिभिः|६१|

Deep incision in the pelvis, abdomen, etc, is sutured. Thus, 6 types of surgical interventions are described, in brief, by the experts in surgery. [60 ½- ½ 61]

Avapidana (Compression)

सूक्ष्माननाः कोषवन्तो ये व्रणास्तान्प्रपीडयेत्||६१||

कलायाश्च मसूराश्च गोधूमाः सहरेणवः| कल्कीकृताः प्रशस्यन्ते निःस्नेहा व्रणपीडने||६२||

For the treatment of ulcers (abscesses) having a fine opening, and expanded base (pouch fomentation), Pidana (compression) therapy is administered.

Application of the paste of kalaya , Masura, Godhuma – wheat – Triticum sativum and Harenu without the addition of any fat is immensely helpful for this compression therapy. [61 ½ – 62]

Nirvapana (Sprinkling Therapy):

शाल्मलीत्वग्बलामूलं तथा न्यग्रोधपल्लवाः| न्यग्रोधादिकमुद्दिष्टं बलादिकमथापि वा||६३||

आलेपनं निर्वपणं तद्विद्व्यातैश्च सेचनम्| सर्पिषा शतधौतेन पयसा मधुकाम्बुना||६४||

निर्वापयेत् सुशीतेन रक्तपितोत्तरान् व्रणान्||६५|

For the external application in paste form, and for sprinkling (affusion) in decoction form, the following recipes are useful:

1. Bark of shalmali – Salmalia malabarica and root of Bala – Country mallow (root) – Sida cordifolia

2. Leaves of Nyagrodha – Ficus benghalensis

3. Group of drugs beginning with Nyagrodha – Ficus benghalensis described in the verse no 46

4. Group of drugs beginning with Bala – Country mallow (root) – Sida cordifolia (Vijaya) described in the verse no 47 and

5. Sprinkling with cold ShataDhauta ghrta (ghee washed with water for 100 times) or with cold milk or with the cold decoction of Madhuka– Licorice – Glycyrrhiza glabra, if the ulcer is caused by the vitiation of Rakta and Pitta 63- ½ 65]

Mamsa Sandhana (restoration of Muscle Tissue):

लम्बानि व्रणमांसानि प्रलिप्य मधुसर्पिषा||६५||
सन्दधीत समं वैद्यो बन्धनैश्चोपपादयेत्| तान्समान्सुस्थिताञ्ज्ञात्वा फलिनी लोध्र कट्फलैः||६६||
समङ्गा धातकी युक्तैश्चूर्णितैरवचूर्णयेत्| पञ्चवल्कलचूर्णैर्वा शुक्तिचूर्णसमायुतैः||६७||
धातकी लोध्रचूर्णैर्वा तथा रोहन्ति ते व्रणाः|६८|

If the muscle tissue over the ulcer is hanging loose, then the physician should smear it with honey and ghee, and appropriately restore it. Thereafter, the wound is bandaged.

After ascertaining its proper and stable restoration, the ulcer is sprinkled with the following:

1. Powder of Phalini – Callicarpa macrophylla, Lodhra – Symplocos racemosa, Katphala – Myrica nagi, Samanga – Rubia cordifolia and Dhataki – Woodfordia fruticosa

2. Powder of the barks of Nyagrodha – Ficus benghalensis, Udumbara – Ficus racemosa, Asvattha – Ficus religiosa, Parisa – Ficus lacor and Plaksa – Ficus lacor taken together, these are called Pancha- Valkala (five barks). To these drugs, powder of Sukti (Badarika) may be added and

3. Powder of Dhataki – Woodfordia fruticosa and Lodhra (Symplocos racemosa).

By the above measures, the ulcer gets healed up. [65 ½ – ½ 68]

Asthi Sandhana (Restoration of Fractured Bones):

अस्थिभग्नं च्युतं सन्धिं सन्दधीत समं पुनः||६८||
समेन सममङ्गेन कृत्वाऽन्येन विचक्षणः| स्थिरैः कवलिकाबन्धैः कुशिकाभिश्च संस्थितम्||६९||
पट्टैः प्रभूत सर्पिष्कैर्बध्नीयादचलं सुखम्| अविदाहिभिरन्नैश्च पैष्टिकैस्तमुपाचरेत्||७०||
ग्लानिर्हि न हिता तस्य सन्धिविश्लेषकारिका| विच्युताभिहताङ्गानां विसर्पादीनुपद्रवान्||७१||
उपाचरेद्यथाकालं कालज्ञः स्वाच्चिकित्सितात्|७२|

Asthi Sandhana (Restoration of Fractured Bones):

If there is fracture or dislocation of bone, it is set (put in appropriate place) correctly by a wise physician keeping the alignment at par with the other unaffected limb or the part of the body. Then it is stabilised by rapping with cotton and splints. It should, thereafter, be bandaged with a cloth profusely smeared with ghee, and made immobile as well as comfortable.

The patient is given food and pastries which do not cause burning sensation (Avidahi). Such a patient should not resort to physical exercise which may cause dislocation of the joints.

If the patient having dislocation of the joints or fracture of bones suffers from complications like erysipelas, then the physician should administer treatment relevant to the concerned ailment (complication) at appropriate time. [68 ½ – ½ 72]

Vrana Svedana (Fomentation)

शुष्का महारुजः स्तब्धा ये व्रणा मारुतोत्तराः| स्वेद्याः सङ्कर कल्पेन ते स्युः कृशर पायसैः||७२||
ग्राम्यबैलाम्बुजानूपैर्वेश्वारैश्च संस्कृतैः| उत्कारिकाभिश्चोष्णाभिः सुखी स्याद्व्रणितस्तथा||७३|

If the ulcer is predominated by aggravated Vayu because of which it is

• Sushka (dry)
• Maha ruja (extremely painful) and
• Stabdha (stiff),

Then the patient is given Sankara type of fomentation therapy (vide Sutra 14: 41) with the help of

• Krsara (Preparation of rice and Mung dal),
• Payasa (preparation of the rice and milk), and
• Sizzled and hot Vesavara (Poultice) prepared of the meat of animals which are domesticated and which live in burrows or water marshy land. This makes the patient comfortable. [2/3 72- 73]

Shamana (Alleviation Therapy):

सदाहा वेदनावन्तो ये व्रणा मारुतोत्तराः| तेषामुमां तिलांश्चैव भृष्टान् पयसि निर्वृतान्||७४||

तेनैव पयसा पिष्ट्वा कुर्यादालेपनं भिषक्| बला गुडूची मधुकं पृश्निपर्णी शतावरी||७५||

जीवन्ती शर्करा क्षीरं तैलं मत्स्यवसा घृतम्| संसिद्धा समधूच्छिष्टा शूलघ्नी स्नेहशर्करा||७६||

द्विपञ्चमूलक्वथितेनाम्भसा पयसाऽथवा | सर्पिषा वा सतैलेन कोष्णेन परिषेचयेत्||७७||

यवचूर्णं समधुकं सतिलं सह सर्पिषा| दद्यादालेपनं कोष्णं दाहशूलोपशान्तये||७८||

उपनाहश्च कर्तव्यः सतिलो मुद्गपायसः| रुग्दाहयोः प्रशमनो व्रणेष्वेष विधिर्हितः||७९||

Roasted Uma and Tila – Sesame (Sesamum indicum) is soaked in milk, and made to a paste by triturating with the same milk. The physician should apply this paste to cure the ulcer caused by aggravated Vayu associated with burning sensation as well as pain.

Oil (1 part) is cooked by adding milk (4 parts), and the paste (1/4th part in total) of Bala – Country mallow (root) – Sida cordifolia, Guduchi – Tinospora cordifolia, Madhuka– Licorice – Glycyrrhiza glabra, Prsniparni, Shatavari – Asparagus racemosus, Jivanti – Leptadenia reticulata, Sarkara (sugar), fat of fish, Ghee and bee's wax (all taken in equal quantities). External application of this preparation (semi- solid in consistency) cures pain in the ulcer.

Sprinkling the ulcer with the decoction, or medicated milk or medicated ghee or medicated oil prepared by boiling with Dasha-Mula (Bilva – Aegle marmelos, Syonaka – Orchis mascula, Gambhari – Gmelina arborea, Patala – Ficus microcarpa, Ganikarika – Premna integrifolia, Shala- Parni, Prsni-parni, Brihati – Solanum indicum, Kantakari – Solanum xanthocarpum and Goksura – Tribulus terrestris) is useful.

Application of Luke warm powder of barley added with Madhuka– Licorice – Glycyrrhiza glabra, Tila or ghee alleviates burning sensation and pain in the ulcer.

Application of the hot poultice prepared of Tila – Sesame (Sesamum indicum), Mudga – Vigna radiate and Payasa (preparation of milk and rice) alleviates pain and burning sensation in the ulcer.

The above mentioned recipes are useful in the treatment of ulcer. [74-79]

Eshana (probing):

सूक्ष्माननना बहुस्रावाः कोषवन्तश्च ये व्रणाः| न च मर्माश्रितास्तेषामेषणं हितमुच्यते||८०||

द्विविधामेषणीं विद्यान्मृद्वीं च कठिनामपि| औद्भिदैर्मृदुभिर्नालैर्लोहानां वा शलाकया||८१||

गम्भीरे मांसले देशे पाट्यं लौह शलाकया| एष्यं विद्याद्व्रणं नालैर्विपरीतमतो भिषक्||८२||

Probing is useful for ulcer having

• Sukshma aanana – narrow opening

• Bahu srava – excessive secretion and

• Kosha vanta – expanded base provided these are not located in vital organs.

Probes are of two types. Viz,

• Soft probes are made of soft stems of plants and

• Hard probes are made of metals if the ulcer is deep- seated and located in a fleshy area, and then it is probed by a metallic probe followed by excision.

If the ulcer is of opposite nature, then probing is done by the stalk or stem of plants [80- 82]

Sodhana (Cleansing of wounds):

पूतिगन्धान् विवर्णांश्च बहुस्रावान्महारुजः| व्रणानशुद्धान् विज्ञाय शोधनैः समुपाचरेत्||८३||

त्रिफला खदिरो दार्वी न्यग्रोधादिर्बला कुशः| निम्ब कोलक पत्राणि कषायाः शोधना मताः||८४||

तिलकल्कः सलवणो द्वे हरिद्रे त्रिवृद्घृतम्| मधुकं निम्बपत्राणि प्रलेपो व्रणशोधनः||८५||

The characteristic features of unclean ulcer which is required to be cleansed:

• Puti gandha – Putrid odour

• Vivarna – discoloration,

• Bahu srava – excessive discharge and

• Maha ruja – excruciating pain

The decoction of Haritaki – Terminalia chebula, Bibhitaka – Terminalia bellerica, Amalaki – Emblica officinalis, Khadira (Acacia catechu), Daruharidra – Berberis aristata, drugs belonging to Nyagrodhadi group (vide verse no .

46), Bala – Country mallow (root) – Sida cordifolia, Kusa (Desmostachya bipinnata) and tender leaves of Nimba – Neem (Azadirachta indica) and Kola helps in the cleansing of ulcer.

Application of the paste of Tila – Sesame (Sesamum indicum), salt, Haridra (turmeric – Curcuma longa), Daru haridra – Berberis aristata, Trivrt – Operculina turpethum, ghee, Madhuka– Licorice – Glycyrrhiza glabra and leaf of Nimba – Neem (Azadirachta indica) cleanses the ulcer. [83-85]

Ropana (healing):

नाति रक्तो नाति पाण्डु नातिश्यावो न चातिरुक्| न चोत्सन्नो न चोत्सङ्गी शुद्धो रोप्यः परं व्रणः||८६||

न्यग्रोधोदुम्बराश्वत्थ कदम्ब प्लक्ष वेतसाः| करवीरार्ककुटजाः कषाया व्रणरोपणाः||८७||

चन्दनं पद्मकिञ्जल्कं दार्वीत्वङ्नीलमुत्पलम्| मेदे मूर्वा समङ्गा च यष्ट्याह्वं व्रणरोपणम्||८८||

प्रपौण्डरीकं जीवन्ती गोजिह्वा धातकी बला| रोपणं सतिलं दद्यात् प्रलेपं सघृतं व्रणे||८९||

कम्पिल्लकं विडङ्गानि वत्सकं त्रिफलां बलाम्| पटोलं पिचुमर्दं च लोध्रं मुस्तं प्रियङ्गुकम्||९०||

खदिरं धातकीं सर्जमेलामगुरु चन्दने| पिष्ट्वा साध्यं भवेत्तैलं तत् परं व्रणरोपणम्||९१||

प्रपौण्डरीकं मधुकं काकोल्यौ द्वे च चन्दने| सिद्धमेतैः समैस्तैलं परं स्याद्व्रणरोपणम्||९२||

दूर्वास्वरससिद्धं वा तैलं कम्पिल्लकेन वा| दार्वीत्वचश्च कल्केन प्रधानं व्रणरोपणम्||९३||

येनैव विधिना तैलं घृतं तेनैव साधयेत्| रक्तपित्तोत्तरं दृष्ट्वा रोपणीयं व्रणं भिषक्||९४||

The ulcer, which is not very red, not very pale, not very brownish black not associated with excruciating pain, not much elevated and not associated with pockets (Utsangi), is suitable for the administration of healing therapy.

The decoctions of Nyagrodha – Ficus benghalensis, Udumbara – Ficus racemosa, Asvattha – Ficus religiosa, Kadamba – Anthocephalus indicus, Plaksa – Ficus lacor, Vetasa, Karavira – Nerium indicum, Arka – Calotropis gigantea and Kutaja – Connessi (Holarrhena antidysenterica Wall.) are useful for healing ulcers.

Similarly, the decoction of Chandana (Sandalwood – Santalum album), Padmakinjalka (filaments of lotus), bark of Daruharidra – Berberis aristata, Nilotpala, Meda, Mahameda – Polygonatum verticllatum, Murva – Marsdenia tenacissima, Samanga – Rubia cordifolia and Yastimadhu – Glycyrrhiza glabra helps in the healing of ulcer.

The paste of prapaundarika, Jivanti – Leptadenia reticulata, Gojihva, Dhataki – Woodfordia fruticosa, Bala – Country mallow (root) – Sida cordifolia and Tila – Sesame (Sesamum indicum), along with ghee is applied on the ulcer (for its healing).

Oil cooked with the paste of Kampillaka – Mallotus philippinensis, Vidanga – Embelia ribes, Vatsaka (Holarrhena antidysenterica Wall.), Haritaki – Terminalia chebula, Bibhitaki – Terminalia bellerica, Amalaki – Emblica officinalis, Bala – Country mallow (root) – Sida cordifolia, atola, Pichumarda – Azadirachta indica, Lodhra - Symplocos racemosa, Musta (Cyperus rotundus), Priyangu – Callicarpa macrophylla, Khadira - Acacia catechu, Dhataki – Woodfordia fruticosa, Sarja - Vateria indica, Ela – Elettaria cardamomum, Aguru – Aquallaria agallocha and Chandana (Sandalwood – Santalum album) is immensely useful for healing ulcers.

Similarly, oil cooked with Prapaundarika (Nymphaea lotus) – red variety, Madhuka– Licorice – Glycyrrhiza glabra, Kakoli – Fritillaria roylei, Ksheerakakoli – Lilium polyphyllum, Chandana (Sandalwood – Santalum album) and Rakta- Chandana (Sandalwood – Santalum album) is especially effective for healing ulcers.

The medicated oils prepared with the ingredients and methods similar to the preparation of medicated oil described above. [86- 94]

Patra – Application of Leaves over Ulcer:

कदम्बार्जुन निम्बानां पाटल्याः पिप्पलस्य च| व्रण प्रच्छादने विद्वान् पत्राण्यर्कस्य चादिशेत्||९५||

A wise physician should cover the ulcer with the leaves of Kadamba – Anthocephalus indicus, Arjuna (terminalia arjuna), Nimba – Neem (Azadirachta indica), Patala , Pippali – Piper longum and Arka – Calotropis gigantea. [95]

Chadana (Padding):

वार्क्षोऽथवाऽऽजिनः क्षौमः पट्टो व्रणहितः स्मृतः|

The Ulcer, [after the application of the above-mentioned leaves] is padded with the barks [fibres] of trees, leather, silk or cotton gauze which is very useful. [½ 96]

Bandha (Bandage):

बन्धश्च द्विविधः शस्तो व्रणानां सव्यदक्षिणः||९६||

The ulcer is tied with a Bandage either clock- wise or anti- clock-wise.

All the 14 types of Bandages described in the book of surgery are covered under the 2 categories described above.

Bhojya (diet and Regimes)

लवणाम्ल कटूष्णानि विदाहीनि गुरूणि च| वर्जयेदन्नपानानि व्रणी मैथुनमेव च||९७||

नातिशीत गुरु स्निग्धमविदाहि यथाव्रणम्| अन्नपानं व्रणहितं हितं चास्वपनं दिवा||९८||

The patient having ulcer should avoid such ingredients of food and drinks which are

• Lavana – saline
• Amla – sour,
• Katu – pungent,
• Ushna – hot, Vidahi (which cause burning sensation) and
• Guru – heavy

He should also avoid sexual intercourse.

Depending upon the nature of [the Doshas in the causation of], the ulcer, the patient should take food and drinks which are not too cold, too heavy, too unctuous and drinks which are not too cold, too heavy, too unctuous and vidahi (which cause burning sensation). He should not sleep during the day. [97 – 98]

Utsadana [Elevation]:

स्तन्यानि जीवनीयानि बृंहणीयानि यानि च| उत्सादनार्थं निम्नानां व्रणानां तानि कल्पयेत्||९९||

For the elevation of depressed ulcer, the paste of drugs belonging to

• Stanya- Varga (group of Galactogogues)
• Jivaniya- Gana (a group of life- promoters) and
• Brmhaniya- Varga (group of nourishing drugs) is used over it. [99]

Avasadana (Removal of excessive Granulation):

भूर्ज ग्रन्थ्यश्म कासीस मधोभागानि गुग्गुलुः| व्रणावसादनं तद्वत् कलविङ्ककपोतविट्||१००||

For the removal of excessive granulation, tissue over the ulcer, the nodes of Bhurja (Betula utilis D. Don.), Asma- Kasisa (dhatu- Kasisa), Purgative drugs (like Trivrt), Guggulu (Commifora mukul Engl.) and the stool of Kalavinka as well as Kapota may, effectively, be applied. [100]

Agni- Karma (cauterization including Heat):

रुधिरेऽतिप्रवृत्ते तु च्छिन्ने च्छेद्येऽधिमांसके| कफग्रन्थिषु गण्डेषु वातस्तम्भानिलार्तिषु||१०१||

गूढपूयलसीकेषु गम्भीरेषु स्थिरेषु च| कप्तेषु चाङ्गदेशेषु कर्माग्नेः सम्प्रशस्यते||१०२||

मधूच्छिष्टेन तैलेन मज्ज क्षौद्र वसा घृतैः| तप्तैर्वा विविधैर्लोहैर्दहेद्दाहविशेषवित्||१०३||

रूक्षाणां सुकुमाराणां गम्भीरान्मारुतोत्तरान्| दहेत् स्नेह मधू च्छिष्टैर्लोहैः क्षौद्रैस्ततोऽन्यथा||१०४||

बाल दुर्बल वृद्धानां गर्भिण्या रक्त पित्तिनाम्| तृष्णा ज्वर परीतानामबलानां विषादिनाम्||१०५||

नाग्निकर्मोपदेष्टव्यं स्नायु मर्म व्रणेषु च| सविषेषु च शल्येषु नेत्र कुष्ठ व्रणेषु च||१०६||

Agni karma (cauterization including application of heat) is useful for ulcer associated with excessive bleeding after excision of the hanging flesh, in muscular over- growth, in glands enlarged because of aggravated kapha, in goitre in stiffness and for such other ailments caused by aggravated Vayu. It is also useful when the ulcer has hidden pockets containing pus and lymph, when the ulcer is deep-seated in the stable part of the body.

This therapy (Agni- karma) may be administered by an expert in this branch of healing with hot bee's wax, oil, bone-marrow, honey, fat or ghee, or with red hot instruments prepared of different types of metals.

If the patient is dry, and is of tender nature, and if the ulcer is deep-seated and is caused by the aggravated Vayu predominantly, then Agni-Karma (cauterization) is done with the help of hot fat, bee's wax, metallic instruments and honey. Such measures are employed otherwise.

Agnikarma (cauterization) is prohibited for

• Bala – infants,

• Durbala – weak and

• Vrdhha – old persons,

• Garbhinya – pregnant women,

• Patients suffering from Rakta- Pitta (ailment characterised by bleeding from various parts of the body),

• Trishna – thirst

• Jvara – fever,

• abalanam – those who are less of strength / women

Vishaditanam – those who are suffering from depression

It is also prohibited if the ulcer is located in ligaments, vital organs, if the ulcer is caused by poisoned weapons (arrows), in ulcers of the eyes and ulcers arising out of Kushta (obstinate skin diseases including Leprosy). [101- 106]

Kshara (application of Alkalies):

रोग दोष बलापेक्षी मात्रा कालाग्नि कोविदः| शस्त्र कर्माग्निकृत्येषु क्षारमप्यवचारयेत्||१०७||

The physician well versed in the dose, time of administration and heat (agni) required by the patient of ulcer on the basis of the strength of the disease and doshas, should also administer Ksara (alkali preparations) to such of the patients for whom surgical intervention and Cauterization are indicated [107]

Dhupana (Fumigation Therapy):

कठिनत्वं व्रणा यान्ति गन्धैः सारैश्च धूपिताः| सर्पि मंज्ज वसा धूपैः शैथिल्यं यान्ति हि व्रणाः||१०८||

रुजः स्रावाश्च गन्धाश्च कृमयश्च व्रणाश्रिताः| शैथिल्यं मार्दवं चापि धूपनेनोपशाम्यति||१०९||

When fumigated with aromatic drugs and the heart- wood of aromatic plants, the ulcerated tissue gets hardened Fumigation with the fumes of ghee, bone- marrow and muscle fat softens the ulcerated tissues. [108 – 109]

Alepa (application of Ointments):

लोध्र न्यग्रोध शुङ्गानि खदिर स्त्रिफला घृतग्| प्रलेपो व्रण शैथिल्य सौकुमार्य प्रसाधनः||११०||

सरुजः कठिनाः स्तब्धा निरास्रावाश्च ये व्रणाः| यवचूर्णैः ससर्पिष्कैर्बहुशस्तान् प्रलेपयेत्||१११||

मुद्ग षष्टिक शालीनां पायसैर्वा यथाक्रमम्| सघृतैर्जीवनीयैर्वा तर्पयेतानभीक्ष्णशः||११२||

Application of ointment prepared of Lodhra (Symplocos racemosa), root of Nyagrodha, (Vata), Khadira (Acacia catechu), Haritaki – Terminalia chebula, Vibhitaka – Terminalia bellerica and Amalaki – Emblica officinalis by adding ghee cures looseness and tenderness of the ulcerated tissues.

If the ulcer is associated with pain, hardness, stiffness and dryness (without any discharge), then it is frequently anointed with barley- flour mixed with ghee.

The ulcer having the above mentioned characteristics is frequently anointed with Payasa (a preparation of milk) of Mudga, Sastika type of rice appropriately. This ulcer is anointed with the medicated ghee prepared by boiling with the drugs belonging to the Jivaniya (life promoting) group of drugs (vide Sutra 4: 19) [110- 112]

Avachurnana (dusting of wounds)

ककुभोदुम्बराश्वत्थ लोध्र जाम्बव कट्फलैः| त्वचमाश्वेव गृह्णन्ति त्वक्चूर्णैश्चूर्णिता व्रणाः||११३||

Dusting over the ulcer with the powder of the bark of Kakubha – Terminalia arjuna, Udumbara – Ficus racemosa, Asvattha – Ficus religiosa, Lodhra (Symplocos racemosa), Jambu – Eugenia jambolana and Katphala – Myrica nagi helps in the formation of new skin over it quickly. [113]

Ropana (Promotion of Healthy Skin):

मनःशिलैला मञ्जिष्ठा लाक्षा च रजनी द्वयम्| प्रलेपः सघृत क्षौद्रस्त्वग्विशुद्धिकरः परः||११४||

Application of the paste of Manahsila, Ela (Elettaria cardamomum Maton), Manjistha – Rubia cordifolia, laksa, Haridra (turmeric – Curcuma longa) and Daruharidra (Berberis aristata) along with ghee and honey helps in the promotion of healthy skin over the ulcer. [114]

Varnya (Restoration of Normal skin colour):

अयोरजः सकासीसं त्रिफला कुसुमानि च| करोति लेपः कृष्णत्वं सद्य एव नवत्वचि||११५||

कालीयकनताम्रास्थि हेमकान्ता रसोत्तमैः | लेपः सगोमयरसः सवर्णीकरणः परः||११६||

ध्यामकाश्वत्थ निचुल मूलं लाक्षा सगैरिका| सहेमश्चामृतासङ्गः कासीसं चेति वर्णकृत्||११७||

Application of the ointment prepared of the Bhasmas of Lauha and Kasisa, and flowers of Haritaki – Terminalia chebula, Vibhitaka – Terminalia bellerica and Amalaki – Phyllanthus officinalis helps in the formation of Pigments (blacksness) instantaneously over the nearly formed skin over the ulcer.

Kaliyaka, Nata (Valeriana wallicii), pulp of the seed of Amra – mango – Mangifera indica, Hema (Mesua ferrea) (Dhustura or the Bhasman of gold), Kanta and Rasottama (mercury or ghee) is made to a paste by triturating with the juice of cow-dung application of this paste over the skin (which has grown over the ulcer) helps in the restoration of its original colour.

Dhyamaka, Asvattha – Ficus religiosa, root of Nicula Laksa and Gairika (red ocher) should be made to a paste and applied over the skin developed over the ulcer which promotes restoration of its natural colou r. Similarly, [application of the paste of] Hema (Mesua ferrea) (Dhustura or the Bhasma of gold], Amrta- Sanga (Khararika Tuttha) and Kasisa promotes the natural colour of the skin. [115- 117]

Loma Rohana (Restoration of Growth of Hair):

चतुष्पदानां त्वग्लोम खुर शृङ्गास्थि भस्मना| तैलाक्ता चूर्णिता भूमिर्भवेल्लोमवती पुनः||११८||

The skin, Hair, hoof, horn and bones of quadruped animals are burnt and reduced to ash. To this ash, oil is added. Application of this medicated oil makes the fresh skin developed over the ulcer full of natural hair. [118]

Treatment of complications:

षोडशोपद्रवा ये च व्रणानां परिकीर्तिताः| तेषां चिकित्सा निर्दिष्टा यथास्वं स्वे चिकित्सिते||११९||

16 ailments which appear as complications of ulcer (vide verse nos. 28-30) are to be treated according to the lines of treatment suggested for each one of them. [119]

Summary:

तत्र श्लोकौ-

द्वौ व्रणौ व्रणभेदाश्च परीक्षा दुष्टिरेव च| स्थानानि गन्धाः स्रावाश्च सोपसर्गाः क्रियाश्च याः||१२०||

व्रणाधिकारे सप्रश्नमेतन्नवकमुक्तवान्| मुनिर्व्यासससमासाभ्यामग्निवेशाय धीमते||१२१||

In this chapter on 'Ulcer', along with Agnivesha's query, the nine topics explained both, in brief and in detail, by the sage (Atreya) are, a follows:

1. 2 categories of ulcer

2. Classification of ulcers

3. Examination of ulcers

4. Morbid effects of ulcers

5. Location of ulcers

6. Odour of ulcer

7. Nature of the discharge from ulcers

8. Complications and method of treatment of ulcers [120- 121]

Colophon

इत्यग्निवेशकृते तन्त्रे चरक प्रतिसंस्कृते दृढबल सम्पूरिते चिकित्सा स्थाने द्विव्रणीय चिकित्सितं नाम पञ्चविंशोऽध्यायः||२५||

Thus, ends the 25th chapter dealing with the treatment of 2 types of ulcers of Chikitsa- sthana (Section on the treatment of diseases) in Agnivesha's work as redacted by Charaka, and supplemented by Drudhabala.

इत्यग्निवेशकृते तन्त्रे चरक प्रतिसंस्कृते दृढबल सम्पूरिते चिकित्सा स्थाने द्विव्रणीय चिकित्सितं नाम पञ्चविंशोऽध्यायः||२५||

9
Chikitsasthana Chapter 26
Trimarmeeya Chikitsitam

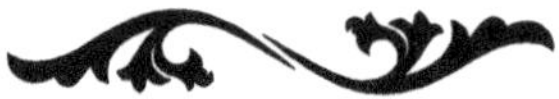

The 26th chapter of Charaka Samhita Chikitsa Sthana, called Trimarmeeya Chikitsa, deals with the treatment of diseases afflicting the urinary system, heart and brain.

अथातस्त्रिमर्मीय चिकित्सितमध्यायं व्याख्यास्यामः||१||

इति ह स्माह भगवानात्रेयः||२||

We shall now explore the chapter on the treatment of the Afflictions of the 3 Vital Organs Marmas. Thus, said Lord Atreya. [1-2]

Prologue:

सप्तोत्तरं मर्मशतं यदुक्तं शरीर सङ्ख्यामधिकृत्य तेभ्यः| मर्माणि बस्तिं हृदयं शिरश्च प्रधान भूतानि वदन्ति तज्ज्ञाः||३||

प्राणाश्रयात्, तानि हि पीड्यन्तो वातादयोऽसूनपि पीड्यन्ति| तत्संश्रितानामनुपालनार्थं महागदानां शृणु सौम्य रक्षाम्||४||

While enumerating different organs and their parts in the body in chapter- 7 (Sarira Sthana), Vital organs are described to be 107 in number (vide Charaka Shareeera Sthana 7/14). Of these, according to the experts in the field, 3 vital organs, viz, –

Basti – Urinary bladder

Hrudaya – Heart and

Shira – Head

These three are the most important because they are the seats of Prana (elan vitae / vital force.)

Their affliction by Vata, etc., endangers life. Thus, the methods of protecting these vital organs from the attacks of diseases, and treatment of the diseases already manifested in them will be described. Listen. [3-4]

Udavarta – Bloating

Etiology and pathogenesis of Udavarta:

कषाय तिक्तोषण रूक्ष भोज्यैः सन्धारणाभोजन मैथुनैश्च | पक्वाशये कुप्यति चेदपानः स्रोतांस्यधोगानि बली स रुद्ध्वा||५||

Because of the intake of

Kashaya (Astringent), Tikta (bitter), Ushna (pungent) and Ruksha (un-unctuous food), and

Sandharana – suppression of natural urges,

Abhojana – skipping food, excessive fasting,

Maithuna – excess sexual intercourse, The Apana Vata gets aggravated in the colon. It obstructs the downward moving channels [like anus and urinary passage] as a result of which the movement of stool, urine and flatus gets gradually obstructed, giving rise to Udavarta (upward movement of the wind in the abdomen) which is a serious ailment. [5- 2/4 6]

Signs and Symptoms of Udavarta:

करोति विण्मारुत मूत्रसङ्गं क्रमादुदावर्तमतः सुघोरम्| रुग्बस्ति हृत्कुक्ष्युदरेष्वभीक्ष्णं सपृष्ठ पार्श्वेष्वतिदारुणा स्यात्||६||

आध्मान हल्लास विकर्तिकाश्च तोदोऽविपाकश्च सबस्तिशोथः| वर्चोऽप्रवृत्तिर्जठरे च गण्डान्यूर्ध्वश्च वायुर्विहतो गुदे स्यात्||७||

कृच्छ्रेण शुष्कस्य चिरात् प्रवृत्तिः स्याद्वा तनुः स्यात् खर रूक्ष शीता| ततश्च रोगा ज्वर मूत्रकृच्छ्र प्रवाहिकाहृद्ग्रहणी प्रदोषाः||८||

वम्यान्ध्य बाधिर्य शिरोऽभिताप वातोदराष्ठील मनोविकाराः| तृष्णास्रपितारुचि गुल्म कास श्वास प्रतिश्यार्दित पार्श्व रोगाः||९||

अन्ये च रोगा बहवोऽनिलोत्था भवन्त्युदावर्तकृताः सुघोराः| चिकित्सितं चास्य यथावदूर्ध्व प्रवक्ष्यते तच्छृणु चाग्निवेश!||१०||

The signs and symptoms of Udavarta are as follows:

Vit Maruta Mutra Sangha – obstruction to gas, faeces (constipation) and Urine (dysurea)

Basti, Hrut, kukshi Udara ruk- Frequent pain in the region of urinary bladder, heart, pelvis and abdomen

Prushta, Parshveshu atidaruna – Excruciating pain in the back side of the chest

Aadhmana (Flatulence), Hrullasa (nausea),

Vikartika (griping pain, cutting type of pain),

Toda (Pricking pain), Vipaka (indigestion) and

Basthi shotha (inflammation of the urinary bladder)

Movement of flatus upwards because of obstruction in the anus

Ejaculation of semen with difficulty and after a long time and

Dryness and coldness of the body

As a result of Udavarta, the serious diseases manifested are

Jwara – fever

Mutrakruchra – difficulty in passing urine

Pravahika – dysentery

Hrud roga – cardiac ailments

Grahani – sprue syndrome

Chardi – vomiting

Aandhya – blindness

Badhirya – deafness

Shiro abhitapa – burning sensation in the head

Vatodara – affliction of abdomen by Vata

Asthila – Tumours

Mano vikara – Mental disorders / Psychic perversion

Trshna – morbid thirst

Rakta pitta – an ailment characterized by bleeding from different parts of the body

Aruchi – anorexia

Gulma – phantom tumour

Kasa – cough

Shvasa – Asthma

Pratishyaya – chronic cold

Ardita – facial paralysis

Parshva roga - diseases in the sides of the chest, and

Anya roga – such other serious diseases caused by the aggravation of Vata.

Agnivesha! You may listen to the treatment of these ailments which will be described hereafter [6 2/4 – 10]

Udavarta Chikitsa Sutra:

तं तैल शीतज्वरनाशनाक्तं स्वेदैर्यथोक्तैः प्रविलीन दोषम्| उपाचरेद्वर्ति निरूह बस्ति स्नेहै विरेकैरनुलोमनान्नैः||११||

Line of treatment of Udavarta:

The Patient suffering from Udavarta is given a massage with oil for the treatment of Sheeta Jvara (fever with coldness in the exterior of the body).

Thereafter, Swedana – sweating therapy is administered for the detachment of the adhered Doshas in the tissue cells. This is followed by the administration of Varti - suppository, Niruha type of medicated enema, and unctuous type of purgative. The patient is given food which helps in the downward movement of Vata [11]

Varti – Suppository:

श्यामात्रिवृन्मागधिकां स दन्तीं गोमूत्र पिष्टां दशभागमाषाम्| सनीलिकां द्विर्लवणां गुडेन वर्तिं कराङ्गुष्ठनिभां विदध्यात्||१२||

पिण्याक सौवर्चल हिङ्गुभिर्वा ससर्षप त्र्यूषण यावशूकैः| क्रिमिघ्न कम्पिल्लक शङ्खिनीभिः सुधार्कजक्षीरगुडैर्युताभिः||१३||

स्यात् पिप्पली सर्षपराढवेश्मधूमैः सगोमूत्रगुडैश्च वर्तिः|

A suppository having the thickness of the thumb is prepared with the following recipes:

1 part of

Syama Trivrt – Operculina turpethum,

Magadhika – Piper longum and

Danti – Baliospermum montanum all taken together, 10 parts of Masha made to a paste by triturating cow's urine, 1 part of Neelika, and 2 parts of salt by adding jaggery in sufficient quantity

Pinyaka, Sauvarcala, Hingu, Sarshapa – Mustard, Sunthi – Ginger, Pippali – Piper longum, Maricha – Black pepper fruit – piper nigrum and Yava Ksara by adding jaggery.

Krimighna – Vidanga,

Kampillaka, Shankini, latex of Sudha (snuhi) and Arka – Calotropis gigantea by adding Jaggery and

Pippali – Long pepper fruit – Piper longum, Sarshapa – mustard, Radha, Madana- phala – Randia dumetorum and house soot by adding cow's urine and jaggery

The above mentioned types of suppository are inserted into the oleated anus of the patient for the downward movement of wind and cure of the retention of stool, flatus and urine [caused by Udavarta or upward movement of wind in the abdomen. [12 – ½ 14]

Pradhamana (Insufflation):

श्यामाफलालाबुक पिप्पलीनां नाड्याऽथवा तत् प्रधमेतु चूर्णम्||१४||

रक्षोघ्न तुम्बी करहाट कृष्णाचूर्ण स जीमूतक सैन्धवं वा|

स्निग्धे गुदे तान्यनुलोमयन्ति नरस्य वर्चोऽनिल मूत्रसङ्गम्||१५||

Anal orifice is applied with ghee or oil. A tube is inserted into it, and through this, the powder of the following recipes is used for Pradhamana (insufflation):

Syama phala (Madana-phala – Randia dumetorum), Alabu and pippali – Piper longum or

Raksoghna (sarsaa), Tumbi –Cucurbita lagenaria, karahata, Madana- Phala – Randia dumetorum, krsna pippali – Piper longum, jimutaka and rock- salt.

These insufflations cause downward movement or voiding of the obstructed stool, flatus and urine. [14 ½ – 15]

Niruha Basti –

तेषां विघाते तु भिषग्विदध्यात् स्वभ्यक्त सुस्विन्नतनो निरूहम्| ऊर्ध्वानुलोमौषध मूत्र तैल क्षाराम्ल वातघ्नयुतं सुतीक्ष्णम्||१६||

वातेऽधिकेऽम्लं लवणं सतैलं, क्षीरेण पित्ते तु, कफे समूत्रम्| स मूत्रवर्चोऽनिलसङ्गमाशु गुदं सिराश्च प्रगुणीकरोति||१७||

If the above mentioned suppositories and Pradhamana therapies fail to produce the desired result, then the patient is given Snehana, Swedana followed by Basti. For the preparation of this enema,

sour herbs and salt along with oil is used if Vata is aggravated in excess;

milk is used if Pitta is aggravated; and

cow's urine is used if Kapha is aggravated.

This Niruha Basti immediately relieves the retention of urine, stool and flatus and promotes the normal functioning of the rectum as well as connected vessels. [16- 17]

Diet for Udavarta – bloating with constipation

त्रिवृत्सुधापत्र तिलादिशाक ग्राम्यौदकानूपरसै यवान्नम्| अन्यैश्च सृष्टानिल मूत्रविड्भिरद्यात् प्रसन्नागुड सीधुपायी||१८||

The patient suffering from Udavarta should take barley, as food along with the following:

Vegetable preparations made out of the aquatic animals, and Snuhi – Euphorbia neriifolia, Tila – Sesame etc.

Soup of the meat of domesticated and aquatic animals, and animals inhabiting marshy land

Such other ingredients which induce voiding of flatus, urine and stool and

Prasanna (clear top portion of alcohol) and Sidhu (type of wine prepared of Jaggery) [18]

Purgation and Anuvasana Basti
भूयोऽनुबन्धे तु भवेद्विरेच्यो मूत्र प्रसन्ना दधिमण्ड शुक्तैः| स्वस्थं तु पश्चादनुवासयेतं रौक्ष्यादिध सङ्गोऽनिलवर्चसोश्चेत्||१९||

If Udavarta continues to exist despite Niruha Basti, then the patient is given Virechana along with cow's urine, Prasanna (clear portion of alcohol), DadhiManda (upper liquid portion of curd) and Sukta (vinegar).

If even after relief from Udavarta, the retention of flatus and stool continues because of dryness, then the patient is given Anuvasana Basti (oil / fat enema) [19]

Dviruttara Hingvadi Churna:
द्विरुत्तरं हिङ्गु वचाग्नि कुष्ठं सुवर्चिका चैव विडङ्ग चूर्णम्| सुखाम्बुनाऽऽनाह विसूचिकार्ति हृद्रोग गुल्मोर्ध्व समीरणघ्नम् ||२०||

The recipe in order contains

1 part Hingu – Asa foetida

2 Parts Vacha – Acorus calamus Linn.

4 parts Agni or Chitraka – Leadword – Plumbago zeylanica,

8 parts Kushta – Saussurea lappa

16 parts Sauvarchala or Svarjika – Ksara and

32 parts Vidanga – Embelia ribes is given along with Luke warm water.

Cures

Anaha – tymphanitis

Visucika – Choloric diarrhea

Hrid roga – heart diseases

Gulma – Phantom tumour and

Urdhva Samirna or Udavarta – upward movement of wind [20]

Vachadi Churna:
वचाभया चित्रक यावशूकान् सपिप्पलीकातिविषान् सकुष्ठान्| उष्णाम्बुनाऽऽनाह विमूढवातान् पीत्वा जयेदाशु रसौदनाशी||२१||

The recipe containing

Vacha – Acorus calamus Linn.

Abhaya – Terminalia chebula

Chitraka – Plumbago zeylanica

Yava Kshara

Pippali – Piper longum

Ativisa – Aconitum heterophyllum and

Kushta – Saussurea lappa is taken with hot water which instantaneously

Cures

Anaha – Constipation and

Vimudha- Vata (arrest of the movement of Vata Dosha in the abdomen)

The patient, while using this recipe should take along with meat- soup. [21]

Hingvadi Churna:
हिङ्गूग्रगन्धा बिड शुण्ठ्यजाजी हरीतकी पुष्करमूल कुष्ठम्| यथोत्तरं भाग विवृद्धमेतत् प्लीहोदराजीर्ण विसूचिकासु||२२||

Intake of recipe containing

1 part Hingu – Asa foetida

2 parts Ugra- gandha or Ajamoda – Ajowan fruit – Trachyspermum roxburghianum,

3 parts Bida type of salt

4 parts Sunthi – Ginger

5 parts Ajaji – Nigella sativa

7 parts Pushkara mula – Inula racemosa and

8 parts Kushta – Saussurea lappa

Cures

Plihodara – Splenomegaly

Vipaka – indigestion and

Visucika – Choloric diarrhea [22]

Sthiradi Ghrita:

स्थिरादि वर्गस्य पुनर्नवायाः शम्पाक पूतीक करञ्जयोश्च| सिद्धः कषाये द्विपलांशिकानां प्रस्थो घृतात् स्यात् प्रतिरुद्धवाते||२३||

1 Prastha of ghee is cooked by adding the decoction of 2 Palas each of

Shalaparni

Prishnaparni – Uraria picta

Brihati – Solanum indicum

Kantakari – Solanum xanthocarpum

Gokshura – Tribulus terrestris

Punarnava – Boerhavia diffusa

Samaka (aragvadha) – Cassia fistula and

Puti-karanja – Holoptelea integrifolia

Intake of this medicated ghee cures

Pratiruddha- vata obstruction of the movement of flatus [23]

Medicine for Virechana:

फलं च मूलं च विरेचनोक्तं हिङ्ग्वर्कमूलं दशमूलमग्र्यम्| स्नुक् चित्रकश्चैव पुनर्नवा च तुल्यानि सर्वैर्लवणानि पञ्च||२४||

स्नेहैः समूत्रैः सह जर्जराणि शरावसन्धौ विपचेत् सुलिप्ते| पक्वं सुपिष्टं लवणं तदन्नैः पानैस्तथाऽऽनाहरुजाघ्नमद्यात्||२५||

Fruits and Roots described in the group of purgative drugs [in Sutra 1: 77-85]

Hingu – Asa foetida,

Root of Arka – Calotropis gigantea,

Bilva – Aegle marmelos

Syonaka

Gambhari – Gmelina arborea

Patali

Ganikarika

Shala Parni

Prishniparni

Brhati – Solanum indicum

Kantakari – Solanum xanthocarpum

Goksura – Tribulus terrestris

Snuhi – Euphobia neerifolia

Chitraka – Leadwort – Plumbago zeylanica and

Punarnava – Boerhavia diffusa is taken in equal quantities.

To this, equal quantity of Pancha lavana (5 types of salt) is added, and made to a coarse powder.

This powder is further triturated by adding fat and Gomutra (cow's urine), and kept inside the earthen saucers having their joints sealed properly [with mud-smeared cloth]. This is then placed over fire. After it is cooked properly, the powder is removed from inside the earthen saucers, and triturated further.

This saline powder is taken along with food and drinks. This cures Anaha (constipation) and pain in the abdomen. [24-25]

Vamana – Emetic Therapy for Anaha:

हृत्स्तम्भ मूर्धामय गौरवाभ्यामुद्गा रसङ्गेन सपीनसेन| आनाहमाम प्रभवं जयेतु प्रच्छर्दनै लङ्घन पाचनैश्च||२६||

Anaha (constipation with bloating) caused by Ama (product of improper digestion), and associated with Hrut stambha (stiffness in the chest), Shiro roga (diseases of the head) Gaurava (heaviness) is treated with Chardana (emesis), Langhana (fasting therapy) and pachana (carminatives) [26]

Use of Castrol Oil for Virechana

गुल्मोदर ब्रध्नार्श:प्लीहोदावर्त योनि शुक्रगदे | मेद:कफसंसृष्टे मारुतरक्तेऽवगाढे च||२७||

गृध्रसि पक्षवधादिषु विरेचनार्हेषु वातरोगेषु| वाते विबद्ध मार्गे मेद:कफ पित्त रक्तेन||२८||

पयसा मांसरसैर्वा त्रिफलारस यूष मूत्र मदिराभि:| दोषानुबन्धयोगात् प्रशस्तमेरण्डजं तैलम्||२९||

तद्वातनुत्स्वभावात् संयोगवशादिविरेचनाच्च जयेत्| मेदोसृक्पित्त कफोन्मिश्रानिलरोगजितस्मात्||३०||

बल कोष्ठ व्याधिवशादापञ्चपला भवेन्मात्रा| मृदुकोष्ठाल्पबलानां सह भोज्यं तत्प्रयोज्यं स्यत्||३१||

इत्युदावर्तचिकित्सा|

If the course of Vata Dosha is obstructed by fat, Kapha, Pitta or Rakta (vitiated blood) in the diseases like

Gulma – phantom tumor

Udara – obstinate abdominal diseases including ascites

Bradhna – Inguinal swelling

Arsha – piles

Pliha – splenic enlargement

Udavarta – upward movement of wind in the abdomen

Yoni Roga – diseases of the female genital tract

Shukra gada – Seminal disorders

Affliction of fat by the vitiated Kapha

Gambhira vata rakta – Deep seated Vata- Rakta (gout)

Gridhrasi – Sciatica

Pakshavadha – Hemiplegia, etc., and in such other Vatika diseases which are curable by Virechana (purgation therapy), castor oil is an excellent remedy.

It is added with such other ingredients as are conducive to the treatment of the aggravated Vata Dosha, and administered along with milk, meat soup,Triphala Kashaya, vegetables soup, cow's urine, alcoholic drink, etc.

Because of its Vata Dosha- alleviating nature, because of the addition of other appropriate drugs, and because of its purgative effects, it cures Vatika diseases associated with the vitiated fat, blood, Pitta and Kapha.

Dosage of castor oil: Upto 5 Palas depending upon the Bala (strength of the patient), the condition of Kostha (thoracic and abdominal visceras), and the nature of the disease, castor oil is administered in the dose

If the patient is of Mrdu- Kostha (laxed bowel) and is weak, then castor oil is given to him along with food.

Thus, ends the treatment of Udavarta (upward movement of wind). [27-31]

Mutra Kricchra – dysuria

Causes of Mutra-Krcchra (Dysuria):

व्यायाम तीक्ष्णौषध रूक्ष मद्य प्रसङ्ग नित्य द्रुत पृष्ठयानात्| आनूप मत्स्याध्यशनादजीर्णात् स्युर्मूत्रकृच्छ्राणि नृणामिहाष्टौ||३२||

Mutrakricchra or dysuria in human beings is of 7 types and these are caused by the following:

Vyayama – Exercise in excess of one's own capacity

Intake of medicaments having Tiksna (sharp) attributes, and Ruksha (ununctuous) ingredients in excess.

Madya sevana – Habitual intake of alcohol

Prushta yanat – Regularly riding over the back of the fast moving animals

Intake of the meat of animals inhabiting marsh land (Anupa mamsa) and Matsya (fish) in excess.

Adhyashana – Intake of food before the previous meal is digested and

Ajirnat -Indigestion (chronic) [32]

Samprapti or pathogenesis of Dysuria:

पृथङ्मलाः स्वैः कुपिता निदानैः सर्वेऽथवा कोपमुपेत्य बस्तौ| मूत्रस्य मार्गं परिपीडयन्ति यदा तदा मूत्रयतीह कृच्छ्रात्||३३||

When, being provoked by their vitiating factors, the 3 Doshas and Malas either individually or jointly get aggravated in the urinary passage, then this gives rise to Mutrakrichra (dysuria). [33]

Signs and Symptoms of Mutrakrichra – Dysuria Caused by Vata Dosha etc:

तीव्रा रुजो वङ्क्षण बस्ति मेढ्रे स्वल्पं मुहुर्मूत्रयतीह वातात्| पीतं सरक्तं सरुजं सदाहं कृच्छ्रान्मुहुर्मूत्रयतीह पित्तात्||३४||

बस्तेः सलिङ्गस्य गुरुत्व शोथौ मूत्रं सपिच्छं कफ मूत्रकृच्छ्रे| सर्वाणि रूपाणि तु सन्निपाताद्भवन्ति तत् कृच्छ्रतमं हि कृच्छ्रम्||३५||

If dysuria is caused by the aggravated Vata, then the signs and symptoms manifested are as follows:

Teevra ruja in Vankshana, Basti, medhra – Excruciating pain in the groins, region of the urinary bladder and genitals and

Muhur muhu mutra visarjana – The patient passes urine very frequently in small quantities

If dysuria is caused by the aggravated Pitta, then the signs and symptoms manifested are as follows:

Pitam mutram – The colour of the urine is yellow

Sa rakta mutram – Blood comes out along with urine

Sa rujam sa daham – Micturation is associated with pain and burning sensation and

Krcchram muhur mutram – The patient passes urine very frequently with difficulty.

If dysuria is caused by the aggravated Kapha, then the signs and symptoms manifested are as follows:

Basthi Sa linga gurutva sotha – Heaviness and oedema in the urinary bladder and phallus; and

Sa piccham kapha mutram – The urine is associated with slimy material.

If all the Doshas are aggravated to cause Sannipatika type of Dysuria, then all the signs and symptoms described above in respect of all the Doshas are manifested. This Sannipatika type of Dysuria is very difficult to cure. [34-35]

Dysuria Caused by Urinary Calculus Ashmari

Pathogenesis:

विशोषयेद्बस्तिगतं सशुक्रं मूत्रं सपित्तं पवनः कफं वा| यदा तदाऽश्मर्युपजायते तु क्रमेण पित्तेष्विव रोचना गोः||३६||

When the aggravated Vata dries up the semen, urine, Pitta and Kapha located in the urinary bladder, then gradually stones are formed there, as Gorochana (gall stone) is formed in bile inside the Gall- Bladder of cattle. [36]

Signs and Symptoms of Urinary Calculus:

कदम्बपुष्पाकृतिरश्मतुल्या श्लक्ष्णा त्रिपुट्यप्यथवाऽपि मृद्वी| मूत्रस्य चेन्मार्गमुपैति रुद्ध्वा मूत्रं रुजं तस्य करोति बस्तौ||३७||

ससेवनी मेहन बस्तिशूलं विशीर्णधारं च करोति मूत्रम्| मृद्नाति मेढ्रं स तु वेदनार्तो मुहुः शकृन्मुञ्चति मेहते च||३८||

क्षोभात् क्षते मूत्रयतीह सासृक् तस्याः सुखं मेहति च व्यपायात्||३९|

The Vataja Ashmari – calculus appears like the flowers of Kadamba – Anthocephalus indicus, and is Triputi (having 3 layers);

Paittika type of calculus is like a stone and smooth; and

Kaphaja as well as Shukraja type of calculus are soft.

If these calculi come into the urinary passage, they cause obstruction of the urine as a result of which there is Basthi shoola (pain in the urinary bladder), Perineum (Sevani [suture] below the pudendum and between to testicles), Phallus and hypogastric region over the urinary bladder.

The stream of the urine flow gets split. Because of pain, the patient squeezes the phallus and frequently voids stool and urine. If, in this process, the urinary passage or bladder gets injured by the calculus, then he passes urine mixed with blood when the calculus passes out, the urine comes out easily. [37- 39½]

Dysuria Caused by Sharkara (Graveluria – urinary gravels):

एषाऽश्मरी मारुतभिन्नमूर्तिः स्याच्छर्करा मूत्रपथात् क्षरन्ती॥३९॥

If the above mentioned calculus gets broken into small particles because of aggravated Vayu, then these sand particles come out through the urinary tract along with the urine. [39 ½]

Dysuria Caused by Semen:

रेतोऽभिघाताभिहतस्य पुंसः प्रवर्तते यस्य तु मूत्रकृच्छ्रम्। स्याद्वेदना वङ्क्षण बस्ति मेढ्रे तस्यातिशूलं वृषणातिवृत्ते॥४०॥

शुक्रेण संरुद्धगतिप्रवाहो मूत्रं स कृच्छ्रेण विमुञ्चतीह। तमण्डयोः स्तब्धमिति ब्रुवन्ति रेतोऽभिघातात् प्रवदन्ति कृच्छ्रम्॥४१॥

If dysuria occurs in a person because of the affliction by the obstruction of semen, then the patient suffers from

Vankshana basti medhre ati shoolam – pain in the groin, urinary bladder and phallus

Vrshana ativrtte – his testicles become enlarged and painful

Since the urinary flow is obstructed by semen, he passes urine with difficulty. This condition is called Anda-stambha or the stiffness of the testicles. The dysuria, thus, manifested is considered to be caused by the seminal obstruction. [41-42]

Dysuria caused by Vitiated Semen:

शुक्रं मलाश्चैव पृथक् पृथग्वा मूत्राशयस्थाः प्रतिवारयन्ति। तद्व्याहतं मेहन बस्ति शूलं मूत्रं सशुक्रं कुरुते विबद्धम्॥४२॥

स्तब्धश्च शूनो भृशवेदनश्च तुद्येत बस्तिर्वृषणौ च तस्य॥४३॥

Malas i.e. aggravated Vayu, Pitta and Kapha individually or all taken together located in the urinary bladder obstructs the passage of semen.

Because of this seminal obstruction, there is pain in the phallus and urinary bladder along with obstruction to the voiding of urine and ejaculation of semen.

Subsequently this leads to

Stabdha – stiffness,

Shuna – swelling,

Bhrsha vedana – excessive pain and

Toda – pricking pain in the region of urinary bladder and testicles. [42- ½ 43]

Dysuria caused by Kshata (Vitiated Blood):

क्षताभिघातात् क्षतजं क्षयाद्वा प्रकोपितं बस्तिगतं विबद्धम्॥४३॥

तीव्रार्ति मूत्रेण सहाश्मरीत्वमायाति तस्मिन्नतिसञ्चिते च। आध्माततां विन्दति गौरवं च बस्तेर्लघुत्वं च विनिःसृतेऽस्मिन्॥४४॥

इति मूत्रकृच्छ्र निदानम्।

If the blood located in the urinary bladder get vitiated by Ksata (trauma) or by Kshaya (emaciation caused by excessive seminal discharge), it causes obstruction and excruciating pain in the urinary bladder, in association with urine, leads to the formation of calculus which causes abdominal distension and heaviness in the region of the urinary bladder. Thus, ends the diagnosis of dysuria [43 2/4 – 44]

Treatment of Vatika Mutrakrichra:

अभ्यञ्जन स्नेह निरूहबस्ति स्नेहोपनाहोत्तरबस्ति सेकान्। स्थिरादिभिर्वातहरैश्च सिद्धान् दद्याद्रसांश्चानिल मूत्रकृच्छ्रे॥४५॥

पुनर्नवैरण्ड शतावरीभिः पत्तूरवृश्चीरबलाश्मभिदिभिः। द्विपञ्चमूलेन कुलत्थ कोल यवैश्च तोयोत्क्वथिते कषाये॥४६॥

तैलं वराहक्षवसा घृतं च तैरेव कल्कै लवणैश्च साध्यम्। तन्मात्रयाऽऽशु प्रतिहन्ति पीतं शूलान्वितं मारुत मूत्रकृच्छ्रम्॥४७॥

एतानि चान्यानि वरौषधानि पिष्टानि शस्तान्यपि चोपनाहे। स्युर्लभतस्तैलफलानि चैव स्नेहाम्लयुक्तानि सुखोष्णवन्ति॥४८॥

To the patient suffering from Vatika type of Mootrakrichra, Massage, oleation, Niruha type of medicated enema, Anuvasana type of medicated enema, Upanaha (application of hot ointment), Uttara- Basti (urethra and vaginal douche), affusion and soup prepared of drugs like those belonging to Sthiradi or Ksudra-panca- Mula group (viz, Shalaparni, Prishnaparni, Brihati – Solanum indicum, Kantakari – Solanum xanthocarpum and Goksura – Tribulus terrestris) is administered.

Oil, fat of bear, and ghee is cooked by adding the decoction and paste of

Punarnava – Boerhavia diffusa,

Eranda – Ricinus communis,

Shatavari – Asparagus racemosus,

Pattura

Vrushceera

Bala – Sida cordifolia,

Pashanabheda – Cyclea peltata

Dashamoola (bilva, Syonaka, Gambhari,, Patala, ganikarika, ShalaParni, Prsniparni, Brihati, Kantakari and Goksura),

Kulattha – horse gram

Kola – Zizyphus jujuba and

Yava – Barley along with

5 types of Salt.

Intake of these medicated oils, etc., in appropriate doses, subdues the Vatika type of Dysuria associated with pain, instantaneously. The above-mentioned drugs and such others having similar properties may also be used in the form of Upanaha (hot poultice) which is very useful in Vatika type of Dysuria.

Intake of oil-seeds like Tila – Sesame (Sesamum indicum), Uma – Linum usitatissimum and Asphota – Jasminum angustifolium along with fat and sour thing in luke-warm form is also useful in this condition Vatika type of Dysuria. [42-48]

Treatment of Paittika Mutrakrichra:

सेकावगाहाः शिशिराः प्रदेहा ग्रैष्मो विधि र्बस्तिपयो विरेकाः| द्राक्षा विदारीक्षु रसै घृतैश्च कृच्छ्रेषु पित्तप्रभवेषु कार्याः||४९||

शतावरी काश कुश श्वदंष्ट्रा विदारि शालीक्षु कशेरुकाणाम्| क्वार्थं सुशीतं मधु शर्कराभ्यां युक्तं पिबेत् पैत्तिक मूत्रकृच्छ्री||५०||

पिबेत् कषायं कमलोत्पलानां शृङ्गाटकानामथवा विदार्याः| दण्डैरकाणामथवाऽपि मूलं पूर्वेण कल्पेन तथाऽम्बु शीतम्||५१||

Treatment of Paittika Dysuria:

To the patient suffering from Paittika type of dysuria,

Seka – cold affusion,

Avagaha – cold bath,

Shishira Pradeha – application of cooling unguentum, regimens prescribed for summer season, medicated enema, medicated milk and purgation therapy prepared of the juice of Draksha – ,vitis viniferaVidari (Pueraria tuberosa), and Sugar-cane solution, and ghee is administered.

The cold decoction of Shatavari –Asparagus racemosus, Kasa – Saccharum spontaneum, Kusha (Desmostachya bipinnata), Svadamstra – Tribulus terrestris, Vidari – Pueraria tuberosa, Shali – rice, Ikshu—Sugarcane and Kaseruka (Scripus grossus), mixed with honey and sugar is administered to the patient suffering from Paittika type of dysuria. The decoctions of Kamala and Utpala (Nymphaea alba) or Srngataka – Tectona grandis or Vidari (Ipomoea paniculata / Pueraria tuberosa) or the root of Dandairaka (Hogaa) along with honey and sugar are useful in Paittika type of dysuria. Simple cold water mixed with honey and sugar is also useful in this type of dysuria. [49- 51]

Medicines for Paittika Mutrakrichra:

एर्वारुबीजं त्रपुषात् कुसुम्भात् सकुङ्कुमः स्याद्वृषकश्च पेयः| द्राक्षारसेनाश्मरि शर्करासु सर्वेषु कृच्छ्रेषु प्रशस्त एषः||५२||

एर्वारुबीजं मधुकं सदारु पैते पिबेतण्डुलधावनेन| दार्वीं तथैवामलकी रसेन समाक्षिकां पित्तकृते तु कृच्छ्रे||५३||

The patient should drink the potion prepared of the seeds of Ervaru – Cucumis melo, Trapusa – Cucumis sativus and Kusumbha – Carthamus tinctorius mixed with the Kunkuma and Vasa along with Grape juice it is exceedingly beneficial for Asmari (urinary Calculus), Sarkara (Graveluria) and all types of dysuria.

In Paittika dysuria, the patient should take the potion prepared of the seeds of Ervaru – Cucumis melo, Madhuka–Licorice and Devadaru (Cedrus deodara) along with Tandulodaka (water used for washing rice).

Similarly, Daruharidra along with the juice of Amalaki – Phyllanthus emblica mixed with honey is useful in curing Paittika type of Dysuria. [52-53]

Treatment of Kaphaja Mutrakrichra:

क्षारोष्ण तीक्ष्णौषधमन्नपानं स्वेदो यवान्नं वमनं निरूहाः| तक्रं सतिक्तौषध सिद्ध तैलमभ्यङ्गपानं कफमूत्रकृच्छ्रे||५४||

व्योषं श्वदंष्ट्रात्रुटिसारसास्थि कोल प्रमाणं मधु मूत्रयुक्तम्| पिबेत्त्रुटिं क्षौद्रयुतां कदल्या रसेन कैडर्यरसेन वाऽपि||५५||

तक्रेण युक्तं शितिवारकस्य बीजं पिबेत् कृच्छ्र विनाश हेतो:| पिबेतथा तण्डुलधावनेन प्रवालचूर्णं कफ मूत्रकृच्छ्रे||५६||

सप्तच्छदारग्वध केबुकैलाधवं करञ्जं कुटजं गुडूचीम्| पक्त्वा जले तेन पिबेद्यवागूं सिद्धं कषायं मधुसंयुतं वा||५७||

For Kaphaja type of Dysuria, following types of therapies are useful:

Medicines, food and drinks containing Alkalis, hot and Sharp (Tikshna) ingredients

Fomentation therapies

Barley

Vamana – Emetic therapy

Niruha Basti (decoction enema)

Butter-milk

Massage with medicated oil prepared by cooking with bitter drugs and

Pana (oral intake) of the above mentioned medicated oil

The following recipes are useful in Kaphaja type of dysuria

One Kola (6 grams) of each of Sunthi – Ginger, Pipalli – Piper longum, Maricha – Black pepper, Svadamstra – Tribulus terrestris, Truti (cardamom) and bone of Sarasa to be taken along with honey and cow's urine.

Truti (ela) mixed with honey along with the juice of Kadali or Kaidarya Maha- Nimba – Neem Azadirachta indica) or Parvata- Nimba – Neem Azadirachta indica)

Seeds of Sitivaraka (Salinca) along with buttermilk

Powder of Pravala (coral) along with Tandulodaka (water used for rice washing)

The decoction of Saptacchada, Aragvadha, Kebuka, Ela – cardamom), Dhava – Anogeissus latifolia, Karanja – Pongamia pinnata, Kutaja – Connessi Holarrhena antidysenterica Wall.) and guduchi – Tinospora cordifolia along with honey and

Yavagu (gruel) prepared of the above mentioned decoction. [54-57]

Treatment of Sannipatika Dysuria

सर्वं त्रिदोष प्रभवे तु वायो: स्थानानुपूर्व्या प्रसमीक्ष्य कार्यम्| त्रिभ्योऽधिके प्राग्वमनं कफे स्यात् पित्ते विरेक: पवने तु बस्ति:||५८||

इति मूत्रकृच्छ्र चिकित्सा|

If the dysuria is caused by Sannipata all the 3 Doshas simultaneously aggravated in equal proportion), then the physician, after proper examination, should, first of all, administer therapies for correcting the location of the aggravated Vayu [and thereafter, of the remaining Doshas].

In this Sannipatika type of Dysuria, the treatment is as follows:

Kapha aggravation – Vamana

Pitta aggravation – Virechana

Vata Aggravation – Basti

Treatment of Dysuria Caused by Calculus (Ashmari) and Gravels (Sharkara)

क्रिया हिता साऽश्मरिशर्कराभ्यां कृच्छ्रे यथैवेह कफानिलाभ्याम्| कार्याऽश्मरी भेदन पातनाय विशेषयुक्तं शृणु कर्म सिद्धम्||५९||

पाषाणभेदं वृषकं श्वदंष्ट्रा पाठाभया व्योष शटी निकुम्भा:| हिंस्राखराश्वाशितिवारकाणामेर्वारुकाणां त्रपुषस्य बीजम्||६०||

उत्कुञ्चिका हिङ्गु सवेतसाम्लं स्याद्द्वे बृहत्यौ हपुषा वचा च| चूर्णं पिबेदश्मरिभेद पक्वं सर्पिश्च गोमूत्र चतुर्गुणं तै:||६१||

मूल श्वदंष्ट्रेक्षुरकोरुबूकात् क्षीरेण पिष्टं बृहती द्वयाच्च| आलोड्य दध्ना मधुरेण पेयं दिनानि सप्ताश्मरिभेदनाय||६२||

पुनर्नवायोरजनी श्वदंष्ट्रा फल्गु प्रवालाश्च स दर्भ पुष्पाः| क्षीराम्बु मद्येक्षुरसैः सुपिष्टं पेयं भवेदश्मरि शर्करासु||६३||

त्रुटिं सुराह्वं लवणानि पञ्च यवाग्रजं कुन्दुरुकाश्मभेदौ| कम्पिल्लकं गोक्षुरकस्य बीजमेर्वारुबीजं त्रपुषस्य बीजम्||६४||

चूर्णीकृतं चित्रक हिङ्गु मासी यवा नितुल्यं त्रिफलादिवभागम्| अम्लैरशुक्तै रस मद्य युषैः पेयं हि गुल्माश्मरि भेदनार्थम्||६५||

बिल्व प्रमाणो घृत तैल भृष्टो यूषः कृतः शिग्रुक मूलकल्कात्| शीतोऽश्मभितः स्याद्दधिमण्डयुक्तः पेयः प्रकामं लवणेन युक्त||६६||

जलेन शोभाञ्जन मूल कल्कः शीतो हितश्चाश्मरि शर्करासु| सितोपला वा समयावशूका कृच्छ्रेषु सर्वेष्वपि भेषजं स्यात्||६७||

पीत्वाऽथ मद्यं निगदं रथेन हयेन वा शीघ्रजवेन यायात्| तैः शर्करा प्रच्यवतेऽश्मरी तु शम्येन्न चेच्छल्यविदुद्धरेताम्||६८||

If dysuria (Mutra Krichra) is caused by Calculus (Asmari) or gravels (Sarkara), then the therapies suggested for Kaphaja and Vatika types of Dysuria are beneficial.

Now, listen to the effective therapies to be administered specifically for the Bhedana (breaking or dissolution) and Patana (expulsion) of Ashmari are being described hereafter:

Pashanabhedadi –Kvatha: Intake of the powder of

Pashana- Bheda – Cyclea peltata,

Vasa – Adhathoda vasica,

Svadamstra – Tribulus terrestris,

Patha – Cissampelos pareira,

Abhaya – Terminalia chebula,

Sunthi – Ginger,

Pippali – Long pepper fruit

Maricha – Black pepper fruit,

Shati – Hedychium spicatum,

Nikumbha – Danti – Baliospermum montanum

seeds of Himsra – Nardostachys jatamamsi,

Kharasva – Apium graveolens,

Ajamoda – Ajowan fruit – Trachyspermum roxburghianum,

Sitivaraka (Salinca),

Ervaruka and

Trapusa

Utkuncika (Krsna- Jiraka – Carum carvi),

Hingu – Asa foetida,

Amla-Vetasa – Garcinia pedunculata,

Brihati – Solanum indicum,

Kantakari – Solanum xanthocarpum,

Hapusa and

Vacha -Acorus calamus Linn) helps in the breaking dissolution of calculus in the urinary tract.

Pasanabhedadi Ghrita: Ghee 4 parts cooked with the paste of the above mentioned drugs (1 part) and 4 parts cow's urine also helps in the breaking & dissolution of calculus in the urinary tract.

Roots of Svadamstra –Tribulus terrestris,

Ikshuraka,

Kokilaksa – Asteracantha longifolia,

Urubuka - eranda – Ricinus communis,

Brihati – Solanum indicum and

Kantakari – Solanum xanthocarpum is mixed by adding sweet curd. Intake of this potion for 7 days helps in the breaking dissolution of calculus in the urinary tract.

Recipes are taken by the patient suffering from Asmari (Calculus) and Sarkara (graveluria):

Punarnava – Boerhavia diffusa,

Lauha- Bhasma,

Rajani – turmeric,

Svadamstra – Tribulus terrestris,

Pravala (adventitious root / tender leaves?) of Phalgu (Kasthodumbara) and

The flowers of Darbha – Desmostachya bipinnata are ground and made into a paste by adding milk, water, alcohol or sugar-cane juice.

Trutyadi Churna: 1 part of each of

Truti (lesser cardamom),

Surahva (Devadaru – Cedrus deodara),

5 types of salt,

Yavakshara,

Kunduru – Boswellia serrata,

Pashana- Bheda – Cyclea peltata,

Kampillaka – Mallotus philippinensis,

Seeds of Goksura – Tribulus terrestris,

Ervaru and

Trapusa

Chitraka – Leadword – Plumbago zeylanica,

Hingu – Asa foetida,

Mamsi – Nordastachys jatamansi and

Yavani – Trachyspermum amami and

2 parts of each of Haritaki – Terminalia chebula, Vibhitaka – Terminalia bellerica and Amalaki – Phyllanthus emblica is made to a powder.

This along with sour drinks excluding Sukta and Vinegar, meat soup, alcohol and vegetable soup helps in the cure of Gulma (phantom tumour) and breaking dissolution) of calculus in the urinary tract.

Root of Shigru – Moringa oliefera is made into a paste. The soup of the measurement of one Bilva of this paste is sizzled with ghee and oil, and cooled. Intake of this cold soup along with Dadhimanda (whey) and adequate quantity of salt helps in the breaking dissolution of the calculus in the urinary tract.

Intake of the root of Sobhanjana along with cold water is useful for curing Asmari (calculus) and Sarkara (Gravels) in the urinary tract.

Sitopala (Sugar of big crystals) mixed with equal quantity of Yavakshara is the remedy for all types of Dysuria.

After taking wholesome alcohol [in large quantities], the patient should ride over a chariot or horse running very fast which causes expulsion of gravels and stones from the urinary tract. If this expulsion does not take place then these stones and gravels are removed surgically by an expert surgeon. [59- 68]

Treatment of Dysuria Caused by Vitiated Semen:

रेतोभिघात प्रभवे तु कृच्छ्रे समीक्ष्य दोषं प्रतिकर्म कुर्यात्| कार्पास मूलं वृषकाश्मभेदौ बला स्थिरादीनि गवेधुका च||६९||

वृश्चीर ऐन्द्री च पुनर्नवा च शतावरी मध्वसनाख्यपण्यौँ| तत्क्वाथ सिद्धः पवने रसः स्यात् पित्तेऽधिके क्षीरमथापि सर्पिः||७०||

कफे च यूषादिकमन्नपानं संसर्गजे सर्वहितः क्रमः स्यात्| एवं न चेच्छाम्यति तस्य युञ्ज्यात् सुरां पुराणां मधुकासवं वा||७१||

विहङ्ग मांसानि च बृंहणाय बस्तींश्च शुक्राशय शोधनार्थम्| शुद्धस्य तृप्तस्य च वृष्ययोगैः प्रियानुकूलाः प्रमदा विधेयाः||७२||

If obstruction by vitiated semen is the cause of dysuria, then the patient is treated with remedies appropriate to the aggravated Doshas responsible for such vitiation.

If dysuria is caused due to the vata type of ashmari, the decoction prepared from the below mentioned shall be administered –

Karpasa – Gossypium herbaceum,

Vasaka – Adhatoda vasica ,

Pashana- Bheda – Cyclea peltata,

Bala – Country mallow,

Shalaparni

Brihati – Solanum indicum,

Kantakari – Solanum xanthocarpum,

Goksura – Tribulus terrestris,

Gavedhuka – Grewia populifolia

Vruscheera (Sveta or white variety of punarnava – Boerhavia diffusa

Aindri – Colocynth – Citrullus colocynthis – indra-Varuni),

Red variety of Punarnava –Boerhavia diffusa

Satavari – Asparagus racemosus,

Madhu-Parni (Guduchi – Tinospora cordifolia) and

Asana-Parni (aparajita – Clitoria ternatea) is useful in dysuria caused by the seminal vitiation of Vatika type.

If dysuria is caused due to the pittaja type of asmari – milk or ghee prepared with the same above said herbs shall be administered.

If dysuria is caused due to kaphaja type of asmari – soup prepared using water processed by the same drugs in Shadanga Paniya method shall be administered along with food. The same water shall be given to drink.

If dysuria is due to ashmari caused by two or three doshas the therapies appropriate to each of these doshas should be administered in a combined form.

If the dysuria caused by the vitiation of semen is not relieved by the above mentioned therapeutic measures, then the patient is given old Sura alcohol or Madhukasava to drink. His body is nourished by the meat of birds, and he is given Uttara Basti (urethral douche) for cleansing the Sukrasaya (seminal vesicle). When he is cleansed, and he is refreshed with aphrodisiac recipes, he is made to stay with lovable ladies and desirable women having erotic disposition [69-72]

Treatment of Raktaja Mutrakrichra:

रक्तोद्भवे तूत्पलनाल तालकासेक्षुबालेक्षु कशेरुकाणि| पिबेत् सिताक्षौद्रयुतानि खादेदिक्षुं विदारीं त्रपुषाणि चैव||७३||

घृतं श्वदंष्ट्रा स्वरसेन सिद्धं क्षीरेण चैवाष्टगुणेन पेयम्| स्थिरादिकानां कनकादिकानामेकैकशो वा विधिनैव तेन||७४||

क्षीरेण बस्तिर्मधुरौषधैः स्यात्तैलेन वा स्वादुफलोत्थितेन| यन्मूत्रकृच्छ्रे विहितं तु पैते कार्यं तु तच्छोणितमूत्रकृच्छ्रे||७५||

Treatment of Dysuria caused by Vitiated Blood:

If dysuria is caused by the vitiation of blood, the following recipes are useful:

The patient should drink the juice of the stalk of Utpala, Tala, Kasa – Saccharum spontaneum, Ikshu – sugarcane, Baleksu and Kaseruka along with sugar and honey

He should eat Ikshu – Saccharum officinarum, Vidari (Pueraria tuberosa) and Trapusa is in uncooked form

The medicated ghee prepared by cooking with juice of Svadamstra – Tribulus terrestris (equal in quantity of ghee) and milk (8 times of the quantity of ghee) is useful in this ailment;

Shalaparni, Prisniparni, Brihati – Solanum indicum, Kantakari – Solanum xanthocarpum, Goksura – Tribulus terrestris and Drugs belonging to the group beginning with Kataka (Kanaka) taken either individually or all together is made to a decoction. Recipes of medicated ghee prepared by cooking with this decoction are useful in this ailment. Medicated milk prepared by cooking with the drugs having sweet taste may be used as urethra douche in this aliment

Medicated oil prepared b cooking with sweet fruits like Madhuka– Licorice – Glycyrrhiza glabra and Aksota – Juglans regia may also be used as urethral douche in this ailment and therapeutic measures described for the treatment of Pattika type of dysuria are also useful in this ailment. [73-75]

Prohibitions in Dysuria

व्यायाम सन्धारण शुष्क रूक्ष पिष्टान्न वातार्ककर व्यवायान्| खर्जूर शालूक कपित्थ जम्बू बिसं कषायं न रसं भजेत्||७६||

इत्यश्मरी चिकित्सा|

The patient suffering from different type of Mutrakruchra (Dysuria) should avoid

Vyayama – exercise,

Vega sandharana – suppression of the manifested natural urges,

Sushka ruksha anna – dry and ununctuous articles of food,

Pistanna – Pastries,

Vata– exposure to strong wind,

Aatapa – strong rays of the sun,

Maithuna – sexual intercourse,

Kharjura – dates, Shaluka, Kapittha – Feronia limonia, Jambu – Sygyzium cumini, Bisa – Nelumbium speciosum and articles having astringent taste.

Thus, ends the description of the treatment of dysuria (Mutrakruchra).

Hrudroga – heart diseases

Causes of Heart Diseases:

व्यायाम तीक्ष्णातिविरेक बस्ति चिन्ता भय त्रासगदातिचाराः| छर्द्याेमसन्धारण कर्शनानि हृद्रोग कर्तृणि तथाऽभिघातः||७७||

Hridroga (heart-disease) is caused by the following factors

Ati vyayama – Excessive Exercise

Excessive use of articles having Teekshna (sharp) attributes

Administration of Virechana (purgation) and Vamana (emetic) therapies, and Basti (enema) in excess

Ati chinta,bhaya, trasa – Excessive worry, fear and stress

Agada atichara – Improper treatment of diseases

Chardi – Emesis,

Ama – product of improper digestion and metabolism

Vega sandharana – suppression of the manifested natural urges

Karshya – Emaciation and

Abhighata – Trauma (physical and mental)

Ailments Associated with Heart disease:

वैवर्ण्य मूर्च्छा ज्वर कास हिक्का श्वासास्यवैरस्य तृषा प्रमोहाः| छर्दिः कफोत्क्लेश रुजोऽरुचिश्च हृद्रोगजाः स्युर्विविधास्तथाऽन्ये||७८||

Ailments manifested in a patient suffering from heart disease:

Vaivarnya – Discoloration of the skin,

Murccha – fainting,

Jwara – fever,

Kasa – cough,

Hikka – hiccup,

Shvasa – Asthma,

Aasya vairasya – bad taste in the mouth,

Trshna – morbid thirst,

Pramoha – unconsciousness,

Chardi – vomiting,

Kapha utklesha – Nausea,

Ruja – pain,

Aruchi – anorexia [78]

Specific features of Different Types of Hridroga:

हृच्छून्यभाव द्रव शोषभेद स्तम्भाः समोहाः पवनादिवशेषः| पित्तातमोद्यन दाह मोहाः सन्त्रास ताप ज्वर पीतभावाः||७९||

स्तब्धं गुरु स्यात् स्तिमितं च मर्म कफात् प्रसेक ज्वर कास तन्द्राः| विद्यात्त्रिदोष त्वपि सर्वलिङ्गं तीव्रार्तितोदं कृमिजं सकण्डूम्||८०||

The specific features of Vatika type of Hridroga :

Hrut shunya bhava – Feeling of emptiness in the heart region,

Hrut drava – tachycardia,

Sosha – atrophy of the cardiac muscles,

Bheda – pricking pain,

Hrut Stambha – heart- block and

Sammoha – unconsciousness

The specific features manifested in Pittaja Hrud roga –

Stabdham – Bradycardia

Guru syat stimitam – heaviness and timidity of the heart,

Praseka – excessive salivation,

Jwara – fever,

Kasa – cough and

Santrasa – drowsiness

In the heart –disease caused by the Sannipata (aggravation of all the 3 Doshas), all the signs and symptoms described above are manifested together.

In the heart-disease caused by krimija (parasitic infestation), the patient gets acute pain, pricking pain and itching. [79- 80]

Treatment of Vatika Hrudroga:

तैलं ससौवीरक मस्तु तक्रं वाते प्रपेयं लवणं सुखोष्णम्| मूत्राम्बु सिद्धं लवणैश्च तैलमानाह गुल्मार्ति हृदामयघ्नम्||८१||

पुनर्नवां दारु स पञ्चमूलं रास्नां यवान् बिल्व कुलत्थ कोलम्| पक्त्वा जले तेन विपाच्य तैलमभ्यङ्गपानेऽनिल हृद्गदघ्नम्||८२||

हरीतकी नागर पुष्कराह्वैर्वय:कयस्थालवणैश्च कल्कैः| सहिङ्गुभिः साधितमग्र्य सर्पि गुल्मे सहृत्पार्श्वगदेऽनिलोत्थे||८३||

सपुष्कराह्वं फलपूरमूलं महौषधं शट्यभया च कल्काः| क्षाराम्बु सर्पि र्लवणै र्विमिश्राः स्युर्वात हृद्रोग विकर्तिकाघ्नाः||८४||

क्वाथः कृतः पौष्कर मातुलुङ्ग पलाश भूतीक शटी सुराह्वैः| सनागराजाजि वचा यवानी क्षारः सुखोष्णो लवणश्च पेयः||८५||

पथ्या शटी पौष्कर पञ्चकोलात् स मातुलुङ्गाद्यमकेन कल्कः| गुड प्रसन्ना लवणैश्च भृष्टो हृत्पार्श्व पृष्ठोदर योनिशूले||८६||

स्यात्र्यूषणं द्वे त्रिफले सपाठे निदिग्धिका गोक्षुरकौ बले द्वे| ऋद्धिस्त्रुटिस्तामलकी स्वगुप्ता मेदे मधूकं मधुकं स्थिरा च||८७||

शतावरी जीवक पृश्निपण्यौँ द्रव्यैरिमैरक्षसमैः सुपिष्टैः| प्रस्थं घृतस्येह पचेद्विधिज्ञः प्रस्थेन दध्ना त्वथ माहिषेण||८८||

मात्रां पलं चार्धपलं पिचुं वा प्रयोजयेन्माक्षिक सम्प्रयुक्ताम्| श्वासे सकासे त्वथ पाण्डुरोगे हलीमके हृद्ग्रहणी प्रदोषे||८९||

Treatment of heart ailment due to Vata imbalance:

Intake of this potion, in luke-warm water cures Vatika type of heart disease:

Oil, Sauviraka, Mastu (whey) and

buttermilk, taken in equal quantities, is added with salt.

Intake of the medicated oil prepared by cooking with cow's urine, water and salt cures flatulence, Gulma (phantom tumour), abdominal pain and heart disease [of Vatika type].

Decoction useful for Abhyanga (massage) and Pana (taking orally) in the Vatika type of heart disease: It may be prepared of

Punarnava, Devadaru, Bilva, Syonaka, Gambhari, Patala, Ganikarika, Rasna, Yava, Kulattha and Kola by boiling with water.

Medicated oil prepared by cooking with the paste of

Haritaki, Nagara, Puskara- Mula, Juice of Vayastha (Guduci), Juice of Kayastha (Amalaki) and salt, and Hingu is immensely effective for curing Gulma (phantom tumour), heart –disease and pain in the chest caused by the aggravated vayu.

Cures Vatika type of heart disease and Vikartika (angina pain): Intake of the paste of Puskara-Mula, root of Phalapura(Bija-Puraka), Mahausadha, Sati and Haritaki mixed with Alkali, ghee and salt

This potion is given in luke-warm form to the patient suffering from Vatika type of heart-disease: The decoction of Puskara-mula, Matulunga, Palasa, Bhutika, Sati and

Devadaru is added as praksepa with the powders of Nagara, Ajaji, Vacha, Yavani, Yava Kshara and Salt

Intake of this potion along with jaggery, Prasanna (scum of alcohol) and salt cures pain in the chest, sides of the chest, back, abdomen and female genital tract: The paste of Patha, Shati, Puskaramoola, Pippali, Pippali mula, Chavya, Chitraka, Shunthi and Matulunga is sizzled by adding oil and ghee.

This medicated ghee is administered in the dose of 1 Pala or 1 pichu by adding honey for curing cough, Asthma,

Anaemia, Halimaka (a serious type of Jaundice), heart disease and sprue syndrome: 1 Aksa of each of Sunthi, Pippali, Maricha, Haritaki, Vibhitaka, Amalaki, Draksha, Kasmarya, Parusaka, Patha, Nidigdhika, Goksura, Bala, Mahameda, Rddhi, Truti (Suksma-ela), Shatavari, Jivaka and Prsniparni is made into a paste.

1 Prastha of ghee is cooked by adding this paste and curd prepared of buffalo- milk [81-89]

Treatment of Paittika Hrudroga:

शीताः प्रदेहाः परिषेचनानि तथा विरेको हृदि पित्तदुष्टे| द्राक्षासिता क्षौद्र परूषकैः स्याच्छुद्धे तु पित्तापहमन्नपानम्||९०||

यष्ट्याह्विका तिक्तकरोहिणीभ्यां कल्कं पिबेच्चापि सिताजलेन| क्षते च सर्पींषि हितानि सर्पि गुंडाश्च ये तान् प्रसमीक्ष्य सम्यक्||९१||

दद्यादिभषग्धन्वरसांश्च गव्यक्षीराशिनां पित्त हृदामयेषु| तैरेव सर्वे प्रशमं प्रयान्ति पित्तामयाः शोणित संश्रया ये||९२||

द्राक्षा बला श्रेयसि शर्कराभिः खर्जूर वीरर्षभकोत्पलैश्च| काकोलिमेदा युग जीवकैश्च क्षीरेण सिद्धं महिषी घृतं स्यात्||९३||

कशेरुका शैवल शृङ्गवेर प्रपौण्डरीकं मधुकं बिसस्य| ग्रन्थिश्च सर्पिः पयसा पचेतैः क्षौद्रान्वितं पित्त हृदामयघ्नम्||९४||

स्थिरादि कल्कैः पयसा च सिद्धं द्राक्षा रसेनेक्षुरसेन वाऽपि| सर्पिर्हितं स्वादुफलेक्षुजाश्च रसाः सुशीता हृदि पित्तदुष्टे||९५||

Treatment for Pittaja Type of Heart Disease:

If the heart disease is caused by aggravated Pitta, then the patient is given cooling Pradeha (application of ointment), affusion and purgation therapy.

After the body is anointed by the administration of purgative therapy, the patient is given food and drinks added with grapes, sugar, honey and parusaka.

The patient may also take the paste of Yastimadhu – Indian licorice and Katukarohini – Picrorhiza kurroa along with sugar mixed water.

If there is ulcer in the chest, then the patient is given medicated ghee and the recipes of Sarpir Guda (Vide Chikitsa 11: 50-77) after proper examination.

In Paittika type of heart disease, the patient is given the soup of the animals inhabiting the arid zone, and food prepared of cow's milk. By this, all types of diseases caused by the aggravation of Pitta, and those located in the blood get cured.

Medicated ghee useful in curing Paittika type of heart disease are prepared by cooking buffalo-ghee with milk and the paste of either

Draksha,Bala,Sreyasi and Sarkara or Kharjura,Veera, Rishabhaka and Utpala, Kakoli, Meda, Maha-Meda and Jivaka.

Intake of this medicated ghee cures heart disease: It is prepared by cooking with the paste of

Kaseruka, Saivala, Shringavera, Prapaundarika, Madhuka and tuber of lotus, milk and Honey (1/4th in quantity of ghee) is added after cooking is over.

Ghee useful in paittika type of cardiac disease is cooked with the paste of - Shalaparni, Prisniparni, Brihati, Kantakari and Goksura and milk or Grape- juice or sugar-cane-juice

Cooling juice of sweet fruits and sugar-cane is useful in paittika type of heart-disease. [90-95]

Treatment of Kaphaja Hrudroga:

स्विन्नस्य वान्तस्य विलङ्घितस्य क्रिया कफघ्नी कफ मर्मरोगे| कौलत्थधान्यैश्च रसैर्ववान्नं पानानि तीक्ष्णानि च शङ्कराणि||९६||

मूत्रे शृताः कट्फल शृङ्गवेर पीतद्रु पथ्यातिविषाः प्रदेयाः| कृष्णा शटी पुष्करमूल रास्ना वचाभया नागर चूर्णकं च||९७||

उदुम्बराश्वत्थ वटार्जुनाख्ये पालाश रौहीतक खादिरे च| क्वाथे त्रिवृत्र्यूषण चूर्ण सिद्धो लेहः कफघ्नोऽशिशिराम्बु युक्तः||९८||

शिलाह्वयं वा भिषग प्रमत्तः प्रयोजयेत् कल्प विधानदिष्टम्| प्राशं तथाऽऽगस्त्यमथापि लेहं रसायनं ब्राह्ममथामलक्याः||९९||

Treatment of Kaphaja Hridroga:

In Kaphaja type of heart-disease, remedies are given after the administration of

Swedana – fomentation,

Vamana – emetic and

Langhana (fasting) therapies.

Intake of barley as food along with the juice soup of Kulattha – horse gram and Dhanyaka – Coriandrum sativum, and drinks having sharp (tiksna) attribute is useful for Kaphaja type of heart disease.

Urine boiled with

Katphala

Shringavera – Ginger,

Pitadru (Daruharidra – Berberis aristata),

Pathya and

Ativisha – Aconitum heterophyllum is useful in this condition

The powder of Krishna Pippali – Long pepper fruit – Piper longum), Shati – Hedychium spicatum, Pushkara- Mula – Inula racemosa, Rasna – Vanda roxburghi / Pluchea lanceolata), Vacha – Acorus calamus Linn.), Abhaya – Terminalia chebula and Nagara – Ginger is useful for this ailment.

Intake of this linctus along with warm water cures Kaphaja type of heart disease: To the decoction (3 parts) of

Udumbara –Ficus race**mosa**

Asvattha – Ficus religiosa

Vata – Ficus bengalensis

Arjuna – terminalia arjuna

Palasha – Butea monosperma

Rohitaka – Tecomela undulata and

Khadira – Acacia catechu, the powder (1 part) of

Trivrt – Operculina turpethum

Sunthi – Ginger

Pippali – Long pepper fruit – Piper longum and

Maricha – Black pepper fruit – piper nigrum is added and made to a linctus

For curing Kaphaja type of cardiac disorder, an expert physician should administer Shilajatu according to the prescribed procedure to get its rejuvenating effect (kalpa—vide Chikitsa 1:3:55-65)

Similarly, ChyavanaPrasa (vide Chikitsa 1:1: 62- 74), Agastya Haritaki or Agastya Rasayana (vide Chikitsa 18: 57-62), Brahma Rasayana (vide Chikitsa 1:1:75) are useful for the patient suffering from Kaphaja type of heart disease. [96-99]

Treatment of Sannipatika Heart Disease

त्रिदोषजे लङ्घनमादितः स्यादन्नं च सर्वेषु हितं विधेयम्।

हीनातिमध्यत्वमवेक्ष्य चैव कार्यं त्रयाणामपि कर्म शस्तम्||१००||

If the heart disease is caused by the simultaneous aggravation of all the 3 Doshas (Sannipata), then at the beginning, langhana (fasting therapy) is administered, and the patient is given such food as are conductive to the alleviation of all the 3 Doshas.

After ascertaining the nature of these aggravated Doshas, i.e. their mid aggravation, moderate aggravation or excessive aggravation, appropriate therapeutic measures are adopted for their alleviation [100]

Treatment of Angina in Sannipatika Heart- disease

भुक्तेऽधिकं जीर्यति शूलमल्पं जीर्णं स्थितं चेत् सुरदारु कुष्ठम्। सतिल्वकं द्वे लवणे विडङ्गमुष्णाम्बुना सातिविषं पिबेत् सः||१०१||

जीर्णेऽधिके स्नेह विरेचनं स्यात् फलै विरेच्यो यदि जीर्यति स्यात्। त्रिष्वेव कालेष्वधिके तु शूले तीक्ष्णं हितं मूल विरेचनं स्यात्||१०२||

प्रायोऽनिलो रुद्धगतिः प्रकुप्यत्यामाशये शोधनमेव तस्मात्।

कार्यं तथा लङ्घन पाचनं च ...|१०३|

If in the Sannipatika type of heart-disease, excruciating pain appears [in the cardiac region] immediately after taking food, is of moderate intensity during the process of digestion, and gets alleviation after the food is digested this happens because of excessive aggravation of kapha, then the patient is given to drink the powder of

Devadaru – Cedrus deodara,

Kushta – Saussurea lappa,

Tilvaka

Saindhava Lavana – rock salt

Sauvarchala Lavana

Vidanga – Embelia ribes and

Ativisa – Aconitum heterophyllum mixed with warm water.

If [in Sannipatika type of heart-disease], excruciating pain [in the cardiac region] appears after the digestion of food this happens because of excessive aggravation of Pitta, then the patient is given Virechana (purgation) therapy containing fruits like

Draksha – Raisin – Vitis vinifera and

Kasmarya – Gmelina arborea

If [in Sannipatika type of heart disease], excruciating pain [in the cardiac region] appears in all the 3 periods, viz, before, during and after digestion this happens because of excessive aggravation of all the 3 Doshas, then the patient is given strong (tiksna) purgation therapy containing roots of Trivrt –Operculina turpethum etc).

Vayu generally gets aggravated because of the obstruction to its movements in the Amasaya stomach including small intestine. Therefore, it is necessary to give Virechana (purgation therapy), Langhana (fasting therapy) and Pachana (carminative therapy) to the patient. [101- ¾ 103]

Treatment of Krumija Heart Disease:

... सर्वं कृमिघ्नं कृमि हृद्गदे च||१०३|| इति हृद्रोग चिकित्सा|

For the treatment of heart disease caused by Krmi (micro- organisms), therapeutic measures for the distribution of these micro –organisms is administered.

Thus, ends the description of the treatment of heart-diseases. [103 ¼]

DISEASES OF HEAD

Pratishyaya – Coryza, rhinitis

सन्धारणाजीर्णरजोतिभाष्य क्रोधर्तु वैषम्य शिरोभितापैः| प्रजागरातिस्वपनाम्बु शीतैरवश्यया मैथुन बाष्प धूमैः||१०४||

संस्त्यानदोषे शिरसि प्रवृद्धो वायु: प्रतिश्यायमुदीरयेतु|

Etiology and Pathogenesis of Pratishyaya (Rhinitis)

Pratishyaya or Rhinitis is caused by the following

Vega sandharana – Suppression of the manifested natural urges

Ajirnat – Indigestion

Excessive exposure to the dust

Ati bhashya – Excessive speech

Krodha – Anger

Vaishamya – Seasonal vagaries

Shiro abhitapa – Excessive exposure of the head to heat

Prajagarana – Remaining awake at night and

Diwa swapna – excessive sleep during day time

Exposure to cold water and forest

Maithuna – Sexual intercourse and

Ati bhaspa – weeping in excess and

Dhuma – Exposure to smoky atmosphere.

The above mentioned factors make the Dosha (mucus) in the head thick, and aggravate Vayu, giving rise to Rhinitis. [104- 1/105]

Signs and symptoms of Vatika Pratishyaya:

घ्राणार्तितोदौ क्षवथुर्जलाभः स्रावोऽनिलात् सस्वरमूर्धरोगः||१०५||

The signs and symptoms of rhinitis caused by the aggravation of Vayu:

Excessive pain and pricking sensation in the nose

Kshavathu jalabha srava – sneezing, watery discharge,

Svara bheda – hoarseness of voice and

murdharoga(Shiro ruk) – headache [105 2/4]

Signs and Symptoms of Paittika Pratishyaya

नासाग्रपाक ज्वर वक्त्रशोष तृष्णोष्ण पीत स्रवणानि पित्तात्|

The signs and symptoms of Paittika type of Rhinitis:

Nasa agra paka – Inflammation of the tip of the nose

Jvara – fever

Vaktra sosha – dryness of the mouth

Trushna – morbid thirst

Pita sravanani pittat – discharge of the hot as well as yellow liquid [2/4 106]

Signs and Symptoms of Kaphaja Rhinitis

कासारुचि स्राव घन प्रसेकाः कफाद्गुरुः स्रोतसि चापि कण्डूः||१०६||

The signs and symptoms of Kaphaja type of Rhinitis:

Kasa – Cough

Aruchi – anorexia

Ghana srava – thick discharge

Praseka – Salivation and

Guru – heaviness as well as

Srotasi kandu – itching sensation in the nasal passage [106 2/4]

Signs and symptoms of Sannipatika Rhinitis:

सर्वाणि रूपाणि तु सन्निपातात् स्युः पीनसे तीव्र रुजेऽतिदुःखे |१०७|

All the above mentioned signs and symptoms along with excruciating pain and discomfort are manifested in Rhinits caused by Sannipata (simultaneous aggravation of a the 3 doshas) [2/4 107]

Dusta Pratishyaya (Pernicious Rhinitis)

सर्वोऽतिवृद्धोऽहितभोजनात्तु दुष्ट प्रतिश्याय उपेक्षितः स्यात्||१०७||

ततस्तु रोगाः क्षवथुश्च नासाशोषः प्रतीनाह परिस्रवौ च| घ्राणस्य पूतित्वमपीनसश्च सपाक शोथार्बुद पूयरक्ताः||१०८||

अरूंषि शीर्ष श्रवणाक्षि रोग खालित्यहर्यर्जुनलोमभावाः| तृट्श्वास कास ज्वर रक्तपित्त वैस्वर्य शोषाश्च ततो भवन्ति||१०९||

If all the above mentioned types of Pratisyaya get excessively aggravated due to neglect of appropriate treatment or due to the intake of unwholesome food, then this leads to Dusta Pratisyaya (pernicious Rhinitis). As a result of this, diseases like

Ksavathu – Sneezing,

Nasa sosha – dryness or atrophy of Nasal mucous membrane,

Pratinaha (nasal obstruction),

Prarisrava (excessive discharge from the nose),

Putighrana (ozena),

Apinasa (chornic Rhinitis),

Nasa-Paka (suppurative Rhinitis),

Nasa-Sotha (Oedematous Rhinitis),

Nasarbuda (Nasal Tumour),

Nasa –Puya-Rakta (discharge of pus and blood)

Arumsi (furunculosis),

Sirsha sravana akshi roga – diseases of the head, ears and eyes,

Khalitya – alopecia,

Kasa – cough,

Jwara – fever,

Rakthapitta – an ailment characterized by bleeding from different parts of the body,

Vaisvarya – hoarseness of voice and

Sosa (Consumption) is caused. [107 2/4 – 109]

Signs and symptoms of Dusta-pratishyaya (Rhinitis with infection):

रोधाभिघात स्रव शोष पाकै घ्राणं युतं यश्च न वेत्ति गन्धम्| दुर्गन्धि चास्यं बहुशःप्रकोपि दुष्टप्रतिश्यायमुदाहरेतम्||११०||

Dusta Pratisyaya is characterized by the following signs and symptoms

Rodha abhighata – Nasal obstruction,

Srava -discharge

Sosha – dryness

Paka – suppression

Na ghrana – Loss of sensation of smell

Durgandhim aasya – Foul smell of the mouth and

Bahushah prakopa – Frequent attack of the ailment [110]

Pathogenesis of Kshavathu (Sneezing):

संस्पृश्य मर्माण्यनिलस्तु मूर्ध्नि विष्वक्पथस्थः क्षवथुं करोति|

Vayu afflicting the vital organs, after pervading all the channels in the head gives rise to sneezing. [2/4- 111]

Pathogenesis of Nasa- Sosa (dryness of Nasal Mucous Membrane):

क्रुद्धः स संशोष्य कफं तु नासा शृङ्गाटक घ्राण विशोषणं च||१११||

The aggravated Vayu dries up the Kapha in the nose and the vital organs (marma) called Srngataka which result in the loss of the sense of smell and dryness of the nasal mucous membranes. [111 2/4]

Pathogenesis of Pratinaha (Nasal Obstruction):

उच्छ्वासमार्गं तु कफः सवातो रुन्ध्यात् प्रतीनाहमुदाहरेतम्|

Obstruction of the channel of Expiration by the aggravated Kapha and Vayu is called Pratinaha. [2/4 112]

Pathogenesis of Parisrava (Nasal Discharge):

यो मस्तुलुङ्गाद्घन पीत पक्वः कफः स्रवेदेष परिस्रवस्तु||११२||

The discharge of thick, yellow and ripe matured Kapha (Mucus) from the brain [Through the nose] is called parisrava.

Pathogenesis of Puti- Nasya (Ozena):

वैवर्ण्य दौर्गन्ध्यमुपेक्षया तु स्यात् पूतिनस्यं श्वयथु भ्रमश्च|

If appropriate treatment of Rhinitis is neglected, then this leads to

Vaivarnya (discoloration),

Daurgandhya (foul smell),

Shavyathu (oedema) and

Bhrama (giddiness) which are called Puti-Nasya. [2/4 113]

Signs and Symptoms of Apeenasa (chronic Rhinitis)

आनह्यते यस्य विशुष्यते च प्रक्लिद्यते धूप्यति चापि नासा||११३||

न वेत्ति यो गन्धरसांश्च जन्तुर्जुष्टं व्यवस्येतमपीनसेन| तं चानिल श्लेष्मभवं विकारं ब्रूयात् प्रतिश्याय समान लिङ्गम्||११४||

The signs and symptoms of Apinasa (chronic Rhinitis):

Anahyate – Obstruction

Visoshana – dryness

Praklidyate – dampness / stickiness

Dhupayati – fuming sensation in the nose and

Gandha rasam cha nasha – inability to recognize taste as well as smell

Caused by: Vayu and Kapha aggravation

It shares the signs and symptoms of Pratisyaya (ordinary Rhinitis). [113 2/4 – 114]

Nasapaka (suppurative Rhinitis):

सदाह रागः श्वयथुः सपाकः स्याद् घ्राणपाकोऽपि च रक्तपित्तात्|

Caused by: Vitiation of Rakta (Blood) and Pitta

It is characterized by the signs and symptoms like

Daha – burning sensation

Raga – redness

Shyvathu – oedema and

Sa paka ghrana – suppuration of the nose. [2/4 115]

Nasa-Sotha (Oedematous Rhinitis):

घ्राणाश्रितासृक्प्रभृतीन् प्रदूष्य कुर्वन्ति नासाश्वयथुं मलाश्च||११५||

The aggravated Doshas vitiate blood, etc, located in the nose giving rise to Nasa- Sotha (oedematous rhinitis) [115 2/4]

Nasa Arbuda (nasal polyp/tumour):

घ्राणे तथोच्छ्वासगतिं निरुध्य मांसासृग्दोषादपि चार्बुदानि|

Nasarbuda (Nasal tumor) is caused by the Vitiation of mamsa and rakta located in the nose, thereby obstructing the course of respiration. [2/4 116]

Puyarakta (Purulent and Sanguinous Rhinitis):

घ्राणात् स्रवेद्वा श्रवणान्मुखाद्वा पित्तासृक्तमसं त्वपि पूय रक्तम्||११६||

In PuyaRakta (purulent and Sanguinous rhinitis), there is discharge of blood mixed with Pitta from the nose, ear or mouth. [116 2/4]

Arumsi (Furuculosis):

कुर्यात् सपित्तः पवनस्त्वगादीन् सन्दूष्य चारूंषि सपाकवन्ति|

Aggravated vayu and Pitta vitiate skin, etc., in the nose to cause Arumshi (furunculosis) which gets suppurated [2/4 117].

Nasa Dipta (Burnt Nose):

नासा प्रदीप्तेव नरस्य यस्य दीप्तं तु तं रोगमुदाहरन्ति||११७||

इति नासारोगनिदानम्|

If the nose looks as if burnt, then the ailment is called NasaDeepta.

Thus, ends the description of the diagnosis of Nasal ailments. [117 2/4]

Shiro Roga (Diseases of Head)

Diagnosis of Shiro Roga (Diseases of Head):

भृशार्तिशूलं स्फुरतीह वातात् पित्तात् सदाहार्ति कफाद्गुरु स्यात्| सर्वैस्त्रिदोषं क्रिमिभिस्तु कण्डू दौर्गन्ध्य तोदार्तियुतं शिरः स्यात्||११८||

इति शिरो रोग निदानम्|

In the Vatika type of Shiro-roga (head diseases) there is

Bhrshaarti – excruciating pain,

Shula – ache and

Spruhati – throbbing sensation.

Paittika type of Shiroroga (headache) is associated with

Daha – burning sensation and

Arti – pain.

Kaphaja type of headache is associated with heaviness.

In the Sannipatika type of Shiro Roga (headache), which is caused by the simultaneous aggravation of all the 3 Doshas, all the above-mentioned signs and symptoms are manifested.

Krimija Shiroroga caused by parasitic infestation gives rise to

Kandu – itching

Daurgandhya – foul smell

Toda – pricking sensation and

Shira ruk – pain in the head.

Thus ends the description of the diagnosis of Shirorog (diseases of the head). [118]

Mukharoga – mouth diseases:

Diagnosis of oral disorders:

मुखामये मारुतजे तु शोषकार्कश्यरौक्ष्याणि चला रुजश्च| कृष्णारुणं निष्पतनं सशीतं प्रसंसन स्पन्दन तोद भेदाः||११९||

तृष्णा ज्वर स्फोटक तालुदाहा धूमायनं चाप्यवदीर्णता च| पित्तात् समूच्छा विविधा रुजश्च वर्णाश्च शुक्लारुणवर्ण वज्याः||१२०||

कण्डू गुरुत्वं सितविज्जलत्वं स्नेहोऽरुचिर्जाड्य कफप्रसेकौ| उत्क्लेश मन्दानलता च तन्द्रा रुजश्च मन्दाः कफवक्रोगे||१२१||

सर्वाणि रूपाणि तु वक्रोगे भवन्ति यस्मिन् स तु सर्वजः स्यात्| संस्थानदूष्याकृतिनामभेदाच्चैते चतुःषष्टिविधा भवन्ति||१२२||

शालाक्यतन्त्रेऽभिहितानि तेषां निमित्त रूपाकृति भेषजानि| यथाप्रदेशं तु चतुर्विधस्य क्रियां प्रवक्ष्यामि मुखामयस्य||१२३||

इति मुखरोग निदानम्|

Mouth –diseases are of 4 types, viz,

Vatika

Paittika

Kaphaja and

Sannipatika

Vatika type of mouth – disease is characterized by:

Krishna aruna pita – dryness and pink coloration

Praseka – excessive salivation

Sa shita – coldness

Nishpatanam – loosening of teeth

Prasamsrana – throbbing sensation and

Toda bheda ruk – pricking as well as breaking pain

Pittaja Mukharoga is characterized by –

Trushna – dry mouth

Jwara – fever,

Sphotaka – boils

Taludaha – burning sensation in pallate

Dhumayana – feeling of smoke

Avadeernata – cracks, degeneration

Murcha – fainting

Kaphaja type of mouth disease is characterized by

White discoloration

Kandu – itching

Guru – heaviness

pallor, Sliminess, dryness

Aruchi – anorexia

Jadya – stiffness

Praseka – excessive salivation

Utklesha – Nausea

Manda analata – suppression of the power of digestion,

Tandra – drowsiness and

Manda ruja – dull pain.

If all the signs and symptoms are manifested, then the ailment is to be diagnosed as Sannipatika, i.e caused by the simultaneous aggravation of all the 3 Doshas.

These oral diseases are described to be of 64 varieties depending upon the varieties in their locations, tissue elements which are vitiated, signs and symptoms, and names. These varieties are described in detail in Shalakya- Tantra specialized branch of Ayurveda, dealing with the diseases of the head and neck with reference to their etiology, signs and symptoms, characteristic features and treatment.

In the present text, however, the treatment of the 4 types of mouth- diseases will be described later.

Thus, ends the description of the diagnosis of mouth- diseases. [199- 123]

Arochaka (Anorexia)

Etiology, Signs and symptoms of Arochaka:

वातादिभिः शोक भयातिलोभ क्रोधै मनोघ्नाशन गन्ध रूपैः| अरोचकाः स्युः परिहृष्टदन्तः कषाय वक्रश्च मतोऽनिलेन||१२४||

कट्वम्लमुष्णं विरसं च पूति पित्तेन विद्याल्लवणं च वक्रम्| माधुर्य पैच्छिल्य गुरुत्व शैत्य विबद्ध सम्बद्धयुतं कफेन||१२५||

अरोचके शोक भयानिलोभ क्रोधा द्यह्हृद्याशन गन्धजे स्यात्| स्वाभाविकं वक्रमथारुचिश्च त्रिदोषजे नैकरसं भवेत्तु||१२६||

इत्यरोचक निदानम्|

Etiology, Signs and symptoms of anorexia:

Arochaka or anorexia is caused by aggravated Vayu, etc. by mental factors like grief, fear, excessive greed and anger, and boy resorting to unpleasant food, smell and sights.

It is of five types, Viz,

Vatika

Paittika

Kaphaja

Manobhighataja and

Sannipatika

The symptoms of Vatika type of Arocaka (anorexia):

Parihrusta danta – Setting teeth on edge and

Kashaya vakra – astringent taste in the mouth

The symptoms of Paittika type of arocaka (anorexia):

Katu amla virasa – Pungent and sour tastes in the mouth,

Ushna – hot sensation,

Virasam – bad taste in the mouth,

Puti vakra – foul smell and

Lavana vakra – Saline taste in the mouth

The symptoms of Kaphaja type of Arocaka (anorexia):

Madhurya – Sweet taste

Paichilya – sliminess

Gurutva – heaviness and

Shaitya – coldness in the mouth and

Vibaddha – knotty mucus

In anorexia caused by mental factors like excessive grief, fear, excessive greed for food), anger and unpleasant food as well as smell, there is dislike for food, even though the condition of the mouth is otherwise normal.

In anorexia caused by Sannipata (when all the 3 Doshas are simultaneously aggravated), different types of taste will appear in the mouth.

Thus, ends the description of the diagnosis of Arocaka (anorexia). [124- 126]

Ear Diseases – Karnaroga

Signs and Symptoms of Ear- Diseases:

नादोऽतिरुक्कर्णमलस्य शोषः स्रावस्तनुश्चाश्रवणं च वातात्| शोफः सरागो दरणं विदाहः स पीत पूति श्रवणं च पित्तात्||१२७||

वैश्रुत्य कण्डू स्थिर शोफ शुक्ल स्निग्ध श्रुतिः श्लेष्मभवेऽल्परुक् च| सर्वाणि रूपाणि तु सन्निपातात् स्रावश्च तत्राधिकदोषवर्णः||१२८||

इति कर्णरोगनिदानम्|

Ear diseases are 4 types, viz.,

Vatika

Paittika

Kaphaja and

Sannipatika (which is caused by the Simultaneous aggravation of all the 3 Doshas)

The signs and symptoms of Vatika type of ear- disease:

Karna nada – Tinnitus

Ruk – excessive pain

Karna mala sosha – drying of ear-wax

Srava – thin discharge and

Ashravanam – inability to hear

The symptoms of Paittika type of ear-disease:

Sopha – Oedema

Raga – Redness

Daranam – ulceration

Vidaha – burning sensation and

Pita puti srava – yellow as well as putrid discharge

The signs and symptoms of Kaphaja type of ear- disease:

Vaisrutya – Defective hearing

Kandu – itching

Sthira – stiffness

Sopha – oedema

Shukla snigdha srava – white and unctuous discharge and

Alpa ruk – dull pain

If the ear disease is caused by Sannipata (simultaneous aggravation of all the 3 Doshas), then all the signs and symptoms described above in respect of each of the three Doshas are manifested. In this case, the discharge from the ear is extremely putrid containing many colors.

Thus ends the description of the diagnosis of ear- diseases. [127- 128]

Eye diseases – Netra Roga

Signs and symptoms of Netra Roga (Eye diseases):

अल्पस्तु रागोऽनुपदेहवांश्च स तोद भेदोऽनिलजाक्षि रोगे| पित्तात् सदाहोऽतिरुजः सरागः पीतोपदेहः सुभृशोष्णवाही||१२९||

शुक्लोपदेहं बहुपिच्छिलाश्रु नेत्रं कफात् स्याद्गुरुता सकण्डुः| सर्वाणि रूपाणि तु सन्निपातान्नेत्रामयाः षण्णवतिस्तु भेदात्||१३०||

तेषामभिव्यक्तिरिभ प्रदिष्टा शालाक्य तन्त्रेषु चिकित्सितं च| पराधिकारे तु न विस्तरोक्तिः शस्तेति तेनात्र न नः प्रयासः||१३१||

इति नेत्ररोगनिदानम्|

Eye diseases are of 4 types, viz,

Vatika

Paittika

Kaphaja and

Sannipatika (caused by the simultaneous aggravation of all the 3 Doshas)

Vatika type of eye disorder is characterized by:

Alpa raga – slight redness

Anupa dehamscha – absences of sticky discharge, and

Toda bheda – pricking as well as cutting pain.

Paittika type of eye disease is characterized by:

Sa daho – burning sensation

Ati ruja – excessive pain

Sa raga – redness

Pitopadeha – discharge of sticky material of yellow color, and

Bhrushoshna vahi – extremely hot lachrymation.

Kaphaja type of eye-disease is characterized by

Shukla upadeham – discharge of sticky material of white color,

Bahu picchila ashru – excessive lachrymation which is slimy, Guru (heaviness) and

Kandu – itching.

In the Sannipatika type of eye disorder (which is caused by the simultaneous aggravation of all the three Doshas), all the signs and symptoms described in respect of each of the Doshas are manifested.

Eye-diseases are 96 varieties. Their signs and symptoms and treatment are described in the Shalakya- Tantra specialized branch of Ayurveda dealing with the description of the diseases of the head and neck).

It is not desirable to delve deep into the field of another specialized branch. Therefore, description of such details are not attempted here.

Thus, ends the description of the diagnosis of eye diseases. [129- 131]

Hair Diseases

Pathogenesis of Baldness and premature graying of hair:

तेजोऽनिलाद्यैः सह केशभूमिं दग्ध्वाऽऽशु कुर्यात् खलितिं नरस्य| किञ्चितु दग्ध्वा पलितानि कुर्याद्धरिप्रभत्वं च शिरोरुहाणाम्||१३२||

The Tejas (heat) of the body in association with Vayu and other Doshas, Scorches up the hair- root (scalp) giving instantaneous rise to alopecia in men.

If there is partial scorching, then this gives rise to premature graying of hair and tawny hair. [132]

Thus, ends the description of the diagnosis of the disease alopecia.

इत्यूर्ध्वजत्रूत्थगदैकदेशस्तन्त्रे निबद्धोऽयमशून्यतार्थम्| अतः परं भेषज सङ्ग्रहं तु निबोध सङ्क्षेपत उच्यमानम्||१३३||

इति खालित्य रोग निदानम्|

Only some of the ailments affecting the organs in the head and neck are described above in order to abviate the allegation of absolute omission of these ailments in this text.

Hereafter, the therapeutic measures for the treatment of these diseases will be described in brief which you may understand properly. [133]

TREATMENT OF PEENASA:

Treatment of Vatika Rhinitis

वातात् स कास वैस्वर्ये सक्षारं पीनसे वृतम्| पिबेद्रसं पयश्चोष्णं स्नैहिकं धूममेव वा||१३४||

शताह्वा त्वग्बला मूलं स्योनाकैरण्ड बिल्वजम्| सारग्वधं पिबेद्वर्ति मधूच्छिष्टवसाघृतैः||१३५||

अथवा सघृतान् सक्तून् कृत्वा मल्लक सम्पुटे| नव प्रतिश्यायवतां धूमं वैद्यः प्रयोजयेत्||१३६||

शङ्ख मूर्ध ललाटार्तौ पाणिस्वेदोपनाहनम्| स्वभ्यक्ते क्षवथु स्राव रोधादौ सङ्करादयः||१३७||

घ्रेयाश्च रोहिषाजाजी वचातक्कारि चोरकाः| त्वक्पत्र मरिचैलानां चूर्णा वा सोपकुञ्चिकाः||१३८||

स्रोतः शृङ्गाट नासाक्षि शोषे तैलं च नावनम्| प्रभाव्याजे तिलान् क्षीरे तेन पिष्टांस्तदुष्मणा||१३९||

मन्दस्विन्नान् सयष्ट्याह्वचूर्णांस्तेनैव पीडयेत्| दशमूलस्य निष्क्वाथे रास्ना मधुक कल्कवत्||१४०||

सिद्धं ससैन्धवं तैलं दशकृत्वोऽणु तत् स्मृतम्| स्निग्धस्यास्थापनैर्दोषं निर्हरेद्वातपीनसे||१४१||

स्निग्धाम्लोष्णैश्च लघ्वन्नं ग्राम्यादीनां रसैर्हितम्| उष्णाम्बुना स्नानपाने निवातोष्णप्रतिश्रयः||१४२||

चिन्ता व्यायाम वाक्चेष्टा व्यवाय विरतो भवेत्| वातजे पीनसे धीमानिच्छन्नेवात्मनो हितम्||१४३||

If Vatika type of Rhinitis is associated with cough and hoarseness of voice, then the patient is given to drink ghee mixed with Ksara (Alkali reparation). He may also be given meat-soup or warm milk to drink. Inhalation of an unctuous type of smoke is also useful for this ailment.

A Varti (cigarette) is prepared of

Satahva

Tvak – cinnamon

root of Bala – Sida cordifolia,

Bark of Syonaka – Orchis mascula

Root of Castor

Bark of Bilva – Aegle marmelos and

Aragvadha (Cassia fistula) by adding bee's wax, fat and ghee.

The patient is given this Varti (cigarette) to smoke.

Alternatively, the physician should keep Saktu (roasted flour of Barley) in an earthen saucer, and cover it with another saucer having a hole in the middle. After sealing the joint of these to earthen saucer, it is kept over the fire. To the hole in the upper saucer, a reed is fixed. The smoke coming out of this reed is inhaled by the patient suffering from freshly occurring rhinitis.

If there is a pain in the temples, head or forehead, then the patient is given fomentation with hot palm or hot poultice (Upanaha).

If there is sneezing, Nasal discharge or nasal obstruction, the patient is given Sankara (Vide Sutra 14: 41) and such other types of fomentation after adequate oleation.

In the above mentioned conditions, the powder of

Rohisa – Cymbopogon martinii

Ajaji – Cuminum cyminum

Sveta Jiraka – Carum carvi

Vacha – Acorus calamus Linn.

Tarkari and

Choraka – Angelica glauca or the order of

Tvak – cinnamon

Patra – Cinnamonum tamala

Maricha – Black pepper fruit – piper nigrum,

Ela – cardamom and

Prakunchika (black cumin) is inhaled.

If there is dryness or atrophy of the channels, Srngataka (name of a vital spot representing the confluence of vessels supplying nourishment to the nose, ears and eyes), nose and eyes, then oil is given for inhalation.

Anu Taila:

Sesame seeds are impregnated with Goat's milk, and made to a paste by triturating with goat's milk. An earthen pot containing goat's milk is heated on fire. A sterile cloth is kept over the opening of the pot and tied to its brim tightly. The sesame paste is kept over this cloth and covered with another earthen pot.

Heat is applied below, and with the steam of the boiling goat's milk the steam-cooked sesame paste is added with the powder of YastiMadhu – Glycyrrhiza glabra (1/4th in quantity of sesame paste). The paste is then squeezed through a cloth by sprinkling with goat's milk so as to extract its oil. The oil which comes out is added with the decoction of Dashamoola and the paste of

Rasa

Madhuka – Madhuca longifolia and

Rock-salt and cooked repeatedly for 10 times.

The oil processed in this manner is called Anu-Taila. This is so named because of its ability to permeate through the Anu-srotas or fine channels. This oil is useful for Snehana (oleation therapy).

After oleation therapy with the above mentioned medicated oil, the patient is given Asthapana type of medicated enema for the elimination of Doshas.

To the patient suffering from Vatika Type of Rhinitis, unctuous, sour, hot and light food is given along with the soup of the meat of domesticated animals. He is given warm water for bath and drinking. He should stay in a place which is warm and free from strong wind.

He should avoid worry, physical exercise, excessive talk and sexual intercourse, if he wants his own well being. [134-143]

Treatment of Paittika Rhinitis:

पैत्ते सर्पिः पिबेत् सिद्धं शृङ्गवेर शृतं पयः| पाचनार्थं पिबेत् पक्वे कार्यं मूर्ध विरेचनम्||१४४||

पाठादिवरजनी मूर्वा पिप्पली जाति पल्लवैः| दन्त्या च साधितं तैलं नस्यं स्यात् पक्वपीनसे||१४५||

पूयास्रे रक्तपितघ्नाः कषाया नावनानि च| पाक दाहाढ्य रूक्षेषु शीता लेपाः ससेचनाः||१४६||

घ्रेय नस्योपचाराश्च कषायाः स्वादु शीतलाः| मन्द पित्ते प्रतिश्याये स्निग्धैः कुर्याद्विरेचनम्||१४७||

घृतं क्षीरं यवाः शालिगोधूमा जाङ्गला रसाः| शीताम्लास्तिक्तशाकानि यूषा मुद्गादिभिर्हिताः||१४८||

For Paittika type of Rhinitis, the patient is given ghee cooked with Shringavera – Ginger, or milk boiled by adding Shringavera – Ginger for the Pachana (ripening) of the morbid matter, and thereafter, he is given Errhines.

Inhalation of medicated oil prepared by cooking with

Patha – Cissampelos pareira

Haridra – turmeric – Curcuma longa

Daruharidra – Berberis aristata

Murva – Marsdenia tenacissima,

Pippali – Long pepper fruit – Piper longum

leaves of Jati – Jasminum grandiflorum and

Danti – Baliospermum montanum is useful for the ripened (Pakva) type of Rhinitis.

If there is discharge of pus and blood from the nose, then the patient is given decoctions and inhalation therapies prescribed for treatment of Rakta-Pitta (an ailment characterized by bleeding from different parts of the body) [vide Chapter 4 of this section].

If there is suppuration and burning sensation in excess, and dryness, then cooling ointments are applied.

Inhalation therapy and other regimes for Paittika type of Rhinits are astringent and sweet in taste and cooling. If Rhinitis is caused by less aggravated Pitta, then purgation therapy with unctuous ingredients is administered.

For the patient suffering from Paittika type of Rhinitis, ghee, milk, barley, rice, wheat, Soup of the meat of animals inhabiting arid zone,

vegetables which are cooling, sour and bitter, and Soup of Mudga etc are useful. [144-148]

Treatment of Kaphaja Peenasa:

गौरवारोचकेष्वादौ लङ्घनं कफ पीनसे| स्वेदाः सेकाश्च पाकार्थं लिप्ते शिरसि सर्पिषा||१४९||

लशुनं मुद्गचूर्णेन व्योष क्षार घृतैर्युतम्| देयं कफघ्न वमनमुत्क्लिष्ट श्लेष्मणे हितम्||१५०||

अपीनसे पूति नस्ये घ्राणास्रावे स कण्डुके| धूमः शस्तोऽवपीडश्च कटुभिः कफपीनसे||१५१||

मनःशिला वचा व्योषं विडङ्गं हिङ्गु गुग्गुलुः| चूर्णो घ्रेयः प्रधमनं कटुभिश्च फलैस्तथा||१५२||

भार्गी मदन तर्कारी सुरसादि विपाचिते| मूत्रे लाक्षा वचा लम्बा विडङ्गं कुष्ठ पिप्पली||१५३||

कृत्वा कल्कं करञ्जं च तैलं तैः सार्षपं पचेत्| पाकान्मुक्ते घने नस्यमेतन्मेदोनिभे कफे||१५४||

स्निग्धस्य व्याहते वेगे च्छर्दनं कफपीनसे| वमनीय शृत क्षीर तिल माष यवागुना||१५५||

वार्ताक कुलक व्योष कुलत्थाढ किमुद्गजाः| यूषाः कफघ्नमन्नं च शस्तमुष्णाम्बुसेचनम्||१५६||

For Kaphaja type of Rhinitis associated with heaviness and anorexia, Langhana (fasting therapy) is administered. For the Paka (ripening of the morbid matter), the head is smeared with ghee, and thereafter, fomentation as well as affusion therapies are administered.

Garlic mixed with the powder of

Mudga – Phaseolus trilobus

Sunthi – Ginger

Pippali – Long pepper fruit

Maricha – Black pepper fruit

Yava Ksara and Ghee is given to the patient, and when Kapha gets dissolved, he is given emetic therapy containing Kapha- alleviating ingredients.

In Kaphaja Rhinitis, chronic Rhinits, ozena and excessive discharge from the nose associated with itching, Dhuma (smoke inhalation therapy) and Avapida pouring of medicated oil with pressure) containing

Sunthi – Ginger,

Pippali – Long pepper fruit and

Maricha – Black pepper fruit – piper nigrum,

Vidanga – Embelia ribes

Hingu – Asafoetida and

Guggulu [In the above mentioned conditions.]

The powder of pungent fruits like

Maricha – Black pepper fruit – piper nigrum and

Pippali – Long pepper fruit – Piper longum) is used for insufflation (Pradhamana) by the patient [in the above mentioned conditions.]

Cow's urine is boiled with

Bhargi – Clerodendrum serratum,

Madana – Randia dumetorum,

Tarkari

Surasa (Tulasi) etc,

Mustard oil is cooked by adding the paste of

Laksa

Vasa – Adhatoda vasica

Jambu – Syzygium cumini,

Katu- Katukarohini – Picrorhiza kurroa),

Vidanga – Embelia ribes,

kustha –Sausserea lappa,

Pippali – Long pepper fruit – Piper longum and

Karanja – Pongamia pinnata

Inhalation therapy with this medicated oil is useful when the Rhinitis has ripened (Pakva) and when there is discharge of thick and fat-like mucus from the nose.

After the Kaphaja type of Rhinitis has become milder, the patient is given oleation therapy followed by emetic therapy. Gruel prepared of Taila and Masa by adding milk boiled with emetic drugs is used in this emetic therapy.

Soup of

Vartaka

Kulaka (a type of Patola—Trichosanthes dioica),

Sunthi – ginger,

Pippali – Long pepper fruit – Piper longum,

Maricha – Black pepper fruit – piper nigrum,

Kulattha – horsegram,

Adhaki – Cajanus cajan and

Mudga – Phaseolus trilobus and

Kapha- alleviating food ingredients and affusion with warm water are useful in Kaphaja type of Rhinitis. [149- 156]

Treatment of Dushta Peenasa:

सर्वजित् पीनसे दुष्टे कार्यं शोफे च शोफजित्| क्षारोऽबुदाधिमांसेषु क्रिया शेषेष्ववेक्ष्य च||१५७||

इति पीनस नासा रोग चिकित्सा|

For Dusta Pratisyaya (Pernicious Rhinitis), Therapeutic measures described above for all the 3 type of Rhinitis is administered.

For edematous Rhinitis, therapeutic measures for the relief of oedema are administered.

If there is a tumor of fleshy growth (Adhi- Mamsa) in the nose, then caustic alkalies are applied.

For the remaining types of nasal ailments, appropriate therapies are administered after proper investigation.

Thus, ends the description of the treatment of nasal ailments including Rhinitis. [157]

Shiroroga Chikitsa – Treatment of head diseases

वातिके शिरसो रोगे स्नेहान् स्वेदान् सनावनान्| पानान्नमुपनाहांश्च कुर्याद्वातामयापहान्||१५८||

For Vatika type of headache, oleation, fomentation and inhalation therapies, and Vayu- alleviating drinks, food and hot poultices are administered. [158]

Upanaha (Hot Poultices):

तैलभृष्टैरगुर्वादयैः सुखोष्णैरुपनाहनम्| जीवनीयैः सुमनसा मत्स्यैर्मांसैश्च शस्यते||१५९||

Luke- warm poultices prepared of the paste of Aguru – Aquallaria agallocha, etc, or of Jivaniya group of drugs or of Sumanas (Jasminum officinale) flowers of Jati or of fish or of meat, all sizzled with oil are useful in Vatika type of headache. [159]

Rasnadi Taila:

रास्ना स्थिरादिभिः सिद्धं सक्षीरं नस्यमर्तिनुत्| तैलं रास्नादिवकाकोली शर्कराभिरथापि वा||१६०||

Medicated oil prepared by cooking with the paste of

Rasna – Vanda roxburghi / Pluchea lanceolata),

Sala- Parni

Brihati – Solanum indicum

Kantakari – Solanum xanthocarpum and

Goksura – Tribulus terrestris is used for Nasya (inhalation therapy) which cures headache. [160]

Baladya Taila:

बला मधूक यष्ट्याह्व विदारी चन्दनोत्पलैः| जीवकर्षभक द्राक्षा शर्कराभिश्च साधितः||१६१||

प्रस्थस्तैलस्य सक्षीरो जाङ्गलार्धतुलारसे| नस्यं सर्वोर्ध्व जत्रूत्थ वात पित्तामयापहम्||१६२||

Ingredients:

1 Prastha (768 ml) of Oil is cooked with

1 Prastha of milk

½ tula of the soup of the meat of animals inhabiting arid zone, and

The paste (¼ Prastha in total) of

Bala – Country mallow root – Sida cordifolia,

Madhuka – Madhuca longifolia

Madhu-Yasti – Glycyrrhiza glabra

Vidari Ipomoea paniculata / Pueraria tuberosa),

Chandana Sandalwood – Santalum album),

Utpala Nymphaea alba),

Jivaka – Malaxis acuminata,

Rishabhaka – Manilkara hexandra,

Draksha – Raisin – Vitis vinifer and

Sugar

Inhalation therapy with this medicated oil cures all the Vatika and Paittika diseases manifested in the head and neck supra-clavicular region) [161-162]

Mayura Ghrita:

दशमूल बला रास्ना त्रिफला मधुकैः सह| मयूरं पक्ष पित्तान्त्र शकृतुण्डाङ्घ्रि वर्जितम्||१६३||

जले पक्त्वा घृतप्रस्थं तस्मिन् क्षीर समं पचेत्| मधुरैः कार्षिकैः कल्कैः शिरोरोगार्दितापहम्||१६४||

कर्णाक्षि नासिका जिह्वा ताल्वास्य गल रोगनुत्| मायूरमितिविख्यातमूर्ध्वजत्रु गदापहम्||१६५||

इति मायूर घृतम्|

Ingredients:

Bilva – Aegle marmelos

Syonaka – Orchis mascula

Gambhari – Gmelina arborea

Patala – Ficus microcarpa

Ganikarika

Salaparni

Prisniparni

Brihati – Solanum indicum

Kantakari – Solanum xanthocarpum

Gokshura – Tribulus terrestris

Bala – Country mallow root) – Sida cordifolia,

Rasna Vanda roxburghi / Pluchea lanceolata),

Haritaki – Terminalia chebula

Vibhitaka – Terminalia bellerica

Amalaki – Phyllanthus emblica and

Madhuka– Licorice – Glycyrrhiza glabra is taken in the quantities of 3 Palas each,

Peacock with its feather, Bile, intestines, fecal matter, beak and feet removed, is taken in quantity equal to all the above mentioned drugs [i.e 48 Tolas in total].

All these ingredients are boiled by adding 1 Drona of water and reduced to 1/4th.

Along with this decoction, 1 prastha of Ghee and 1 Karsa of each of drugs belonging to Madhuradi- Gana or the Group of drugs havin sweet taste viz,

Jivaka – Malaxis acuminata,

Rishabhaka – Manilkara hexandra,

Meda – Polygonatum cirrhifolium,

Maha- meda

Kakoli – Fritillaria roylei,

Mudgaparni – Phaseolus trilobus

Masha-parni – Teramnus labialis

Jivanti – Leptadenia reticulata and

Madhuka– Licorice – Glycyrrhiza glabra

This medicated ghee cures

head diseases, facial paralysis,

Diseases of the ears, eyes, nose, tongue, palates, mouth and throat.

This recipe is well known as Mayura ghrta which cures the diseases of the head and neck.

Thus, ends the description of Mayura-Ghrta [163-165]

Mahamayura Ghrta:

एतेनैव कषायेण घृत प्रस्थं विपाचयेत्| चतुर्गुणेन पयसा कल्कैरेभिश्च कार्षिकैः||१६६||

जीवन्ती त्रिफला मेदा मृद्वीकर्धि परूषकैः| समङ्गा चविका भार्गी काश्मरी सुरदारुभिः||१६७||

आत्मगुप्ता महामेदा ताल खर्जूर मस्तकैः| मृणाल बिस शालूक शृङ्गी जीवक पद्मकैः ||१६८||

शतावरी विदारीक्षु बृहती सारिवा युगैः| मूर्वा श्वदंष्ट्रर्षभक शृङ्गाटक कसेरुकैः||१६९||

रास्ना स्थिरा तामलकी सूक्ष्मैला शटि पौष्करैः| पुनर्नवा तुगाक्षीरी काकोली धन्वयासकैः||१७०||

खर्जूराक्षोट वाताममुञ्जाताभिषुकैरपि | द्रव्यैरेभिर्यथालाभं पूर्वकल्पेन साधितम्||१७१||

नस्ये पाने तथाऽभ्यङ्गे बस्तौ चैव प्रयोजयेत्| शिरो रोगेषु सर्वेषु कासे श्वासे च दारुणे||१७२||

मन्यापृष्ठग्रहे शोषे स्वरभेदे तथाऽर्दिते| योन्यसृक्शुक्र दोषेषु शस्तं वन्ध्या सुतप्रदम्||१७३||

ऋतुस्नाता तथा नारी पीत्वा पुत्रं प्रसूयते| महा मायूरमित्येतद्घृतमात्रेय पूजितम्||१७४||

इति महामायूर घृतम्|

To the decoction of Bilva – Aegle marmelos, etc., described above, 1 Prastha of ghee and 4 Prasthas of water is added.

This is cooked by adding the paste of one Karsa of each of

Jivanti ,Haritaki,Vibhitaka, Amalaki, Meda, Mrdvika, Rddhi, Parusaka, Samana, Cavika, Bhargi, Kasari, Sura-daru, Atmagupta, Maha meda, Tala, Kharjura, Mrinala, Bisa, Saluka, Srngi, Jivaka, Padmaka, Shatavari, Vidari, Iksu, Brihati, Sveta- Sariva, Krsna- Sariva, Murva, Svadamstra, Rishabhaka, Srngataka, Kaseruka, Rasna, Sthira, Tamalaki, Suksma-ela, Sati, Puskara- Mula, Punarnava, Tuga-Ksiri, Kakoli, Dhanvayasaka, Kharjura, Aksota, Vatama, Mujata and Abhisuka or as many of these drugs as are available. Cooking is done according to the above mentioned procedure.

This medicated ghee is used for Nasya (inhalation therapy), pana (drinking), enema and massage. It is very useful for all types of head- diseases, serious types of cough and asthma, torticollis, stiffness of the back, consumption, hoarseness of voice, facial paralysis, diseases of the female genital tract, menstrual disorders and seminal vitiation. It helps in the procreation of offerings even by a barren woman. Drinking this ghee, after the bath at the end of the menstrual period, will help in the procreation of a male offspring

This medicated ghee is called MahaMayura Ghruta, and is held in high esteem by Lord Atreya.

Thus, ends the description of MahaMayura Ghrita. [166-174]

Ghee prepared of Rat etc.

आखुभिः कुक्कुटैर्हंसैः शशैश्चापि हि बुद्धिमान्| कल्पेनानेन विपचेत् सर्पिरूर्ध्व गदापहम्||१७५||

With the above mentioned ingredients and following the same procedure, a wise physician may also prepare medicated ghee by replacing peacock with a rat, cock, swan and rabbit which also cure the diseases of the head and neck. [175]

Treatment of Paittika Headache:

पैत्ते घृतं पयः सेकाः शीता लेपाः स नावनाः| जीवनीयानि सर्पींषि पानान्नं चापि पित्तनुत्||१७६||

चन्दनोशीर यष्ट्याह्व बला व्याघ्रनखोत्पलैः| क्षीरपिष्टैः प्रदेहः स्याच्छृतैर्वा परिषेचनम्||१७७||

त्वक्पत्र शर्करा कल्कः सुपिष्टस्तण्डुलाम्बुना| कार्योऽवपीडः सर्पिश्च नस्यं तस्यानु पैत्तिके||१७८||

यष्ट्याह्व चन्दनानन्ता क्षीर सिद्धं घृत हितम्| नावनं शर्करा द्राक्षा मधूकैर्वाऽपि पित्तजे||१७९||

In Paittika type of headache, ghee, milk, affusion, cold poultice, inhalation therapy prepared of cooling drugs, medicated ghee prepared with drugs belonging to Jivaniya group vide Sutra 4:9), and Pitta- alleviating food and drinks are useful.

Recipe –

Chandana – Sandalwood

Ushira – Vetiveria zizanioides,

YastiMadhu – Glycyrrhiza glabra

Bala – Country mallow root) – Sida cordifolia,

Vyaghra-Nakha – Capparis zeylanica and

Utpala – Nymphaea alba is made to a paste by triturating with milk which is applied over the head, the decoction of the above mentioned drugs may also be used for effusion in Paittika type of headache.

Tvak, Patra – Cinnamomum tamala Nees and Eberum and sugar is made to a paste by adding Tandulambu (rice-wash). This paste is kept inside a cloth, and the liquid is squeezed into the nostrils (avapida). Thereafter, ghee is given for inhalation to alleviate Paittika type of headache.

Medicated ghee prepared by boiling with

Yastimadhu – Glycyrrhiza glabra

Chandana – Sandalwood – Santalum album),

Ananta and milk are useful for inhalation.

Similarly, inhalation of the medicated ghee prepared by boiling with

Sugar,

Draksha – Raisin – Vitis vinifera and

Madhuka – Glycyrrhiza glabra is useful in Paittika type of Headache. [176- 179]

Treatment of Kaphaja Headache

कफजे स्वेदितं धूम नस्य प्रधमनादिभिः| शुद्धं प्रलेपपानान्नैः कफघ्नैः समुपाचरेत्||१८०||

पुराण सर्पिषः पानैस्तीक्ष्णै बस्तिभिरेव च| कफानिलोत्थिते दाहः शेषयो रक्त मोक्षणम्||१८१||

एरण्ड नल दक्षौम गुग्गुल्वगुरु चन्दनैः| धूमवर्ति पिबेद्गन्धैरकुष्ठ तगरैस्तथा||१८२||

In Kaphaja type of headache, fomentation therapy, smoking therapy, inhalation therapy, Pradhamana (Insufflations of powders into the nostrils) Etc, is administered for cleaning the morbid matter from the head. Thereafter, Kapha-alleviating pralepa (application of drugs in a paste form), drinks and food are given to the patient. He is given old ghee to drink to such patients. Medicated enema prepared of drugs having Tiksna (sharp) attributes is administered. In Kaphaja and Vatika types of headache, Daha - cauterization in the fore-head and temples (vide Susruta: Sutra 12: 9) is useful. In the remaining types of headache, Blood-letting therapy is administered.

Dhuma varti (cigar) prepared of

Eranda – Ricinus communis

Nalanda

Kshauma

Guggulu – Commifora mukul Engl.

Aguru – Aquallaria agallocha

Chandana Sandalwood – Santalum album) and other aromatic drugs, except Kushta – Saussurea lappa and Tagara – Valerian walichii , is used for smoking in Kaphaja type of headache [180- 182]

Treatment of Sannipatika Headache

सन्निपातभवे कार्या सन्निपातहिता क्रिया|

In the Sannipatika type of headache (which is caused by the simultaneous aggravation of all the 3 Doshas), therapeutic measures prescribed above for all the 3 types of headaches caused by Vayu, Pitta and Kapha) are administered together. [1/2 – 183]

Treatment of Krimija Headache:

क्रिमिजे चैव कर्तव्यं तीक्ष्णं मूर्ध विरेचनम्||१८३||

त्वग्दन्ती व्याघ्रकरज विडङ्ग नवमालिकाः|

अपामार्गफलं बीजं नक्तमाल शिरीषयोः| क्षवकोऽश्मन्तको बिल्वं हरिद्रा हिङ्गु यूथिका||१८४||

फणिज्झकश्च तैस्तैलमविमूत्रे चतुर्गुणे| सिद्धं स्यान्नावनं चूर्णं चैषां प्रधमनं हितम्||१८५||

फलं शिग्रु करञ्जाभ्यां सव्योषं चावपीडकः| कषायः स्वरसः क्षारश्चूर्णं कल्कोऽवपीडकः||१८६||

इति शिरोरोग चिकित्सा|

For the headache caused by Krimi (parasitic infestation), strong errhines having sharp (Tiksna) ingredients are administered.

Medicated oil prepared by cooking with

4 times of sheep's urine, and the paste of

Tvak – Cinnamonum zeylanica

Danti – Baliospermum montanum

Vyaghra Nakhi – Capparis zeylanica

Vidanga – Embelia ribes

Nava-Mallika

Fruits seeds of Apamarga – Achyranthes aspera

Seeds of Nakta-Mala – Pongamia glabra and

Phanijjhaka [in total 1/4th in quantity of oil] is useful for the headache (head disease) caused by Krimi (Parasitic infestation).

Insufflation of the nostrils with the powder of the drugs mentioned above beginning with Tvak – Cinnamonum zeylanica and ending with Phanijjhaka is also useful in Krimija type of headache.

The paste of the fruits of Sigru – Moringa oliefera and Karanja – Pongamia glabra added with Sunthi – Ginger, Pippali – Long pepper fruit – Piper longum and Maricha – Black pepper fruit – piper nigrum is [tied in a piece of cloth and] squeezed into the Nostrils (Avapida). The decoction, juice, alkali preparation, powder including paste of these drugs may also be used for Avapida.

Thus, ends the description of the treatment of headache. [183 ½- 186]

Mukharoga Chikitsa: Treatment of oral disorders:

Line of Treatment:

शुक्त तिक्त कटु क्षौद्र कषायैः कवलग्रहः| धूमः प्रधमनं शुद्धिरधश्छर्दन लङ्घनम्||१८७||

भोज्यं च मुखरोगेषु यथास्वं दोषनुद्धितम्|

Kavala- Graha (holding the paste of drugs in the mouth) containing vinegar, paste of bitter and pungent drugs, honey and decoction of bitter and pungent drugs is useful for mouth- diseases.

Similarly, smoking pradhamana (insufflations), purgation, emetic and fasting therapies, and food containing ingredients which alleviate the aggravated Doshas are useful in mouth – diseases [187- ½ 188]

Pipalyadi Churna:

पिप्पल्यगुरु दार्वीत्वग्यवक्षार रसाञ्जनम्||१८८||

पाठां तेजोवतीं पथ्यां समभागं विचूर्णयेत्| मुख रोगेषु सर्वेषु सक्षौद्रं तद्विधारयेत्||१८९||

सीधु माधव माध्वीकैः श्रेष्ठोऽयं कवलग्रहः|

Ingredients: All taken equal quantities is made to a powder

Pippali – Piper longum

Aguru – Aquallaria agallocha

bark of Daruharidra – Berberis aristata

Yava Ksara,

Rasanjana (Aqueous extract of Berberis aristata),

Patha – Cissampelos parriera

Tejovati – Zanthoxylum alatum and

Pathya – Terminalia Chebula

This is mixed with honey, and kept in the mouth which is useful in all types of mouth- diseases.

Adding Sidhu (a type of wine prepared of sugar-cane juice), Madhava (a type of wine prepared of honey) and Madhvika (a type of wine prepared of Madhuka– Licorice – Glycyrrhiza glabra) to the above mentioned powder, and holding it in the mouth (Kavala – Graha) is immensely useful for curing all types of mouth –diseases. [188 ½ –190½]

Tejovatyadi Tooth powder:
तेजोह्वामभयामेलां समङ्गां कटुकां घनम्||१९०||
पाठां ज्योतिष्मतीं लोध्रं दार्वीं कुष्ठं च चूर्णयेत्| दन्तानां घर्षणं रक्त स्राव कण्डू रुजापहम्||१९१||
Ingredients:
Tejohva (tejabala) – Zanthoxylum alatum
Abhaya – Terminalia chebula,
Ela (Elettaria cardamomum) ,
Samanga – Rubia cordifolia,
Katuka – Myrica carifera
Ghana
Patha – Cissampelos parriera
Jyotismati – Celastrus paniculatus
Lodhra – Symplocos racemosa
Darvi – Berberis aristata and
Kushta – Saussurea lappa is made to a powder
Brushing teeth with this powder cures bleeding, itching and pain in the teeth [190 ½ – 191]

Kshara Gutika:
पञ्चकोलक तालीसपत्रैला मरिच त्वचः| पलाश मुष्कक क्षार यवक्षाराश्च चूर्णिताः||१९२||
गुडे पुराणे द्विगुणे क्वथिते गुटिकाः कृताः| कर्कन्धुमात्राः सप्ताहं स्थिता मुष्ककभस्मनि||१९३||
कण्ठ रोगेषु सर्वेषु धार्याः स्युरमृतोपमाः|
Ingredients: The powder of [1 part of each of]
Pippali – Long pepper fruit – Piper longum,
Pippali Mula
Chavya – Piper retrofractum,
Chitraka – Leadword,
Nagara – Ginger
Talisa-patra – Abies webbiana
Ela – Elattaria cardamum
Maricha – Black pepper fruit – piper nigrum,
Tvak – Cinnamonum zeylanica
Palasa – Butea monosperma
Muskaka- Ksara and is cooked by adding double the quantity of old jaggery 24 parts in syrup form), and pills the size of Karkandhu (bear fruit) are made out of this paste. These pills are kept inside a heap of ash or Ksara (alkali preparation) of Muskaka. Gradually sucking the part of this pill dissolved in the mouth [and gradually sucking the part of this pills dissolved in saliva] is useful like ambrosia in all types of throats- diseases [192 –194½]

Kalaka Curna:
गृहधूमो यवक्षारः पाठा व्योषं रसाञ्जनम्||१९४||
तेजोह्वा त्रिफला लोध्रं चित्रकश्चेति चूर्णितम्| सक्षौद्रं धारयेदेतद्गलरोग विनाशनम्||१९५||
कालकं नाम तच्चूर्णं दन्तास्य गल रोगनुत्|
इति कालकचूर्णम्|

Ingredients:

Grha-Dhuma (Kitchen- Soot or carbon deposited in the chimney in the house)

Yava Ksara

Patha – Cissampelos parriera

Ela – Elattaria cardamum

Maricha – Black pepper fruit – piper nigrum,

Tvak – Cinnamon

Palasa – Butea monosperma

Muskaka- Ksara is cooked by adding double the quantity of old jaggery (24 parts in syrup form), and pills the size of Karkandhu (bear fruit) are made out of this paste. These pills are kept inside a heap of ash or Ksara (alkali preparation) of Muskaka for 7 days.

Keeping this pill in the mouth [and gradually sucking the part of this pill dissolved in Saliva] is useful like ambrosia in all types of throat diseases. [192- 194½]

Thus, ends the description of Kalaka-Churna [194 ½- 196½]

Peetaka Churna:

मनःशिला यवक्षारो हरितालं ससैन्धवम्||१९६||

दार्वीत्वक् चेति तच्चूर्णं माक्षिकेण समायुतम्| मूर्च्छितं घृतमण्डेन कण्ठ रोगेषु धारयेत्||१९७||

मुख रोगेषु च श्रेष्ठं पीतकं नाम कीर्तितम्|

इति पीतक चूर्णम्|

Manah –Sila, Yava -Ksara, Haritala, Saindhava and bark of Daru Haridra – Berberis aristata is made into powder mixed with honey and Ghrta-Manda (upper part of ghee). This powder is kept in the mouth for the cure of mouth-diseases. Known as Pitaka- Curna, this is an excellent remedy for mouth – diseases.

Thus, ends the description of Peetaka Churna [192 ½ – ½ 198]

Mrudvikadi Churna

मृद्वीका कटुका व्योषं दार्वी त्वक् त्रिफला घनम्||१९८||

मूर्च्छितं घृतमण्डेन कण्ठ रोगेषु धारयेत्| पाठा रसाञ्जनं मूर्वा तेजोह्वेति च चूर्णितम्||१९९||

क्षौद्रयुक्तं विधातव्यं गल रोगे भिषग्जितम्| योगास्त्वेते त्रयः प्रोक्ता वात पित्त कफापहाः||२००||

The powder of

Mrdvika – Vitis vinifera

Katuka – Myrica carifera

katu- Katukarohini – Picrorhiza kurroa),

Sunthi – Ginger

Pippali – Long pepper fruit – Piper longum,

Maricha – Black pepper fruit – piper nigrum,

Bark of Daru- Haridra – Berberis aristata

Haritaki – Terminalia chebula

Vibhitaka – Terminalia bellerica

Amalaki – Phyllanthus emblica

Ghana

Patha – Cissampelos parriera

Rasanjana (Aqueous extract of Berberis aristata),

Murva – Marsedenia tenacissima and

Tejohva is mixed with honey, and kept in the mouth for the treatment of throat-diseases

These 3 recipes Viz,

Kalaka Churna – Vatika types of Throat disease

Pitaka Churna – Paittika types of Throat disease and

Mrdvikadi Churna – Kaphaja types of Throat disease [190 ½ – 200]

Katukadi Kvatha:

कटुकातिविषा पाठा दार्वी मुस्त कलिङ्गकाः| गोमूत्रक्वथिताः पेयाः कण्ठ रोग विनाशनाः||२०१||

Cow's urine is boiled by adding

Katuka – Myrica carifera,

Ativisa – Aconitum heterophyllum

Patha – Cissampelos parriera

Daru- Haridra – Berberis aristata

Musta – Cyperus rotundus and

Kalinaka

Intake of this decoction cures Throat- diseases. [201]

Darvi Rasakriya:

स्वरसः क्वथितो दार्व्या घनीभूतो रसक्रिया| सक्षौद्रा मुखरोगासृग्दोष नाडीव्रणापहा||२०२||

The juice of decoction of Daru- Haridra (berberis aristata) is boiled in order to make it thick which is called Rasa- Kriya. Use of this with honey cures mouth- diseases, diseases caused by the vitiation of blood and Nadi- Vrana (sinus). [202]

Administration of Ghee:

तालुशोषे त्वतृष्णस्य सर्पिरौतरभक्तिकम्| नावनं मधुराः स्निग्धाः शीताश्चैव रसा हिताः||२०३||

If there is dryness of the palate in a patient who is not suffering from morbid thirst (Atrsna), then he is given ghee to drink after the intake of food (Uttara- Bhakitka) he is given inhalation therapy, and meat- soup which is sweet, unctuous and cooling. [203]

Venesection (Sirakarma) etc in Stomatitis:

मुखपाके सिराकर्म शिरःकाय विरेचनम्| मूत्र तैल घृत क्षौद्र क्षीरैश्च कवलग्रहाः||२०४||

सक्षौद्रास्त्रिफला पाठा मृद्वीका जातिपल्लवाः| कषाय तिक्तकाः शीताः क्वाथाश्च मुखधावनाः||२०५||

If thcrc is stomatitis, the patient is given venesection (Rakta- Moksana) therapy, errhines and purgatives. Kavala- Graha therapy (keeping in mouth drugs in paste form) prepared of cow's urine, oil, ghee, honey and milk is administered to him. Mouth- wash (Mukha- Dhavana) with cold decoction of drugs having astringent and bitter tastes is useful in this condition. [204- 205]

Khadiradi Gutika and Khadiradi Taila

तुलां खदिरसारस्य द्विगुणामरिमेदसः| प्रक्षाल्य जर्जरीकृत्य चतुर्द्रोणेऽम्भसः पचेत्||२०६||

द्रोण शेषं कषायं तं पूत्वा भूयः पचेच्छनैः| ततस्तस्मिन् घनीभूते चूर्णीकृत्याक्षभागिकम्||२०७||

चन्दनं पद्मकोशीरं मञ्जिष्ठा धातकी घनम्| प्रपौण्डरीकं यष्ट्याह्वत्वगेला पद्म केशरम्||२०८||

लाक्षां रसाञ्जनं मांसी त्रिफला लोध्र वालकम्| रजन्यौ फलिनीमेलां समङ्गां कट्फल वचाम्||२०९||

यवासागुरु पत्तङ्ग गैरिकाञ्जनमावपेत्| लवङ्ग नखकक्कोलजातिकोशान् पलोन्मितान्||२१०||

कर्पूर कुडवं चापि क्षिपेच्छीतेऽवतारिते| ततस्तु गुटिकाःकार्याःशुष्काश्चास्येन धारयेत्||२११||

तैलं चानेन कल्केन कषायेण च साधयेत्| दन्तानां चलन भ्रंश शौशिर्य क्रिमि रोगनुत्||२१२||

मुखपाकास्य दौर्गन्ध्य जाड्यारोचक नाशनम्| स्रावोपलेप पैच्छिल्य वैस्वर्य गल शोषनुत्||२१३||

दन्तास्य गल रोगेषु सर्वेष्वेतत् परायणम्| खदिरादि गुटीकेयं तैलं च खदिरादिकम्||२१४||

इति खदिरादि गुटिका तैलं च|

1 Tula of the heartwood of Khadira (Acacia catechu) and two Tulas of Arimeda – Acacia leucophloea is washed well, and made to a coarse powder which is boiled by adding 4 Dronas of water till 1 Drona remains. The decoction after

filtering the wood – powder which is boiled by adding 4 Dronas of water till 1 Drona remains the decoction after filtering the wood-powder) is boiled again till it becomes thick.

To this paste, the powder of the Aksa of each of

Chandana – Sandalwood – Santalum album),

Padmaka – Prunus cerasoides,

Ushira – Vetiver – Vetiveria zizanioides,

Manjistha – Rubia cordifolia

Dhataki – Woodfordia fruticosa,

Ghana –

Prapaundarika Nymphaea lotus) – red variety,

Yastimadhu – Glycyrrhiza glabra

Tvak – Cinnamonum zeylanica

Ela – Elettaria cardamomum Maton) ,

Padmakesara,

Laksa

Rasanjana (Aqueous extract of Berberis aristata),

Mamsi – Nordostachys jatamamsi

Haritaki – Terminalia chebula

Vibhitaka – Terminalia bellerica

Amalaki – Phyllanthus emblica

Lodhra – Symplocos racemosa

Balaka – Coleus vettiveroides

Haridra – turmeric – Curcuma longa),

Daru Haridra – Berberis aristata

Phalini (Priyangu Callicarpa macrophylla),

Ela – Elettaria cardamomum Maton) ,

Samanga – Mimosa pudica

Katphala – Myrica nagi,

Vacha – Acorus calamus Linn.

Yavasa – Alhagi pseudalhagi

Aguru – Aquallaria agallocha

Pattanga – Caesalpinia sappan

Gairika and

Anjana is added after the cooking is over; the pan is removed from the oven and allowed to become cool.

Thereafter, the powder of 1 Pala of each of

Lavanga – Syzygium aromaticum

Nakha, Kakoli and

Jatipatra along with 1 Kudava of

Karpura – Cinnamonum camphora is added [and mixed well]. From out of this paste, pills are prepared and dried. These pills are kept in the mouth and sucked.

With the above mentioned decoction and paste of drugs Chandana Sandalwood – Santalum album), etc, which mentioned above to be used in the form of powder), oil is cooked.

Use of these pills and medicated oil cures

Chalana – looseness,

Bhramsha – displacement and

Saushirya – porosity of teeth,

Caries (teeth parasitic infestation of teeth),

Mukha paka – stomatitis,

Daurgandhya – foul odor emanating from the mouth,

Jadya – stiffness of the mouth,

Aruchi – anorexia

ptyalism,

Srava upalepa – stickiness and sliminess of the mouth,

Vaisvarya – hoarseness of the voice and

Gala sosha – Dryness of the throat.

This pill is an excellent remedy for all the diseases of teeth, mouth and throat. The pill described above is called Khadiradi- gutika, and the medicated oil is called Khadiradi – Taila.

Thus ends the description of Khadiradi – Gutika and Khadiradi – Taila. Here ends description of the treatment of mouth- diseases [206-214]

Aruchi Chikitsa – Treatment of Anorexia

Line of Treatment of Anorexia

अरुचौ कवलग्राहा धूमाः समुखधावनाः| मनोज्ञमन्नपानं च हर्षणाश्वासनानि च||२१५||

In Aruchi, Kavalagraha (keeping thin paste of drugs in the mouth), Dhuma (Smoking therapy), Mukha Dhavana (mouth wash), pleasing food and drinks, and cheering as well as consulting / assuring measures are useful. [215]

Kavala Graha for Different Types of Anorexia

कुष्ठ सौवर्चलाजाजी शर्करा मरिचं बिडम्| धात्र्येला पद्मकोशीर पिप्पल्युत्पल चन्दनम्||२१६||

लोध्रं तेजोवती पथ्या त्र्यूषणं सयवाग्रजम्| आर्द्रं दाडिम निर्यासश्चाजाजी शर्करायुतः||२१७||

सतैल माक्षिकास्त्वेते चत्वारः कवलग्रहाः| चतुरोऽरोचकान् हन्युर्वाताद्येकज सर्वजान्||२१८||

For the cure of Vatika Aruchi –

Kushta – Saussurea lappa

Sauvarcala

Ajaji – Cuminum cyminum

Sugar

Maricha – Black pepper fruit – piper nigrum and

Vida along with oil and honey is given as Kavala- graham (to keep the thin paste of drugs in the mouth).

For the cure of Pittaja Aruchi:

Dhatri – Emblica officinalis

Ela – Cardamom

Padmaka – Prunus cerasoides,

Ushira – Vetiver – Vetiveria zizanioides

Pippali – Long pepper fruit – Piper longum

Utpala – Nymphaea alba and

Chandana – Sandalwood – Santalum album along with oil and honey are given as Kavala- Graha.

For the cure of Kaphaja Aruchi:

Lodhra – Symplocos racemosa

Tejovati – Zanthoxylum alatum

Pathya – Terminalia chebula

Sunthi – Ginger

Pippali – Long pepper fruit – Piper longum,

Maricha – Black pepper fruit – piper nigrum and

Yava Ksara along with oil and honey is given as Kavala-Graha (to keep the thin paste of drugs in the mouth).

For the cure of Paittika Aruchi –

Dhatri – Emblica officinalis

Ela – Elettaria cardamomum Maton

Tejovati – Zanthoxylum alatum
Pathya – Terminalia chebula
Sunthi – Ginger
Pippali – Long pepper fruit – Piper longum,
Maricha – Black pepper fruit – piper nigrum and
YavaKshara along with oil and honey is given as Kavala-Graha.
For Sannipataja Aruchi:
Juice of green Dadima – Pomegranate – Punica granatum,
Ajaji – Cuminum cyminum, and
Sugar along with honey is given as Kavala Graha. [216- 218]

Karavyadi Yoga:

कारवी मरिचाजाजी द्राक्षा वृक्षाम्ल दाडिमम्| सौवर्चलं गुडः क्षौद्रं सर्वारोचक नाशनम्||२१९||

Use of the recipes containing
Karavi – Carum roxburghianum,
Maricha – Black pepper fruit – piper nigrum,
Ajaji – Cuminum cyminum,
Draksha – Raisin – Vitis vinifera,
Vrksamla – Rhus parviflora
Dadima – Pomegranate – Punica granatum,
Sauvarcala
Jaggery and
Honey cures all the types of anorexia. [219]

PanchaKarma Therapy, etc:

बस्तिं समीरणे, पित्ते विरेकं, वमनं कफे| कुर्याद्धृद्यानुकूलानि हर्षणं च मनोघ्नजे||२२०||
इत्यरोचक चिकित्सा|

In Vatika type of anorexia – Basti (medicated enema) is useful;
In Paittika Type of anorexia – Virekam (purgation) therapyis useful; and
In Kaphaja type of anorexia – Vamana (emetic) therapy is useful.
In anorexia caused by mental afflictions, measures for easing the heart and cheering the mind of the patient are adopted.
Thus, ends the description of the treatment of Arocaka (anorexia). [220]

Karnaroga Chikitsa – Treatment of ear diseases:
Line of treatment:

कर्णशूले तु वातघ्नी हिता पीनसवत् क्रिया| प्रदेहाः पूरणं नस्यं पाकस्रावे व्रणक्रियाः||२२१||
भोज्यानि च यथादोषं कुर्यात् स्नेहांश्च पूरणान्|

In Karna Shoola (earache), Vayu-alleviating treatment on the lines suggested for [Vatika type of] rhinitis is administered application of ointment; ear- drops and inhalation therapy [containing Vayu- alleviating ingredients] are beneficial for this ailment.
If there is KarnaPaka (otitis) and Karna-Srava (Otorrhea), then the line of treatment prescribed for ulcers is adopted.
Depending upon the Doshas involved, suitable food and ear- drops is used. [221- 222½]

Hingvadi-Taila:

हिङ्गु तुम्बरु शुण्ठीभिस्तैलं तु सार्षपं पचेत्||२२२||
एतद्दि पूरणं श्रेष्ठं कर्णशूल निवारणम्|

Mustard oil is cooked by adding Hingu – Asafoetida, Tumburu – Zanthoxylum alatum and Sunthi – Ginger. Use of this medicated oil as ear-drop is immensely useful for curing earache. [222 ½ –223½]

Devadarvadi Taila:

देवदारु वचा शुण्ठी शताह्वा कुष्ठ सैन्धवैः||२२३||
तैलं सिद्धं बस्तमूत्रे कर्णशूल निवारणम्|

Oil cooked with

Deva- Daru – Cedrs deodara,

Vacha (Acorus calamus Linn.),

Sunthi – Ginger,

Satahva – Saccharum munja

Kushta – Saussurea lappa and

Saindhava along with Goat's urine cures earache. [223 ½- ½ 224]

Gandha Taila:

वराटकान् समाहृत्य दहेन्मृद्भाजने नवे||२२४||
तद्भस्म श्च्योतयेतेन गन्धतैलं विपाचयेत्| रसाञ्जनस्य शुण्ठ्याश्च कल्काभ्यां कर्णशूलनुत्||२२५||

In a new earthen pot, corie- shells are kept [with a cover], and burnt over fire. The Bhasma (ash), thus, obtained, is decanted. By adding water with this alkaline water and the paste of Rasanjana (Aqueous extract of Berberis aristata) and Sunthi – Ginger, Gandha Taila (aromatic oil) is cooked. Ear- drop with this medicated oil cures earache. [224 ½ – 225]

Kshara Taila:

शुष्क मूलक शुण्ठानां क्षारो हिङ्गु महौषधम्| शतपुष्पा वचा कुष्ठं दारु शिगु रसाञ्जनम्||२२६||
सौवर्चल यव क्षार स्वर्जिकोद्भिद सैन्धवम्| भूर्ज ग्रन्थि बिडं मुस्तं मधुशुक्तं चतुर्गुणम्||२२७||
मातुलुङ्गरसश्चैव कदल्या रस एव च| सर्वैरितैर्यथोद्दिष्टैः क्षारतैलं विपाचयेत्||२२८||
बाधिर्य कर्णनादश्च पूयस्रावश्च दारुणः| क्रिमयः कर्णशूलं च पूरणादस्य नश्यति ||२२९||

Ingredients and method:

Dry radish is cut into pieces and burnt to prepare ash.

Oil is cooked by adding the paste of this alkali preparation.

Hingu – Asa foetida,

Mahausadha – Ginger

Satapuspa – Anethum sowa

Vacha (Acorus calamus Linn.),

Kushta – Saussurea lappa,

Deva- daru – Cedrus deodara

Sigru – Moringa oleifera,

Rasanjana (Aqueous extract of Berberis aristata),

Sauvarcala

Yava Ksara

Svarji- Ksara

Audbhida-Lavana

Saindhava

Knots of Bhurja Betula utilis D. Don

Bida and

Mustra [all taken in equal quantities: in total 1/4th of the quantity of oil]

Madhu- Sukta (4 times of the quantity of oil),

Juice of Matulunga – Lemon variety – Citrus decumana / Citrus limon (equal to the quantity of oil).
This Ksara-Taila is dropped into the ears, which cures
Badhirya – Deafness
Tinitus
Serious type of Pus- discharge from ears,
Parasitic infestation of the ears and Ear ache. [226- 229]

Treatment of Diseases of Mouth, etc in General:

मुख कर्णाक्षि रोगेषु यथोक्तं पीनसे विधिम्| कुर्याद्भिषक् समीक्ष्यादौ दोष काल बलाबलम्||२३०||
इति कर्ण रोग चिकित्सा |

In the case of the diseases of the mouth, ears and eyes, the physician should first of all, ascertain the strength or weakness of the aggravated Doshas and the nature of the season, and thereafter administer therapies as described for different types of Pinasa (Rhinitis).
Thus, ends the description of the treatment of ear-diseases. [230]
Akshiroga Chikitsa – Treatment of eye disorders:

Line of Treatment:

उत्पन्न मात्रे तरुणे नेत्ररोगे बिडालकः| कार्यो दाहोपदेहाश्रु शोफ राग निवारणः||२३१||

In the critical stage of the freshly occurring eye disorder, Bidalaka (application of drugs in paste form over the closed eye-lids excluding eyelashes) is applied to relieve
Daha (burning sensation),
stickiness (Mucous discharge),
Ashru (lachrymation),
Sopha (swelling) and
Raga (redness) [231]

Bidalaka for Vatika Eye Diseases:

नागरं सैन्धवं सर्पि मण्डेन च रसक्रिया| निघृष्टं वातिके तद्वन्मधु सैन्धव गैरिकम्||२३२||
तथा शावरकं लोध्रं घृतभृष्टं बिडालकः| तद्वत् कार्यो हरीतक्या घृतभृष्टो रुजापहः||२३३||

Nagara, Saindhava and Supernatant part of ghee is triturated and made to a paste (Rasa-kriya). This paste is used as Bidalaka (application of drugs in Paste form over the closed eyelids excluding eye-lashes) for the cure of Vatika type of eye-disease. Similarly, the paste of honey, Saindhava and Gairika can be in this condition.
The paste of Savara- Lodhra Symplocos racemosa) or Haritaki – Terminalia chebula may be sizzled with ghee, and used as Bidalaka for the cure of pain in the eyes. [232-233]

Bidalaka for paittika Eye-Diseases:

पैतिके चन्दनानन्ता मञ्जिष्ठाभिर्बिडालकः| कार्यः पद्मक यष्ट्याह्व मांसी कालीयकैस्तथा||२३४||

The paste of Chandana (Sandalwood – Santalum album), Ananta – Cynodon dactylon and Manjistha – Rubia cordifolia or the paste of Padmaka – Prunus puddum,Yastimadhu – Glycyrrhiza glabra, Jata- Mamsi – Nordostachys jatamamsi and Kaliyaka is used as Bidalaka in Paittika type of eye diseases. [234]

Bidalaka for Kaphaja Eye Diseases [Gairikadya Bidalaka]:

गैरिकं सैन्धवं मुस्तं रोचना च रसक्रिया| कफे कार्या तथा क्षौद्रं प्रियङ्गुः समनःशिला||२३५||

The Rasa- Kriya (sticky paste) of Gairika, Saindhava, Musta (Cyperus rotundus) and Gorocana, or the Paste of Priyangu (Callicarpa macrophylla), Manah- shila, and honey is used as Bidalaka in Kaphaja type of eye disorders. [235]

Bidalaka for Sannipatika Eye Diseases:

सन्निपाते तु सर्वैः स्याद्बहिरक्ष्णोः प्रलेपनम्| पक्ष्माण्यस्पृश्यता कार्यं सम्पक्वे त्वञ्जनं त्र्यहात्||२३६||

For eye diseases caused by Sannipata (Simultaneous aggravation of all the 3 Doshas), the paste of all the above-mentioned ingredients described in verse nos. 232- 235) may be used by Bidalaka. While applying the paste over the [closed] eyelids, the eye- lashes are not to be touched. After 3 days when the eye—disease is matured (sampakva), collyrium (anjana) may be applied. [236]

Aschyotana for Vatika eye diseases:

आश्च्योतनं मारुतजे क्वाथो बिल्वादिभिर्हितः| कोष्णः सैरण्ड तर्कारी बृहती मधुशिगुभिः||२३७||

In Vatika type of eye-disease, Ascyotana (sprinkling therapy or eye-douche) with the Luke-warm decoction of

Bilva – Aegle marmelos

Syonaka – Orchis mascula

Gambhari – Gmelina arborea

Patala – Ficus microcarpa and

Ganikarika along with

Eranda – Ricinus communis

Tarkari

Brihati – Solanum indicum and sweet varieties [237]

Eye Drop for Paittika Eye Diseases:

पृथ्वीकादार्वि मञ्जिष्ठा लाक्षादिवमधुकोत्पलैः| क्वाथः सशर्करः शीतः पूरणं रक्तपितनुत्||२३८||

In Paittika type of eye disorder, the cold decoction of Prthvika, Daru-Haridra – Berberis aristata, Manjistha – Rubia cordifolia, Laksha, both the types of Yasti-Madhu – Glycyrrhiza glabra and Utpala along with sugar is used as eye-drop. [238]

Aschyotana for Kaphaja and Sannipatika types of Eye Diseases:

नागर त्रिफला मुस्त निम्ब वासा रसः कफे| कोष्णमाश्च्योतनं मिश्रैरोषधैः सान्निपातके||२३९||

Use of Lukewarm decoction or juice of

Nagara – Ginger,

Haritaki – Terminalia chebula,

Vibhitaka – Terminalia bellerica,

Amalaki – Phyllanthus emblica,

Musta (Cyperus rotundus),

Nimba – Neem Azadirachta indica), and

Vasaka – Adhatoda vasaka

Used as – Ascyotana (eye- douche) is useful in Kaphaja type of eye diseases.

In eye-diseases caused by Sannipata (Simultaneous aggravation of all the three Doshas), all the above mentioned drugs (vide verse nos 237- 239) are used as Ascyotana eye douche). [239]

Varti (wick – bougie) for Vatika Type of Eye diseases [Brihatadi Varti]:

बृहत्येरण्डमूलत्वक् शिग्रोः पुष्पं ससैन्धवम्|

अजाक्षीरेण पिष्टं स्याद्वर्तिर्वाताक्षिरोगनुत्||२४०||

Brihati – Solanum indicum, root-bark of eranda- Ricinus communis, flower of Sigru – Moringa oliefera and Saindhava is triturated by adding goat's milk, and made to a paste Varti (bougie) is made out of this paste application of this Varti cures Vatika type of eye-diseases. [240]

Varti for Paittika Type of Eye-diseases [Sumana koradi Varti]:

सुमनःकोरकाः शङ्ख स्त्रिफला मधुकं बला| पित्त रक्तापहा वर्तिः पिष्टा दिव्येन वारिणा||२४१||

Buds of sumanas (Jati-Puspa), Sankha, Haritaka – Terminalia chebula, Vibhitaka – Terminalia bellerica, Amalaki – Phyllanthus emblica, Madhuka– Licorice – Glycyrrhiza glabra and Bala – Country mallow root – Sida cordifolia is triturated by adding clean rain- water and varti (bougie) is made out of this paste. Application of this Varti (bougie) cures eye diseases caused by the vitiation of Pitta and Raktha (blood). [241]

Varti for Kaphaja Type of Eye diseases [Saindhavadi Varti]:

सैन्धवं त्रिफला व्योषं शङ्खनाभिः समुद्रजः| फेनः शैलेयकं सर्जो वर्तिः श्लेष्माक्षि रोगनुत्||२४२||

Application of the Varti (bougie) containing

Saindhava – rock salt

Haritaki – Terminalia chebula

Vibhitaka – Terminalia bellerica

Amalaki – Phyllanthus emblica

Sunthi – Zingiber officinale

Pippali – Long pepper fruit – Piper longum,

Maricha – Black pepper fruit – piper nigrum,

Sankha,

Samudra- Phena,

Saireyaka and

Sarja (Vateria indica) cures Kaphaja type of eye diseases. [242]

Varti for Sannipatika Eye diseases [Amrtahvadi –Varti]:

अमृताह्वा बिसं बिल्वं पटोलं छागलं शकृत्| प्रपौण्डरीकं यष्ट्याह्वं दार्वी कालानु सारिवा||२४३||
एषामष्टपलान् भागान् सुधौताञ्जर्जरीकृतान्| तोये पक्त्वा रसे पूते भूयः पक्वे रसे घने||२४४||
कर्षं च श्वेतमरिचाज्जातीपुष्पान्नवात् पलम्| चूर्णं क्षिप्त्वा कृता वर्तिः सर्वघ्नी दृक्प्रसादनी||२४५||

8 palas of each of

Amrtahva – Guduci – Tinospora cordifloia

Bisa – Nelumbium speciosum

Bilva – Aegle marmelos

Patola – Trichosanthes dioica

Stool of goat,

Prapaundarika – Nymphaea lotus) – red variety,

Yasti-Madhu – Glychriza glabra

Daru-Haridra – Berberis aristata and

Kalanusariva are washed well and made to a coarse powder, and cooked by adding water.

This decoction is further boiled till it becomes thick. To this paste, 1 Karsa of

Sveta- Maricha – Black pepper fruit – piper nigrum

seeds of Sobhanjana and

1 Pala fresh Jatipuspa (dried) is added in powder form.

Varti (bougie) is made out of this paste.

Application of this Varti cures eye diseases caused by Sannipata (simultaneous aggravation of all the 3 Doshas). It also promotes eye- sight [243-245]

Recipes of other Eye Diseases:

शङ्ख प्रवाल वैदूर्य लौह ताम्र प्लवास्थिभिः| स्रोतोजश्वेतमरिचैं वर्तिः सर्वाक्षि रोगनुत्||२४६||
शाणार्धं मरिचाद्द्वौ च पिप्पल्यर्णवफेनयोः| शाणार्धं सैन्धवाच्छाणा नव सौवीरकाञ्जनात्||२४७||
पिष्टं सुसूक्ष्मं चित्रायां चूर्णाञ्जनमिदं शुभम्| कण्डूकाचकफार्तानां मलानां च विशोधनम्||२४८||

बस्तमूत्रे त्र्यहं स्थाप्यमेलाचूर्णं सुभावितम्| चूर्णाञ्जनं हि तैमिर्य क्रिमि पिल्ल मलापहम्||२४९||

सौवीरमञ्जनं तुत्थं ताप्यो धातुर्मनःशिला| चक्षुष्या मधुकं लोहा मणयः पौष्पमञ्जनम्||२५०||

सैन्धवं शौकरी दंष्ट्रा कतकं चाञ्जनं शुभम्| तिमिरादिषु चूर्णं वा वर्तिर्वेयमनुत्तमा||२५१||

Shankhadi Varti:

Varti (bougie) prepared of Sankha bhasma, Pravala Bhasma, Vaidurya Pisti, Lauha Bhasma, Tamra Bhasma, Bhasma of the bone of Plava, Srotonjana and Sveta- Maricha – Black pepper fruit – piper nigrum cures all types of eye diseases.

Churnanjana:

Half Sana of Maricha – Black pepper fruit – piper nigrum, 2 Sanas of Pipali – Piper longum, 2 Sanas of Samudra-Phena, ½ Sana of Saindhava and 9 Sanas of Sauviranjana shoud be triturated and made to a fine powder during the constellation of Chitra.

This powder is used as colyrium which is useful in itching, Kaca (cataract) and eye disorders caused by Kapha. It cleanses the eyes of its purulent discharge.

Seeds of Ela – Elattaria cardamum is well impregnated with goat's urine and made to a powder. Application of this powder in the form of collyrium cures Timira (a type of cataract), Krimi (parasitic infestation), Patala (another type of cataract) and discharge of mucoid matter from the eyes.

Sauviranjana, Tuttha, Tapya-dhatu (maksika), Manah- Sila, Caksusya (variety of Kulattha), Madhuka– Licorice – Glycyrrhiza glabra, Loha Bhasma (iron), precious stones, puspanjana, Saindhava, Tusk of boar, and Kataka – Strychnos potatorum may be used in the form of either powder or Varti (bougie) as collyrium which are unsurpassable remedies for Timira Cataract) and such other eye-diseases. [246- 251]

Sukhavati- Varti:

कतकस्य फलं शङ्खः सैन्धवं त्र्यूषणं सिता| फेनो रसाञ्जनं क्षौद्रं विडङ्गानि मनःशिला||२५२||

कुक्कुटाण्डकपालानि वर्तिरेषा व्यपोहति| तिमिरं पटलं काचं मलं चाशु सुखावती||२५३||

इति सुखावती वर्तिः |

Varti (Bougie) prepared of the

fruit of Kataka – Strychnos potatorum

Sankha

Saindhava – rock salt

Sunthi – Ginger

Pippali – Long pepper fruit,

Maricha – Black pepper fruit,

Sugar

Samudraphena

Rasanjana (Aqueous extract of Berberis aristata),

honey

Vidanga – Embelia ribes

Manah- Sila and

shell of hen's egg

Instantaneously cures

Timira (cataract)

Patala

Kaca (another type of cataract) and

putrid discharge from the eyes

This is called Sukhavati- Varti

Thus, ends the description of Sukhavati- Varti [252-253]

Drushtiprada Varti:

त्रिफला कुक्कुटाण्ड त्वक्कासीसमयसो रजः| नीलोत्पलं विडङ्गानि फेनं च सरितां पतेः||२५४||
आजेन पयसा पिष्ट्वा भावयेताम्रभाजने| सप्तरात्रं स्थितं भूयः पिष्ट्वा क्षीरेण वर्तयेत्||२५५||
एषा दृष्टिप्रदा वर्तिरन्धस्याभिन्नचक्षुषः||२५६||
इति दृष्टिप्रदा वर्तिः |

Ingredients and Method:

Haritaki – Terminalia chebula,

Vibhitaka – Terminalia bellerica,

Amalaki – Phyllanthus emblica,

shell of hen's egg,

Kasisa,

Lauha bhasma – Iron calx

Nilotpala,

Vidanga – Embelia ribes, and

Samudra-phena is made to a paste by triturating them with goat's milk], and smeared over a cover pot. This is kept for 7 nights.

This paste is scraped out the copper plate, triturated with goat's milk again, and rolled into the form of Varti (bougie). This is called Dristi Prada-Varti.

Benefit: Application of this bougie bestows eye-sight even to a blind person, provided the pupils of his eyes have not undergone any physical change or been damaged.

Thus, ends the description of Drshti- Prasada- Varti [254 -1/4 256]

Collyrium for Timira:

वदने कृष्ण सर्पस्य निहितं मास मञ्जनम्||२५६||
ततस्तस्मात् समृद्धृत्य सुशुष्कं चूर्णयेद्बुधः| सुमनःकोरकैः शुष्कैरर्धांशैः सैन्धवेन च||२५७||
एतन्नेत्राञ्जनं कार्यं तिमिरघ्नमनुत्तमम्|

A wise physician should keep Anjana inside the buccal cavity of a dead black snake cobra for one month. Thereafter, this is removed, added with half the quantity of each of the dry buds of Sumanas (Jasminum officinale – jati- Puspa and Saindhava, and made to a fine powder. This is an unsurpassable recipe for the cure of Timira (cataract). [256 ½ – ½ 258]

Pippalyadi Rasakriya:

पिप्पल्यः किंशुकरसो वसा सर्पस्य सैन्धवम्||२५८||
जीर्णं घृतं च सर्वाक्षि रोगघ्नी स्याद्रसक्रिया|

Rasa-Kriya (thin paste) prepared of pippali – Piper longum, Juice of Kimsuka – Butea monosperma, fat of snake, Saindhva and old ghee cures all types of eye-diseases. [258 ½ – ½ 259]

Krishna sarpa Vasadi –Rasakriya:

कृष्णसर्प वसा क्षौद्रं रसो धात्र्या रसक्रियाः||२५९||
शस्ता सर्वाक्षि रोगेषु काचार्बुदमलेषु च|

RasaKriya (thin paste) prepared of the fat of black snake cobra, honey and the juice of Amalaki – Phyllanthus emblica is useful in curing all eye-diseases like Kaca (Cataract), Arbuda (Tumor in the eyes) and discharge of excreta from the eyes. [259 ½- ½ 260]

Other recipes for eye diseases:

धात्री रसाञ्जन क्षौद्रि सर्पिर्भिस्तु रसक्रिया||२६०||
पित्तरक्ताक्षि रोगघ्नी तैमिर्यपटलापहा| धात्री सैन्धव पिप्पल्यः स्युरल्प मरिचाः समाः||२६१||
क्षौद्रियुक्ता निहन्त्यान्ध्यं पटलं च रसक्रिया|२६२|

इति नेत्र रोग चिकित्सा |

The Rasa-Kriya (thin paste) prepared of Dhatri, Rasanjana (Aqueous extract of Berberis aristata), honey and ghee cures eye-diseases caused by the vitiation of Pitta and Raktha (blood), Timira (cataract) and Patala (another type of Cataract).

Thus, ends the description of the treatment of eye diseases. [260 ½ – ½ 262]

Kesha roga Chikitsa – Treatment of hair diseases:

Line of Treatment:

खालित्ये पलिते वल्यां हरिलोम्नि च शोधितम्||२६२||

नस्यैस्तैलैः शिरोवक्रप्रलेपैश्चाप्युपाचरेत्|

In Khalitya (alopecia), Palitya (Graying of the hair), Vali (appearance of wrinkles over the face) and Hari- Loman (Tawny hair), the patient should, in the beginning, be given elimination therapies, emetic, Purgation etc and thereafter, be given Nasya (inhalation therapy) with medicated oil, and application of paste of drugs over the head and face. [262 1/- ½ 263]

Medicated Oil and other medicines:

सिद्धं विदारीगन्धाद्यै जीवनीयैरथापि च||२६३||

नस्यं स्यादणुतैलं वा खालित्य पलितापहम्| क्षीरात् सहचराद्भृङ्गराजाच्च सौरसाद्रसात्||२६४||

प्रस्थैस्तु कुडवस्तैलाद्यष्ट्याह्वपलकल्कितः| सिद्धः शिलासमे भाण्डे मेषशृङ्गादिषु स्थितः||२६५||

नस्यं स्यादिभषजा सम्यग्योजितं पलितापहम्| भिषजा क्षीरपिष्टौ वा दुग्धिका करवीरकौ||२६६||

उत्पाट्य पलिते देयौ तावुभौ पलितापहौ| मार्कव स्वरसात् क्षीरादिद्वप्रस्थं मधुकात् पलम्||२६७||

तैः पचेत् कुडवं तैलात्तन्नस्यं पलितापहम्|

Recipe 1: Medicated oil is prepared by cooking with

Vidari- Gandha—Pueraria tuberosa

Shala- parni

Prishnaparni

Brhati – Solanum indicum

Kantakari – Garcinia Morella and

Goksura – Tribulus terrestris

Or with Jivaniya group of drugs, viz, Jivaka – Malaxiz acuminata, Rsabhaka – Manilkara hexandra, Meda – Polygonatum cirrhifolium, Maha-meda – Polygonatum verticillatum , Kakoli – Fritillaria roylei , Mudga – Green gram- Parni and Masa-Parni – Teramnus labialis.

Inhalation therapy with these medicated oils or with Anu Taila cures alopecia and graying of the hair.

Recipe 2:

1 Prastha – 768 ml of each of milk and

juice of Sahacara – Barleria prionitis,

Bhrnga-Raja – Eclipta alba and

Surasa –Cinnamonum zeylanica,

1 Kudava – 192 g of oil and

The paste of 1 Pala of

Yasti –Madhu – Glychrizza glabra is cooked, and kept inside a pot of stone or

the horn of sheep.

Appropriately administered by the physician for inhalation therapy, this medicated oil cures graying of hair.

Recipe 3: Dugdhika – Euphorbia hirta and Karavira – Nerium indicum are made to a paste by triturating them with milk. After pulling out gray hairs, the physician should apply this paste over the head of the patient for curing graying of hair.

Recipe 4: 1 Kudava – 192 g of oil is cooked by adding 1 Prastha – 768 ml of the Juice of markava (Bhrnga- Raja –

Eclipta alba) and milk and 1 Pala of Yasti-Madhu – Glychriza glabra.

Administration of this medicated oil for inhalation therapy cures graying of hair. [263 ½- 268½)

Mahaneela taila:

आदित्यवल्ल्या मूलानि कृष्णशैरेयकस्य च||२६८||

सुरसस्य च पत्राणि पत्रं कृष्णशणस्य च| मार्कवः काकमाची च मधुकं देवदारु च||२६९||

पृथग्दशपलांशानि पिप्पल्यस्त्रिफलाऽञ्जनम्| प्रपौण्डरीकं मञ्जिष्ठा लोध्रं कृष्णागुरूत्पलम्||२७०||

आम्रास्थि कर्दमः कृष्णो मृणालं रक्तचन्दनम्| नीली भल्लातकास्थीनि कासीसं मदयन्तिका||२७१||

सोमराज्यसनः शस्त्रं कृष्णौ पिण्डीत चित्रकौ| पुष्करार्जुन काश्मर्याण्याम्र जम्बूफलानि च||२७२||

पृथक् पञ्चपलांशानि तैः पिष्टैराढकं पचेत्| बैभीतकस्य तैलस्य धात्री रस चतुर्गुणम्||२७३||

कुर्यादादित्यपाकं वा यावच्छुष्को भवेद्रसः| लोहपात्रे ततः पूतं संशुद्धमुपयोजयेत्||२७४||

पाने नस्यक्रियायां च शिरोभ्यङ्गे तथैव च| एतच्चक्षुष्यमायुष्यं शिरसः सर्वरोगनुत्||२७५||

महानीलमिति ख्यातं पलितध्नमनुत्तमम्|

इति महानीलतैलम्|

Ingredients:

1 Adhaka of oil extracted from the seeds of Vibhitaka – Terminalia bellerica

4 Adhakas of juice of Amalaki – Phyllanthus emblica is added with the

Paste of 10 palas of each of the

Root of Adityavalli and

Black variety of Saireyaka – Barleria prionitis,

leaves of Surasa – Cinnamonum zeylanica and

Black variety of Sana – Brassica alba,

Markava (Bhrnga-Raja – Eclipta alba),

Kakamaci – Solanum nigrum,

Yastimadhu –Glycrrhiza glabra and

Devadaru – Cedrus deodara

5 Palas of each of

Pippali – Piper longum

Haritaki – Terminalia chebula

Vibhitaka – Terminalia bellerica

Amalaki – Phyllanthus emblica

Anjana

Prapaundarika

Manjistha – Rubia cordifolia

Lodhra – Symplocos racemosa

black variety of Aguru – Aquallaria agallocha

Utpala – Nymphaea alba

Amrasthi (seeds of Mango –Mangifera indica),

Krishna – Kardama (black mud),

Mrinala – Lotus stalk

Rakta Chandana – red sandalwood

Nili – Indigofera tinctoria

Seeds of Bhallataka – Semecarpus anacardium Linn.

Kasisa

Madayantika – Lawsonia alba,

Somaraji – Psorelea corylifolia,

Asana – Terminalia crenulata,

Sastra Bhasma of Tiksna (type of iron),
black variety of Pinditaka (Madana –Randia dumetorum) and
Chitraka – Leadword – Plumbago zeylanica
Puskara – Inula racemosa
Arjuna – Terminalia arjuna
Kasmarya – Gmelina arborea and
fruits of Amra – mango – Mangifera indica as well as
Jambu – Syzmium cumini, and
Cooked in an iron pot by solar heat till the water is evaporated
This medicated oil is given to a patient whose body is cleansed by purgation therapy, etc], in the form of inhalation therapy or massage over the head.
Promotes: eye-sight and longevity
Cures: All the diseases of the head
This is called MahaNila Taila which is the best remedy for those suffering from gray hairs.
Thus, ends the description of Mahaneela taila. [268 ½ – ½ 276]

Prapaundarikadya Taila
प्रपौण्डरीक मधुक पिप्पली चन्दनोत्पलै:||२७६||
कार्षिकैस्तैलकुडवो द्विगुणामलकीरस:| सिद्ध: स प्रतिमर्श: स्यात् सर्व मूर्धगदापह:||२७७||
पलितघ्नो विशेषेण कृष्णात्रेयेण भाषित:|
Ingredients:
1 Kudava of oil and
2 Kudavas of the juice of Amalaki – Phyllanthus emblica is cooked by adding
Paste of 1 Karsa of each
Prapaundarika,
Yasti- Madhu – Glycrrhiza glabra
Pippali – Long pepper fruit – Piper longum,
Chandana – Sandalwood – Santalum album and
Utpala – Nymphaea alba
Administration: Pratimarsa Nasya (a type of inhalation therapy)
Cures: All the diseases of the head
According to Krsnatreya, this therapy is especially useful for curing graying of hair. [276 ½- 278½]

Ointment for Tawny hair:
क्षीरं प्रियाल यष्ट्याह्वे जीवकाद्यो गणस्तिला:||२७८||
कृष्णा वक्त्रे प्रलेप: स्याद्धरिलोम निवारण:|
Application of the paste prepared of
Milk
Priyala (Buchanania lanzan),
Yasti- Madhu – Glycrrchiza glabra
Jivaka – Malaxis acuminata,
Rishabhaka – Manilkara hexandra,
Meda – Polygonatum cirrhifolium,
Maha- Meda – Polygonatum cirrhifolium,
Kakoli – Fritillaria roylei, Ksira-Kakoli,
Mudga-Parni – Phaseolus trilobus,
Masa-Parni – Teramnus labialis,

Jivanti – Leptadenia reticulata,
Madhuka– Licorice – Glycyrrhiza glabra,
Honey,
Tila – Sesame Sesamum indicum) and
Pippali – Piper longum over the face cures Tawny hair. [278 ½- ½ 279]

Recipe for restoration of hair:

तिलाः सामलकाश्चैव किञ्जल्को मधुकं मधु||२७९||
बृंहयेद्रञ्जयेचैतत् केशान्मूर्ध प्रलेपनात्

Application of the paste of Tila – Sesame Sesamum indicum), Amalaki – Phyllanthus emblica, Kinjalka, Madhuka– Licorice – Glycyrrhiza glabra and honey over the head restores the color of hair, and promotes hair growth. [279 ½- ½ 280]

Recipes for dyeing and softening hair:

पचेत्सैन्धव शुक्ताम्लैरयश्चूर्ण सतण्डुलम्||२८०||
तेनालिप्तं शिरः शुद्धमस्निग्धमुषितं निशि| तत् प्रातस्त्रिफलाधौतं स्यात् कृष्ण मृदु मूर्धजम्||२८१||
अयश्चूर्णोऽम्लपिष्टश्च रागः सत्रिफलो वरः|

Lauha powder (bhasma) is cooked with Saindhava, Suktama (sour vinegar) and rice [all taken in equal quantities]. After washing the head well to make it free from oily matter, this paste is applied over the scalp, and kept overnight. In the morning, the head is washed with the decoction of Haritaki – Terminalia chebula, Vibhitaka – Terminalia bellerica and Amalaki – Phyllanthus emblica with this therapy, the hair becomes black and soft.
Lauha powder (bhasma) triturated with sour articles and Haritaki – Terminalia cheula, Vibhitaka – Terminalia bellerica and Amalaki – Phyllanthus emblica and Amalaki is an excellent hair-dye. [280 ½- 1/3 282]

Treatment of remaining Shiroroga – head diseases:

कुर्याच्छेषेषु रोगेषु क्रियां स्वां स्वाच्चिकित्सितात्| शेषेष्वादौ च निर्दिष्टा सिद्धौ चान्या प्रवक्ष्यते||२८२||
इति खालित्यादि चिकित्सा|

For the remaining ailments which appear as complications of the diseases described above, the treatment suitable for these ailments is given for the diseases of the three vital spots not described here. The lines of treatment have been described earlier in this chapter, and some others are going to be described in Siddhi section [which are to be followed keeping in view the Doshas involved in the manifestation of these diseases]. Thus, ends the treatment of alopecia etc. [282 2/3]

Svarabheda Chikitsa – Treatment of hoarseness of voice:

Treatment of Vatika Svara-Bheda

सर्पींष्युपरिभक्तानि स्वरभेदेऽनिलात्मके| तैलैश्चतुष्प्रयोगैश्च बला रास्नामृताह्वयैः||२८३||
बर्हि तित्तिरि दक्षाणां पञ्चमूलशृतान् रसान्| मायूरं क्षीर सर्पिर्वा पिबेत्र्यूषणमेव वा||२८४||

In Vatika type of Svarabheda (hoarseness of voice):
Dosage: medicated ghee is given after the intake of food
Recipes:
Medicated oil prepared by cooking with
Bala – Country mallow root – Sida cordifolia, etc),
Rasna (Vanda roxburghi / Pluchea lanceolata) etc), and
Guduci – Tinospora cordifolia etc., is administered in 4 ways viz,
Pana or drinking,
Abhyanga – massage,
Gargle and

Basti – enema

Meat-soup of peacock, partridge and cock prepared by cooking with Bilva- Aegle marmelos, Syonaka – Orchis mascula, Gambhari – Gmelina arborea, Patala – Ficus microcarpa and Ganikarika

Or medicated milk and

Medicated ghee prepared by boiling with the meat of peacock or Tryusana (Sunthi – Ginger, Pippali – Long pepper fruit and Maricha – Black pepper) are beneficial in this condition. [283- 284]

Treatment of Paittika SvaraBheda:

पैत्तिके तु विरेकः स्यात् पयश्च मधुरैः शृतम्| सर्पि गुडा घृतं तिक्तं जीवनीयं वृषस्य वा||२८५||

For the Paittika type of Svara-Bheda (hoarseness of voice), purgation therapy is useful. In addition, following recipes are useful in this condition:

Milk boiled with drugs having sweet taste (vide Vimana 8 : 139)

Sarpirguda vide Chikitsa (11:50-69)

Tiktaka ghrita vide Chikitsa (7:140- 150)

Jivaniya Ghrta vide Chikitsa (29: 61-70) and

Vrusha Ghrita vide Chikitsa (5:126-127) [285]

Treatment of Kaphaja Svarabheda:

कफजे स्वरभेदे तु तीक्ष्णं मूर्धविरेचनम्| विरेको वमनं धूमो यवान्न कटु सेवनम्||२८६||

चव्य भार्ग्यभया व्योष क्षार माक्षिक चित्रकान्| लिह्याद्वा पिप्पलीपथ्ये तीक्ष्णं मद्यं पिबेच्च सः||२८७||

In Kaphaja type of Svarabheda (hoarseness of voice), the patient is given strong errhine, purgation, emetic and smoking therapies.

He should eat a barley diet added with pungent ingredients.

He should take the linctus prepared of Chavya – Piper retrofractum, Bharngi – Clerodendrum serratum, Abhaya, Sunthi – Ginger, Pippali – Long pepper, Maricha – Black pepper fruit – piper nigrum, Yava Ksara, and Chitraka – Plumbago zeylanica, or the linctus prepared of Pippali – Long pepper fruit – Piper longum and Pathya (Haritaki – Terminalia chebula)

He should drink strong wine. [286- 287]

Treatment of Raktaja Svara Bheda:

रक्तजे स्वरभेदे तु सघृता जाङ्गला रसाः| द्राक्षा विदारीक्षु रसा· सगृत क्षौद्र शर्कराः||२८८||

यच्चोक्तं क्षय कासघ्नं तच्च सर्व चिकित्सितम्| पित्तज स्वरभेदघ्नं सिरावेधश्च रक्तजे||२८९||

If Svara Bheda (hoarseness of voice) is caused by the vitiated blood (Raktaja), then the patient is given

The soup of the meat of animals living in arid zone sizzled with ghee.

The juice of Draksha – Raisin – Vitis vinifera, Vidari (Ipomoea paniculata / Pueraria tuberosa) and sugar- cane added with ghee and sugar are beautiful for such patients.

All the therapeutic measures prescribed for the treatment of Ksayaja type of Kasa are useful in this condition similarly , the therapeutic measures prescribed in this chapter of treatment of Paittika type of Svara Bheda, and venesection therapy are useful for the treatment of Raktaja type of svara-Bheda (hoarseness of voice). [288-289]

Treatment of Sannipatika Svara-Bheda:

सन्निपाते हिताः सर्वाः क्रिया न तु सिराव्यधः| इत्युक्तं स्वरभेदस्य समासेन चिकित्सितम्||२९०||

इति स्वरभेद चिकित्सा|

Svara Bheda (hoarseness of voice) caused by Sannipata (simultaneous vitiation of all the 3 Doshas) is treated with all the therapeutic measures prescribed above for the Vatika, Paittika and Kaphaja type of Svara Bheda, except vensection therapy (siravyadha).

Thus, in brief, the treatment of Svara-Bheda is described.

Thus, ends the description of the treatment of Svara-Bheda (hoarseness of voice) [290]

भवन्ति चात्र-
वात पित्त कफा नृणां बस्ति हृन्मूर्ध संश्रयाः| तस्मातत्स्थान सामीप्याद्धर्तव्या वमनादिभिः||२९१||
In human beings, Vata, Pitta and Kapha are located in the basti region of the urinary bladder, i.e Pelvic region, Hrt (cardiac region) and Murdhan (head) respectively. Therefore, the morbid matter located in these places are eliminated from the nearby region appropriately by emetic therapy etc [291]
Microcosm and macrocosm:
As the Loka (macrocosm) is afflicted or maintained respectively by the morbidity and normalcy of the wind, sun and moon, so also the Adhyatma-loka (sentiment world or micro-cosm) is either afflicted or maintained respectively by the morbidity and normal state of Vayu, Pitta and Kapha. [292]

Dosha balance:
अध्यात्मलोको वातादयैर्लोको वातरवीन्दुभिः| पीड्यते धार्यते चैव विकृताविकृतैस्तथा||२९२||
The Doshas Viz, Vayu, Pitta and Kapha never destroy each other. They coexist in a harmonious state, even though they are of mutually contradictory attributes. This happens because of their Sahaja- Satmya (natural wholesome disposition of coexistence), on the analogy of the virulent poison not causing any harm to the snake which contains it (poison). [293]

To sum up:
विरुद्धैरपि न त्वेते गुणैर्घ्नन्ति परस्परम्| दोषाः सहज सात्म्यत्वादिवष घोरमहीनिव||२९३||
In this chapter on "the Treatment of diseases of the Three Vital Organs", the etiology, signs and symptoms, and treatment of the body of the individual diseases afflicting the three vital organs of the body are described in detail.

इत्यग्निवेशकृते तन्त्रे चरकप्रतिसंस्कृतेऽप्राप्ते दृढबलसम्पूरिते चिकित्सास्थाने त्रिमर्मीयचिकित्सितं नाम षड्विंशोऽध्यायः||२६||
Thus, ends the 26th chapter of Chikitsa sthana section dealing with the treatment of diseases of the three vital organs in Agnivesha's work as redacted by Charaka and supplemented by Drudhabala.

10

Chikitsasthana Chapter 27
Urustambha Chikitsitam

The 27th Chapter of Charaka Samhita deals with Urustambha Chikitsa – a rather rare medical condition correlated with thigh stiffness or spasticity of the thigh.

अथात ऊरुस्तम्भ चिकित्सितं व्याख्यास्यामः||१||
इति ह स्माह भगवानात्रेयः||२||

Now, we shall expound the chapter on the "treatment of Urustambha (Spasticity of the thigh)" Thus, said Lord Atreya [1-2]

Prologue:

श्रिया परमया ब्राह्मया परया च तपःश्रिया| अहीनं चन्द्र सूर्याभ्यां सुमेरुमिव पर्वतम्||३||
धी धृति स्मृति विज्ञान ज्ञान कीर्ति क्षमालयम्| अग्निवेशो गुरुं काले संशयं परिपृष्टवान्||४||

Once, Agnivesha asked Lord Punarvasu, who was endowed with both Brahminical knowledge as well as elegance, who was like the Mt. Sumeru flanked by the sun and the moon, and who was also the abode of wisdom, memory, mundane knowledge, spiritual knowledge, frame and forgiveness, the following questions. [3-4]

Agnivesa's question: What is the disease contraindicated for Panchakarma?

भगवन् पञ्च कर्माणि समस्तानि पृथक् तथा| निर्दि ष्टान्यामयनां हि सर्तेषामेत भेषजम्||५||
दोषजोऽस्त्यामयः कश्चिद्यस्य तानि भिषग्वर! | न स्युः शक्तानि शमने साध्यस्य क्रियया सतः||६||

Oh! Lord, all the 5 purification therapies (Pancha Karma) are described in many instances of disease treatment. Is there any curable disease caused by doshas for the alleviation of which these 5 elimination therapies (Pancha-Karma) are contra-indicated? [5-6]

Dialogue:

अस्त्यूरुस्तम्भ इत्युक्ते गुरुणा तस्य कारणम्| सलिङ्गभेषजं भूयः पृष्टस्तेनाब्रवीद्गुरुः||७||

To the above query of Agnivesha, Master Punarvasu replied, "there is such a disease for which PanchaKarma is contra-indicated and it is called Urustambha (spasticity of the thighs)".
Agnivesha again enquired about the aetiology, symptomatology and treatment of this aliment. The preceptor again replied as follows. [7]

Urustambha nidana and Samprapti:

स्निग्धोष्ण लघु शीतानि जीर्णाजीर्ण समश्नतः| द्रव शुष्क दधि क्षीर ग्राम्यानूपौदकामिषैः||८||
पिष्ट व्यापन्न मद्यानि दिवास्वप्न प्रजागरैः| लङ्घनाध्यशनायास भय वेग विधारणैः||९||
स्नेहाच्चामं चितं कोष्ठे वातादीन्मेदसा सह| रुद्ध्वाऽऽशु गौरवादूरू यात्यधोगैः सिरादिभिः||१०||

पूरयन् सक्थिजङ्घोरु दोषो मेदोबलोत्कटः| अविधेय परिस्पन्दं जनयत्यल्प विक्रमम्||११||

Urustambha (spasticity of the thighs) is caused by the following factors:

Intake of Snigdha (unctuous), Ushna (hot), Laghu (light) and Shita (cold) ingredients when the ingested food is partially digested and partially undigested

Intake of Drava (liquid) and Sushka (dry) ingredients

Intake of Dadhi (yoghurt), Kshira (milk) and meat of animals who are Gramya (domesticated animals), Anupa (animals inhabiting marshy land) and Audaka (aquatic animals)

Intake of Pistanna (pastries) and Madya (alcohol)

Divaswapna – Excessive sleep during the day time and

Prajagraih – keeping awake at night for a long time

Langhana (Fasting) or Adhyashana (taking food while the previous meal is not digested)

Aayasa (Overexertion) and Bhaya – exposure to fearful situations; and

Vega vidharana – Suppression of the manifested natural urges.

Pathology of Urustambha:

Because of unctuousness, the Ama (a product of altered digestion and metabolism) located in the gastro-intestinal tract, along with fat, causes obstruction to the movement of Vata, etc. Because of heaviness, it immediately reaches the thighs through the downward moving vessels. Etc and being provoked by the powerful fat, these Doshas (morbid material) fill up the lower limbs including the thighs and calf regions to cause involuntary spasms and immobility in these parts. [8-11]

Simile of Pond:

महासरसि गम्भीरे पूर्णेsम्बु स्तिमितं यथा| तिष्ठति स्थिरमक्षोभ्यं तद्वदूरुगतः कफः||१२||

As in a pond which is large, deep and full, the water remains motionless, stable and un-agitated, similarly the Kapha shifted to the thighs remains motionless, stable and un-agitated [in Urustambha] [12]

Further complications:

गौर वायास सङ्कोच दाह रुक्सुप्ति कम्पनैः | भेद स्फुरण तोदैश्च युक्तो देहं निहन्त्यसून्||१३||

This ailment (urustambha or spasticity of the thighs) thereafter, gets associated with

Gaura – heaviness

Aayasa – fatigue

Sankocha – contracture

Daha – burning sensation

Ruk – pain

Supti – numbness

Kampana – tremor and

Bheda – breaking,

Sphurana – itching and

Bheda – pricking types of pain leading to the death of the patient [13]

Urustambha Nirukti:

ऊरू श्लेष्मा समेदस्को वात पित्तेऽभिभूय तु| स्तम्भयेत्स्थैर्य शैत्याभ्यामूरुस्तम्भस्ततस्तु सः||१४||

Definition of Urustambha:

Kapha associated with Medas affects Vata and Pitta to cause spasticity (Stambha) of the thighs (uru) characterized by their stiffness and coldness because of which the ailment is called Uru-Stambha (Spasticity of the thighs) [14]

Premonitory Signs and Symptoms:

ध्यान निद्राति स्तैमित्यारोचक ज्वराः| लोम हर्षश्च छर्दिश्च जङ्घोर्वोः सदनं तथा||१५||

The premonitory signs and symptoms of Urustambha (spasticity of the thighs):

Dhyana – Fixed Gaze

Ati nidra – excessive sleep

Staimitya – excessive indolence

Aruchi – anorexia

Jwara – fever

Loma harsha – horripilation

Chardi – vomiting and

Jangha uru sadana – Asthenia of the calf region as well as thighs [15]

Mistaken identity:

वात शङ्किभिरज्ञानातस्य स्यात् स्नेहनात् पुनः| पादयोः सदनं सुप्तिः कृच्छ्रादुद्धरणं तथा||१६||

Mistaking it as an ailment caused by aggravated Vata Dosha, because of ignorance, if oleation therapy is administered, then these results in asthenia as well as numbness of the legs, and the lifting of the legs becomes difficult. [16]

Urustambha Lakshana:

जङ्घोरु ग्लानिरत्यर्थं शश्वच्चादाह वेदना| पदं च व्यथते न्यस्तं शीत स्पर्शं न वेत्ति च||१७||

संस्थाने पीडने गत्यां चालने चाप्यनीश्वरः| अन्यनेयौ हि सम्भग्नावूरू पादौ च मन्यते||१८||

Signs and symptoms of Urustambha:

Jangha uru glani – Excessive fatigue of the calf muscles and thighs

Daha vedana – Constant pain with slight burning sensation

Feeling of pain while putting the feet on the ground

Sheetam sparsham na vetti cha – Insensitivity to cold touch

Lack of control over the functions like standing, pressing the feet on the ground, walking and movement of the lower limbs and

Feeling as if limbs are propelled by someone else (not by himself) and as if these are broken [17-18]

Prognosis:

यदा दाहार्ति तोदार्तो वेपनः पुरुषो भवेत्| ऊरुस्तम्भस्तदा हन्यात् साधयेदन्यथा नवम्||१९||

If the patient is further afflicted with burning sensation, pain and tremors, then this disease Urustambha (spasticity of the thighs) leads to his death i.e he is incurable. If such signs and symptoms are absent, and if the ailment is of recent origin, then such a patient is treated, i.e. he is curable. [19]

Reasons for prohibiting Panchakarma in Urustambha:

तस्य न स्नेहनं कार्यं न बस्तिर्न विरेचनम्| न चैव वमनं यस्मात् न्निबोधत कारणम्||२०||

वृद्धये श्लेष्मणो नित्यं स्नेहनं बस्ति कर्म च| तत्स्थस्योद्धरणे चैव न समर्थं विरेचनम्||२१||

कफं कफस्थानगतं पित्तं च वमनात् सुखम्| हर्तुमामाशयस्थौ च संसनातावुभावपि||२२||

पक्वाशयस्थाः सर्वेऽपि बस्तिभिर्मूलनिर्जयात्| शक्या न त्वाममेदोभ्यां स्तब्धा जङ्घोरुसंस्थिताः||२३||

वातस्थाने हि तच्छैत्याद्द्वयोः स्तम्भाच्च तद्गताः| न शक्याः सुखमुद्धर्तुं जलं निम्नादिव स्थलात्||२४||

Why Panchakarma is not indicated in Urustambha:

The reason for which Snehakarma, Vamana, Virechana and Basti are contra-indicated in the treatment of Urustambha is being explained.

Snehana and Basti therapies aggravate Kapha. Purgation therapy is also too ineffective to remove Kapha localized in the thighs).

Kapha is located in its own place (i.e Amashaya or stomach), and pitta can be easily removed by emesis. Both of these, viz, Kapha and Pitta, located in the Amashaya or stomach can be eliminated by purgation. When located in Pakvashaya (Colon) all the 3 Doshas, viz, Vata Dosha, Pitta and Kapha can be rooted out by enema therapy. But when associated with Ama (product of improper digestion) and fat, and especially when these are firmly located in the thighs, it is impossible to eliminate them by the above mentioned therapies.

Since the Ama and Medas are lodged in the abode of Vayu which is cold by nature and since these are firmly localized there, it is not easy to eliminate them just as it is difficult to lift water located at a lower level. [20-24]

Line of treatment:

तस्य संशमनं नित्यं क्षपणं शोषणं तथा| युक्त्यपेक्षी भिषक् कुर्यादधिकत्वात्कफामयोः||२५||

Since Kapha and Ama (product of improper digestion) are predominant in the pathogenesis of Urustambha, the physician should constantly administer appropriate alleviation therapies for their

Kshapana (complete extraction) and

Shoshana (Absorption / drying of the liquid fraction) [25]

Food and Vegetables:

सदा रूक्षोपचाराय यव श्यामाक कोद्रवान्|

शाकैरलवणैर्दद्याज्जल तैलोपसाधितैः||२६||

सुनिषण्णक निम्बार्कवेत्रारग्वध पल्लवैः|

वायसी वास्तुकैरन्यैस्तिक्तैश्च कुलकादिभिः||२७||

The patient of Urustambha is constantly given un-unctuous regimes, So, Yava – Barley (Hordeum vulgare) (barley), Syamaka (Millet) and Kodrava along with Vegetables cooked with water and oil without adding salt, Leaves of Sunisannaka, Nimba – Neem (Azadirachta indica), Aragvadha (Cassia fistula), Vayasi (Kakamachi – Solanum xanthocarpum), Vastuka and bitter Vegetables like Kulaka (karavellaka – Momordica charantia) are useful for the patient. [26-27]

Drinks:

क्षारारिष्ट प्रयोगाश्च हरीतक्यास्तथैव च| मधूदकस्य पिप्पल्या ऊरुस्तम्भ विनाशनाः||२८||

Administration of Alkali preparations, Arista (medicated wines), Haritaki—Terminalia chebula, after added with honey and Pippali – Long pepper cures Urustambha. [28]

Samangadi Yoga:

समङ्गां शाल्मली बिल्वं मधुना सह ना पिबेत्|

The patient suffering from Urustambha should take

Samanga – Rubia cordifolia,

Shalmali – Salmalia malabarica (Gum- resin) and

Bilva – Aegle marmelos along with honey. [1/2 29]

Srivestakadi Yoga:

तथा श्रीवेष्टकोदीच्य देवदारुनतान्यपि||२९|| चन्दनं धातकीं कुष्ठं तालीसं नलदं तथा|३०|

The patient may also be given

Srivestaka

Udicya

Devadaru (Cedrus deodara),

Nata (Valeriana wallichii),

Chandana (Sandalwood – Santalum album),

Dhataki – Woodfordia fruticosa,

Kushta – Saussurea lappa,

Talisa – Taxus baccata and

Nalada – Nordastachys jatamansi along with honey [29 ½ – ½ 30]

Kalkas (recipes in the form of Paste):

मुस्तं हरीतकीं लोध्रं पद्मकं तिक्त रोहिणीम्||३०||

देवदारु हरिद्रे द्वे वचां कटुक रोहिणीम्| पिप्पलीं पिप्पलीमूलं सरलं देवदारु च||३१||

चव्यं चित्रकमूलानि देवदारु हरीतकीम्| भल्लातकं समूलां च पिप्पलीं पञ्च तान् पिबेत्||३२||

सक्षौद्रानर्ध श्लोकोक्तान् कल्कानूरुग्रहापहान्|३३|

The following 5 recipes cure Urustambha (spasticity of thighs):

Musta (Cyperus rotundus), Haritaki – Terminalia chebula, Lodhra (Symplocos racemosa), Padmaka and Tikta-Katukarohini – Picrorhiza kurroa

Devadaru – Cedrus deodara, Haridra (turmeric – Curcuma longa), Daru-Haridra – Berberis aristata, Vacha (Acorus calamus Linn.) And Katuka- Katukarohini –Picrorhiza kurroa

Pippali – Long pepper fruit – Piper longum, Pippali Mula, Sarala and Deva-Daru – Cedrus deodara

Chavya – Piper chaba , root of Chitraka – Plumbago zeylanica, Deva- Daru – Cedrus deodara and Haritaki – Terminalia chebula and

Bhallataka (Semecarpus anacardium Linn.), Pippali Mula and Pippali – Long pepper fruit – Piper longum.

All the above mentioned recipes in the form of paste are to be taken along with honey. [30 ½ – ½ 33]

Churna Yoga:

शाङ्गैष्टां मदनं दन्तीं वत्सकस्य फलं वचाम् ||३३||

मूर्वामारग्वधं पाठां करञ्जं कुलकं तथा| पिबेन्मधुयुतं तुल्यं चूर्णं वा वारिणाऽऽप्लुतम्||३४||

सक्षौद्रं दधिमण्डैर्वाऽप्यूरुस्तम्भ विनाशनम्| मूर्वामतिविषां कुष्ठं चित्रकं कटुरोहिणीम्||३५||

पूर्ववद्गुग्गुलुं मूत्रे रात्रिस्थितमथापि वा| स्वर्णक्षीरीमतिविषां मुस्तं तेजोवर्तीं वचाम्||३६||

सुराह्वं चित्रकं कुष्ठं पाठां कटुक रोहिणीम्| लेहयेन्मधुना चूर्णं सक्षौद्रं वा जला प्लुतम्||३७||

फलीं व्याघ्रनखं हेम पिबेद्वा मधुसंयुतम्| त्रिफलां पिप्पलीं मुस्तं चव्यं कटुक रोहिणीम्||३८||

लिह्याद्वा मधुना चूर्णमूरुस्तम्भार्दितो नरः|३९|

The patient suffering from Urustambha should take the following recipes:

Sarngestadi Yoga: All these ingredients taken in equal quantities is made to a powder:

Sarngesta (Gunja) – Abrus precatorius

Madana – Randia dumetorum

Danti – Baliospermum montanum

Fruits (seeds) of Vatsaka (Holarrhena antidysenterica Wall.),

Vacha (Acorus calamus Linn.),

Murva – Marsdenia tenacissima

Aragvadha (Cassia fistula),

Patha – Cissampelos parriera

Karnja – Pongamia pinnata and

Kulaka (Karavellaka – Momordica chirantia).

Adjuvant: honey added with water or with honey and whey

Murvadi Yoga:

In the above mentioned manner the powder of

Murva – Marsdenia tenacissima

Ativisa – Aconitum heterophyllum

Kushta – Saussurea lappa,

Chitraka – Leadword – Plumbago zeylanica and

Katu-Katukarohini – Picrorhiza kurroa may be taken.

Guggulu – Commiphora mukul is soaked overnight in cow's urine and taken.

Svarnaksiryadi Yoga: The powder of

Svarna-Ksiri

Ativisa – Aconitum heterophyllum

Musta - Cyperus rotundus

Tejovati

Vacha - Acorus calamus Linn.

Surahva

Chitraka – Leadwort – Plumbago zeylanica,

Kushta – Saussurea lappa

Patha – Cissampelos parriera and

Katuka- Katukarohini – Picrorhiza kurroa is made by adding honey.

Alternatively, the powder may be mixed with water and honey, and taken.

The Powder of Phali (Nyagrodha – Ficus bengalensis), Vyaghra-Nakha and Hema (Mesua ferrea) (Naga-Kesara) may be taken by the patient.

The powder of Triphala (Haritaki – Terminalia chebula, Vibhitaka – Terminalia bellerica and Amalaki – Phyllanthus emblica), Pippali – Long pepper fruit – Piper longum, Musta (Cyperus rotundus),Cavya and Katuka- Katukarohini – Picrorhiza kurroa may be made to a Linctus, and taken. [33 ½ – ½ 39]

Nourishing Therapy:

अपतर्पणजश्चेत् स्याद्दोषः सन्तर्पयेदिद्ध तम्||३९||

युक्त्या जाङ्गलजैर्मांसैः पुराणैश्चैव शालिभिः|

If the diseases Urustambha is caused by Apatarpana (depletion of tissues), then the patient is appropriately given Santarpana (nourishing) therapy consisting of the meat of animals inhabiting Jangala Desha (the land with shrubs and small trees) and old Shali rice. [39 ½ – ½ 40]

Oleation and Fomentation Therapies

रूक्षणाद्वातकोपश्चेन्निद्रानाशार्ति पूर्वकः||४०||

स्नेह स्वेद क्रमस्तत्र कार्यो वातामयापहः|

If because [of excessive use] of un-unctuous therapies, Vata Dosha gets aggravated thereby causing insomnia and pain, then the patient is given oleation and fomentation therapies for the alleviation of the ailments caused by Vata Dosha. [40 ½ –41½]

Piluparnyadi Taila

पीलुपर्णी पयस्या च रास्ना गोक्षुरको वचा||४१||

सरलागुरु पाठाश्च तैलमेभिर्विपाचयेत्| सक्षौद्रं प्रसृतं तस्मादञ्जलिं वाऽपि ना पिबेत्||४२||

Oil is cooked by adding

Piluparni (Morata – Chonemorpha fragrans)

Payasya – Impomoea paniculata,

Rasna (Vanda roxburghi / Pluchea lanceolata),

Goksuraka – Tribulus terrestris

Vacha (Acorus calamus Linn.),

Sarala,

Aguru – Aquilaria agallocha and

Patha – Cissampelos pariera

Adjuvant: 1 Prasta or 1 Anjali of this medicated oil is taken by adding honey (1/4th in quantity of the medicated oil). [41 ½ – 42]

Kusthadya Taila:

कुष्ठ श्रीवेष्टकोदीच्य सरलं दारु केशरम्| अजगन्धाऽश्वगन्धा च तैलं तैः सार्षपं पचेत्||४३||
सक्षौद्रं मात्रया तच्चाप्यूरुस्तम्भार्दितः पिबेत्|
(रौक्ष्यान्मुक्त ऊरुस्तम्भात्ततश्च स विमुच्यते)||४४||
Mustard oil is cooked by adding

Kushta – Saussurea lappa

Srivestaka

Udicya

Sarala,

Devadaru - Cedrus deodara

Kesara,

Ajagandha (Ajamoda – Ajowan (fruit) – Trachyspermum roxburghianum and

Ashwagandha – Winter Cherry / Indian ginseng (root) – Withania somnifera

The patient suffering from Urustambha (spasticity should take this medicated oil in appropriate quantities by adding honey. This recipe makes the patient free from un-unctuousness leading to the cure of Urustambha [43-44]

Saindhavadya Taila:

द्वे पले सैन्धवात् पञ्च शुण्ठ्या ग्रन्थिक चित्रकात्| द्वे द्वे भल्लातकास्थीनि विंशतिर्द्वे तथाऽऽढके||४५||
आरनालात् पचेत् प्रस्थं तैलस्यैतैरपत्यदम्| गृध्रस्यूरुग्रहार्शोर्ति सर्ववात विकारनुत्||४६||
1 Prastha of oil is cooked by adding 2 Palas of Saindhava, 5 palas of Sunthi – Zingiber officinale, 2 Palas of Granthika, 2 Palas of Chitraka – Leadwort – Plumbago zeylanica, 20 fruits of Bhallataka (Semecarpus anacardium Linn.) and 2 Adhakas of Aranala (sour vinegar). Intake of this medicated oil helps in the procreation of offspring.

It cures

Grdhrasi – sciatica,

Urugraha (spasticity of the thighs),

Arshas – Piles,

Arti – pain and

Sarva vata vikara – all types of diseases causes by the aggravated Vayu. [45-46]

Astakatvara Taila

पलाभ्यां पिप्पलीमूल नागरादष्टकट्वरः| तैलप्रस्थः समो दध्ना गृध्रस्यूरुग्रहापहः||४७||
इत्यष्टकट्वरतैलम्|
1 Prastha of oil is cooked by adding 2 Palas of Pipali-Mula and Nagara – Zingiber officinale taken together, 8 Prasthas of Katvara (takra or butter- milk) and 1 Prastha of yogurt. This medicated oil cures sciatica and Urustambha (spasticity of thighs).

Thus, ends the description of Astakatvara Taila. [47]

External Therapy:

इत्याभ्यन्तरमुद्दिष्टमूरुस्तम्भस्य भेषजम्| श्लेष्मणः क्षपणं त्वन्यद्बाह्यं शृणु चिकित्सितम्||४८||
वल्मीक मृत्तिका मूलं करञ्जस्य फलं त्वचम्| इष्टकानां ततश्चूर्णैः कुर्यादुत्सादनं भृशम्||४९||
मूलैर्वाऽप्यश्वगन्धाया मूलैरर्कस्य वा भिषक्| पिचुमर्दस्य वा मूलैरथवा देवदारुणः||५०||
क्षौद्र सर्षप वल्मीक मृत्तिका संयुतै भिषक्| गाढमुत्सादनं कुर्यादूरुस्तम्भे प्रलेपनम्||५१||
दन्ती द्रवन्ती सुरसा सर्षपैश्चापि बुद्धिमान्| तर्कारी शिग्रु सुरसाविश्व वत्सक निम्बजैः||५२||
पत्रमूलफलैस्तोयं शृतमुष्णं च सेचनम्| पिष्टं तु सर्षपं मूत्रेऽध्युषितं स्यात् प्रलेपनम्||५३||
वत्सकः सुरसं कुष्ठं गन्धास्तुम्बुरु शिग्रुकौ| हिंस्रार्क मूल वल्मीक मृत्तिकाः सकुठेरकाः||५४||
दधि सैन्धव संयुक्तं कार्यमेतैः प्रलेपनम्| (ऊरुस्तम्भ विनाशाय भिषजा जानता क्रमम्)||५५||
श्योनाकं खदिरं बिल्वं बृहत्यौ सरलासनौ| शोभाञ्जनक तर्कारी श्वदंष्ट्रा सुरसार्जकान्||५६||

अग्निमन्थ करञ्जौ च जलेनोत्क्वाथ्य सेचयेत्| प्रलेपो मूत्रपिष्टैर्वाऽप्यूरुस्तम्भ निवारणः||५७||
कफ क्षयार्थं शक्येषु व्यायामेष्वनुयोजयेत्| स्थलान्याक्रामयेत् कल्यं शर्कराः सिकतास्तथा||५८||
प्रतारयेत् प्रतिस्रोतो नदीं शीतजलां शिवाम्| सरश्च विमलं शीतं स्थिरतोयं पुनः पुनः||५९||
तथा विशुष्केऽस्य कफे शान्तिमूरुग्रहो व्रजेत्|६०|

In the above mentioned verses (nos. 25-47), the recipes to be used internally for the cure of Urustambha are described in brief .Hereafter, recipes to be administered externally for the diminution of kapha will be described which you (addressed to Agnivesha by the preceptor) may hear.

Valmika- Mrttikadyutsasana:

The mud of Ant-hill, the root, fruits and barks of Karanja (Pongamia pinnata), and bricks is made into a powder. This is used for Utsadana (dry rubbing) frequently.

Alternatively, the physician should administer this. Utsadana therapy with the help of the root of Ashwagandha – Winter Cherry / Indian ginseng (root) – Withania somnifera, Arka – Calotropis gigantea, Picumarda (Nimba – Neem (Azadirachta indica)) or Devadaru (Cedrus deodara), any one of these drugs may be mixed with honey, Sarsapa – Brassica campestris and mud of ant-hill before being used as thick Utsasana (dry rubbing or massage) or Pralepana (external application).

A wise physician may also apply the paste of Danti – Baliospermum montanum, Dravanti (a variety of Danti), Surasa – Cinnamonum zeylanica and Sarsapa – Brassica campestris for the cure of Urustambha (Spasticity of the thighs).

The warm decoction prepared by boiling water with the leaves, roots and fruits of Tarkari (Jayanti – Sesbania egyptica), Sigru – Moringa oliefera, Surasa – Cinnamonum zeylanica, Visva, Vatsaka (Holarrhena antidysenterica Wall.) And Nimba – Neem (Azadirachta indica) may be sprinkled over the affected part.

Mustard is made to a paste by triturating with cow's urine kept overnight and used for external application.

Vatsakadi Pralepa:

Vatsaka (Holarrhena antidysenterica Wall.), Surasa – Cinnamonum zeylanica, Kushta – Saussurea lappa, aromatic drugs (like Aguru – Aquallaria agallocha), Tumburu – Zanthoxylum alatum, Sigru – Moringa oleifera, Himsra – Nordastachys jatamamsi, Root of Arka – Calotropis gigantea, mud of ant- hill and Kutheraka (Parnasa – Ocimum basilicum) is made to a paste by adding Yoghurt and Rock-salt. A physician conversant with the line of treatment should administer this paste for external application for the cure of Urustambha (Spasticity of the thighs).

Shyonakadi Pariseka Pralepa:

Shyonaka – Orchis mascula, Khadira (Acacia catechu), Bilva – Aegle marmelos, Brihati – Solanum indicum, Kantakari – Solanum xanthocarpum, Sarala, Asana – Pterocarpus marsupium, Sobhanjana, Tarkari – Sesbania aegyptica, Svadamstra – Tribulus terrestris, Surasa – Cinnamonum zeylanica, Arjaka, Agnimantha – Premna integrifolia and Karanja (Pongamia pinnata) is boiled in water. This decoction is used for sprinkling over the affected part.

The above mentioned drugs may be made to a paste by triturating them with cow's urine, and applied eternally for the cure of Urustambha (spasticity of the thighs).

To alleviate Kapha, the able bodied patients are engaged in physical exercise, and they are made to walk over the ground covered with gravel and sand in the morning.

The Patient is made to swim frequently against the current of a river with cold water but harmless (free from dangerous aquatic animals). He may also be advised to swim frequently in a pond having clean cold and stable water. [48- ½ 60]

Urustambha – Line of treatment:

श्लेष्मणः क्षपणं यत् स्यान्न च मारुतमावहेत् ||६०||
तत् सर्वं सर्वदा कार्यमूरुस्तम्भस्य भेषजम्| शरीरं बलमग्निं च कार्यैषा रक्षता क्रिया||६१||

All the therapeutic measures which alleviate Kapha but do not aggravate Vata should always be employed for the treatment of Urustambha. These therapeutic measures should however, be administered to the patient while protecting his physical strength and Agni (power of digestion and metabolism) [60 ½ – 61]

Summary:

तत्र श्लोकः-

हेतुः प्रागूप लिङ्गानि कर्मायोग्यत्वकारणम्|

द्विविधं भेषजं चोक्तमूरुस्तम्भ चिकित्सिते||६२||

In this chapter on the treatment of Urustambha (spasticity of the thighs), the following topics are discussed:

Aetiology of the disease

Premonitory signs and symptoms of the disease

Signs and symptoms of the disease

Unsuitable therapeutic measures, and the reason for their unsuitability and

Two categories of therapeutic measures (viz, internal and external therapies) [62]

इत्यग्निवेशकृते तन्त्रे चरक प्रतिसंस्कृतेऽप्राप्ते दृढबल सम्पूरिते चिकित्सा स्थाने ऊरुस्तम्भ चिकित्सितं नाम सप्तविंशोऽध्यायः||२७||

Thus, ends the 27th chapter with the treatment of Urustambha in the section on treatment of diseases (Chikitsa-Sthana) of Agnivesha's work as redacted by Charaka and supplemented by Dridhabala.

11

Chikitsasthana Chapter 28
Vatavyadhi Chikitsitam

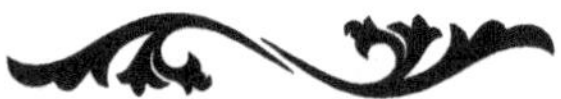

The 28th Chapter of Charaka Samhita Chikitsa Sthana is called Vatavyadhi Chikitsa Adhyaya. It deals with treatment for various disorders caused due to Vata Imbalance.

अथातो वात व्याधि चिकित्सितं व्याख्यास्यामः||१||
इति ह स्माह भगवानात्रेयः||२||

We shall now expound the chapter on the "Treatment of Diseases caused by Vata". Thus said Lord Atreya [1-2]

Importance of Vata Dosha:
वायुरायु बलं वायु र्वायु र्धाता शरीरिणाम्|
वायुर्विश्वमिदं सर्वं प्रभुर्वायुश्च कीर्तितः||३||

Vata Dosha is life, it is strength, it sustains the body, it holds the body and life together.
Vata is all- pervasive, and Vata is the controller of everything in the universe [3]

Longevity and Vata Dosha:
अव्याहत गतिर्यस्य स्थानस्थः प्रकृतौ स्थितः| वायुः स्यात्सोऽधिकं जीवेद्वीतरोगः समाः शतम्||४||

If a person Vata moves unimpaired, if Vata is located in its own site, and it is in its natural state, then the person lives for more than 100 years free from any disease. [4]

Five types of Vata Dosha:
प्राणोदान समानाख्य व्यानापानैः स पञ्चधा| देहं तन्त्रयते सम्यक् स्थानेष्व व्याहतश्चरन्||५||

With its 5-fold divisions, Viz,
Prana, Udana, Samana, Vyana and Apana Vata appropriately control and sustain the functions of the body by its unimpaired movement in the locations concerned. [5]

Prana Vata Sthana and karma:
स्थानं प्राणस्य मूर्धोरःकण्ठ जिह्वास्य नासिकाः | ष्ठीवन क्षवथूद्गार श्वासाहारादि कर्म च||६||

Location and function of Prana Vata:
Prana Vata is located in the
Murdha – head, Ura – chest, Kantha – throat, Jihva – tongue, Aasya – mouth and Nasa – nose
Its functions are:
Sthivana – spitting, Kshvathu – sneezing, Udgara – eructation, Shvasa – respiration, Aahara karma – deglutition of food. Etc. [6]

Location and function of Udana Vata:

उदानस्य पुनः स्थानं नाभ्युरः कण्ठ एव च| वाक्प्रवृतिः प्रयत्नौर्जोबल वर्णादि कर्म च||७||

Udana Vata Dosha is located in the -

Nabhi – umbilicus, Ura – chest and, Kantha – throat.

Its functions are -

Vak pravritti – manifestation of speech,, Prayatna – effort, Urja – enthusiasm, Bala – strength and Varna – complexion. [7]

Location and Function of Samana Vayu:

स्वेद दोषाम्बु वाहिनि स्रोतांसि समधिष्ठितः| अन्तरग्नेश्च पार्श्वस्थः समानोऽग्नि बलप्रदः||८||

Samana Vata is situated in

Sveda Vaha Srotas (channels carrying seat),

DoshaVaha Srotas (channels carrying Doshas) and

Ambu Vaha Srotas (channels carrying aqueous material)

It is located near to the Antaragni (digestive fire / enzymes). It promotes the power of digestion. [8]

Location and Function of Vyana Vayu:

देहं व्याप्नोति सर्व तु व्यानः शीघ्र गतिर्नृणाम्| गति प्रसारणाक्षेप निमेषादि क्रियः सदा||९||

The Vyana Vayu moves very swiftly throughout the entire body.

It always functions in the form of

Gati – motion

Prasarana – extension,

Aakshepa – sudden movements

Nimeshadi kriya – Blinking of the eyes and similar other movements (contractions, relaxation, etc). [9]

Location and Function of Apana Vayu:

वृषणौ बस्ति मेढ्रं च नाभ्यूरू वङ्क्षणौ गुदम्| अपान स्थान मन्त्रस्थः शुक्र मूत्र शकृन्ति च||१०||

सृजत्यार्तवगर्भौ च युक्ताः स्थान स्थिताश्च ते| स्वकर्म कुर्वते देहो धार्यते तैरनामयः||११||

Apana Vata is located in the- Vrushana – two testicles, Basti – urinary bladder, Medhra – Phalus, Nabhi – umbilicus, Uru – thighs, Vankshana- groins, Guda – anus and Colon

Its functions are the- ejaculation of semen, voiding of urine and stool elimination of menstrual blood and Parturition of foetus.

These 5 types of Vata, located in their respective abodes in normal state, perform their functions properly in order to sustain the physique in a healthy state. [10- 11]

Functions of Impaired Vata Dosha:

विमार्गस्था ह्ययुक्ता वा रोगैः स्व स्थान कर्मजैः| शरीरं पीडयन्त्येते प्राणानाशु हरन्ति च||१२||

These 5 types of Vata Dosha get located in a place which is different from the normal and then impaired, they afflict the body with diseases, specific to their locations and functions. This may also lead to instantaneous death. [12]

Number of Vata imbalance disorders:

सङ्ख्यामप्यतिवृतानां तज्जानां हि प्रधानतः| अशीतिर्नखभेदाद्या रोगाः सूत्रे निदर्शिताः||१३||

तानुच्यमानान् पर्यायैः सहेतूपक्रमाञ्छृणु| केवलं वायुमुद्दिश्य स्थानभेदातथाऽऽवृतम्||१४||

Diseases caused by these 5 varieties of Vata dosha are innumerable. However, the principal ailments caused by them are 80 in number, viz, Nakha Bheda (cracking of nails) etc., which enumerated in the Sutra section (vide Charaka Sutrasthana 20/11).

Now, Listen! To the description of the synonyms, aetiology and treatment of these ailments caused by Vata Dosha alone which are classified on the basis of their different locations, and those caused by the occlusion of Vata [by other Doshas] [13-14]

Causes for Vata Dosh imbalance:

रूक्ष शीताल्प लघ्वन्न व्यवायाति प्रजागरैः| विषमादुपचाराच्च दोषासृक्स्रवणादति||१५||

लङ्घन प्लवनात्यध्व व्यायामातिविचेष्टितैः| धातूनां सङ्क्षयाच्चिन्ता शोक रोगातिकर्षणात्||१६||

दुःख शय्यासनात् क्रोधादिदिवास्वप्नादभयादपि| वेगसन्धारणादामादभिघातादभोजनात्||१७||

मर्माघातादगजोष्ट्राश्व शीघ्र यानापतंसनात्| देहे स्रोतांसि रिक्तानि पूरयित्वाऽनिलो बली||१८||

करोति विविधान् व्याधीन् सर्वाङ्गैकाङ्ग संश्रितान्|१९|

Vata gets aggravated by the following:

Intake of Ruksha (dryness), Sheeta (cold), Alpa (less quantity) and Laghu anna (light-to-digest food)

Ati vyavaya – Excessive sexual indulgence

Prajagara – Remaining awake at night in excess

Vishamat upachara – Inappropriate Panchakarma / other therapies

Ati Dosha Sravana – excess of Panchakarma therapies

Ati Asruk Sravana – excess Raktamokshana treatment or excess bleeding

Ati plavana – Excessive swimming

Ati langhana – Excessive fasting

Atyadhva – walking for long distance

Ati vyayama – Resorting to wayfaring, exercise and other physical activities in excess.

Dhatu Samkshayaat – depletion of body tissues, loss of Dhatus

Chinta Shoka karshana – weakening due to excess stress, grief and worries

Roga Ati karshana – Excessive emaciation because of affliction of diseases

Dukha Shayyasana – Sleeping over uncomfortable beds and sitting

Vega vidharana – suppression of natural urges

Krodha (Anger), Diwa swapna (sleep during day time), Bhaya (fear)

Formation of Ama (product of improper digestion and metabolism), suffering from trauma and abstinence from food.

Marmaghata – Injuries to Marmas (vital spots) and riding over an elephant, camel, horse or fast moving vehicles, and vehicles.

Because of the above mentioned factors, the aggravated Vata, fills up the empty body channels (Srotas). Thus it produces different ailments affecting the whole body or a part of it. [15- ½ 19]

Vataroga Purvaroopa – Premonitory Signs:

अव्यक्तं लक्षणं तेषां पूर्वरूपमिति स्मृतम्||१९||

आत्मरूपं तु तद्व्यक्तमपायो लघुता पुनः|२०|

Purva Rupa (premonitory signs):

Avyakta Lakshana – Indistinct manifestations of the signs and symptoms of these ailments

When these signs and symptoms get distinctly manifested, they are called Roopa (actual signs and symptoms).

Diminution (laghuta) of these signs and symptoms indicates that the diseases are going to be cured (Apaya) [19 ½ – ½ 20]

Vatavyadhi Lakshana –

सङ्कोचः पर्वणां स्तम्भो भेदोऽस्थ्नां पर्वणामपि||२०||

लोमहर्षः प्रलापश्च पाणि पृष्ठ शिरोग्रहः| खाञ्ज्य पाङ्गुल्य कुब्जत्वं शोषोऽङ्गानामनिद्रता||२१||

गर्भ शुक्ररजो नाशः स्पन्दनं गात्र सुप्तता| शिरो नासाक्षि जत्रूणां ग्रीवायाश्चापि हुण्डनम्||२२||

भेदस्तोदार्तिराक्षेपो मोहश्चायास एव च| एवंविधानि रूपाणि करोति कुपितोऽनिलः||२३||

हेतु स्थान विशेषाच्च भवेद्रोग विशेषकृत्|२४|

Signs and Symptoms of Vata imbalance disorders:

Aggravation of Vata gives rise to the following –

Sankocha – Contraction,

Parvanam stambha bheda – stiffness of joints and pain

Loma harsha – horripilation

Pralapa – irrelevant talk and

Pani prushta shiro graha – stiffness of hands, back and head.

Khanjya Pangulya Kubjatva- Numbness of hands and feet, and hunch-back, shortness

Anganam sosha – Atrophy, emaciation of limbs,

Anidra – insomnia

Garbha shukra rajo nasha – Destruction of foetus, semen and periods (female reproductive system)

Spandanam gatra suptata – Twitching sensation and numbness in the body

Shiro nasa akshi jatrunam griva hundanam – Shrinking of the head, nose, eyes, clavicular region and neck

Bheda- Splitting pain,

Toda – pricking pain,

Arti- excruciating pain,

Aakshepa – convulsions,

Moha – unconsciousness and

Aayasa -excess tiredness and similar other signs and symptoms.

The aggravated Vata Dosha produces specific diseases because of the specific nature of the causative factors and the seats of manifestation. [20 ½ – ½ 24]

Koshtashrita Vata Dosha:

तत्र कोष्ठाश्रिते दुष्टे निग्रहो मूत्र वर्चसो:||२४||

ब्रध्नहृद्रोग गुल्मार्श:पार्श्वशूलं च मारुते|

Aggravation of Vata located in Kostha (abdominal and thoracic visceras) leads to –

Nigraha mutra varchasa – Retention of urine and faeces (constipation)

Bradhna – prolapsed rectum and

Hrud roga – Heart diseases,

Gulma (tumour),

Arshas (Piles) and

Parshva Shula (pain in flanks). [24 ½ – ½ 25]

Sarvanga Kupita Vata Lakshana:

सर्वाङ्ग कुपिते वाते गात्र स्फुरण भञ्जने||२५||

वेदनाभि: परीतश्च स्फुटन्तीवास्य सन्धय:|

Aggravation of Vayu all over the body causes

Gatra sphurana bhanjana – Twitching sensation and breaking pain in the body

Vedana – Affliction of the entire body with different types of pain and

Paritascha spuhtana – A feeling as if the joints are getting cracked.[25 ½ – ½ 26]

Gudagata Vata lakshana:

ग्रहो विण्मूत्र वातानां शूलाध्मानाश्म शर्करा:||२६||

जङ्घोरु त्रिक पात्पृष्ठ रोग शोषौ गुद स्थिते

Aggravation of the Vayu in rectum causes

Vit mutra vata graha – Retention of stool, urine and flatus

Shoola adhmana – Colic pain, flatulence, bloating

Ashma sharkara – Formation of stone and gravels in the urinary tract and

Jangha uru trika pat prstha sosha – emaciation and stiffness in calf-region, thighs, Trika (Sacroiliac joint), legs and back. [26 ½ – ½ 27]

Amashayagata Vata Lakshana:

हृन्नाभि पार्श्वोदर रुक्तृष्णोद्गार विसूचिकाः||२७||

कासः कण्ठास्य शोषश्च श्वासश्चामाशय स्थिते|

Aggravation of Vata in stomach leads to

Hrut nabhi parshva udara ruk – Pain in the cardiac region, umbilicus, sides of the chest and abdomen.

Trushna – Thirst,

Udgara – eructation and Visuchika – choleric diarrhoea and

Kasa – Cough,

Kanta aasya shosha – dryness of the throat as well as mouth and

Shvasa – dyspnoea. [27 ½ – ½ 28]

Pakvashayagata Vata:

पक्वाशयस्थोऽन्त्रकूजं शूलाटोपौ करोति च||२८||

कृच्छ्रमूत्र पुरीषत्वमानाहं त्रिक वेदनाम्|

Aggravation of Vata located in the colon causes:

Aantra kujana – rumbling sound in the intestine, Shoola – colic pain, Aatopa – gurgling sound in stomach, Mutra krichra – dysuria, constipation, Aanaha – flatulence and Trika vedanam – pain in the lumbar region. [28 ½ – ½ 29]

Aggravation of Vata in sense organs:

श्रोत्रादिष्विन्द्रियवधं कुर्याद्दुष्ट समीरणः||२९||

Vayu, aggravated in the ears and other sense organs, causes impairment (destruction) of the functions of the respective sense organs. [29 ½]

Tvak Gata Vata lakshana:

त्वग्रूक्षा स्फुटिता सुप्ता कृशा कृष्णा च तुद्यते| आतन्यते सरागा च पर्वरुक् त्वक्स्थितेऽनिले||३०||

Vata Dosha aggravated in skin causes

Tvak ruksha- Dryness, Sphutita – cracking,

Supta – numbness, Krusha – shrivelling and Krushna – black coloration of the skin

Tudhyate – Pricking pain in the skin

Aatanyate -Stretching and Sa raga – redness of the skin and

Parva ruk – pain in the joints [30]

Raktagata Vata Lakshana:

रुजस्तीव्राः स सन्तापा वैवर्ण्य कृशताऽरुचिः| गात्रे चारूंषि भुक्तस्य स्तम्भश्चासृग्गतेऽनिले||३१||

Aggravation of Vata Dosha in blood causes –

Teevra ruja – acute pain, Santapa- burning sensation, Vaivarnya – discoloration of skin, Krushata – emaciation and Aruchi – anorexia, Arumshi – Appearance of rashes on the body and Bhuktasya stambha- Stiffness of the body after taking food. [31]

Mamsa Medogata Vata:

गुर्वङ्गं तुद्यतेऽत्यर्थं दण्डमुष्टिहतं तथा| सरुक् श्रमितमत्यर्थं मांस मेदोगतेऽनिले||३२||

Imbalance of Vata in muscles and fat tissues causes:

Anga gaurava – Heaviness of the body
Excessive pain in the body as if the person had been beaten with a stick or with fist,
Excessive fatigue along with pain. [32]

Asthi Majjagata Vata:
भेदोऽस्थि पर्वणां सन्धि शूलं मांस बल क्षयः| अस्वप्नः सन्तता रुक् च मज्जास्थि कुपितेऽनिले||३३||
Increase of Vayu in the bones and bone marrow causes
Asthi bheda – Cracking of the bones and joints
Parvanam sandhi shoola – Piercing pain in the joints
Bala kshaya – Diminution of muscle tissue and strength
Asvapna – Insomnia and
Santata ruk – Constant pain [33]

Shukragata Anila Lakshana:
क्षिप्रं मुञ्चति बध्नाति शुक्रं गर्भमथापि वा| विकृतिं जनयेच्चापि शुक्रस्थः कुपितोऽनिलः||३४||
Aggravation of Vayu in the semen and ovum (Sukra) causes
Premature ejaculation and undue retention of the semen.
Premature expulsion and undue retention of the foetus and
disorders of the semen, ovum and foetus. [34]

Snayugata Vata:
बाह्याभ्यन्तरमायामं खल्लिं कुब्जत्वमेव च| सर्वाङ्गैकाङ्गरोगांश्च कुर्यात् स्नायुगतोऽनिलः||३५||
Aggravation of Vayu in tendons and ligaments causes
Bahya abhyanatara aayama- Opisthotonus and emprosthotonos- backward or forward bending of body
Khalli (neuralgic pain in feet, shoulders, etc)
Kubjatva – Hunchback and other Vatika diseases pertaining to the entire body or a part thereof. [35]

Siragata Vata Lakshana:
शरीरं मन्द रुक्शोफं शुष्यति स्पन्दते तथा| सुप्तास्तन्व्यो महत्यो वा सिरा वाते सिरागते||३६||
Aggravation of Vata Dosha in Siras (vessels) gives rise to
Manda ruk -- Mild pain
Sopham – oedema in the body
Shushyate spandayate- Emaciation and throbbing pain
Lack of pulsation in the vessels and
Thinness or excessive thickness of the vessels. [36]

Sandhivata Lakshana:
वातपूर्ण दृतिस्पर्शः शोथः सन्धिगतेऽनिले| प्रसारणाकुञ्चनयोः प्रवृत्तिश्च सवेदना||३७||
(इत्युक्तं स्थानभेदेन वायोर्लक्षणमेव च)|३८|
Aggravation of Vata Dosha in the joints gives rise to –
Vata purna Druti sparsha shotha – Oedema of the joints which, on palpation, appears as if it is a leather bag inflated with air; and
Prasarana aakunchana pravritti vedana – Pain while making efforts for extensions and contraction of the joints.
Thus, the signs and symptoms caused by aggravated Vayu, on the basis of its location in different parts of the body, are described. [37]

Ardita – Facial paralysis:

अतिवृद्धः शरीरार्धमेकं वायुः प्रपद्यते| यदा तदोपशोष्यासृग्बाहुं पादं च जानु च||३८||
तस्मिन् सङ्कोचयत्यर्धे मुखं जिह्मं करोति च| वक्री करोति नासाभ्रू ललाटाक्षि हनूस्तथा||३९||
ततो वक्रं व्रजत्यास्ये भोजनं वक्र नासिकम् | स्तब्धं नेत्रं कथयतः क्षवथुश्च निगृह्यते||४०||
दीना जिह्मा समुत्क्षिप्ता कला सज्जति चास्य वाक्| दन्ताश्चलन्ति बाध्येते श्रवणौ भिद्यते स्वरः||४१||
पाद हस्ताक्षि जङ्घोरु शङ्ख श्रवण गण्ड रुक् | अर्धे तस्मिन्मुखार्धे वा केवले स्यात्तदर्दितम्||४२||

Facial Paralysis – Ardita Roga:

When excessively aggravated Vayu afflicts half of the body, it dries up Rakta dhatu, and causes excessive contraction of the arm, foot and knee of that part.

It causes distortion in half of the face and curvature of the nose, eye brow, forehead, eye and mandible.

Because of this, ingested food moves tortuously to one side of the mouth, instead of going straight to the oesophagus.

While speaking, the nose becomes curved and eyes remain fixed. There is suppression of sneezing.

His speech becomes faint, distorted, imperceptible and interrupted.

His teeth become loose, deafness, and hoarseness of voice.

There is pain in the foot, hand, eye, calf, thigh, temple, ear and cheek.

These signs and symptoms appear in the half of his body or in the half of his face only. This ailment is called Ardita (Facial paralysis). [38-42]

Antarayama (Emprosthotonous) – Forward bending:

मन्ये संश्रित्य वातोऽन्तर्यदा नाडीः प्रपद्यते| मन्यास्तम्भं तदा कुर्यादन्तरायाम सञ्ज्ञितम्||४३||
अन्तरायम्यते ग्रीवा मन्या च स्तभ्यते भृशम्| दन्तानां दंशनं लाला पृष्ठायामः शिरोग्रहः||४४||
जृम्भा वदन सङ्गश्चाप्यन्तरायाम लक्षणम्|
(इत्युक्तस्त्वन्तरायामो...|४५|

When aggravated Vayu located in the sterno-mastoid area afflicts the internal channels (nerves) of this region, it causes

Manya Stambha – neck rigidness.

Neck becomes bent forward and the sterno-mastoid region becomes exceedingly stiff. There is

Dantanam damshanm – clenching of the teeth, Lala Praseka – salivation, Prstha aayama – contraction of the back, Shiro graha -stiffness of the head, Jrumbha – yawning and Vadana sangha – rigidity of the face.

This ailment is called Antarayanama. [43- ¾ 45]

Bahirayama (Opisthotonus): Backward bending:

...बहिरायाम उच्यते)||४५||
पृष्ठ मन्याश्रिता बाह्याः शोषयित्वा सिरा बली| वायुः कुर्याद्धनुस्तम्भं बहिरायाम सञ्ज्ञकम्||४६||
चापवन्नाम्यमानस्य पृष्ठतो नीयते शिरः| उर उत्क्षिप्यते मन्या स्तब्धा ग्रीवाऽवमृद्यते||४७||
दन्तानां दशनं जृम्भा लालास्रावश्च वाग्ग्रहः| जातवेगो निहन्त्येष वैकल्यं वा प्रयच्छति||४८||

The aggravated Vata located in the back side of the neck causes constriction of Siras (vessels or nerves) as a result of which the body bends like a bow which is called Bahirayama or opisthotonus.

While bending backwards like a bow, the head moves towards the back, the chest is protruded, the Manyas (Sterno-mastoid muscles) become rigid, the neck is squeezed, and the teeth become clenched.

There is yawning, salivation and aphasia (absence of speech). When the attack becomes acute, it either leads to the death of the patient or causes serious deformity in his body. [45 ¼ -48]

Hanu Graha (locked jaw)

हनुमूले स्थितो बन्धात् संस्रयत्यनिलो हनू| विवृतास्यत्वमथवा कुर्यात् स्तब्धमवेदनम्||४९||
हनुग्रहं च संस्तभ्य हनुं(नू)संवृत वक्रताम्|५०|

The aggravated Vata located at the root of the jaw causes dislocation of jaw bones. It may cause

Vivruta Asya – constant opening of mouth with stiffness.

Alternatively, it may cause lock-jaw because of the stiffness of its joints when the mouth remains closed, and cannot be opened. [49- ½ 50]

Akshepaka (convulsions):

मुहुराक्षिपति क्रुद्धो गात्राण्याक्षेपकोऽनिलः||५०||
पाणिपादं च संशोष्य सिराः स स्नायु कण्डराः|५१|

When the aggravated Vata causes frequent convulsions in different parts of the body, then ailment is caused by the constriction of hands and legs as well as vessels, ligament and tendons. Thus it causes Aksepaka. [50 ½- ½ 51]

Dandaka (staff-like Spasticity of the Body):

पाणि पाद शिरःपृष्ठ श्रोणीः स्तभ्नाति मारुतः||५१||
दण्डवत्स्तब्धगात्रस्य दण्डकः सोऽनुपक्रमः|५२|

When the aggravated Vata causes rigidity of hands, legs, head, back and hips in a person resulting in stiffness of body like a stick, then the ailment is called Dandaka (stick-like stiffness). This condition is incurable. [51 ½ – ½ 52]

Specific features of Ardita Etc:

स्वस्थः स्यादर्दितादीनां मुहुर्वेगे गतेऽगते||५२||
पीड्यते पीडनैस्तैस्तैर्भिषगेतान् विवर्जयेत्|५३|

When the frequent Vega (affliction) of diseases like Ardita (Facial paralysis) subside, the patient becomes normal. However, if these paroxysms do not subside, the patient continuously remains afflicted with the signs and symptoms and of respective diseases, leading to incurability. The physicians should not treat such patients. [52 ½ -1/2 53]

Pakshavadha (Hemiplegia), Ekanga roga (Monoplegia) and Sarvanga Roga (Paralysis of the Entire Body):

हत्वैकं मारुतः पक्षं दक्षिणं वाममेव वा||५३||
कुर्याच्चेष्टा निवृत्तिं हि रुजं वाक्स्तम्भमेव च| गृहीत्वाऽर्धं शरीरस्य सिराः स्नायू विशोष्य च||५४||
पादं सङ्कोचयत्येकं हस्तं वा तोद शूल कृत्| एकाङ्ग रोगं तं विद्यात् सर्वाङ्गं सर्व देहजम्||५५||

When the aggravated Vata paralyzes one side of the body, it causes immobility of that side along with pain, loss of speech. This condition is called Paksa Vadha.

By afflicting half of the body, the aggravated Vata may cause constriction of the vessels and ligaments as a result of which there will be contracture, either of one leg or one hand along with aching or piercing pain. This is called Ekanga Roga (monoplegia).

If, however, the above mentioned morbidity pervades the entire body, then the ailment is called Sarvanga Roga (Paralysis of the entire body). [53 ½- 55]

Gridhrasi (Sciatica)

स्फिक्पूर्वा कटि पृष्ठोरुजानु जङ्घा पदं क्रमात्|
गृध्रसी स्तम्भ रुक्तोदैर्गृह्णाति स्पन्दते मुहुः||५६||
वातादवात कफातन्द्रा गौरवारोचकान्विता|

Gridhrasi, caused by aggravated Vata Dosha, the hip is afflicted with

Stambha – stiffness,

pain and pricking sensation in the waist, back, thigh, knee and calf region.

All these organs get a twitching sensation frequently.

If the ailment is caused by both, the aggravated Vata Dosha and Kapha, then the patient suffers from drowsiness, heaviness and anorexia in addition to the above symptoms. [56 – ½ 57]

Read more about sciatica and Ayurvedic treatment

Khalli (Twisting Pain in Upper and lower Limbs):

खल्ली तु पाद जङ्घोरुकरमूलावमोटनी||५७||

Khalli is characterized by the twisting pain of the feet, calf regions, thighs and shoulders. [57 ½]

Other Vatika Diseases

स्थानानामनुरूपैश्च लिङ्गैः शेषान् विनिर्दिशेत्|५८|
सर्वेष्वेतेषु संसर्गं पित्तादयैरुपलक्षयेत्||५८||

Other Vatic diseases can be determined on the basis of the signs and symptoms commensurate with their locations. In all these ailments, the combination of aggravated Pitta, etc, may also be observed. [58]

Vata Avarana – obstruction of body channels by Vata Dosha:

वायोर्धातु क्षयात् कोपो मार्गस्यावरणेन च (वा)| वात पित्त कफा देहे सर्व स्रोतोऽनुसारिणः||५९||
वायुरेव हि सूक्ष्मत्वाद्द्वयोस्तत्राप्युदीरणः | कुपितस्तौ समुद्धूय तत्र तत्र क्षिपन् गदान्||६०||
करोत्यावृतमार्गत्वाद्रसादींश्चोप शोषयेत्|६१|

Vata Dosha gets aggravated in 2 different ways, viz,

By Dhatu Kshaya – depletion of tissue elements and

Marga Avarana – Occlusion of its channel of circulation.

Vata, Pitta and Kapha move through all the channels of circulation. Because of its subtle nature, Vata Dosha provokes and pulls Pitta and Kapha Doshas. The aggravated Vata spreads Pitta and Kapha into different places of the body and obstructs the channels of circulation leading to the manifestation of various diseases, and drying up of tissue elements like Rasa Dhatu, Rakta Dhatu etc [59- ½ 61]

Pittavruta Vata Occlusion of Vata Dosha by Pitta

लिङ्गं पित्तावृते दाहस्तृष्णा शूलं भ्रमस्तमः ||६१||
कट्वम्ल लवणोष्णैश्च विदाहः शीत कामिता|

Occlusion of Vayu by Pitta causes:

Daha – Burning sensation, Trushna – morbid thirst, Shoolam – colic pain and Bhrama – giddiness

Tamas (a feeling as if entering into darkness)

Katu amla lavana ushna vidaha – Burning sensation by taking pungent, sour, saline and hot ingredients of food and

Shita kamita – Craving for cold things. [61 ½ – ½ 62]

Kaphavruta Vata – Occlusion of Vayu by Kapha

शैत्य गौरव शूलानि कट्वाद्युपशयोऽधिकम्||६२||
लङ्घनायास रूक्षोष्ण कामिता च कफावृते|

Occlusion of Vayu by Kapha gives rise to –

Shaitya – Feeling of cold and Gaurava – heaviness

Shoola – Colic pain

Katvadi upashayo adhikam – Considerable relief by the intake of pungent and such other ingredients and

Langhana, Aayasa, Ruksha ushna kamita – Desire for fasting, exercise and unctuous as well as hot ingredients. [62 ½ – ½ 63]

Raktavrita Vata – Occlusion of Vata Dosha by Rakta (Blood):

रक्तावृते स दाहार्तिस्त्वङ्मांसान्तरजो भृशम्||६३||
भवेत् सरागः श्वयथुर्जायन्ते मण्डलानि च|

Occlusion of Vata Dosha by Rakta (blood) gives rise to –

Daha arti tvak mamsa antarajo – Excessive pain and burning sensation in the area between the skin and muscle tissue.

Sa raga Shyavathu – Oedema with redness and

Mandala (Circular type of rash – ringworm infection). [63 ½ – ½ 64]

Mamsavrita Vata – Occlusion of Vata Dosha by mamsa (Muscle Tissue):

कठिनाश्च विवर्णाश्च पिडकाः श्वयथुस्तथा||६४||
हर्षः पिपीलिकानां च सञ्चार इव मांसगे|

Occlusion of Vata by mamsa (Muscle tissue) gives rise to –
Kathinascha vivarnascha pidaka – Appearance of hard and discoloured pimples and swellings
Harshah – horripilation and
Pipilikanam – Formiculation (a feeling as if ants are moving in the body) [64 ½- ½ 65]

Medavruta Vata – Occlusion of Vata by medas (fat):

चलः स्निग्धो मृदुः शीतः शोफोऽङ्गेष्वरुचिस्तथा||६५||
आढ्यवात इति ज्ञेयः स कृच्छ्रो मेदसाऽऽवृतः|

Occlusion of Vata by Medas (fat) gives rise to –
Chala snigdha mrudu sheeta shopha – Appearance of oedema in the limbs, the oedema is mobile, unctuous and smooth which is mobile
This condition is called Adhya Vata which is difficult to cure. [65 ½ – ½ 66]

Asthi Avrita Vata – Occlusion of Vata Dosha by Bone Tissue:

स्पर्शमस्थ्नाऽऽवृते तूष्णं पीडनं चाभिनन्दति||६६||
सम्भज्यते सीदति च सूचीभिरिव तुद्यते|

Obstruction of Vata by the bone tissue gives rise to –
Liking for hot touch, and pressure (kneading)
breaking type of pain and depression and
Soochibhiriva tudyate – A feeling as if pricked with needles. [66 ½ – ½ 67]

Majjavrita Vata – Vata obstructed by bone marrow:

मज्जावृते विनामः स्याज्जृम्भणं परिवेष्टनम्||६७||
शूलं तु पीड्यमाने च पाणिभ्यां लभते सुखम्|

Occlusion of Vata Dosha by bone marrow gives rise to –
Vinamah – Bending of the body
Jrumbha – Yawning
Pariveshtanam – Twisting pain
Shula – Colic pain and
Panibhyam labhate sukham – The patient gets relief if pressed by hand. [67 ½- ½ 68]

Shukravrita Vata – Occlusion of Vata by Shukra dhatu:

शुक्रावेगोऽतिवेगो वा निष्फलत्वं च शुक्रगे||६८||

Occlusion of Vata by semen gives rise to –
Shukra avega -Non-ejaculation or Ati vega – excessive ejaculation (premature ejaculation) of semen and
Nishphalatvam – Sterility [68 ½]

Annavruta Vata – Occlusion of Vata by Food:

भुक्ते कुक्षौ च रुग्जीर्णे शाम्यत्यन्नावृतेऽनिले|

Occlusion of the Vata by food gives rise to –
Kuksha ruk jeerne – Pain in the pelvic region after the intake of food and
Alleviation of pain after the digestion of food. [1/2 69]

Mutravrita Vata – Occlusion of Vata by Urine:

मूत्रप्रवृतिराध्मानं बस्तौ मूत्रावृतेऽनिले||६९||

Obstruction of Vata by urine results in –

Mutra apravritti – Retention of urine and

Adhmanam – Distension of urinary bladder [69 ½]

Pureesha avrita Vata – Occlusion of Vata by stool:

वर्चसोऽतिविबन्धोऽधः स्वे स्थाने परिकृन्तति| व्रजत्याशु जरां स्नेहो भुक्ते चानह्यते नरः||७०||

चिरात् पीडितमन्नेन दुःखं शुष्कं शकृत् सृजेत्| श्रोणी वङ्क्षण पृष्ठेषु रुग्विलोमश्च मारुतः||७१||

अस्वस्थं हृदयं चैव वर्चसा त्वावृतेऽनिले|७२|

Occlusion of Vata by stool gives rise to –

Absolute constipation

Parikartana – Griping pain in the colon (abode of stool)

Instantaneous digestion of the ingested fat

Abdominal distension after the digestion of food

Because of the pressure of the [undigested] food, the patient voids after a long time. The voiding is painful and the stool is dry.

Shroni Vankshana prstha ruk – Pain in the hips, groin and back

Vilomascha maruta – Upward movement of Vata (flatus or gas) in the abdomen and

Asvastham hrdayam – Uncomfortable sensation in chest region. [70 – 1/ 72]

Prognosis

सन्धि च्युति हनुस्तम्भः कुञ्चनं कुब्जताऽर्दितः||७२||

पक्षाघातोऽङ्ग संशोषः पङ्गुत्वं खुडवातता| स्तम्भनं चाढ्यवातश्च रोगा मज्जास्थिगाश्च ये||७३||

एते स्थानस्य गाम्भीर्यादयत्नात् सिध्यन्ति वा न वा| नवान् बलवतस्त्वेतान् साधयेन्निरुपद्रवान्||७४||

The following diseases (because of their deep-seated and chronic nature) may get cured only by careful treatment; otherwise these diseases cannot be cured at all:

Sandhi chyuti – Joint dislocation, Hanu stambha – Lock-jaw, Kunchanam -Contraction, Kubjata (Hunch-Back), Ardita – Facial paralysis, Pakshaghata – Hemiplegia, Anga samsosha – Atrophy of limbs, Pangutva (inability to walk because of muscular dystrophy), Khuda Vatata (affliction of the ankle joint by Vata Dosha or arthritis), Stambha – Stiffness, Adhya Vata (an ailment caused by the occlusion of Vata Dosha by fat- vide verse no. 66) and Majja asthi gata roga – Diseases located in the bone marrow and bones

The above mentioned diseases could be treated only under the following circumstances:

If these ailment are of recent origin

If the patient is strong and

If these are not associated with complications. [72 ½ – 74]

Vata Roga Chikitsa: Snehana

क्रियामतः परं सिद्धां वातरोगापहां शृणु| केवलं निरुपस्तम्भमादौ स्नेहैरुपाचरेत्||७५||

वायुं सर्पि वसा तैल मज्ज पानैनरं ततः| स्नेह क्लान्तं समाश्वास्य पयोभिः स्नेहयेत् पुनः||७६||

यूषै ग्राम्याम्बुजानूपरसैर्वा स्नेह संयुतैः| पायसैः कृशरैः साम्ल लवणैरनुवासनैः||७७||

नावनैस्तर्पणैश्चान्नैः

Treatment for Vata imbalance:

Now, listen to the exposition on the effective line of treatment for the cure of the diseases caused by Vata, which will be described hereafter.

Snehana – oleation treatment:

If the diseases are caused by Vata exclusively, and if no Avarana (occlusion) is involved, then in the beginning, the patient is treated by oleation therapy for which ghee, muscle fat, oil and bone marrow are administered.

Thereafter, when the patient gets disgusted or tired with the intake of oleation therapy, he is rested and again oleation therapy is administered with –

– milk,

vegetable soup and

Gramya, Ambuja, Anupa Mamsarasa – soup of the meat of animals inhabiting domesticated (Gramya), aquatic (Ambuja) and marshy land (Anupa) after adding fat.

He may be given Payasa (preparation of rice and milk) and Krishara (a preparation of rice, legumes, etc) added with sour ingredients as well as salt. He may also be given Anuvasana type of medicated enema, inhalation therapy and refreshing food. [75- ¼ 78]

Swedana – Fomentation Therapy:

सुस्निग्धं स्वेदयेततः|

स्वभ्यक्तं स्नेह संयुक्तै र्नाडी प्रस्तर सङ्करैः||७८||

तथाऽन्यैर्विविधैः स्वेदैर्यथायोगमुपाचरेत्|

After the patient is properly oleated, he is given fomentation therapy before the administration of fomentation therapy, the body of patient is properly oleated and thereafter, fomentation therapies viz Nadi Sveda, Prastara Sveda, Sankara Sveda as well as other types of appropriate fomentation therapies are administered. [78 ¾ – ½ 7]

Effects of Snehana and Swedana in Vatavyadhi:

स्नेहाक्तं स्विन्नमङ्गं तु वक्रं स्तब्धमथापि वा||७९||

शनैर्नामयितुं शक्यं यथेष्टं शुष्कदारुवत्| हर्ष तोदरुगायाम शोथ स्तम्भ ग्रहादयः||८०||

स्विन्नस्याशु प्रशाम्यन्ति मार्दवं चोपजायते| स्नेहश्च धातून्संशुष्कान् पुष्णात्याशु प्रयोजितः||८१||

बलमग्निबलं पुष्टिं प्राणांश्चाप्यभिवर्धयेत्| असकृत्तं पुनः स्नेहैः स्वेदैश्चाप्युपपादयेत्||८२||

तथा स्नेहमृदौ कोष्ठे न तिष्ठन्त्यनिलामयाः|८३|

Oleation and Fomentation Therapies:

As a dry wood can be slowly bent, as desired, by the application of oily substance and fomentation, similarly even a curved / crooked or stiff limb can be slowly brought back to health by the administration of oleation and fomentation therapies.

Swedana – Fomentation therapy immediately relieves – Harsha (tingling sensation), Toda (pricking pain), Ruk (ache), Aayama (contracture), Sotha (oedema), Stambha (stiffness), Graha (spasticity), etc.

Snehana – Oleation therapy, when administered, instantaneously provides nourishment to the emaciated tissue elements. Snehana promotes strength, Agni (digestion strength), nourishment, and Prana (Vital force).

The patient is given repeated Sneha and Sweda treatment, as a result of which the Kostha (Viscera in the abdomen and thorax) becomes soft and the diseases of Vayu do not get an opportunity to get lodged there permanently. [79 ½ – ½ 83]

Shodhana treatment for Vata:

यद्यनेन सदोषत्वात् कर्मणा न प्रशाम्यति||८३||

मृदुभिः स्नेह संयुक्तैरौषधैस्तं विशोधयेत्| घृतं तिल्वक सिद्धं वा सातलासिद्धमेव वा||८४||

पयसैरण्डतैलं वा पिबेद्दोषहरं शिवम्| स्निग्धाम्ल लवणोष्णाद्यैराहारैर्हि मलश्चितः||८५||

स्रोतो बद्ध्वाऽनिलं रुन्ध्यात्स्मात्तमनुलोमयेत्| दुर्बलो योऽविरेच्यः स्यात्तं निरूहैरुपाचरेत्||८६||

पाचनै र्दीपनीयैर्वा भोजनैस्तद्युतैर्नरम्| संशुद्धस्योत्थिते चाग्नौ स्नेह स्वेदौ पुनर्हितौ||८७||

स्वाद्वम्ल लवण स्निग्धैराहारैः सततं पुनः| नावनै र्धूमपानैश्च सर्वानेवोपपादयेत्||८८||

इति सामान्यतः प्रोक्तं वातरोग चिकित्सितम्|८९|

Elimination Therapy for Vata disorders:

If because of inappropriate administration of [the above mentioned] therapies (oleation and fomentation) the ailments [caused by Vayu] do not subside, then the patient is given elimination therapy with the help of mild herbs added with oily (unctuous) ingredients.

For this purpose, the patient should take medicated ghee prepared by boiling, either with Tilvaka or Saptala – Hibiscus cannibus or he may take castor oil with milk. They help in the elimination of morbid material, and produce beneficial effects.

Because of intake of food which is unctuous, sour, salt, hot etc the morbid material gets accumulated and it obstructs the channels of circulation leading to obstruction of Vata movement. Therefore, the patient is given Anulomana – mild purgation treatment.

If the patient is weak, and is therefore, unsuitable for Anulomana -Virechana treatment, then he is given Niruha Basti (decoction enema) with Pachana (carminative) and Deepana (digestion promoting) herbs.

He should also be given food added with ingredients which are Pachana (carminative) and Dipana (digestive stimulants).

After elimination of morbid matters and stimulation of Agni (enzymes), it is beneficial to administer oleation and fomentation therapies again.

In addition, all the patients suffering from diseases caused by Vayu are continuously given a diet containing ingredients which are sweet, sour, saline and unctuous. All of them should also be treated with inhalation (Navana) and Dhumapana – smoking therapies.

Thus, the general line of treatment for Vata imbalance disorders is explained. [83 ½ – ½ 89]

Treatment for specific Ailments

विशेषतस्तु कोष्ठस्थे वाते क्षारं पिबेन्नरः||८९||
पाचनै दीपनैर्युक्तैरम्लैर्वा पाचयेन्मलान्|

Koshtagata Vata Chikitsa:

Treatment of Vata Located in Gastro- intestinal Tract

If Vata is located in the Kostha (digestive tract), then

Kshara medicines such as Yavakshara are administered.

Mala Pachana – digestion and elimination of waste products is done with the help of medicines having – Pachana (carminative), Deepana (digestive) and sour properties. [89 ½ – ½ 90]

Guda Pakvashayagata Vata:

गुद पक्वाशयस्थे तु कर्मोदावर्तनुद्दिधतम्||९०||

If the vitiation Vayu is located in the anus or colon, then therapies prescribed for the treatment of Udavarta (upward movement of wind in the abdomen) are to be used. [90 ½]

Amashaya Gata Vata Chikitsa:

आमाशयस्थे शुद्धस्य यथा दोषहरीः क्रियाः|

If the Vitiated Vayu is located in stomach, then –

Shodhana – Vamana, Virechana treatments are administered, based on predominant Dosha. [1/2 91]

Sarvanga Vata Chikitsa:

सर्वाङ्ग कुपितेऽभ्यङ्गो बस्तयः सानुवासनाः||९१||

If the whole body is afflicted by vitiated Vayu, then

Abhaynga – oil massage and

Niruha and Anuvasana Basti are administered. [91 ½]

Twak Gata Vata Chikitsa:

स्वेदाभ्यङ्गावगाहाश्च हृद्यं चान्नं त्वगाश्रिते|

If the vitiated Vayu is located in skin, then
Sweda – fomentation,
Abhyanga – massage and
Avagaha medicated bath
Hurdya Anna – food pleasing to the heart are administered. [1/2 92]

Rakta Gata Vata Chikitsa:

शीताः प्रदेहा रक्तस्थे विरेको रक्त मोक्षणम्||९२||

If the vitiated Vata is located in the blood, then
Sheeta Pradeha – coolant ointments
Vireka – purgation and
Rakta mokshana (blood-letting) therapies are administered. [92 ½]

Mamsa Medogata Vata Chikitsa:

विरेको मांस मेदःस्थे निरूहाः शमनानि च|

If the vitiated Vata is situated in the muscle and fat tissues, then
Vireka (purgation) and
Niruha Basti treatment
Shamana – Vata alleviating medicines are administered. [1/2 93]

Asthi Majjagata Vata Chikitsa:

बाह्याभ्यन्तरतः स्नेहैरस्थि मज्जगतं जयेत्||९३||

If the vitiated Vayu is located in the bone and bone marrow, then
Bahya Abhyantara Sneha – internal and external oleation therapies are administered. [93 ½]

Shukragata Vata Chikitsa:

हर्षोऽन्नपानं शुक्रस्थे बल शुक्रकरं हितम्| विबद्ध मार्गं दृष्ट्वा वा शुक्रं दद्यादिवरेचनम्||९४||
विरिक्त प्रतिभुक्तस्य पूर्वोक्तां कारयेत् क्रियाम्|

If the vitiated Vayu is located in the semen, then
Harsha Annapana – aphrodisiac foods and drinks are administered.
If there is obstruction in the seminal channel, then Virechana – purgation therapy is administered. After Virechana, the patient is given food, and thereafter, the earlier mentioned therapies (for sexual excitement and promotion of strength as well as semen) is administered (Charaka Chikitsa -2nd chapter) [94- ½ 95]

Garbhagata Vata Chikitsa:

गर्भ शुष्के तु वातेन बालानां चापि शुष्यताम्||९५||
सिता काश्मर्य मधुकैर्हितमुत्थापने पयः|

Treatment of foetal afflictions by Vayu:
If the fetus or the child (after delivery) gets emaciated by Vata Dosha, then milk boiled with sugar candy, Kashmarya – Gmelina arborea and Madhuka– Licorice is administered for the restoration of normal growth. [95 ½ – ½ 96]

Hrudayagata Vata Chikitsa:

हृदि प्रकुपिते सिद्धमंशुमत्या पयो हितम्||९६||

If Vata is aggravated in the heart, then milk boiled by adding Amsumati (Shalaparni) is useful. [96 ½]

Nabhigata Vata Chikitsa:

मत्स्यान्नाभि प्रदेशस्थे सिद्धान् बिल्व शलाटुभिः|

If Vayu is aggravated in umbilical region, the patient is given fish prepared with slices of Bilva (bael).

Treatment of Cramps and Contractures:

वायुना वेष्ट्यमाने तु गात्रे स्यादुपनाहनम्||९७||
तैलं सङ्कुचितेऽभ्यङ्गो माष सैन्धव साधितम्|

If there are cramps because of aggravated Vayu, then

Upanaha – hot poultice [prepared of Vayu-alleviating herbs] is applied all over the body.

If there are contractures because of Vata, then Abhyanga with medicated oil or ghee prepared with black gram and rock salt is done.

Treatment of Vayu Located in Arms, Head Etc:

बाहु शीर्षगते नस्यं पानं चौतरभक्तिकम्||९८||
बस्ति कर्म त्वधो नाभेः शस्यते चावपीडकः|९९|

If arms and head get afflicted by aggravated Vayu, then

Nasya – nasal drops treatment is administered with the medicated oil prepared by boiling it with black gram and rock salt.

The same medicated oil is administered internally after the intake of food (Uttara Bhauktika).

If the abdomen below the umbilical region is afflicted by the aggravated Vayu, then the above-mentioned oil prepared by boiling with Masha and rock-salt is used for medicated enema. This oil is given internally just before the intake of food (avapidaka). [98 ½ – ½ 99]

Treatment of Ardita (Facial Paralysis):

अर्दिते नावनं मूर्ध्नि तैलं तर्पणमेव च||९९||
नाडी स्वेदोपनाहश्चाप्यानूप पिशितैर्हिताः|

For the treatment of facial paralysis,

Navana – nourishing type of nasal drops

Murdhni Taila – head is anointed with medicated oil.

Tarpana – nourishing treatment

Nadi Sveda (a type of fomentation therapy) and

Upanaha (application of hot ointment or poultice) prepared with the meat of animals inhabiting marshy lands (Anupa) are useful. [99 ½ – ½ 100]

Treatment of Ardhanga Vata (Hemiplegia):

स्वेदनं स्नेह संयुक्तं पक्षाघाते विरेचनम्||१००||

Fomentation accompanied with oleation and purgation therapy is useful for the treatment of hemiplegia. [100 ½]

Treatment of Gridhrasi (Sciatica):

अन्तरा कण्डरा गुल्फं सिरा बस्त्यग्निकर्म च|
गृध्रसीषु प्रयुञ्जीत खल्ल्यां तूष्णोपनाहनम्||१०१||

For sciatica, Siravyadha – venesection is performed over the Antara Kandara Gulpha Sira – vein located between the tendo- Achilles and ankle joint (medial side).

The patient is given

Basti – enema treatment and

Agni – cauterization therapies [3/4 101]

Treatment of Khalli

गृध्रसीषु प्रयुञ्जीत खल्ल्यां तूष्णोपनाहनम्||१०१||

पायसैः कृशरै र्मांसैः शस्तं तैल घृतान्वितैः|

For Khalli (twisting pain of the feet, calf regions, thighs and shoulders), hot poultice prepared of milk pudding, Krishara (a preparation of rice and pulses) and meat added with oil and ghee are beneficial. [101 ¼ – ½ 102]

Treatment of Hanu Graha (Lock Jaw)

व्यात्तानने हनुं स्विन्नामङ्गुष्ठाभ्यां प्रपीड्य च||१०२||

प्रदेशिनीभ्यां चोन्नाभ्य चिबुकोन्नामनं हितम्| स्रस्तं स्वं गमयेत्स्थानं स्तब्धं स्विन्नं विनामयेत्||१०३|

In Lock-Jaw, if the mouth remains open, the mandibular joints are fomented (Swedana). Thereafter, with the help of thumbs inserted into the mouth the mandibular joints are pressed, and with the help of index fingers (kept outside) the mandibles and chin is elevated. The dislocated mandibular bone will then slide into its normal position. If there is stiffness of the mandibular joint, then it is fomented, and then pressed downwards to ensure mobility of the joint. [102 ½ – 103]

Therapies for Hanu Graha:

प्रत्येकं स्थानदूष्यादि क्रिया वैशेष्यमाचरेत्|१०४|

Depending upon the location of Vata (in stomach etc), tissue elements vitiated by Vata and such other factors (occlusion of Vata etc) each patient is given specific therapies. [1/2 104]

Vataroga Samanya Chikitsa Sutra:

सर्पिस्तैल वसा मज्ज सेकाभ्यञ्जन बस्तयः ||१०४||

स्निग्धाः स्वेदा निवातं च स्थानं प्रावरणानि च| रसाः पयांसि भोज्यानि स्वाद्वम्ल लवणानि च||१०५||

बृंहणं यच्च तत् सर्वं प्रशस्तं वात रोगिणाम्|१०६|

General line of treatment for Vata imbalance disorders:

Ghee, oil, muscle fat, marrow,

Swedana, Abhyanga (massage) ,

Basti – medicated enema,

Residing in windless place, covering the body with blankets, meat soup, different types of milk, food ingredients which are sweet, sour and saline, and such other measures which are nourishing- all these are beneficial for the patient suffering from diseases caused by the aggravated Vata. [104 ½ – ½ 106]

Meat Soup for Vatika Diseases

बलायाः पञ्चमूलस्य दशमूलस्य वा रसे||१०६||

अज शीर्षाम्बुजानूपमांसाद पिशितैः पृथक्| साधयित्वा रसान् स्निग्धान्दध्यम्ल व्योष संस्कृतान्||१०७||

भोजयेद्वातरोगार्तं तैर्व्यक्त लवणै नरम्|

Soup of meat of head of a goat or meat of aquatic (ambuja), marshy land (Anupa) or carnivorous (Pishita) animals are prepared separately by boiling it with the decoctions of

Bala – Country mallow (root) or Pancha Mula or Dasha Mula.

These soups are added with fat (ghee), and sizzled with yoghurt, sour ingredients and Trikatu (Ginger, pepper and long pepper fruit) added with small quantities of Salt. These soups are given to the patient suffering from diseases caused by Vata. [106 ½ – ½ 108]

Upanaha – Hot Poultice

एतैरेवोपनाहांश्च पिशितैः सम्प्रकल्पयेत्||१०८||

घृत तैलयुतैः साम्लैः क्षुण्ण स्विन्नैरनस्थिभिः|

The above mentioned types of meat are made free from bones, cut into small pieces, steam- boiled and added with ghee, oil and sour ingredients. These recipes are applied in the form of hot poultice for the cure of diseases caused by Vata Dosha. [108 ½- ½ 109]

Medicated Bath:

पत्रोत्क्वाथ पयस्तैल द्रोण्यः स्युरवगाहने||१०९||

The patient suffering from Vataroga should take a bath in a bath-tub filled with the decoction of Vata-alleviating leaves, milk and oil. [109½]

Seka – Affusion:

स्वभ्यक्तानां प्रशस्यन्ते सेकाश्चानिल रोगिणाम्|

For the patient suffering from Vatika diseases, affusion (dripping) after proper oleation is useful. [1/2 110]

Nadi Sveda and Upanaha

आनूपौदक मांसानि दशमूलं शतावरीम्||११०||

कुलत्थान् बदरान्माषांस्तिलान्रास्नां यवान् बलाम्| वसादध्यारनालाम्लैः सह कुम्भ्यां विपाचयेत्||१११||

नाडीस्वेदं प्रयुञ्जीत पिष्टैश्चाप्युपनाहनम्| तैश्च सिद्धं घृतं तैलमभ्यङ्गं पानमेव च||११२||

In a pot, the meat of marshy land- inhabiting (Anupa) and aquatic animals (Varija), Dasha Mula, Satavari –Asparagus racemosus,

Kulattha – Horse gram,

Badara – Zizyphus jujuba,

Masha – Black gram

Tila

Rasna (Vanda roxburghi / Pluchea lanceolata),

Yava – Barley (Hordeum vulgare) and

Bala – Sida cordifolia is cooked by adding muscle fat, yogurt and sour vinger (Amla Aranala).

Nadi sveda is given with this decoction.

Upanaha (hot poultice) is applied with the paste of the above mentioned ingredients. Medicated ghee and medicated oil prepared by boiling with the above mentioned ingredients may be used for massage and Pana (internal intake). [110 ½- 112]

Recipes for Upanaha (hot Poultice):

मुस्तं किण्वं तिलाः कुष्ठं सुराह्वं लवणं नतम्| दधि क्षीर चतुःस्नेहैः सिद्धं स्यादुपनाहनम्||११३||

Musta (Cyperus rotundus),

Kinva – sour enzymes,

Kushta – Saussurea lappa,

Surahva – Devadaru, Salt and Nata (Valeriana wallicii) is cooked with yoghurt, milk and 4 types of fat (oil, ghee, muscle fat and bone marrow). This recipe is used as hot poultice. [113]

Application of Thick paste – Alepana

उत्कारिका वेसवार क्षीर माष तिलौदनैः| एरण्डबीज गोधूम यव कोलस्थिरादिभिः||११४||

सस्नेहैः सरुजं गात्रमालिप्य बहलं भिषक्| एरण्डपत्रै र्बध्नीयाद्रात्रौ कल्यं विमोक्षयेत्||११५||

क्षीराम्बुना ततः सिक्तं पुनश्चैवोपनाहितम्| मुञ्चेद्रात्रौ दिवाबद्धं चर्मभिश्च सलोमभिः||११६||

Application of Thick paste – Alepana

Utkarika (pan-cake), Vesavara (a type of meat preparation with hot spices), milk, Masha – black gram, , Tila – Sesame, boiled rice, seeds of castor, wheat, barley, Kola, Sthira , etc. is added with fat, [and made to a paste] the physician should apply a thick layer of this paste over the painful part of the body at night. It is bandaged with castor leaves.

The next morning, the bandage, along with the paste, is removed. Thereafter, the affected part is sprinkled with milk. Again, during the day time, hot poultice is applied and bandaged by leather containing fur. This bandage [along with the paste] is removed at night. [114-116]

Pradeha and Upanaha:

फलानां तैलयोनीनामम्ल पिष्टान् सुशीतलान्| प्रदेहानुपनाहांश्च गन्धैर्वातहरैरपि||११७||

पायसैः कृशरैश्चैव कारयेत् स्नेह संयुतैः|११८|

Oil bearing fruits (seeds) – such as castor, sesame seeds, mustard seeds, are made to a paste by triturating them with sour ingredients, and are allowed to cool down before application. This paste is applied in the form of a Pradeha (thin poultice).

Vata balancing aromatic herbs like Aguru, cardamom, camphor etc), milk pudding (Payasa) and Krishara (a preparation of rice and pulses) is added with fat and is applied in the form of Upanaha (thick poultice). These are used to prepare ointment and are applied over affected areas. [117- ½ 118]

Medicated Ghee for Vatika Diseases:

रूक्ष शुद्धानिलार्तानामतः स्नेहान् प्रचक्ष्महे||११८||

विविधान् विविध व्याधि प्रशमायामृतोपमान्| द्रोणेऽम्भसः पचेद्भागान् दशमूलाच्चतुष्पलान्||११९||

यव कोल कुलत्थानां भागैः प्रस्थोन्मितैः सह| पादशेषे रसे पिष्टैर्जीवनीयैः सशर्करैः||१२०||

तथा खर्जूर काश्मर्य द्राक्षा बदर फल्गुभिः| सक्षीरैः सर्पिषः प्रस्थः सिद्धः केवलवातनुत्||१२१||

निरत्ययः प्रयोक्तव्यः पानाभ्यञ्जन बस्तिषु|

For the treatment of different diseases caused by Vayu alone, we shall now describe preparations of medicated fat which are like Amruta – ambrosia:

In 1 Drona of water, 4 Palas of Dasha Mula, and 1 Prastha of each of Yava – Barley, Kola- ber and Kulattha – horse gram is boiled till 1/4th of it remains.

To this decoction, the paste of the herbs belonging to Jivaniya group, sugar, Kharjura – dates, Kashmarya – Gmelina arborea, Draksha – Raisin, Badara – Zizyphus jujuba and Phalgu – Bauhinia tomentosa is cooked.

This medicated ghee cures diseases caused by Vayu alone (not associated with other Doshas). This medicated ghee has no adverse effects. It is taken internally and used for massage as well as medicated enema. [118 ½ – ½ 122]

Chitrakadi Ghrita for Vata roga:

चित्रकं नागरं रास्नां पौष्करं पिप्पली शटीम्||१२२||

पिष्ट्वा विपाचयेत् सर्पि र्वात रोगहरं परम्|

Ghee cooked with the paste of Chitraka – Leadword – Plumbago zeylanica, nagara – Zingiber officinale, Rasna (Vanda roxburghi / Pluchea lanceolata), Puskara Mula, Pippali – Long pepper fruit – Piper longum, and Sati – Hedychium spicatum cures Vata vyadhis. [122 ½ -1/2 123]

Bala-Bilva ghrita for Nasya:

बला बिल्व शृते क्षीरे घृत मण्डं विपाचयेत्||१२३||

तस्य शुक्तिः प्रकुञ्चो वा नस्यं मूर्धगतेऽनिले|

Milk is boiled by adding Bala – Country mallow (root) – Sida cordifolia and Bilva – Aegle marmelos. Ghrita Manda (upper Part of the ghee) is cooked by adding this milk to it. 1 Sukti (1/2 Pala) or Prakuncha (1 Pala) of this medicated ghee is used for inhalation therapy which cures diseases caused by the aggravated Vayu afflicting the head. [123 ½- ½ 124]

Medicated Bone Marrow:

ग्राम्यानूपौदकानां तु भित्वाऽस्थीनि पचेज्जले||१२४||

तं स्नेहं दशमूलस्य कषायेण पुनः पचेत्| जीवकर्षभका स्फोता विदारी कपिकच्छुभिः||१२५||

वातघ्नै र्जीवनीयैश्च कल्कैर्दिर्वक्षीरभागिकम्| तत्सिद्धं नावनाभ्यङ्गात्तथा पानानुवासनात्||१२६||

सिरा पर्वास्थि कोष्ठस्थं प्रणुदत्याशु मारुतम्| ये स्युः प्रक्षीणमज्जानः क्षीण शुक्रौजसश्च ये||१२७||

बल पुष्टिकरं तेषामेतत् स्यादमृतोपमम्‌।

Bones of the domesticated (Gramya), Marshy-land (Anupa) and aquatic animals is crushed and cooked by adding Dashamoola Kashaya the paste of

Jivaka – Malaxis acuminata,

Rishabhaka – Manilkara hexandra,

Asphota – Jasminum angustifolium,

Vidari (Ipomoea paniculata / Pueraria tuberosa),

Kapikacchu – Mucuna pruriens, group of Vata-alleviating herbs (vide Vimanasthana 8th chapter) and jeevaneeya gana herbs, and double the quantity of milk.

This medicated bone marrow should be used for

Nasya – inhalation,

Abhyanga – massage and

Basti – medicated enema, and

Taken internally which instantaneously cures diseases of vessels, joints, bone and gastrointestinal tract caused by their affliction with aggravated Vata.

In the patients having diminished bone marrow, semen and Ojas (elan Vitae), this recipe promotes strength and nourishment like ambrosia. [123 -127]

Siddha Vasa – medicated muscle fat

तद्वत्सिद्धा वसा नक्र मत्स्य कूर्म चुलूकजा||१२८||

प्रत्यग्रा विधिनाऽनेन नस्य पानेषु शस्यते।

In the same, above mentioned method, the Vasa – muscle fat of Nakra – crocodile, fish, tortoise and owl are cooked and used for Nasya and oral administration. [128]

Maha sneha – combination of medicated oil, fat, ghee and bone marrow

प्रस्थः स्यात्रिफलायास्तु कुलत्थ कुडव द्वयम्‌||१२९||

कृष्णगन्धात्वगाढक्योः पृथक् पञ्चपलं भवेत्‌। रास्ना चित्रकयोर्द्वे द्वे दशमूलं पलोन्मितम्‌||१३०||

जलद्रोणे पचेत् पाद शेषे प्रस्थोन्मितं पृथक्‌। सुराराम्ल दध्यम्ल सौवीरक तुषोदकम्‌||१३१||

कोल दाडिम वृक्षाम्ल रसं तैलं वसां घृतम्‌। मज्जानं च पयश्चैव जीवनीय पलानि षट्‌||१३२||

कल्कं दत्त्वा महा स्नेहं सम्यगेनं विपाचयेत्‌। सिरा मज्जास्थिगे वाते सर्वाङ्गैकाङ्ग रोगिषु||१३३||

वेपनाक्षेप शूलेषु तदभ्यङ्गे प्रयोजयेत्‌।

Mahasneha –

Ingredients:

In 1 Drona of water,

1 Prastha of Triphala,

2 Kudavas of Kulattha – horse gram,

5 Palas of each of bark of Krishna Gandha (sobhanjana) and Adhaki,

2 Palas of each Rasna and Chitraka – Plumbago zeylanica , and

1 Pala of Dashamula is cooked till 1/4th of it remains. To this decoction,

1 prastha of each of Sura (alcohol), Aranala (preparation of sour gruel), sour Yoghurt, Sauviraka (Vinegar), Tushodaka (a sour preparation of paddy), juice of Kola, Dadima – Pomegranate and Vrukshodaka,

oil, muscle fat, ghee, bone marrow and milk, and the paste of 6 palas of herbs of Jeevaniya group is added and properly cooked.

This Maha Sneha (Preparation of ghee, oil, muscle fat and bone marrow taken together) is used for massage which cures diseases caused by the affliction of Vessels, bones and bone marrow by aggravated Vata, Sarvanga roga, Ekanga roga, tremors, convulsions and colic pain. [129 ½ – ½ 134]

Nirgundi Taila:

निर्गुण्ड्या मूल पत्राभ्यां गृहीत्वा स्वरसं ततः||१३४||

तेन सिद्धं समं तैलं नाडी कुष्ठानिलार्तिषु| हितं पामापचीनां च पानाभ्यञ्जन पूरणम्||१३५||

Oil is cooked by adding equal quantities of –

juice of the roots and leaves of Nirgundi (Vitex negundo).

Oral administration of this taila and massage and as ear drops is useful in fistula, Kushta – skin diseases, diseases caused by Vata, Scabies and Apachi (adenitis in the submandibular and axillary regions). 134 ½ – 135]

कार्पासास्थि कुलत्थानां रसे सिद्धं च वातनुत्|१३६|

Oil cooked with the decoction of cotton seed and Kulattha cures diseases caused by the aggravated Vata. [½ 136]

Mulaka Taila:

मूलक स्वरसे क्षीर समे स्थाप्यं त्र्यहं दधि||१३६||

तस्याम्लस्य त्रिभिः प्रस्थैस्तैल प्रस्थं विपाचयेत्| यष्ट्याह्व शर्करा रास्ना लवणार्द्रक नागरैः||१३७||

सुपिष्टैः पलिकैः पानात्तदभ्यङ्गाच्च वातनुत्|१३८|

1 Prastha of the juice of Mulaka – radish and 1 prastha of milk is added with 1 Prastha of Yoghurt and kept for 3 days. One Prastha of oil is prepared by adding 3 prasthas of this sour preparation, and the fine paste of 1 Pala of each of Yashtimadhu – Glycyhrriza glabra, Sugar, Rasna (Vanda roxburghi / Pluchea lanceolata), Salt, fresh ginger (Ardraka) and dry ginger.

This medicated oil is taken internally, and used for massage to treat Vata disorders. [136 ½- ½ 138]

Panchamuladi taila:

पञ्चमूल कषायेण पिण्याकं बहु वार्षिकम्||१३८||

पक्त्वा तस्य रसं पूत्वा तैल प्रस्थं विपाचयेत्| पयसाऽष्टगुणेनैतत् सर्व वात विकारनुत्||१३९||

संसृष्टे श्लेष्मणा चैतद्वाते शस्तं विशेषतः|

In the decoction of Pancha Mula, many-years-old pinyaka (oil cake of paste of seed from which oil has been extracted) is cooked and the decoction is strained.

In this decoction, 1 Prastha of oil is cooked by adding 8 times of milk. This medicated oil cures all the Vatik diseases.This oil is especially useful when Vayu is associated with vitiated Kapha to produce the ailment. [138 ½ – ½ 140]

Yava Koladi taila:

यव कोल कुलत्थानां श्रेयस्याः शुष्क मूलकात्||१४०||

बिल्वाच्चाञ्जलिमेकैकं द्रवैरम्लै विपाचयेत्| तेन तैलं कषायेण फलाम्लैः कटुभिस्तथा||१४१||

पिष्टैः सिद्धं महावातैरार्तः शीते प्रयोजयेत्|१४२|

1 Anjali of each of Yava – Barley (Hordeum vulgare), Kola- ber, Kulattha – horse gram, Sreyasi (Gaja pippali), dry Radish – Raphanus sativus and Bilva – Aegle marmelos are cooked by adding sour liquids (like sour gruel and curd) and decoction is prepared. Oil is cooked by adding this decoction and the paste of sour fruits (like pomegranate, etc) and pungent ingredients. This medicated oil, while cool, is used for the treatment of patients suffering from serious types of Vatika diseases. [140½ – ½ 142]

Sahachara Taila:

सर्व वात विकाराणां तैलान्यन्यान्यतः शृणु||१४२||

चतुष्प्रयोगाण्यायुष्य बल वर्णकराणि च| रजःशुक्र प्रदोषघ्नान्यपत्यजननानि च||१४३||

निरत्ययानि सिद्धानि सर्व दोषहराणि च| सहाचरतुलायाश्च रसे तैलाढकं पचेत्||१४४||

मूल कल्काद्दशपलं पयो दत्त्वा चतुर्गुणम्| सिद्धेऽस्मिञ्छर्कराचूर्णादष्टादशपलं भिषक्||१४५||

विनीय दारुणेष्वेतद्वातव्याधिषु योजयेत्|

Now listen to the description of other types of medicated oil useful for the treatment of all varieties of Vatika diseases. These oils can be used in 4 different modes (viz., oral intake, massage, nasya and enema).

They promote longevity, strength and complexion. They cure morbidities of menstruations (ovulation) and semen, and help in the procreation of offspring. These are harmless, therapeutically effective and alleviators of all the [3] Doshas.

1 Adhaka of oil is cooked by adding the decoction of 1 Tula of whole plant of Sahachara, the paste of 10 Palas of the root of Sahachar and 4 Adhakas of milk after the oil is cooked, 18 palas of sugar-powder is added to it by the physician. This medicated oil is useful for serious types of Vatika diseases. [142 ½- ½ 146]

Svadamshtradi Taila:

शवदंष्ट्रा स्वरस प्रस्थौ द्वौ समौ पयसा सह||१४६||

षट्पलं शृङ्गवेरस्य गुडस्याष्टपलं तथा| तैल प्रस्थं विपक्वं तैर्ददयात् सर्वानिलार्तिषु||१४७||

जीर्णे तैले च दुग्धेन पेयाकल्पः प्रशस्यते|

1 Prastha of oil is cooked by adding 2 Prasthas of each of the juice (decoction) of Svadamstra – Tribulus and milk, 6 palas of Sringavera- fresh ginger, and 8 palas of Jaggery.

This medicated oil can be used for the types of Vatika diseases. When the oil is digested after its intake, the patient is given Peya (thin gruel) reared by adding milk. [146 ½ – ½ 148]

Baladi Taila

बला शतं गुडूच्याश्च पादं रास्नाष्टभागिकम्||१४८||

जलाढकशते पक्त्वा दश भाग स्थिते रसे| दधिमस्त्विक्षु निर्यास शुक्तैस्तैलाढकं समैः||१४९||

पचेत् साजपयोऽर्धांशैः कल्कैरेभिः पलोन्मितैः| शटी सरल दार्वेला मञ्जिष्ठागुरु चन्दनैः||१५०||

पद्मकातिविषा मुस्त सूर्पपर्णी हरेणुभिः| यष्टयाह्व सुरस व्याघ्रनखर्षभक जीवकैः||१५१||

पलाश रस कस्तूरी नलिका जाति कोषकैः| स्पृक्का कुङ्कुम शैलेय जाती कटुफलाम्बुभिः||१५२||

त्वचा कुन्दुरु कर्पूर तुरुष्क श्रीनि वासकैः| लवङ्ग नखकक्कोल कुष्ठ मांसी प्रियङ्गुभिः||१५३||

स्थौणेय तगर ध्याम वचा मदन पल्लवैः| स नागकेशरैः सिद्धे क्षिपेच्चात्रावतारिते||१५४||

पत्र कल्कं ततः पूतं विधिना तत् प्रयोजयेत्| श्वासं कासं ज्वरं हिक्कां छर्दिं गुल्मान् क्षतं क्षयम्||१५५||

प्लीह शोषावपस्मारमलक्ष्मीं च प्रणाशयेत्| बला तैलमिदं श्रेष्ठं वातव्याधि विनाशनम्||१५६||

(अग्निवेशाय गुरुणा कृष्णात्रेयेण भाषितम्)|

इति बलातैलम्|

Baladi taila:

100 Adhakas of water is boiled by adding 100 palas of

Bala – Country mallow (root) – Sida cordifolia, 25 Palas of guduchi – Tinospora cordifolia and 12 ½ Palas of Rasna (Vanda roxburghi / Pluchea lanceolata) till 1/10th (ten Adhakas) of water remains.

1 Adhaka of oil is cooked by adding the above mentioned decoction, 10 Adhakas of each of

whey,

sugar- cane juice and

vinegar,

5 Adhakas of goat milk, and the paste of 1 pala of each of

Sati – Hedychium spicatum,

Sarala,

Devadaru (Cedrus deodara),

Ela (Elettaria cardamomum Maton) ,

Manjistha – Rubia cordifolia,

Aguru – Aquallaria agallocha,

Chandana (Sandalwood – Santalum album),

Padmaka – Prunus cerasoides,
Ativisa – Aconitum heterophyllum,
Musta (Cyperus rotundus),
Suraparni (Masa parni – Teramnus labialis and mudga parni – Phaseolus trilobus),
Harenu
Yasti Madhu – Glycyhrrhiza glabra,
Surasa – Cinnamonum zeylanica,
Vyaghra Nakha
Rishabhaka – Manilkara hexandra,
Jivaka – Malaxis acuminata,
Juice of Palasa – Butea monosperma,
Kasturi, Nalika, JatiKosa (Mace),
Sprikka, Kunkuma, Shaileya,
Jatiphala – Myristica fragrans,
Katu Phala(Lata Kasturi),
Ambu – pavonia odorata Willd. (Netra Bala – Country mallow (root) – Sida cordifolia),
Tvak – cinnamon
Kunduru – Cassia fistula
Karura, Turaska (Silhaka),
Srinivasaka,
Lavanga – Syzygium aromaticum,
Nakha (Svalpa Nakhi), Kakkola,
Kushta – Saussurea lappa,
Mamsi,
priyangu—Callicarpa macrophylla,
Sthauneya
Tagara – Valerian walichii,
Dhyama
Vaca (Acorus calamus Linn.),
leaves of madana – Randia dumetorum and
Naga Kesara – Mesua ferrea.
When the oil is fully cooked, the container (oil can) is taken out of the fire, and the oil is added with Patra Kalka (Paste of aromatic herbs) and filtered.
Indication:
Shvasa – Bronchial asthma,
Kasa – bronchitis,
Jwara – fever,
Hikka – hiccup,
Chardi – vomiting,
Gulma (Phantom tumor),
phthisis,
Sosha – consumption,
Pliha – splenic disorders,
cachexia,
epilepsy and
inauspiciousness
This is called BalaTaila which is the best for curing Vatika diseases. This recipe was taught to Agnivesha by his preceptor Krsnatreya.

Thus, ends the description of Bala Taila. [148 ½ – ½ 157]

Amrtadya Taila:

अमृतायास्तुलाः पञ्च द्रोणेष्वष्टस्वपां पचेत्||१५७||

पाद शेषे समक्षीरं तैलस्य द्व्याढकं पचेत्| एला मांसी नतोशीर सारिवा कुष्ठ चन्दनैः||१५८||

बला तामलकी मेदा शतपुष्पर्धि जीवकैः | काकोली क्षीरकाकोली श्रावण्यति बला नखैः||१५९||

महाश्रावणि जीवन्ती विदारी कपिकच्छुभिः| शतावरी महामेदा कर्कटाख्या हरेणुभिः||१६०||

वचागोक्षुरकैरण्ड रास्ना काला सहाचरैः| वीरा शल्लकि मुस्तत्वक्पत्रर्षभक बालकैः||१६१||

सहैला कुङ्कुम स्पृक्का त्रिदशाह्वैश्च कार्षिकैः| मञ्जिष्ठायास्त्रिकर्षेण मधुकाष्टपलेन च||१६२||

कल्कैस्तत् क्षीण वीर्याग्नि बल सम्मूढ चेतसः| उन्मादारत्यपस्मारैरार्तांश्च प्रकृतिं नयेत्||१६३||

वातव्याधि हरं श्रेष्ठं तैलाग्र्यममृताह्वयम्| (कृष्णात्रेयेण गुरुणा भाषितं वैद्यपूजितम्)||१६४||

इत्यमृताद्यं तैलम्|

Ingredients and Method:

8 Dronas of water is boiled by adding

5 Tulas of Amrta (Guduchi – Tonospora cordifolia) till 1/4th of water remains.

2 Adhakas of oil is cooked by adding this decoction ,

2 Dronas of milk and the paste of 1 Karsa of each of

ela (brhadela) – Elattaria cardamum

Mamsi – Nardostachys jatamamsi,

Nata (Valeriana wallicii),

Ushira – Vetiver – Vetiveria zizanioides,

Sariva – Indian Sarsaparilla – Hemidesmus indicus,

kustha – Saussera lappa,

Chandana (Sandalwood – Santalum album),

Bala – Country mallow (root) – Sida cordifolia,

Tamalaki – Phyllanthus niruri,

Meda –

Satapuspa – Anethum sowa,

Rddhi,

Jivaka – Malaxis acuminata,

Kakoli – Fritillaria roylei,

Ksira Kakoli

Sravani,

Atibala – Abutilon indicum,

Nakha,

maha sravani, (maha Munditika),

Jivanti – Leptadenia reticulata,

Vidari (Ipomoea paniculata / Pueraria tuberosa),

Kapikacchu – Mucuna pruriens

Satavari – Asparagus racemosus

Mahameda – Polygonatum verticillatum,

karkatakhya

Harenu

Vacha – Acorus calamus

Goksuraka – Tribulus terrestris

Eranda – Ricinus communis

Rasna (Vanda roxburghi / Pluchea lanceolata)

Kala (Kalanusariva)

Sahacara

Vira

Sallaki – Boswellia serrate

Musta (Cyperus rotundus),

Tvak – cinnamon

Patra – Cinnamomum tamala,

Rishabhaka – Manilkara hexandra,

Blaka,

Saha,

Kunkuma

Sprkka and

TriDashahva (deva Daru – Cedrus deodara)

3 Karsas of Manjistha –Rubia cordifolia and

8 palas of Madhuka– Licorice – Glycyrrhiza glabra (yasti Madhu)

This medicated oil causes restoration of normal health of patients who have less of potency, less of digestion, less of strength, less of potency, less power of digestion, less of strength, less of intelligence, and those suffering from insanity, depression (Arati), and epilepsy. It is the foremost among the medicated oils used for curing Vatika diseases. This is called Amrta Taila which is held in high esteem by physicians. It was propounded by the preceptor Krsnatreya. Thus ends description of Amrtadya Taila. [157 ½ – 164]

Rasna Taila:

रास्ना सहस्र निर्यूहे तैल द्रोणं विपाचयेत्| गन्धै हैमवतैः पिष्टैरेलाद्यैश्चानिलार्तिनुत्||१६५||

कल्पोऽयमश्वगन्धायां प्रसारण्यां बलाद्वये| क्वाथ कल्क पयोभिर्वा बलादीनां पचेत् पृथक्||१६६||

इति रास्ना तैलम्|

1 Drona of oil is cooked by adding the decoction of 1000 Palas of Rasna (Vanda roxburghi / Pluchea lanceolata), and the paste of aromatic herbs available in the Himalayas (like Aguru – Aquallaria agallocha, Kushta – Saussurea lappa and Ksemaka) and Ela (Elettaria cardamomum Maton), etc. This medicated oil cures Vatika diseases.

Following the above mentioned procedure, medicated oil is prepared of Ashwagandha – Winter Cherry / Indian ginseng (root) or Prasarani – Paederia foetida or 2 types of Bala – Country mallow (root) – Sida cordifolia.

Similarly, medicated oil can be prepared of Bala – Country mallow (root) – Sida cordifolia, Prasarani – Paedaria foetida and Ashwagandha – Withania somnifera seperetely by adding the decoction and Paste of these herbs along with milk.

Thus, ends the description of Rasna Taila. [165- 166]

Mulakadya Taila:

मूलक स्वरसं क्षीरं तैलं दध्यम्ल काञ्जिकम्| तुल्यं विपाचयेत् कल्कै बला चित्रक सैन्धवैः||१६७||

पिप्पल्यतिविषा रास्ना चविकागुरु शिग्रुकैः| भल्लातक वचा कुष्ठ श्वदंष्ट्रा विश्वभेषजैः||१६८||

पुष्कराह्व शटी बिल्व शताह्वा नत दारुभिः| तत्सिद्धं पीतमत्युग्रान् हन्ति वातात्मकान् गदान्||१६९||

इति मूलकाद्यं तैलम्|

Ingredients and Method of preparing:

Juice of Mulaka – Raphanus sativus,

Ksiram – milk,

Tailam -oil,

Dadhi – curd and

sour Kanji (a preparation of sour gruel) taken in equal quantities is cooked by adding the paste of

bala – Sida cordifolia,

Chitraka – Plumbago zeylanica,

saindhava – rock salt

Pippali – Long pepper fruit – Piper longum,

Ativisa – Aconitum heterophyllum,

Rasna - Vanda roxburghi / Pluchea lanceolata),

Cavika –Piper chaba,

Aguru – Aquillaria agallocha,

Sigru – Moringa oleifera,

Bhallataka - Semecarpus anacardium Linn.

Vaca (Acorus calamus Linn.),

Kushta – Saussurea lappa,

Svadamstra – Tribulus terrestris

Visva Bhesaja,

Puskara Mula – Inula racemosa ,

Sati – Hedychium spicatum,

Bilva – Aegle marmelos,

Satahva,

Nata (Valeriana wallicii) and

Deva daru – Cedrus deodara.

Internal intake of this medicated oil cures even serious types of Vatika diseases. Thus, ends the description of Mulakadya Taila. [167- 169]

Vrusgamuladi Taila:

वृषमूल गुडूच्योश्च द्विशतस्य शतस्य च| चित्रकात् साश्वगन्धाच्च क्वाथे तैलाढकं पचेत्||१७०||

सक्षीरं वायुना भग्ने दद्याज्जर्जरिते तथा| प्राक्तै लावापसिद्धं च भवेदेतद्गुणोत्तरम्||१७१||

इति वृषमूलादि तैलम्|

One Adhaka of oil is cooked by adding the decoction of 200 Palas of each of the root of Vasaka –Adhatoda vasaka and Guduchi – Tinospora cordifolia, and 100 palas of Chitraka – Plumbago zeylanica and Ashwagandha – Withania somnifera (taken together), and milk. This medicated oil is used for the treatment of bone fracture and osteoporosis caused by Vayu

If this medicated oil is cooked by adding the Paste of ingredients mentioned in connection with the medicated oils described before, and then it becomes very effective

Thus, ends the descriptions of Vrsa Mulakadya Taila [170-171]

Mulaka Taila:

रास्ना शिरीष यष्ट्याह्व शुण्ठी सहचरामृताः||१७२||

स्योनाक दारु शम्पाक हयगन्धा त्रिकण्टकाः| एषां दशपलान् भागान् कषायमुपकल्पयेत्||१७३||

ततस्तेन कषायेण सर्वगन्धैश्च कार्षिकैः| दध्यारनाल माषाम्बु मूलकेक्षुरसैः शुभैः||१७४||

पृथक् प्रस्थोन्मितैः सार्धं तैलप्रस्थं विपाचयेत्| प्लीह मूत्रग्रह श्वास कास मारुत रोगनुत्||१७५||

एतन्मूलकतैलाख्यं वर्णायुर्बल वर्धनम्|

इति मूलक तैलम्|

Decoction is prepared of 10 Palas of each of the (root of)

Rasna (Vanda roxburghi / Pluchea lanceolata),

Sirisha (Albizzi lebbeck Benth.),

Yasti Madhu – Glycyhrrhiza glabra

Sunthi – Zingiber officnale

Sahacara – Barleria prionitis

Amrta – Tinospora cordifolia
Syonaka
Deva daru – Cedrus deodara
Samaka
Haya Gandha (Asvagandha – Withania somnifera) and
Tri Kantaka – Tribulus terrestris
1 prastha of oil is cooked by adding this decoction, 1 Prastha of each of Yogurt, Aranala (sour gruel), decoction of Masa, juice of radish and sugar-cane juice, and [the paste of] 1 Karsa of each of Sarva Gandha (group of aromatic herbs).
This medicated oil cures
Pliha (splenic disorders),
Mutra krchrra – retention of urine,
Shvasa – asthma,
Kasa – bronchitis, and
diseases caused by Vayu
This is called Mulaka Taila. It promotes complexion, longevity and strength.
Thus, ends the descriptions of Mulaka Taila [172-175]

Yavadi taila:

यव कोल कुलत्थानां मत्स्यानां शिग्रु बिल्वयोः| रसेन मूलकानां च तैलं दधि पयोन्वितम्||१७६||
साधयित्वा भिषग्दद्यात् सर्व वातामयापहम्| लशुन स्वरसे सिद्धं तैलमेभिश्च वातनुत्||१७७||
तैलान्येतान्यृतुस्नातामङ्गनां पाययेत च| पीत्वाऽन्यतममेषां हि वन्ध्याऽपि जनयेत् सुतम्||१७८||

Oil is cooked with the decoction of Yava – Barley (Hordeum vulgare), Kola, Kulattha –horse gram, fish, Sigru – Moringa oliefera, Bilva – Aegle marmelos and radish by adding yoghurt and milk. The physician should administer this medicated oil for the cure of all Vatika diseases.
These medicated oils are administered internally after the purificatory bath on the cessation of menstruation, to a woman. By drinking these medicated oils, even a sterile woman becomes capable of giving birth to a son [176-178]

Agurvadi Taila:

यच्च शीतज्वरे तैलमगुर्वाद्यमुदाहृतम्| अनेक शत शस्तच्च सिद्धं स्याद्वातरोगनुत्||१७९||
वक्ष्यन्ते यानि तैलानि वात शोणितकेऽपि च| तानि चानिलशान्त्यर्थं सिद्धिकागः प्रयोजयेत्||१८०||

Agurvadya Taila described for the treatment of Sita – white variety of Cynodon dactylon-Jvara or cold fever (vide Chikitsa 3: 267) is cooked 100 times (by using the same ingredients and same method). This medicated oil cures Vatika diseases.
Medicated oils to be described in the next chapter dealing with the treatment of VayuRakta or gout (vide Chikitsa 29: 88-129) may also be used for the alleviation of Vayu by a physician desirous of professional excellence. [179-180]

Importance of Oil in curing Vatika diseases

नास्ति तैलात् परं किञ्चिदौषधं मारुतापहम्| व्यवाय्युष्ण गुरु स्नेहात् संस्काराद्वलवत्तरम्||१८१||
गणैर्वातहरैस्तस्माच्छतशोऽथ सहस्रशः| सिद्धं क्षिप्रतरं हन्ति सूक्ष्म मार्ग स्थितान् गदान्||१८२||

There is no medication which excels oil in curing Vatika diseases because of its Vyavayi (which pervades the body before going through the Process of digestion), hot, heavy and unctuous properties. When cooked or processed with other herbs, it becomes more powerful therapeutically.
Therefore, oil is cooked for 100 and 1000 times with the group of herbs which all alleviate Vayu. Such medicated oils cure diseases located in the minutest channels of the body quickly. [181-182]

Treatment of diseases caused by Vayu in association with other Doshas:

क्रिया साधारणी सर्वा संसृष्टे चापि शस्यते| वाते पित्तादिभिः स्रोतःस्वावृतेषु विशेषतः||१८३||

All the general therapies described above (for the treatment of diseases caused by Vata alone) are also useful when Vata is associated with other Doshas, and especially when it is occluded by Pitta, etc., in the channels of circulation [183]

Treatment of Pittavruta Vata – Vata Occluded by Pitta:

पित्तावृते विशेषेण शीतामुष्णां तथा क्रियाम्| व्यत्यासात् कारयेत् सर्पि जीवनीयं च शस्यते||१८४||

धन्व मांसं यवाः शालियार्यापना क्षीर बस्तयः| विरेकः क्षीरपानं च पञ्च मूली बला शृतम्||१८५||

मधुयष्टि बला तैल घृत क्षीरैश्च सेचनम्| पञ्चमूल कषायेण कुर्याद्वा शीतवारिणा||१८६||

If the ailment is caused by the aggravated Vayu occluded by Pitta, then the patient is specially given cooling and heating therapies alternatively administration of Jeevaniya Ghrita (ghee cooked by adding Jivaniya group of herbs). The patient is given the meat of animals inhabiting arid one, barley and Sali type of rice as food. He is give YApana Basti, Ksira Basti (2 types of medicated enema to be described later- vide Siddhi 12: 16), purgation therapy and milk boiled by adding Pancha Mula as well as Bala – Country mallow (root) – Sida cordifolia to drink.

His body is sprinkled with the oil, ghee or milk boiled by adding the decoction of YastiMadhu, Bala – Country mallow (root) – Sida cordifolia or Pancha Mula, or by simple cold water. [184- 186]

Treatment of Vata Occluded by Kapha:

कफावृते यवान्नानि जाङ्गला मृग पक्षिणः| स्वेदास्तीक्ष्णा निरूहाश्च वमनं स विरेचनम्||१८७||

जीर्णं सर्पिस्तथा तैलं तिल सर्षपजं हितम्|

If the ailment is caused by the occlusion of Vayu by Kapha then the patient is given barley and meat of the animals as well as birds inhabiting arid one as food.

He is given strong Swedana (fomentation), Niruha Basti and Vamana as well as Virechana therapies. Old ghee, sesame oil and mustard oil are useful in this condition. [187- ½ 188]

Association of Kapha and Pitta:

संसृष्टे कफपित्ताभ्यां पित्तमादौ विनिर्जयेत्||१८८||

If Kapha and Pitta both are associated with Vata to cause the disease, then in the beginning, therapies are given for the alleviation of Pitta [and Kapha is subdued latter]. [188 ½]

Treatment of Vata Associated with Kapha and Pitta:

आमाशयगतं मत्वा कफं वमनमाचरेत्||१८९||

पक्वाशये विरेकं तु पित्ते सर्वत्रगे तथा| स्वेदे विष्यन्दितः श्लेष्मा यदा पक्वाशये स्थितः||१९०||

पित्तं वा दर्शयेल्लिङ्गं बस्तिभिस्तौ विनिर्हरेत्| श्लेष्मणाऽनुगतं वातमुष्णै र्गोमूत्र संयुतैः||१९१||

निरूहैः पित्त संसृष्टं निर्हरेत् क्षीर संयुतैः| मधुरौषध सिद्धैश्च तैलैस्तमनुवासयेत्||१९२||

शिरोगते तु सकफे धूम नस्यादि कारयेत्| हृते पित्ते कफे यः स्यादुरःस्रोतोऽनुगोऽनिलः||१९३||

सशेषः स्यात् क्रिया तत्र कार्या केवल वातिकी|

If the aggravated Vata, in association with Kapha, gets located in the stomach, then the patient is given emetic therapy.

If they are located in the colon, then the patient is given purgation therapy.

If Vata, in association with Pitta, pervades the entire body (including the stomach and colon), then also purgation therapy is given.

If Kapha liquefied by fomentation therapy gets located in the colon or if the signs and symptoms of Pitta are manifested, then both these morbidities are to be eliminated by enema therapy.

If Vata is associated with Kapha, then Niruha type of medicated enema is administered with a recipe added with cow's urine.

If Vayu is associated with Pitta, then Niruha Basti is administered with a recipe added with milk.

To such a patient (Vayu associated with Pitta), Anuvasana Basti prepared by boiling with a group of sweet herbs is used.

If Vayu associated with Kapha gets located in the head, then the patient is given Dhuma (fumigation therapy) and inhalation therapies

If after the elimination of Pitta and Kapha, the residual Vayu gets located in the channels of the chest, then therapies prescribed for Vayu alone is administered [189- ½ 194]

Raktavrita Vata Chikitsa:

शोणितेनावृते कुर्याद्वात शोणितकीं क्रियाम्||१९४||

If Vata is occluded by Rakta (blood), then the therapies prescribed for the treatment of vata Rakta or gout (in the next chapter) are to be administered. [194 ½]

Amavata Chikitsa: Treatment of Vata Associated with Ama:

प्रमेह वात मेदोघ्नीमामवाते प्रयोजयेत्|

If Vata is associated with Ama (uncooked product of digestion and metabolism), then therapies prescribed for Prameha (obstinate urinary disorders including diabetes), Vatika disorders and adiposity are to be administered. [1/2 195]

Treatment of Mamsavruta Vata Dosha – Vata Occluded by Muscle tissue:

स्वेदाभ्यङ्ग रस क्षीर स्नेहा मांसावृते हिताः||१९५||

If Vayu is occluded by Mamsa (muscle tissue), then fomentation, massage, meat-soup, milk and fat are useful [195]

Occlusion of Vayu by Bone marrow and Semen:

महा स्नेहोऽस्थि मज्जस्थे पूर्ववद्रेतसाऽऽवृते|

If Vayu is occluded by bone and bone marrow, then the patient is given Maha Sneha (vide description in verse nos. [129 ½ – 133]

If Vayu is located by semen, then the therapies prescribed earlier for the treatment of affliction of semen by Vayu (vide verse no. 94) is given [½ 196]

Occlusion of Vayu by Food:

अन्नावृते तदुल्लेखः पाचनं दीपनं लघु||१९६||

If Vayu is occluded by food, then emesis, Pachana (carminative) Dipana (digestive Stimulant) and light diet is given. [196 ½]

Occlusion of Vayu by Urine:

मूत्रलानि तु मूत्रेण स्वेदाः सोत्तरबस्तयः|

If Vata is occluded by urine then diuretics, fomentation and Uttara Basti (urethral Douches) is given. [½ 197]

Occlusion of Vata by Feces:

शकृता तैलमैरण्डं स्निग्धोदावर्तवत्क्रिया ||१९७||

If Vata is occluded by feces, then castor oil and oleation therapy as indicated for Udavarta (upward movement of wind in the abdomen – vide Chikitsa 26: 11-44) is given. [197 ½]

Treatment of Doshas Located in Their Own Habitat:

स्वस्थानस्थो बली दोषः प्राक् तं स्वैरौषधैर्जयेत्| वमनैर्वा विरेकैर्वा बस्तिभिः शमनेन वा||१९८||

(इत्युक्तमावृते वाते पित्तादिभिर्यथायथम्)|१९९|

A morbid Dosha located in its own habitat becomes more powerful. Therefore, first of all such Doshas are subdued by the administration of appropriate therapies like emesis, purgation, medicated enema and alleviation therapies. Thus, ends the treatment of diseases caused by Vata being occluded by Pitta, etc. [198- ½ 199]

Mutual Occlusion of Five Varieties of Vata:

मारुतानां हि पञ्चानामन्योन्यावरणे शृणु||१९९||

लिङ्गं व्याससमासाभ्यामुच्यमानं मयाऽनघ!| प्राणो वृणोत्युदानादीन् प्राणं वृण्वन्ति तेऽपि च||२००||

उदानाद्यास्तथाऽन्योन्यं सर्व एव यथाक्रमम्| विंशतिर्वरणान्येतान्युल्बणानां परस्परम्||२०१||

मारुतानां हि पञ्चानां तानि सम्यक् प्रतर्कयेत्|

The signs and symptoms of the mutual occlusion of 5 varities of Vata will be described hereafter in extensor as well as in brief. O! Sinless one (addressed to the disciple Agnivesha), Listen to these descriptions.

Prana Vata occludes other 4 varieties of Vayu, Viz.., Udana Vayu, etc.., and they in turn occlude Prana Vayu. These 4 types of Vayu (viz. Udana, Samana, Vyana and Apana) also occlude each other. These 5 types of Vayu, when aggravated, occlude each other, thus resulting in 20 types of occlusions. The physician should properly understand these conditions. [199 ½ – ½ 202]

Pranavrita Vyana vata –

सर्वेन्द्रियाणां शून्यत्वं ज्ञात्वा स्मृति बल क्षयम्||२०२||

व्याने प्राणावृते लिङ्गं कर्म तत्रोर्ध्वजत्रुकम्|

Signs and treatment of Vyana Vayu Occluded by Prana Vayu:

If Vyana Vayu is occluded by Prana Vayu, then there will be loss of the functions of all the senses, and there will be loss of memory as well as strength. This condition is treated by the administration of therapies prescribed for supra clavicular diseases. [202 ½ – ½ 203]

Vyanavrita Prana –

स्वेदोऽत्यर्थं लोमहर्षस्त्वग्दोषः सुप्त गात्रता||२०३||

प्राणे व्यानावृते तत्र स्नेहयुक्तं विरेचनम्|

Signs and Treatment of Prana Vayu Occluded by Vyana Vayu:

If Prana Vayu is occluded by Vyana Vayu, then there will be

Ati sveda – excessive sweating,

Loma harsha – horripilation,

Tvak dosha – skin- diseases and

Supta gatrata – Numbness in the body.

To such patients, purgation therapy with medicated oil is administered. [203 ½- ½ 204]

Pranavrita Samana Vata:

प्राणावृते समाने स्युर्जडगद्गद मूकताः||२०४||

चतुष्प्रयोगाः शस्यन्ते स्नेहास्तत्र सयापनाः|

Signs and treatment of Samana Vayu Occluded by PranaVata

If Samana Vata is occluded by Prana Vata, then there will be differences in speech, slurring speech and even dumbness.

For such patients, Yapana Basti (a type of medicated enema) and administration of medicated fat in 4 different ways are beneficial. [204 ½- ½ 205]

Samanavrita Apana –

समानेनावृतेऽपाने ग्रहणी पार्श्व हृद्गदाः||२०५||

शूलं चामाशये तत्र दीपनं सर्पिरिष्यते|२०६|

Signs and Treatment of Apana Vayu Occluded by Samana Vayu:

If Apana Vayu is occluded by Samana Vayu, then there will be diseases of
Grahani (duodenum),
Parshva hrud gadah – diseases of the sides of the chest and heart, and
Aamshaya shoolam – colic Pain in the stomach.
To such patients, Dipana Sarpis (medicated ghee prepared by boiling it with digestive stimulants) is given [205 ½ – ½ 206]

Pranavrita Udana: Signs and Treatment of Udana Vata occulated by Prana Vata:

शिरोग्रहः प्रतिश्यायो निःश्वासोच्छ्वास सङ्ग्रहः||२०६||
हृद्रोगो मुखशोषश्चाप्युदाने प्राणसंवृते| तत्रोर्ध्वभागिकं कर्म कार्यमाश्वासनं तथा||२०७||

If Udana Vata is located by Prana Vata, then there will be
Shiro graha – stiffness of the head,
Pratishyaya – rhinitis,
Nihshvasa ucchshvasa – obstruction to inspiration and expiration,
Hrud roga – heart- diseases and
Mukha sosha – dryness of the mouth.
For such patients prescribed for the treatment of the diseases of head and neck is given, and the patient is comforted [206 ½ – 207]

Udanavrita Prana: Signs and Treatment of Prana Vayu Occluded by Udana Vayu:

कर्मैंजो बल वर्णानां नाशो मृत्युर्थापि वा| उदानेनावृते प्राणे तं शनैः शीत वारिणा||२०८||
सिञ्चेदाश्वासयेच्चैनं सुखं चैवोपपादयेत्|

If Prana Vayu is occulated by Udana Vata, then there will be loss of the functions (of Different parts of the body). Ojas (vital essence), strength and complexion there may even be the death of the patient. He is slowly sprinkled with cold water, consoled and comforted. [208- ½ 209]

Udanavrita Apana: Signs and Treatment of Apana Occluded By Udana Vata:

उर्ध्वगेनावृतेऽपाने छर्दि श्वासादयो गदाः||२०९||
स्युर्वाते तत्र बस्त्यादि भोज्यं चैवानुलोमनम्|

If Apana Vayu is occluded by Udana Vata, then there will be vomiting and diseases like Asthma. To such patients, medicated enema and such food as would cause downward movement of Vata is given. [209 ½ – ½ 210]

Apanavrita udana: Signs and treatment of Udana Vata Occluded by Apana Vayu

मोहोऽल्पोऽग्निरतीसार ऊर्ध्वगेऽपानसंवृते||२१०||
वाते स्याद्वमनं तत्र दीपनं ग्राहि चाशनम्|

If Udana Vata is occluded by Apana Vata, then there will be
Moho – unconsciousness
Alpa agni – suppression of the power of digestion and
Atisara – diarrhoea.
To such patients, emetic therapy, digestive stimulants and astringent ingredients is giving for the downward movement of the wind in the stomach. [210 ½ – ½ 211]

Vyanavrita Apana: Signs and Treatment of Apana Vata Occluded by Vyana Vata:

वम्याध्मानमुदावर्त गुल्मार्ति परिकर्तिकाः||२११||
लिङ्गं व्यानावृतेऽपाने तं स्निग्धैरनुलोमयेत्|

If Apana Vata is occluded by Vyana Vata, then there will be
Vamya – vomiting

Aadhmana – abdominal distension
Udavarta – upward movement of Vata
Gulma – phantom tumor and
Parikartika – sawing pain in the abdomen [211 ½ – ½ 212]

Apanavrita Vyana: Signs and Treatment of Vyana Vata Occluded By Apana Vata

अपानेनावृते व्याने भवेद्विण्मूत्र रेतसाम्||२१२||

अतिप्रवृत्तिस्तत्रापि सर्वं सङ्ग्रहणं मतम्|

If Vyana Vata is occluded by Apana Vayu, then there will be excessive discharge of stool, urine and semen

For such patients, all types of astringent are given. [212 ½- ½ 213]

Samanavrita Vyana: Signs and Treatment of Vyana Vayu Occluded by Samana Vata:

मूर्च्छा तन्द्रा प्रलापोऽङ्गसादोऽग्न्योजो बल क्षयः||२१३||

समानेनावृते व्याने व्यायामो लघु भोजनम्|

If Vyana –Vata is occluded by Samana Vata, then there will be unconsciousness / fainting, sleepiness / drowsiness, delirium, weakness in body parts, deterioration of digestive power, strength and ojus.
For such patients, exercise and light foods shall be advocated. [213 ½ – ½ 214]

Udanavrita Vyana: Signs and treatment of Vyana Vata Occluded by Udana Vata

स्तब्धताऽल्पाग्निताऽस्वेदश्चेष्टाहानि निर्मीलनम्||२१४||

उदानेनावृते व्याने तत्र पथ्यं मितं लघु|

If Vyana Vata is occluded by Udana Vayu, then there will be
Stabdhata – stiffness,
Alpa agni – less of Agni (digestive enzymes),
Alpa sweda – less of sweating,
Alpa chesta – lack of efforts and
Nirmilinam – closure of the eyes
To such patients, a wholesome and light diet is given in limited quantities. [214 ½ – ½ 215]

Effects of Occlusion in General:

पञ्चान्योन्यावृतानेवं वातान् बुध्येत लक्षणैः||२१५||

एषां स्व कर्मणां हानिवृद्धिर्वाऽऽवरणे मता| यथास्थूलं समुद्दिष्टमेतदावरणेऽष्टकम्||२१६||

सलिङ्ग भेषजं सम्यग्बुधानां बुद्धि वृद्धये|२१७|

Thus, mutual occlusions of 5 types of Vata are diagnosed from their signs and symptoms. In the event of such an occlusion, there is either increase or decrease of the functions (actions) of the particular type of Vayu.
These 8 types of occlusion along with their signs and treatment are described for the proper understanding of intelligent physicians. [215 ½ – ½ 217]

Remaining Twelve Types of Occlusions:

स्थानान्यवेक्ष्य वातानां वृद्धिं हानिं च कर्मणाम्||२१७||

द्वादशावरणान्यन्यान्यभिलक्ष्य भिषग्जितम्| कुर्यादभ्यञ्जन स्नेहपान बस्त्यादि सर्वशः||२१८||

क्रममुष्णमनुष्णं वा व्यत्यासादवचारयेत्|२१९|

After examining the locations and increase as well as decrease of the functions, the remaining 12 types of occlusions are ascertained. For their treatment, massage, drinking of unctuous potions, medicated enema, etc., are used in their entirety. Hot and cold therapies are administered to such patients alternatively. [217 ½ – ½ 219]

General line of treatment of five types of Vata Dosha:

उदानं योजयेदूर्ध्वमपानं चानुलोमयेत्||२१९||

समानं शमयेच्चैव त्रिधा व्यानं तु योजयेत्| प्राणो रक्ष्यश्चतुर्भ्योऽपि स्थाने ह्यस्य स्थितिर्ध्रुवा||२२०||

स्वं स्थानं गमयेदेवं वृतानेतान् विमार्गगान्|२२१|

For the morbidity of Udana Vata, upward moving therapy (emesis) is administered.

For the morbidity of Apana Vata, downward moving therapy (purgation and medicated enema) is employed.

For the morbidity of Samana Vata, the therapy which causes stability in the abdomen (by alleviation) is used.

For the morbidity of Vyana Vata, all the above mentioned 3 categories of therapies are employed.

Prana Vata is more important than these 4 types of Vata; hence it is protected with priority. Its state of equilibrium helps in the sustenance of life.

These Vayus, when occluded, go Astray (move in different channels). Therefore, they are brought to their own habitat. [219 ½ – ½ 221]

Occlusion of Prana Vata by Pitta:

मूर्च्छा दाहो भ्रमः शूलं विदाहः शीतकामिता||२२१||

छर्दनं च विदग्धस्य प्राणे पित्त समावृते|

If Prana Vayu is occluded by Pitta, then this gives rise to

Murcha – fainting

Daha – burning sensation

Bhrama – giddiness

Shoola – colic pain

Vidaha – indigestion,

Sheeta kamita – desire for cold things and

Vidagdha chardana – vomiting of undigested food. [221 ½ – ½ 222]

Occlusion of Prana Vayu by Kapha:

ष्ठीवनं क्षवथूद्गार निःश्वासोच्छ्वास सङ्ग्रहः||२२२||

प्राणे कफावृते रूपाण्यरुचिश्छर्दिरेव च|

If Prana Vayu is occluded by Kapha, then there will be

Sthivanam – excessive spitting of Saliva

Kshavathu – sneezing

Udgara – eructation

Nihshvasa ucchvasa nigraha – obstruction to inspiration and expiration,

Aruchi – anorexia and

Chardi – vomiting [222 ½- ½ 223]

Occlusion of Udana Vata by Pitta

मूर्च्छाद्यानि च रूपाणि दाहो नाभ्युरसः क्लमः||२२३||

ओजोभ्रंशश्च सादश्चाप्युदाने पित्तसंवृते|

If Udana Vayu is occluded by Pitta, then there will be fainting etc, was described in verse no 221 ½ above), burning sensation in the umbilical region and chest, exhaustion, loss of Ojas (vital essence) and prostration. [223 ½ – ½ 224]

Occlusion of Udana Vata by Kapha:

आवृते श्लेष्मणोदाने वैवर्ण्य वाक्स्वरग्रहः||२२४||

दौर्बल्यं गुरुगात्रत्वमरुचिश्चोपजायते|

If Udana Vayu is occluded by Kapha, then there will be

Vaivarnyam – discoloration of the skin,

Vak svara graha – obstruction to speech and voice,

Daurbala – weakness and

Guru gatratva – heaviness of the body and

Aruchi – anorexia.

Occlusion of Samana Vata by Pitta:

अतिस्वेदस्तृषा दाहो मूर्च्छा चारुचिरेव च||२२५||

पित्तावृते समाने स्यादुपघातस्तथोष्मणः|

If Samana Vata is occluded by Pitta, then there will be

Ati sveda – excessive sweating

Ati trsha – thirst,

Daha – burning sensation

Murchha – fainting,

Aruchi – anorexia and

loss of body- heat. [225 ½ – ½ 226]

Occlusion of Samana Vayu by Kapha:

अस्वेदो वह्निमान्द्यं च लोमहर्षस्तथैव च||२२६||

कफावृते समाने स्याद्गात्राणां चातिशीतता|

If Samana Vayu gets occlude by Kapha, then there will be

Asveda – absence of sweating

Vahni mandya – suppression of the power of digestion

Loma harsha – horriplation and

Ati shitata – excessive cold feeling in the body. [226 ½ – 227]

Obstruction of Vyana Vayu by Pitta

व्याने पित्तावृते तु स्याद्दाहः सर्वाङ्गगगः क्लमः||२२७||

गात्र विक्षेप सङ्गश्च स सन्तापः स वेदनः|

If Vyana Vata is occluded by Pitta, then there is

Sarvanga daha – burning sensation all over the body,

Klamah – exhaustion and

Gatra vikshepa sanga – arrest of the mobility in different parts of the body accompanied with Sa santapa, Sa vedana - burning sensation and pain. [227 ½ – ½ 228]

Obstruction of Vyana Vata by Kapha:

गुरुता सर्वगात्राणां सर्व सन्ध्यस्थिजा रुजः||२२८||

व्याने कफावृते लिङ्गं गति सङ्गस्तथाऽधिकः |

If Vyana Vayu is located by Kapha, then there is

Gurugatrata – heaviness all over the body and

arrest of the mobility in different parts of the body accompanied with burning sensation and pain.[228 ½- ½ 229]

Occlusion of Apana Vayu by Pitta:

हारिद्र मूत्र वर्चस्त्वं तापश्च गुद मेढ्योः||२२९||

लिङ्गं पित्तावृतेऽपाने रजसश्चातिवर्तनम्|

If Apana Vayu is occluded by Pitta, then there is yellow coloration of the urine and stool, sensation of heat in the anus and phallus, and menorrhagia. [229 ½- ½ 230]

Occlusion of Apana Vayu by Kapha

भिन्नामश्लेष्म संसृष्ट गुरुवर्चःप्रवर्तनम्||२३०||
श्लेष्मणा संवृतेऽपाने कफमेहस्य चागमः|२३१|

If Apana Vata is occluded by Kapha, then the patient will avoid stool which is loose, mixed with Ama (mucus or undigested food) and heavy. There will be Kaphaja Meha (obstinate urinary disorders caused by Kapha). [230 ½ – ½ 231]

Occlusion by Both Pitta and Kapha:

लक्षणानां तु मिश्रत्वं पित्तस्य च कफस्य च||२३१||
उपलक्ष्य भिषग्विद्वान् मिश्रमावरणं वदेत्|

When any one of these varieties of Vata is occluded by both Pitta and Kapha together, then the wise physician should ascertain this condition from the signs and symptoms of both Pitta and Kapha as described before. [231 ½ -1/2 232]

Location of Pitta and Kapha in the Habitat of Vata:

यद्यस्य वायो निर्दिष्टं स्थानं तत्रेतरौ स्थितौ||२३२||
दोषौ बहु विधान् व्याधीन् दर्शयेतां यथानिजान्|

If Pitta and Kapha get located in the habitats of Vata, then this causes manifestation of various disorders, characteristic of each one or both of them. [232 ½ – ½ 233]

Prognosis of Occlusions: Avarana Upashaya:

आवृतं श्लेष्म पित्ताभ्यां प्राणं चोदानमेव च||२३३||
गरीयस्त्वेन पश्यन्ति भिषजः शास्त्र चक्षुषः| विशेषाज्जीवितं प्राणे उदाने संश्रितं बलम्||२३४||
स्यातयोः पीडनाद्धानिरायुषश्च बलस्य च| सर्वेऽप्येतेऽपरिज्ञाताः परि संवत्सरास्तथा||२३५||
उपेक्षणादसाध्याः स्युरथवा दुरुपक्रमाः |२३६|

Expert physicians view the obstruction (occlusion) of Prana Vata and Udana Vata by both Kapha and Pitta as a serious condition. Therefore, these occlusions lead to loss of life and vitality.
If undiagnosed or if diagnosed correctly but not treated properly or if the treatment is neglected for more than a year, then all these ailments become incurable or difficult to cure. [233 ½- ½ 236]

Complications of Avarana – Occlusion:

हृद्रोगो विद्रधिः प्लीहा गुल्मोऽतीसार एव च||२३६||
भवन्त्युपद्रवास्तेषामावृतानामुपेक्षणात्| तस्मादावरणं वैद्यः पवनस्योपलक्षयेत्||२३७||
पञ्चात्मकस्य वातेन पित्तेन श्लेष्मणाऽपि वा|

Neglect of these occlusions leads to complications like

Hrud roga – heart disease

Vidradhi – abscesses

Pliha – splenic disorders

Gulma (phantom tumor) and

Atisara – diarrhoea.

Therefore, the physician should properly examine and ascertain the occlusion of these 5 Varieties of Vayu by other varieties of Vayu, Pitta and Kapha. [236 ½- ½ 238]

Avarana Chikitsa Sutra: Line of Treatment of Occlusion:

भिषग्जितमतः सम्यगुपलक्ष्य समाचरेत्||२३८||
अनभिष्यन्दिभिः स्निग्धैः स्रोतसां शुद्धिकारकैः| कफ पित्ताविरुद्धं यद्यच्च वातानुलोमनम्||२३९||
सर्वस्थानावृतेऽप्याशु तत् कार्यं मारुते हितम्| यापना बस्तयः प्रायो मधुराः सानुवासनाः||२४०||
प्रसमीक्ष्य बलाधिक्यं मृदु वा स्रंसनं हितम्| रसायनानां सर्वेषामुपयोगः प्रशस्यते||२४१||

शैलस्य जतुनोऽत्यर्थं पयसा गुग्गुलोस्तथा| लेहं वा भार्गव प्रोक्तमभ्यसेत् क्षीर भुड्नरः||२४२||

अभयामलकीयोक्तमेकादश सिताशतम्| अपानेनावृते सर्व दीपनं ग्राहि भेषजम्||२४३||

वातानुलोमनं यच्च पक्वाशय विशोधनम्| इति सङ्क्षेपतः प्रोक्तमावृतानां चिकित्सितम्||२४४||

प्राणादीनां भिषक् कुर्यादिवतर्क्य स्वयमेव तत्| पित्तावृते तु पित्तघ्नैर्मारुतस्याविरोधिभिः|

कफावृते कफघ्नैस्तु मारुतस्यानुलोमनैः||२४५||

Avarana Chikitsa Sutra: Line of Treatment of Occlusion:

After proper examination, the patient is treated with therapies which are Anabhisyandi (do not cause obstruction to the channels of circulation), which are unctuous and which help in the cleansing of the channels of circulation.

If Vayu is occluded in all its locations, then prompt administration of therapies which are not antagonistic of Kapha and Pitta, but which causes downward movement of Vata is beneficial.

Yapana Basti prepared with sweet herbs accompanied with Anuvasana type of medicated enema is generally useful. If the patient is strong, then mild laxative is beneficial.

Administration of all types of rejuvenating recipes, Shilajatu and Guggulu (Commifora mukul Engl.) along with milk is useful in this ailment.

The patient should take Chyavana Prasa (described in Chikitsa 1:1:62-74) prepared with 100 Palas of Sugar, regularly along with milk as food.

If the occlusion occurs due to Apana Vata, then all therapies which are stimulants of digestion, which are astringent, which cause downward movement of Vata, and which cleanse the colon are given.

Thus, in brief, the treatment of various types of occlusions by Prana Vayu, etc. is described. The physician himself should use his own discretion to find out the details of the relevant therapeutic measures.

If there is occlusion of Vata by Pitta, then therapy which alleviates Pitta does not work against Vayu. If the occlusion of vayu by Kapha takes place, then therapies which alleviate Kapha and one which cause downward movement of Vata is administered. [238 ½ -245]

Need for Proper Examination:

लोके वाय्वर्कसोमानां दुर्विज्ञेया यथा गतिः| तथा शरीरे वातस्य पित्तस्य च कफस्य च||२४६||

As the movements of the wind, sun and moon in the macrocosm are difficult to comprehend, similarly, the activities of Vata, Pitta and Kapha in the body (microcosm) are difficult to ascertain.

The physician, who after ascertaining the states of diminution, aggravation, equilibrium and occlusion of these Doshas, administers [appropriate] therapies, never fails to be successful in his efforts. [246-247]

Summary:

तत्र श्लोकौ-

पञ्चात्मनः स्थानवशाच्छरीरे स्थानानि कर्माणि च देहधातोः| प्रकोप हेतुः कुपितश्च रोगान् स्थानेषु चान्येषु वृतोऽवृतश्च||२४८||

प्राणेश्वरः प्राणभृतां करोति क्रिया च तेषामखिला निरुक्ता| तां देश सात्म्यर्तुबलान्यवेक्ष्य प्रयोजयेच्छास्त्रमतानुसारी||२४९||

In this chapter, in view of contextual property, the following aspects of the sustainer of life, i.e Vata with its 5 varieties are described:

The locations and functions

Cause of their aggravation

The diseases caused in living beings by these aggravated varieties of Vata in their own locations or in other locations, and while being occluded or otherwise (not being occluded) and

Details of the therapeutic measures for the treatment of these diseases.

For the treatment of these diseases, the physician should administer appropriate therapies guided by the description in Ayurvedic scriptures after examining the habitat, wholesomeness, seasonal effects and the strength of the patient. [248-249]

इत्यग्निवेशकृते तन्त्रे चरक प्रति संस्कृतेऽप्राप्ते दृढबल सम्पूरिते चिकित्सा स्थाने वातव्याधि चिकित्सितं नामाष्टाविंशोऽध्यायः||२८||

Thus, ends the 28th chapter dealing with the "Treatment of Vatika Diseases" in the Chikitsa section of the text by Agnivesha, redacted by Charaka and supplemented by Dridhabala.

12

Chikitsasthana Chapter 29
Vatarakta Chikitsitam

The 29th chapter of Charaka Samhita Chikitsa Sthana deals with causes, types and treatment for Vatarakta, a condition often correlated with Gout.

अथातो वात शोणित चिकित्सितं व्याख्यास्यामः||१||

इति ह स्माह भगवानात्रेयः||२||

We shall now expound the chapter on "the treatment of Vata Shonita. Thus, said Lord Atreya. [1-2]

Agnivesha's Query and Atreya's Reply:

हुताग्निहोत्र मासीनमृषि मध्ये पुनर्वसुम्| पृष्टवान् गुरुमेकाग्रमग्निवेशोऽग्नि वर्चसम्||३||

अग्नि मारुत तुल्यस्य संसर्गस्यानिलासृजोः| हेतु लक्षण भैषज्यान्यथास्मै गुरुरब्रवीत्||४||

While the preceptor Atreya Punarvasu, glowing like fire, was seated in an attentive mood surrounded by saints after completing his Agnihotra (ritual of offering oblation to fire), Agnivesha requested him to explain the etiology, symptoms and treatment of the ailment caused by the simultaneous aggravation of both Vata and Rakta (blood) which is like the combination of the wind and fire. The Guru answered as below:[3-4]

Vatarakta Nidana and Samprapti

लवणाम्ल कटु क्षार स्निग्धोष्णाजीर्ण भोजनैः| क्लिन्न शुष्काम्बुजानूप मांस पिण्याक मूलकैः||५||

कुलत्थ माष निष्पाव शाकादि पललेक्षुभिः| दध्यारनाल सौवीर शुक्त तक्र सुरासवैः||६||

विरुद्धाध्यशन क्रोध दिवास्वप्न प्रजागरैः| प्रायशः सुकुमाराणां मिष्टान्न सुखभोजिनाम्||७||

अचङ्क्रमणशीलानां कुप्यते वातशोणितम्| अभिघातादशुद्ध्या च प्रदुष्टे शोणिते नृणाम्||८||

कषाय कटु तिक्ताल्प रूक्षाहारादभोजनात्| हयोष्ट्रयानयानाम्बु क्रीडा प्लवन लङ्घनैः||९||

उष्ण चात्यध्व वैषम्याद्व्यवायाद्वेग निग्रहात्| वायु विवृद्धो वृद्धेन रक्तेनावारितः पथि||१०||

कृत्स्नं सन्दूषयेद्रक्तं तज्ज्ञेयं वातशोणितम्| खुडं वात बलासाख्यमाढ्यवातं च नामभिः||११||

Causes and pathophysiology of Vatarakta:

Generally people of tender health who indulge in sweet food, leisurely eating and sedentary habits get afflicted by Vatarakta because of the following:

lavaṇāmla kaṭu kṣāra snigdhoṣṇājīrṇa bhojanaihi – Excessive intake of salt, sour, pungent, alkaline, unctuous, hot and uncooked food.

klinna śuṣkāmbujānūpa māmsa piṇyāka mūlakaiḥ – Intake of putrefied or dry meat of aquatic (Ambuja) or marshy land (Anupa) inhabiting animals

kulattha māṣa niṣpāva śākādipalalekṣubhiḥ – Excessive intake of oil-cake preparation or radish, excessive intake of Kulattha – horse gram, black gram, Nisava, Leafy vegetables, etc. meat and sugarcane

dadhyāranāla sauvīra śukta takra surāsavaiḥ – Excessive intake of curd, Aranala(Kanji), Sauvira (sour preparation of

• 246 •

dehusked barley), Sukta (vinegar), Buttermilk, alcohol and wine,

Virudhha ahara – Intake of mutually contradictory food.

Adhyashana – Intake of food before the previous meal is digested

Ati Krodha – Resorting to anger in excess

Divasvapna – Sleeping during day time and

Prajagara – remaining awake at night.

miṣṭānna sukhabhojinām – sweet food, leisurely eating

achankramanashila – sedentary habits

Pathogenesis of Vatarakta - The blood gets vitiated due to Abhighata (injury) and Ashuddhi (skipping seasonal Panchakarma therapies)

Following this when the person gets indulged in the below mentioned, vata would get aggravated –

Kashaya katu tikta alpa ruksha aharat na bhojanat – excessive consumption of astringent, pungent, bitter foods, foods in less quantity, dry foods and not taking food at all,

hayoṣṭrayānayānāmbu krīḍā – Riding over horses, camels or on vehicles drawn by them

plavana laṅghanaiḥ – Resorting to aquatic games, swimming and jumping

vaiṣamyādvyavāyādvega nigrahāt – Excessive wayfaring in hot season, which disturbs the equilibrium of Vata

Ati maithuna – Indulgence in sexual intercourse and

Vega nigrahat – Suppression of the manifested natural urges.

Being obstructed in its course by the vitiated blood, the excessively aggravated Vata vitiates the entire blood. The disease thus caused is called Vata-Rakta (gout).

It is also known by the synonyms like Kuddha, Vata Balasa and Adya Vata. [5-11]

Parts of Body Affected By Vatarakta:

तस्य स्थानं करौ पादावङ्गुल्यः सर्व सन्धयः| कृत्वाऽऽदौ हस्त पादे तु मूलं देहे विधावति||१२||

सौक्ष्म्यात् सर्व सरत्वाच्च पवनस्यासृजस्तथा| तद्द्रवत्वात् सरत्वाच्च देहं गच्छन् सिरायनैः||१३||

पर्व स्वभिहतं क्षुब्धं वक्रत्वादवतिष्ठते| स्थितं पित्तादि संसृष्टं तास्ताः सृजति वेदनाः||१४||

करोति दुःखं तेष्वेव तस्मात् प्रायेण सन्धिषु| भवन्ति वेदनास्तास्ता अत्यर्थं दुःसहा नृणाम्||१५||

The sites where Vatarakta is manifested are –

hands, feet, fingers including toes and all joints. In the beginning, the hands and feet are afflicted. From this base, it spreads to all other body parts because of the subtle (Sookshma) pervasive nature of Vata and Rakta.

Because of thcir fluidity (Dravatvaat) and mobility (Saratvaat), they (Vata and Rakta), while moving through the vessels; get obstructed in the joints which makes them further aggravated. Because of the tortuous nature of the course in the joints, the morbid matter gets lodged there.

Being localized in joints, they get further associated with Pitta, etc., (i.e., Rakta and Vata Dosha are associated with Pitta and Kapha, the disease produces different types of pain characterized by the nature of these elements. Therefore, in general, the disease gives rise to pain in all these joints. These different types of pain become excessively unbearable for the patients. [12-15]

Vatarakta Poorvaroopa: Premonitory Signs and Symptoms:

स्वेदोऽत्यर्थं न वा काष्ण्र्य स्पर्शाज्ञत्वं क्षतेऽतिरुक्| सन्धि शैथिल्यमालस्यं सदनं पिडकोद्गमः||१६||

जानु जङ्घोरु कट्यंस हस्त पादाङ्ग सन्धिषु| निस्तोदः स्फुरणं भेदो गुरुत्वं सुप्तिरेव च||१७||

कण्डूः सन्धिषु रुग्भूत्वा भूत्वा नश्यति चासकृत्| वैवर्ण्य मण्डलोत्पत्तिर्वातासृक्पूर्वलक्षणम्||१८||

The premonitory signs and symptoms of Vatarakta:

Svedo atyartham na va – Excess or absence of perspiration.

Karshnyam – Black coloration of the joints

Sparsha ajnatvam – Insensibility to touch, and

Kshate ati ruk – excessive pain if there is injury to the afflicted part

Sandhi shaithilya – fragile joints

Aalasyam – indolence and

Sadanam – asthenia

Pidaka udgamah – Appearance of pimples

Janu jangha uru kati amsha hasta pada anga sandhi nistoda – Pricking pain, twitching sensation, splitting pain, heaviness and numbness in the knees, calf, thighs, umbilical region, shoulders, hands, feet and joints in the body.

Kandu – Itching

Sandhishu ruk bhutva nashyati – Frequently, the pain while appearing in the joints disappears [suddenly] and

Vaivarnyam – Discoloration of the skin and

Mandala utpatti – Appearance of circular patches over the body. [16-18]

Types of Vatarakta:

उत्तानमथ गम्भीरं द्विव विधं तत् प्रचक्षते| त्वङ्मांसाश्रयमुत्तानं गम्भीरं त्वन्तराश्रयम्||१९||

Vatarakta is of 2 types:

Uthana Vatarakta (superficial) – located in the skin as well as muscle tissues and

Gambheera Vatarakta (deep seated) – located in deeper tissues

Uttana Vatarakta Lakshana:

कण्डू दाह रुगायामतोद स्फुरणकुञ्चनैः| अन्विता श्याव रक्ता त्वग्बाह्ये ताम्रा तथेष्यते||२०||

The superficial or external (Uthana or Bahya) varieties of Vatarakta gives rise to the following signs and symptoms:

Kandu – Itching

Daha – burning sensation

Ruk – ache

Aayama – extension

Toda – pricking pain

Sphurana – throbbing sensation and

Aakunchana – contraction and

Shyava rakta tvak – The skin becomes brownish black, red or coppery in color

Signs and Symptom of Gambhira Vatarakta:

गम्भीरे श्वयथुः स्तब्धः कठिनोऽन्तर्भृशार्तिमान्| श्यावस्ताम्रोऽथवा दाह तोद स्फुरण पाकवान्||२१||

रुग्विदाहान्वितोऽभीक्ष्णं वायुः सन्ध्यस्थि मज्जसु| छिन्दन्निव चरत्यन्तर्वक्रीकुर्वंश्च वेगवान्||२२||

करोति खञ्जं पङ्गुं वा शरीरे सर्वतश्चरन्| सर्वैर्लिङ्गैश्च विज्ञेयं वातासृग्भयाश्रयम्||२३||

The deep seated (gambhira) Vatarakta gives rise following signs and symptoms:

Shvayathu – Oedema

Stabdha – stiffness

Kathina – hardness and

Antar bhrusha arti – excruciating pain in the interior of the body

Shyava tamra tvak – Blackish brown or coppery coloration [of the skin] and

Daha – Burning sensation

Toda – pricking pain

Sphurana – twitching sensation and

Pakavan – suppuration of the joints.

If Vatarakta is located both in exterior (Uthana) and interior (gambhira) of the body, then the following signs and symptoms are manifested:

Aggravated Vata while causing pain and burning sensation constantly, moves with high speed through the joints, bones and bone marrow as if cutting them to make the joints curved inwards

While moving all over the body, this aggravated Vata Dosha makes the person lame and paraplegic and all the signs and symptoms described above (in respect of Uthana and Gambhira types of Vatarakta) are manifested. [20-23]

Classification of Vatarakta:

तत्र वातेऽधिके वा स्याद्रक्ते पित्ते कफेऽपि वा| संसृष्टेषु समस्तेषु यच्च तच्छृणु लक्षणम्||२४||

Now listen to the signs and symptoms of Vatarakta classified on the basis of the following:

Vataja, Pittaja, Kaphaja and Raktaja.

Caused by the predominance of 2 or 3 or all of the above-mentioned factors. [24]

Vataja Vatarakta Lakshana:

विशेषतः सिरायाम शूल स्फुरण तोदनम् | शोथस्य काष्ण्र्य रौक्ष्यं च श्यावता वृद्धिह्रानयः||२५||

धमन्यङ्गुलि सन्धीनां सङ्कोचोऽङ्गग्रहोऽतिरुक्| कुञ्चन स्तम्भने शीत प्रद्वेषश्चानिलेऽधिके||२६||

Symptoms of Vatarakta by aggravated Vata Dosha

Sira aayama – Dilatation of veins

Shula – Colic pain

Sphurana – throbbing pain and

Todanam – pricking pain

Karshnyam raukshyam shyavata sotha – Blackness, dryness and brownish coloration of oedema

Vriddhi haanayah sotha – Increase and decrease of the oedema

Dhamani anguli sandhinam sankocha – Contraction of vessels, fingers (including toes) and joints

Anga graha – Stiffness of the limbs & body parts

Ati ruk – Excessive pain

Sandhi kunchana stambhana – Contractures and stiffness [of joints] and

Shita pradvesha – Disliking for cold things [25-26]

Raktaja Vatarakta Lakshana:

श्वयथु भृश रुक् तोदस्तामश्चिमिचिमायते| स्निग्ध रूक्षैः शमं नैति कण्डू क्लेदान्वितोऽसृजि ||२७||

Vatarakta dominated by vitiated blood is characterized by:

Shyvathu – Oedema,

Bhrsha ruk – excessive pain and

Toda – pricking pain

Tamra tvak – Coppery coloration of the skin

Chimchimayana – Tingling sensation

Snigdha ruksha shamam – Not yielding to therapies which are either unctuous or ununctuous and

Kandu – Itching and

Kleda – sloughing. [27]

Pittaja Vatarakta Lakshana:

विदाहो वेदना मूच्छीं स्वेदस्तृष्णा मदो भ्रमः| रागः पाकश्च भेदश्च शोषश्चोक्तानि पैत्तिके||२८||

Vatarakta dominated by increased Pitta causes:

Vidaha – Burning sensation

Vedana – pain

Murccha – fainting

Sweda – sweating

Trushna – morbid thirst

Mada – intoxication and

Bhrama – dizziness

Raga – Redness

Paka – suppuration

Shosha – Emaciation of the afflicted limb [28]

Kaphaja Vatarakta Lakshana:

स्तैमित्यं गौरवं स्नेहः सुप्ति मन्दा च रुक् कफे|

Vatarakta dominated by Kapha is characterized by the following signs and symptoms in special:

Staimitya – Indolence

Gaurava – heaviness

Sneha – unctuousness

Supti – numbness and

Manda ruk – Less of pain

Signs and symptoms of Vatarakta Dominated by 2 or 3 Doshas

हेतु लक्षण संसर्गादि्वद्याद्द्वन्द्व त्रिदोषजम्||२९||

Vatarakta dominated by 2 or 3 of the aggravated Doshas is characterized by the etiological factors as well as signs of 2-3 Doshas together as described above. [26 ½]

Upashaya – Prognosis:

एकदोषानुगं साध्यं नवं, याप्यं दि्व दोषजम्|

त्रिदोषजमसाध्यं स्याद्यस्य च स्युरुपद्रवाः||३०||

If Vatarakta is caused by:

Only 1 Dosha, and if it is of recent origin, then it is curable.

The combination of 2 Doshas, then it is only Palliable.

All the 3 Doshas (including the 4th one i.e Rakta vide commentary above), then it is incurable.

If the curable varieties are attended with (associated with) complications (to be described hereafter), then they also become incurable. [30]

Vatarakta Upadrava – Complications:

अस्वप्नारोचक श्वास मांसकोथ शिरोग्रहाः| मूच्छर्ायमदरुक्तृष्णा ज्वर मोह प्रवेपकाः||३१||

हिक्का पाङ्गुल्य वीसर्प पाक तोद भ्रम क्लमाः| अङ्गुली वक्रता स्फोटा दाह मर्म ग्रहाबुर्दाः||३२||

एतैरुपद्रवैर्वर्ज्यं मोहेनैकेन वाऽपि यत्| सम्प्रस्रावि विवर्ण च स्तब्धमर्बुदकृच्च यत्||३३||

वर्जयेच्चैव सङ्कोचकरमिन्द्रियतापनम्| अकृत्स्नोपद्रवं याप्यं साध्यं स्यान्निरुपद्रवम्||३४||

Patients of Vatarakta having complications like these are not to be treated:

Asvapna – sleepless

Arochaka – anorexia

Shvasa – asthma

Mamsa kotha – sloughing of muscles

Shiro graha – stiffness of the head

Murccha – fainting

Mada – Intoxication

Ruk – pain

Trshna – morbid thirst

Jwara – fever

Moha – unconsciousness

Vepana – trembling

Hikka – hiccup

Pangulya – lameness

Visarpa – erysipelas

Paka – suppuration

Toda – pricking pain

Bhrama – giddiness

Klamah – mental fatigue

Anguli vakrata – curvature of fingers and toes

Sphota – pustule eruptions

Daha – burning sensation

Marma graha – affliction of vital parts and

Arbuda upadrava – tumour is not to be treated.

Even association of Moha (unconsciousness) alone as a complication renders the patient of Vatarakta incurable.

If Vata is associated with these symptoms then such patients are treated:

Srava – exudation [from the afflicted joint]

Vivarna – manifestation of opposite color of the skin

Stabdha – stiffness

Arbuda – tumour

Sankocha – contraction and

Indriyatāpanam – affliction of the senses

If the ailment is associated with only some of the aforesaid complications, then the patient is palliable, and if there is none of these complications, then the patient is curable. [31-34]

Raktamokshana in Vatarakta:

रक्तमार्गं निहन्त्याशु शाखा सन्धिषु मारुतः| निविश्यान्योन्यमावार्य वेदनाभिर्हरेदसून्||३५||

तत्र मुञ्चेदसृक् शृङ्ग जलौकःसूच्यलाबुभिः| प्रच्छनैर्वा सिराभिर्वा यथादोषं यथाबलम्||३६||

Need for blood-letting treatment in Vatarakt:

The aggravated Vata located in the Shakha (peripheral tissues) and joints cause obstruction to the channels of blood instantaneously. Then the Vata and blood enter into, and cause obstruction of each other giving rise to pain and even death. Therefore, depending upon the Doshas involved and the strength of the patient, blood-letting is done with the help of horn, leech, needle, and gourd or by vensection.

Jalauka Raktamokshana:

रुग्दाह शूल तोदार्तादसृक् स्राव्यं जलौकसा|

Indication for Jalauka – leech therapy for bloodletting:

Ruk – pain

Daha – burning sensation

Shula – colic pain and

Toda – pricking pain

Shrunga, Pracchanna, Siravyadha:

शृङ्गैस्तुम्बैर्हरेत् सुप्ति कण्डू चिमिचिमायनात्||३७||

देशाद्देशं व्रजत् स्राव्यं सिराभिः प्रच्छनेन वा| अङ्ग ग्लानौ न तु स्राव्यं रूक्षे वातोत्तरे च यत्||३८||

गम्भीरं श्वयथुं स्तम्भं कम्पं स्नायु सिरामयान्| ग्लानिं चापि स सङ्कोचां कुर्याद्वायुरसृक्क्षयात्||३९||

खाञ्ज्यादीन् वातरोगांश्च मृत्युं चात्यवसेचनात्| कुर्यात्तस्मात् प्रमाणेन स्निग्धाद्रक्तं विनिर्हरेत्||४०||

If the pain moves from one part of the body to the other, then blood-letting is done by Siravyadha or Pracchana (scratching with rough surface leaves or instruments).

However, blood-letting is not to be done if there is emaciation of the limbs and if there is dryness of the body because of predominance of the aggravated Vata Dosha. Blood-letting is avoided in such cases because as a result of the depletion of blood.

The aggravated Vata gives rise to

Sotha – deep-seated oedema

Stabdhata – stiffness

Kampa – trembling

Snāyu sirāmayā – diseases of the vessels and ligaments

Glani – Asthenia and

Sankocha – Contractures

Excessive bloodletting gives rise to

Pangulya – lameness

Vata vyadhi – diseases of Vata and

Even death

Therefore, it is done in appropriate measure only in persons having unctuousness. [35-40]

Vatarakta Samanya Chikitsa Sutra:

विरेच्यः स्नेहयित्वाऽऽदौ स्नेहयुक्तै विरेचनैः| रूक्षैर्वा मृदुभिः शस्तमसकृद्वस्तिकर्म च||४१||

सेकाभ्यङ्ग प्रदेहान्न स्नेहाः प्रायोऽविदाहिनः|

वातरक्ते प्रशस्यन्त ...|४२|

Line of treatment in general:

In the beginning, Snehana – oleation therapy is given to the patient suffering from Vatarakta.

Thereafter, he is given

Sneha virechana – purgation therapy with unctuous ingredients (if the patient is slightly unctuous) or Rooksha Virechana – if the patient has excess oiliness.

These purgatives are of mild nature. [Sharp purgative may excessively provoke Vayu for which these are contraindicated for the treatment of patients suffering from Vatarakta].

The patient is given medicated enema therapies (both Niruha and Anuvasana) frequently.

He is given

Seka – affusion

Abhyanga – massage

Pradeha – application of thick ointments

Food and unctuous substances which do not cause burning sensation. [41- ¾ 42]

Specific Treatment:

Hereafter, specific treatment of various types of Vatarakta will be described which may be listened to. [42 ¼]

Specific Treatment of Uthana Vatarakta:

बाह्यमालेपनाभ्यङ्ग परिषेकोपनाहनैः|

Uthana (superficial) type of Vatarakta (gout) is treated with

Alepana – application of ointments

Abyanga – Massage

Seka – affusion and

Upanaha – application of hot poultice [1/2 43]

Specific Treatment of Gambhira Vatarakta:

विरेकास्थापन स्नेहपानै गम्भीरमाचरेत्||४३||

Gambhira (deep seated) type of Vatarakta is treated with

Vireka – purgation

Asthapana – a type of medicated enema containing decoction of drugs among others and
Snehapana – intake of unctuous potions. [43 ½]

Specific Treatment of Vatarakta Dominated by Vata:
सर्पिस्तैल वसा मज्जापानाभ्यञ्जन बस्तिभिः| सुखोष्णैरुपनाहैश्च वातोत्तरमुपाचरेत्||४४||
Vatarakta caused by the predominance of aggravated Vata is treated with potions containing
Sarpi – ghee
Taila – oil
Vasa – muscle fat and
Majja – bone marrow
Abhyanga – massage
Basti – medicated enema and
Sukhoshna upanaha – application of lukewarm Upanaha (poultices). [44]

Specific Treatment of Vatarakta Dominated by Pitta and Rakta:
विरेचनै घृत क्षीरपानैः सेकैः स बस्तिभिः| शीतै निर्वापणैश्चापि रक्तपित्तोत्तरं जयेत्||४५||
If Vatarakta is dominated by vitiated Rakta (blood), and aggravated Pitta, then the patient is treated with
Vireka – purgation
Kshirapana – potions containing ghee and milk
Seka – affusion
Basti – medicated enema and
Cooling Nirvapana – application of ointment for the alleviation of burning sensation [45]

Specific Treatment of Kaphaja Vatarakta:
वमनं मृदु नात्यर्थं स्नेह सेकौ विलङ्घनम्| कोष्णा लेपाश्च शस्यन्ते वातरक्ते कफोत्तरे||४६||
If Vatarakta is dominated by aggravated Kapha, then the patient is treated by emetics.
He is not given Sneha and Seka in excess. He should keep fast, and lukewarm ointment – Lepa is applied over his body. [46]

Specific Management of Vatarakta Dominated by Kapha and Vayu:
कफ वातोत्तरे शीतैः प्रलिप्ते वातशोणिते| दाह शोथ रूजा कण्डू विवृद्धिः स्तम्भनाद्भवेत्||४७||
If Vatarakta is caused by the dominance of Kapha and Vata, then application of cold poultice will cause Stambhana (astringent action) as a result of which there will be aggravation of
Daha – burning sensation
Sotha – oedema
Ruja – pain and
Knadu – itching sensation [47]

Precaution in treatment of Vatarakta dominated by Rakta and Pitta:
रक्त पित्तोत्तरे चोष्णै र्दाहः क्लेदोऽवदारणम्| भवेत्स्मादिभिषग्दोषबलं बुद्ध्वाऽऽचरेत्क्रियाम्||४८||
If Vata Rakta is caused by the predominance of vitiated Rakta and aggravated Pitta, then the use of heating therapies may cause
Daha – burning sensation
Kleda – softness of tissues and
Avadarana – bursting of the wounds.
Therefore, the physician should administer appropriate therapies after determining the strength (aggravated nature) of the Doshas. [48]

Prohibitions in VataRakta

दिवास्वप्नं स सन्तापं व्यायामं मैथुनं तथा| कटूष्णं गुर्वभिष्यन्दि लवणाम्लं च वर्जयेत्||४९||

Things to be avoided by the patient suffering from Vata Rakta (gout):

Diva svapna – Sleep during day time

Santapa – exposure to heat

Vyayama – exercise

Maithuna – sexual intercourse and

intake of Katu (pungent), Ushna (hot), Guru (heavy), abhisyandi (ingredients which cause obstruction to the channels of circulation), Lavana (saline) and Amla (sour) ingredients [49]

Pathya for Vata Rakta

पुराणा यवगोधूम निवाराः शालि षष्टिकाः| भोजनार्थं रसार्थं वा विष्किर प्रतुदा हिताः||५०||

आढक्यश्चणका मुद्गा मसूराः समकुष्ठकाः| यूषार्थं बहु सर्पिष्काः प्रशस्ता वात शोणिते||५१||

सुनिषण्णक वेत्राग्र काकमाची शतावरी| वास्तुकोपोदिकाशाकं शाकं सौवर्चलं तथा||५२||

घृत मांस रसैर्भृष्टं शाक सात्म्याय दापयेत्| व्यञ्जनार्थं, तथा गव्यं माहिषाजं पयो हितम्||५३||

इति सङ्क्षेपतः प्रोक्तं वात रक्त चिकित्सितम्| एतदेव पुनः सर्वं व्यासतः सम्प्रवक्ष्यते||५४||

Wholesome food and drinks for Gout:

Cereals like old barley, wheat, Nivara (a type of wild rice), and Sali as Sastika types of rice.

Soup of the meat of Viskira (Gallinaceous) and Pratuda (Pecker) birds

Soup of Adhaki – Cajanus cajan, Chanaka – Chickpea,

Mudga – Green gram, Masura – Lens esculenta and Makustha – Phaseolus aconitifolius added with ghee in liberal quantity

Leafy vegetables like Sunisannaka, tender branches of Vetra (Salix caprea), Kakamachi – Solanum nigrum, Shatavari – Asparagus racemosus, Vastuka – Chenopodium album, Upodika and Sauvarcala (suryavartta) sizzled with ghee and meat-soup. These are to be given for making side dishes. Milk of cow, buffalo and goat too shall be given.

Thus, the treatment of Vatarakta is described in brief. These are to be elaborated hereafter. [50-54]

Shravanyadi Ghrita:

श्रावणी क्षीरकाकोली जीवकर्षभकैः समैः| सिद्धं समधुकैः सर्पिः सक्षीरं वातरक्तनुत्||५५||

Ghee cooked by adding milk – 4 times of ghee and the paste of

Munditika (Sravani)

Ksira Kakoli – Fritillaria roylei

Jivaka – Malaxis acuminata

Rishabhaka – Manilkara hexandra and

Madhuka– Licorice – Glycyrrhiza glabra all taken in equal quantities [in total 1/4th in quantity of ghee] cures Vatarakta (gout). [55]

Bala Ghrita:

बलामतिबलां मेदामात्मगुप्तां शतावरीम्| काकोलीं क्षीरकाकोलीं रास्नामृद्धिं च पेषयेत्||५६||

घृतं चतुर्गुण क्षीरं तैः सिद्धं वातरक्तनुत्| हृत्पाण्डुरोग वीसर्प कामला ज्वर नाशनम्||५७||

A paste is prepared of:

Bala – Sida cordifolia

Atibala – Abutilon indicum

Meda

Atma Gupta – Mucuna pruriens

Shatavari – Asparagus racemosus

Kakoli – Fritillaria roylei

Ksheera Kakoli

Rasna (Vanda roxburghi / Pluchea lanceolata) and

Riddhi.

Ghee is cooked by adding milk, 4 times in quantity of ghee, and the aforesaid paste.

This medicated ghee cures

Vatarakta – gout

Hrud roga – heart disease

Pandu – anemia

Visarpa – erysipelas

Kamala – Jaundice and

Jwara – fever. [56-57]

Parushaka Ghrita:

त्रायन्तिका तामलकी द्विकाकोली शतावरी| कशेरुका कषायेण कल्कैरेभिः पचेद्धृतम्||५८||

दत्वा परूषका द्राक्षा काश्मर्येक्षुरसान् समान्| पृथग्विदार्याः स्वरसं तथा क्षीरं चतुर्गुणम्||५९||

एतत् प्रायोगिकं सर्पिः पारूषकमिति स्मृतम्| वातरक्ते क्षते क्षीणे वीसर्पे पैत्तिके ज्वरे||६०||

इति पारूषकं घृतम्|

Ghee is cooked be cooked with the paste of

Trayantika

Tamalaki – Phyllanthus niruri

Kakoli – Fritillaria roylei

Ksira Kakoli and

Shatavari – Asparagus racemosus and the decoction of

Kaseruka - by adding the juice of

Parusaka – Grewia asiatica

Draksha – Raisin – Vitis vinifera

Kashmarya – Gmelina arborea

Sugarcane and

Vidari (Pueraria tuberosa), taken in equal quantities, separately, and 4 times of milk.

This medicated ghee is taken regularly (prayogika) which cures

Vatarakta – gout

Kshata kshina – Phthisis

Visarpa – erysipelas and

Paittika jware – Paittika type of fever.

Thus ends the description of Parushaka ghrta [58-60]

Jeevaneeya Ghrta:

द्वे पञ्चमूले वर्षाभूमेरण्डं सपुनर्नवम्| मुद्गपर्णीं महामेदां माषपर्णीं शतावरीम्||६१||

शङ्खपुष्पीमिवाकपुष्पीं रास्नामतिबलां बलाम्| पृथग्विदपलिकं कृत्वा जलद्रोणे विपाचयेत्||६२||

पादशेषे समान् क्षीर धात्रीक्षुच्छागलान् रसान्| घृताढकेन संयोज्य शनैमृद्वग्निना पचेत्||६३||

कल्कानावाप्य मेदे द्वे काश्मर्यफलमुत्पलम्| त्वक्क्षीरीं पिप्पलीं द्राक्षां पद्मबीजं पुनर्नवम्||६४||

नागरं क्षीरकाकोलीं पद्मकं बृहतीद्वयम्| वीरां शृङ्गाटकं भव्यमुरुमाणं निकोचकम्||६५||

खर्जूराक्षोट वाताममुञ्जाताभिषुकांस्तथा| एतैर्घृताढके सिद्धे क्षौद्रं शीते प्रदापयेत्||६६||

सम्यक् सिद्धं च विज्ञाय सुगुप्तं सन्निधापयेत्| कृत रक्षा विधिं चौक्षे प्राशयेदक्ष सम्मितम्||६७||

पाण्डुरोगं ज्वरं हिक्कां स्वरभेदं भगन्दरम्| पार्श्वशूलं क्षयं कासं प्लीहानं वात शोणितम्||६८||

क्षत शोषमपस्मारमश्मरीं शर्करां तथा| सर्वाङ्गैकाङ्गरोगांश्च मूत्रसङ्गं च नाशयेत्||६९||

बलवर्णकरं धन्यं वली पलित नाशनम्‌| जीवनीयमिदं सर्पिर्वृष्यं वन्ध्या सुतप्रदम्‌||७०||

2 Palas of each of

Bilva – Aegle marmelos

Syonaka

Gambhari – Gmelina arborea

Patali

Ganikarika

Shalaparni – Desmodium gangeticum

Prishniparni – Uraria picta

Brihati – Solanum indicum

Kantakari – Solanum xanthocarpum

Goksura – Tribulus terrestris

Varsabhu (white variety of Punarnava – Boerhavia diffusa)

Eranda – Ricinus communis

Mudga Parni – Phaseolus trilobus

Mahameda

Masha Parni – Teramnus labialis

Shatavari – Asparagus racemosus

Sankha Pushpi

Avak-Puspi (adhah-Puspi)

Rasna (Pluchea lanceolata)

Atibala – Abutilon indicum and

Bala – Country mallow (root) is added with 1 Drona of water and boiled till $1/4^{th}$ of water remains.

Along with this decoction, equal quantities (1 Adhaka) of each of milk, juice of Dhatri, Sugar-cane juice and soup of the meat of goat is added to 1 Adhaka of ghee, and cooked over mild fire, this 1 Adhaka of ghee is cooked by adding the paste of

Meda

Mahameda

fruit of Kasmarya – Gmelina arborea

Utpala – Nymphaea alba

Tvak-Ksiri (Vamsa Locana)

Pippali – Long pepper fruit – Piper longum

Draksha – Raisin – Vitis vinifera

Seeds of lotus

Punarnava – Boerhavia diffusa

Nagara – Zingiber officinale

Ksira Kakoli

Padmaka – Prunus cerasoides

Brihati – Solanum indium

Kantakari – Solanum xanthocarpum

Vira(vrddhi), Srngataka, Bhavya, Urumana, Nikochaka , Kharjura – Phoenix slyvestris, Aksota, Vatama Munjaka and Abhisuka (Pista)

After it is properly cooked and cooled, honey ($1/4^{th}$ in quantity of ghee) is added. This recipe is kept in a clean pot in a well protected place (free from wind) after performing protective rituals (Raksa Vidhi).

This medicated ghee is taken in the dose of 1 Aksa which cures

Pandu – anemia

Jwara – fever

Hikka – hiccup

Svara bheda – hoarseness of voice

Bhagandara – anal fistula

Parshva shoola – pain in the sides of the chest

Sosha – consumption

Kasa – cough

Pliha – splenic disorders

Vatarakta

Kshata – Phthsis

Karshya – emaciation

Apsmara – epilepsy

Asmari, sarkara – urinary stone and gravel

Paralysis of the whole body or only one part of it, and urinary obstruction.

It is an excellent promoter of strength and complexion. It destroys wrinkles and grey hair. This Jivaniya Ghrta promotes virility, and helps in the fertility of sterile women. [61-70]

Drakshadi Ghruta:

द्राक्षा मधु(धू)क तोयाभ्यां सिद्धं वा ससितोपलम्| पिबेद्धृतं तथा क्षीरं गुडूची स्वरसे शृतम्||७१||

The patient suffering from Vatarakta may take the following recipes containing 4 Types of Fat

Ghee cooked by adding the juice of Draksha – Raisin – Vitis vinifera or the decoction of Madhuka– Licorice – Glycyrrhiza glabra, and added with Sitopala (sugar of big crystals);or

Milk boiled by adding the juice of Guduchi – Tinospora cordifolia, and added with sitopala. [71]

Mahasneha Yoga:

जीवकर्षभकौ मेदामृष्यप्रोक्तां शतावरीम्| मधुकं मधुपर्णी च काकोलीद्वयमेव च||७२||

मुद्ग माषाख्यपर्णिन्यौ दशमूलं पुनर्नवाम्| बलामृता विदारीश्च साश्वगन्धाश्मभेदकाः||७३||

एषां कषाय कल्काभ्यां सर्पिस्तैलं च साधयेत्| लाभतश्च वसा मज्ज धान्व प्रातुद वैष्किरम्||७४||

चतुर्गुणेन पयसा तत् सिद्धं वात शोणितम्| सर्व देहाश्रितं हन्ति व्याधीन् घोरांश्च वातजान्||७५||

Muscle fat as well as bone marrow of animals belonging to the group of dhanva (inhabiting dry land forests or deserts), Pratuda (Pecker birds) and Viskira (gallinaceous birds) are collected.

Ghee and oil along with the aforesaid muscle fat and bone marrow is cooked by adding the decoction and paste of

Jivaka – Malaxis acuminata

Rishabhaka

Meda

Rsya Prokta (Atibala – Abutilon indicum)

Shatavari – Asparagus racemosus

Madhuka– Licorice – Glycyrrhiza glabra

Madhu Parni (Vikankata)

Kakoli – Fritillaria roylei

Ksira Kakoli

Mudga Parni – Phaseolus trilobus

Masha Parni – Termnus labialis

Bilva – Aegle marmelos

Synonaka

Gambhari – Gmelina arborea

Patala

Ganikarika

Sala Parni

Prishniparni – Uraria picta

Brihati – Solanum indicum

Kantakari – Solanum xanthocarpum

Goksura – Tribulus terrestris

Punarnava – Boerhavia diffusa

Bala – Country mallow (root) – Sida cordifolia

Amrta – Tinospora cordifolia

Vidari - Pueraria tuberos

Ashwagandha – Winter Cherry / Indian ginseng (root) – Withania somnifera and

Ashmabhedaka by adding milk (4 times in quantity of ghee).

This recipe of medicated fat (containing 4 types of fat) cures Vatarakta pervading the whole body, and other serious diseases caused by the aggravated Vata. [72-75]

Sthiradya Ghrita and Taila:

स्थिरा श्वदंष्ट्रा बृहती सारिवा स शतावरी| काश्मर्याण्यात्मगुप्ता च वृश्चीरो द्वे बले तथा||७६||

एषां क्वाथे चतुःक्षीरं पृथक् तैलं पृथग्घृतम्| मेदा शतावरी यष्टि जीवन्ती जीवकर्षभैः||७७||

पक्त्वा मात्रा ततः क्षीर त्रिगुणाऽध्यर्ध शर्करा| खजेन मथिता पेया वातरक्ते त्रिदोषजे||७८||

Oil or ghee is cooked by adding the decoction of

Sthira

Svadamstra – Tribulus terrestris

Brihati – Solanum indicum

Sariva – Indian Sarsaparilla – Hemidesmus indicus

Shatavari – Asparagus racemosus

Kasmarya – Gmelina arborea

Atmagupta – Mucuna pruriens

Vruscheera

Bala – Country mallow (root) – Sida cordifolia and

Maha bala and milk (4 times in quantity of ghee or oil) along with the paste of

Meda

Shatavari – Asparagus racemosus

Yashtimadhu – Glycyhrrhiza glabra

Jivanti – Leptadenia reticulata,

Jivaka – Malaxis acuminata and

Rishabhaka

1 dose of this medicated ghee and medicated oil (both taken together according to Chakrapani) is added with 3 times in quantity of milk, and 1 ½ times in quantity of sugar. This recipe is then churned with the help of a Khaja (churning stick or hand with fingers spread out).

Intake of this recipe cures Vatarakta caused by the simultaneous aggravation of all the 3 Doshas. [76-78]

Ksheera Yoga – medicated milk:

तैलं पयः शर्करां च पाययेद्वा सुमूच्छितम्| सर्पिस्तैल सिता क्षौद्रै र्मिश्रं वाऽपि पिबेत् पयः||७९||

अंशुमत्या शृतः प्रस्थः पयसो दिव सितोपलः| पाने प्रशस्यते तद्वत् पिप्पली नागरैः शृतः||८०||

बला शतावली रास्ना दशमूलैः सपीलुभिः| श्यामैरण्डस्थिराभिश्च वातार्तिघ्नं शृतं पयः||८१||

The patient suffering from Vatarakta is given the following recipes which alleviate Vayu:

tailaṃ payaḥ śarkarāṃ payam – Oil, milk and sugar mixed together

Milk added with ghee, oil, sugar and honey

1 Prastha of milk boiled by adding Amsumati (shala parni), and added with 2 Palas of Sugar

1 Prastha of milk boiled by adding

Pippali – Long pepper fruit – Piper longum, and

Sunthi – Zingiber officinale and added with 2 Palas of Sugar

Milk Boiled by adding

Bala – Country mallow (root) – Sida cordifolia

Shatavari – Asparagus racemosus

Rasna (Vanda roxburghi / Pluchea lanceolata)

Bilva – Aegle marmelos

Syonaka

Gambhari – Gmelina arborea

Patala

Ganikarika

Sala Parni

Prishniparni – Uraria picta

Brihati – Solanum indicum

Kantakari – Solanum xanthocarpum

Goksura – Tribulus terrestris and

Pilu and

Milk boiled by adding

Syama – Operculina ipomoea

Eranda – Ricinus communis and

Sthira (Sala Parni). [79-81]

Virechana Yogas:

धारोष्णं मूत्र युक्तं वा क्षीरं दोषानुलोमनम्| पिबेद्वा स त्रिवृच्चूर्णं पित रक्तावृतानिलः||८२||

क्षीरेणैरण्डतैलं वा प्रयोगेण पिबेन्नरः| बहु दोषो विरेकार्थं जीर्णे क्षीरौद नाशनः||८३||

कषायमभयानां वा घृत भृष्टं पिबेन्नरः| क्षीरानुपानं त्रिवृता चूर्णं द्राक्षा रसेन वा||८४||

काश्मर्य त्रिवृतां द्राक्षां त्रिफलां स परूषकाम्| शृतं पिबेद्विरेकाय लवण क्षौद्र संयुतम्||८५||

त्रिफलायाः कषायं वा पिबेत् क्षौद्रेण संयुतम्| धात्री हरिद्रा मुस्तानां कषायं वा कफाधिकः||८६||

योगैश्च कल्प विहितै रसकृतं विरेचयेत्| मृदुभिः स्नेह संयुक्तैर्जीत्वा वातं मलावृतम्||८७||

The Vatarakta patient is given the following Virechana Yoga:

Milk which is Dharosna (freshly collected and still warm) is added with cow's urine (in equal quantity), and taken which causes downward movement of morbid matter from the colon.

The powder of Trivrt – Operculina turpethum may also be taken along with Dharosna milk.

Eranda Taila (castor oil) may be taken habitually with milk for the purgation (elimination) of morbid mater. After the digestion of this potion, the patient is given rice with milk to eat

The decoction of Abhaya – Terminalia chebula sizzled with ghee

The powder of Trivrit should be given along with grape juice or milk used as post-prandial drink,

The decoction of these drugs are taken after adding salt and honey for purgation:

Kasmarya – Gmelina arborea

Trivrt – Operculina turpethum

Draksha – Raisin – Vitis vinifera

Haritaki – Terminalia chebula

Vibhitaka – Terminalia bellerica

Amalaki – Phylanthus emblica and

Parusaka – Grewia asiatica

The decoction of these drugs are taken mixed with honey:

Haritaki , Vibhitaki and Amalaki

Decoction of

Dhatri – Emblica officinalis

Haridra (turmeric – Curcuma longa) and Musta (Cyperus rotundus)

The above cited 2 recipes (no. 8 & 9) are useful in the treatment of Vatarakta if it is caused by the predominance of Kapha.

The recipes to be described in Kalpa section which are mild are administered after adding fat, to the patient suffering fom Vatarakta frequently for purgation if Vata is occluded by faeces. [82-87]

Basti Yoga: Medicated Enema

निर्हरेद्वा मलं तस्य सघृतैः क्षीर बस्तिभिः| न हि बस्तिसमं किञ्चिद्वातरक्त चिकित्सितम्||८८||

बस्ति वङ्क्षण पार्श्वोरु पर्वास्थि जठरार्तिषु| उदावर्ते च शस्यन्ते निरूहाः सानुवासनाः||८९||

दद्यात्तैलानि चेमानि बस्तिकर्मणि बुद्धिमान्| नस्याभ्यञ्जन सेकेषु दाह शूलोप शान्तये||९०||

If in Vatarakta (gout), Vayu is occluded by faeces, then the faecal matter is eliminated by Ksheera Basti (a recipe of medicated enema containing milk in large quantity) prepared by adding ghee. There is no therapeutic measure comparable to Basti (medicated enema) for the cure of Vatarakta (gout).

Niruha Basti (Decoction mix enema) along with Anuvasana (oil enema) is useful for pain in the urinary bladder, groin, sides of the chest, thighs, joints, bones and abdomen, and in Udavarta (upward movement of the wind in the abdomen).

For the cure of burning sensation and colic pain, a wise physician should use the medicated oils to be described hereafter, for medicated enema, inhalation, massage and affusion. [88-90]

Madhuparnyadi Taila

मधुकस्य शतं द्राक्षा खर्जूराणि परूषकम्| मधूकौदनपाक्यौ च प्रस्थं मुञ्जातकस्य च||९६||

काश्मर्याढकमित्येतच्चतुर्द्रोणे पचेदपाम्| शेषेऽष्टभागे पूते च तस्मिंस्तैलाढकं पचेत्||९७||

तथाऽऽमलक काश्मर्य विदारीक्षु रसैः समैः| चतुर्द्रोणेन पयसा कल्कं दत्वा पलोन्मितम्||९८||

कदम्बामलकाक्षोट पद्म बीज कशेरुकम्| शृङ्गाटकं शृङ्गवेरं लवणं पिप्पलीं सिताम्||९९||

जीवनीयैश्च संसिद्धं क्षौद्र प्रस्थेन संसृजेत्| नस्याभ्यञ्जन पानेषु बस्तौ चापि नियोजयेत्||१००||

वातव्याधिषु सर्वेषु मन्यास्तम्भे हनुग्रहे| सर्वाङ्गैकाङ्गवाते च क्षतक्षीणे क्षतज्वरे||१०१||

सुकुमारकमित्येतद्वातासाामय नाशनम्| स्वरवर्णकरं तैलमारोग्य बल पुष्टिदम्||१०२||

इति सुकुमारक तैलम्|

1 Tula of Madhu Yasti – Glycyhrrhiza glabra is boiled (by adding 1 drona of water), and reduced to 1/4th. To this (1 Adhaka) decoction, 1 Adhaka of oil and 1 Adhaka of milk is added, and cooked by adding the paste of 1 pala of each of

Shata Puspa – Anethum sowa

Shatavari – Asparagus racemosus

Murva – Marsdenia tenacissima

Payasya – Impomoea paniculata

Aguru – Aquillaria agallocha

Chandana – Santalum album

Sthira – Desmodium gangeticum

Hamsa Padi

Mamsi – Nordastachys jatamansi

Meda

Mahameda

Madhu Parni – Glycyrrhiza glabra

Kakoli – Fritillaria roylei

Ksira Kakoli

Tamalaki – Phyllanthus niruri

Riddhi

Padmaka – Prunus cerasoides

Jivaka – Malaxis acuminata

Rishabhaka – Manilkara hexandra

Jivanti – Leptadenia reticulata

Tvak – Cinnamonum zeylanica

Patra – Cinnamomum tamala Nees and Eberum.,

Nakha

Balaka

Prapaundarika (Nymphaea lotus) – red variety

Manjistha – Rubia cordifolia

Sariva – Indian Sarsaparilla – Hemidesmus indicus,

Aindri – Colocynth – Citrullus colocynthis and

Vitunnaka(Dhanyaka) – Coriandrum sativum

Use of this medicated oil in 4 different ways (internal intake, Massage, medicated enema and inhalation) cures Vatarakta accompanied with complications, pain in the limbs and affliction of the whole body.

It also cures diseases caused by

Vata

Rakta (vitiated blood) and

Pitta

Daha – burning sensation

Ruja – pain and

Jvara – fever.

It promotes strength and complexion.

Thus ends the description of Madhuparnyadi Taila [91-95]

Sukumaraka Taila:

मधुकस्य शतं द्राक्षा खर्जूराणि परूषकम्| मधूकौदनपाक्यौ च प्रस्थं मुञ्जातकस्य च||९६||

काश्मर्याढकमित्येतच्चतुर्द्रोणे पचेदपाम्| शेषेऽष्टभागे पूते च तस्मिंस्तैलाढकं पचेत्||९७||

तथाऽऽमलक काश्मर्य विदारीक्षुरसैः समैः| चतुर्द्रोणेन पयसा कल्कं दत्त्वा पलोन्मितम्||९८||

कदम्बामलकाक्षोट पद्म बीज कशेरुकम्| शृङ्गाटकं शृङ्गवेरं लवाणं पिप्पलीं सिताम्||९९||

जीवनीयैश्च संसिद्धं क्षौद्रप्रस्थेन संसृजेत्| नस्याभ्यञ्जनपानेषु बस्तौ चापि नियोजयेत्||१००||

वातव्याधिषु सर्वेषु मन्यास्तम्भे हनुग्रहे| सर्वाङ्गैकाङ्गवाते च क्षतक्षीणे क्षत ज्वरे||१०१||

सुकुमारकमित्येतद्वातासामयनाशनम्| स्वर वर्णकरं तैलमारोग्य बल पुष्टिदम्||१०२||

इति सुकुमारक तैलम्|

Sukumaraka Tailam:

100 Palas of Madhuka– Licorice – Glycyrrhiza glabra, 1 Prastha of each of

Draksha – Raisin – Vitis vinifera

Kharjura – Phoenix slyvestris

Parusaka – Grewia asiatica

Madhuka– Licorice – Glycyrrhiza glabra,

Odana Paki (Atibala – Abutilon indicum) and

Munjataka – Orchis latifolia and

1 Adhaka of Kashmarya – Gmelina arborea is boiled until one eighth of it remains.

The decoction is filtered.

1 Adhaka of oil is cooked by adding the aforesaid decoction, 4 Adhakas of milk, 1 Adhaka of each juice of the

Amalaki – Emblica officinalis/Phyllanthus emblica

Kashmarya – Gmelina arborea

Vidari (Ipomoea paniculata / Pueraria tuberosa) and sugar-cane, and

The paste of 1 Pala of each of

Kadamba – Anthocephlus indicus

Amalaka – Emblica officinalis/ Phyllanthus emblica

Aksota

Lotus-seed

Kaseruka

Srngataka

Srngavera – Zingiber officinale

Lavana

Pippali – Long pepper fruit – Piper longum

Sita – white variety of Cynodon dactylon and

10 drugs belonging to Jivaniya group (Jivaka – Malaxis acuminata, Rishabhaka – Manilkara hexandra, Meda, Mahameda – Polygonatum cirrhifolium, Kakoli – Fritillaria roylei, Ksira Kakoli – Fritillaria roylei, Mudga Parni –Phaseolus trilobus, Masha Parni – Teramnus labialis, Jivanti – Leptadenia reticulata and Madhuka– Licorice – Glycyrrhiza glabra).

After the oil is properly cooked, 1 Prastha of honey is added to it.

This medicated oil is used for

Nasya (inhalation)

Abhyanga (massage)

Potion (internal intake) for Manyastambha (torticollis),

Hanu graha – lock-jaw,

Sarvanga vata – Paralysis of the whole body or one part of it,

Ksata kshina – phthisis and

Kshate jware – fever caused by phthisis.

This is called Sukumaraka Taila, and it cures Vatarakta (gout).

This medicated oil promotes

Svara – voice

Varna – complexion

Aarogya – positive health and

Bala – robustness of the body.

Thus, ends the description of Sukumaraka Taila. [96-102]

Amritadya Taila:

गुडूची मधुकं ह्रस्वं पञ्चमूलं पुनर्नवाम्| रास्नामेरण्ड मूलं च जीवनीयानि लाभतः||१०३||

पलानां शतकैर्भागै बला पञ्चशतं तथा| कोल बिल्व यवान्माषान्कुलत्थांश्चाढकोन्मितान्||१०४||

काश्मर्याणां सुशुष्काणां द्रोणं द्रोणशतेऽम्भसि| साधयेज्जर्जरं धौतं चतुर्द्रोणं च शेषयेत्||१०५||

तैलद्रोणं पचेतेन दत्वा पञ्चगुणं पयः| पिष्ट्वा त्रिपलिकं चैव चन्दनोशीर केशरम्||१०६||

पत्रैलागुरु कुष्ठानि तगरं मधुयष्टिकाम्| मञ्जिष्ठाष्ट पलं चैव तत् सिद्धं सार्वयौगिकम्||१०७||

वातरक्ते क्षतक्षीणे भारार्ते क्षीण रेतसि| वेपनाक्षेप भग्नानां सर्वाङ्गैकाङ्ग रोगिणाम्||१०८||

योनिदोषमपस्मारमुन्मादं खञ्ज पङ्गुताम्| हन्यात् प्रसवनं चैत तैलाब्यममृताह्वयम्||१०९||

इत्यमृताद्यं तैलम्|

100 Palas of each of

Guduchi – Tinospora cordifolia

Madhuka– Licorice – Glycyrrhiza glabra,

Shala Parni

Prishniparni – Uraria picta

Brihati – Solanum indicum

Kantakari – Solanum xanthocarpum

Goksura – Tribulus terrestris

Punarnava – Boerhavia diffusa

Rasna (Vanda roxburghi / Pluchea lanceolata)

Root of Eranda – Ricinus communis and

Available drugs belonging to Jivaniya group (viz., Jivaka – Malaxis acuminata, Rishabhaka – Manilkara hexandra, Meda – Polygonatum cirrhifolium, Maha medha, Kakoli – Fritillaria roylei, Ksira Kakoli – Fritillaria roylei, Mudga Parni – Phaseolus trilobus, Masha Parni – Teramnus labialis, Jivanti – Leptadenia reticulata and Madhuka—Madhuca longifolia),

500 Palas of Bala – Country mallow (root) – Sida cordifolia

1 Adhaka of each of

Kola – Zizyphus jujuba

Bilva – Aegle marmelos

Yava – Barley (Hordeum vulgare),

Masha – Phaseolus mungo and

Kulattha – horse gram and

1 Drona of well dried fruits of Kasmari – Gmelina arborea is coarsely pounded and washed with water.

This coarse powder is boiled by adding 100 Dronas of water till 4 Dronas of water remain.

1 Drona of oil is cooked by adding the aforesaid decoction, 5 Dronas of milk and the paste of 3 Palas of each of

Chandana – Sandalwood – Santalum album

Ushira – Vetiver – Vetiveria zizanioides

Kesara

Patra – Cinnamomum tamala Nees and Eberum.,

Ela – Elattaria cardamomum

Aguru – Aquillaria agallocha

Kushta – Saussurea lappa

Tagara – and

Yashtimadhu – Glycyrrhiza glabra and

8 Palas of Manjistha – Rubia cordifolia

This medicated oil is used in the form of

Pana – Potion for internal intake

Abhyanga – massage

Nasya – inhalation and

Basti – medicated enema.

It cures

Vatarakta – gout

Kshata kshina – Phthis

Ailments caused by carrying heavy load

seminal defieciency treatment

Vepana – tremors

Aakshepa – convulsions

Bhanga – fractures

Sarvanga vata – Paralysis of the whole body or a part of it

Yoni dosha – Ailments of the female genital organs

Apasmara – epilepsy

Unmada – insanity

Pangu Khanja - Lameness of hands and legs, and

Prasava roga – ailments caused during parturition.

This is an excellent recipe of medicated oil and it is called Amrtadya Taila.

Thus, ends the description of Amrtadya Taila. [103- 109]

Mahapadma Taila:

पद्म वेतस यष्ट्याह्व फेनिला पद्मकोत्पलैः| पृथक्पञ्चपलै दर्भ बला चन्दन किंशुकैः||११०||

जले शृतैः पचेतैलप्रस्थं सौवीर सम्मितम्| लोध्र कालीयकोशीर जीवकर्षभ केशरैः||१११||

मदयन्ती लतापत्र पद्म केशर पद्मकैः| प्रपौण्डरीक काश्मर्य मांसी मेदा प्रियङ्गुभिः||११२||

कुङ्कुमस्य पलार्धन मञ्जिष्ठायाः पलेन च| महापद्ममिदं तैलं वातासृग्ज्वर नाशनम्||११३||

इति महापद्मं तैलम्|

5 Palas of each of

Padma – Lotus (Nelumbo nucifera),

Vetasa

Yastimadhu – Glycyhrrhiza glabra

Phenila (upodika)

Padmaka – Prunus cerasoides

Utpala – Nymphaea alba

Darbha – Desmostachya bipinnata

Bala – Sida cordifolia

Chandana (Sandalwood – Santalum album) and

Kimsuka – Butea monosperma is boiled by adding water.

1 Prastha of oil is cooked by adding the aforesaid decoction, 1 Prastha of Sauvira, and the paste of each of

Lodhra

Kaliyaka – Berberis aristata

Ushira – Vetiver – Vetiveria zizanioides

Jivaka – Malaxis acuminata

Rishabhaka – Manilkara hexandra

Kesara

Madayanti

Lata

Patra – Cinnamomum tamala Nees and Eberum

Padma Kesara

Padmaka – Prunus cerasoides

Prapaundaraika

Kasmarya – Gmelina arborea

Mamsi – Nordastachya jatamansi

Meda

Priyangu – Callicarpa macrophylla and

Kunkuma – Crocus sativus and

1 Pala of Manjistha – Rubia cordifolia.

This is called Mahapadma – taila which cures Vatarakta and fever. Thus ends the description of Mahapadma Taila. [110-113]

Khuddaka Taila:

पद्मकोशीर यष्ट्याह्व रजनी क्वाथ साधितम्| स्यात् पिष्टैः सर्ज मञ्जिष्ठा वीरा काकोलि चन्दनैः||११४||
खुड्डाक पद्मकमिदं तैलं वातास्र दाहनुत्|११५|
इति खुड्डाक पद्मकं तैलम्|

Oil is cooked by adding the decoction of

Padmaka – Prunus cerasoides

Ushira – Vetiver – Vetiveria zizanioides

Yastimadhu – Glycyrrhiza glabra and

Haridra – turmeric – Curcuma longa and the paste of

Sarja – Vateria indica

Manjistha – Rubia cordifolia

Vira – Ksira Kakoli and

Chandana – Sandalwood – Santalum album

This medicated oil is called Khuddaka Padmaka Taila, and

It cures

Vatarakta and

Daha – burning sensation.

Thus, ends the description of Khuddhaka Padmaka Taila. [114- ½ 115]

Madhuka Taila:

शतेन यष्टिमधुकात् साध्यं दशगुणं पयः||११५||
तस्मिंस्तैले चतुर्द्रोणे मधुकस्य पलेन तु|
सिद्धं मधुक काश्मर्य सैर्वा वातरक्तनुत्||११६||

100 Palas of Yastimadhu – Glycyrrhiza glabra is boiled by adding 10 times (1000 Palas) of milk (till 1/4th of milk remains). In 4 dronas of oil, the aforesaid medicated milk and 1 Pala of Madhuka – Madhuca longifolia (in paste form) is added and cooked.

Similarly, oil may be cooked by adding the decoction or juice of Madhuka – Madhuca longifolia or Kasmari – Gmelina arborea [and the paste of Madhuka– Licorice – Glycyrrhiza glabra].

These medicated oils cure Vatarakta (gout). [115 ½ – 116]

Satapaka Madhuka Taila:

मधुपर्ण्याः पलं पिष्ट्वा तैल प्रस्थं चतुर्गुणे| क्षीरे साध्यं शतं कृत्वा तदेवं मधुकाच्छते||११७||
सिद्धं देयं त्रिदोष स्याद्वातास्रे श्वास कासनुत्| हृत्पाण्डुरोग वीसर्प कामला दाह नाशनम्||११८||
इति शतपाकं मधुकतैलम्|

1 Prastha of oil is added with 4 Prasthas of milk, and 1 Pala of the Paste of MadhuParni – Indian tinospora (stem) – Tinospora cordifolia, this medicated oil is again added with 4 times of milk, and the paste of 1 Pala of MadhuParni – Indian tinospora (stem) – Tinospora cordifolia (Yashti Madhu) is repeated for 100 times in total. As a result of this repeated cooking with the paste of 100 Palas of paste of Yastimadhu,

This medicated oil cures

Shvasa – asthma and

Kasa – cough in Tridoshaja Vatarakta

Hrud roga – heart diseases

Pandu – anemia

Visarpa – erysipelas

Kamala – jaundice and

Daha – burning sensation.

Thus, ends the description of Satapaka Madhuka -Taila. [117-118]

Sahasrapaka and Shatapaka Bala Taila:

बला कषाय कल्काभ्यां तैलं क्षीर समं पचेत्| सहस्रं शतवारं वा वातासृग्वात रोगनुत्||११९||

रसायनमिदं श्रेष्ठमिन्द्रियाणां प्रसादनम्| जीवनं बृंहणं स्वर्यं शुक्रासृग्दोष नाशनम्||१२०||

इति सहस्र पाकं शत पाकं वा बलातैलम्|

Oil is cooked by adding the decoction of bala (4 times in quantity of oil), paste of Bala – Country mallow (root) (1/4th in quantity of oil), and milk (in equal quantity of oil) for 1000 or 100 times.

This medicated oil cures both the rejuvenation of the body, promotion of clarity of sense perception, longevity, robustness and voice. It cures morbidities in semen and menstruation.

Thus, ends the description of Sahasra Paka bala Taila and Satapaka Bala Taila. [119-120]

Guduchyadi taila:

गुडूची रस दुग्धाभ्यां तैलं द्राक्षा रसेन वा| सिद्धं मधुक काश्मर्य रसैर्वा वात रक्तनुत्||१२१||

Oil is cooked with the

Juice of Guduchi – Tinospora cordifolia and milk or

With juice of Draksha – Raisin – Vitis vinifera or

With the decoction of Madhuka– Licorice – Glycyrrhiza glabra and

The juice of Kasmari – Gmelina arborea.

These medicated oils cure Vatarakta (gout). [121]

Aranaladi taila:

आरनालाढके तैलं पाद सर्ज रसं शृतम्| प्रभूते खजितं तोये ज्वर दाहार्तिनुत् परम्||१२२||

Oil (1 Prastha) is cooked by adding 1 Adhaka of Aranala (sour vinegar) and 1/4th of a Prastha of Sarja (Vateria indica)-Rasa. This medicated oil is then added with liberal quantity of water, and churned.

This is an excellent recipe for the cure of

Jwara – fever

Daha – burning sensation and

Arti – pain. [122]

Pinda Taila

स मधूच्छिष्ट माञ्जिष्ठं स सर्जरस सारिवम्| पिण्डतैलं तदभ्यङ्गाद्बातरक्त रुजापहम्||१२३||

इति पिण्ड तैलम्|

Oil is cooked with the paste of

Madhucchista (bee's wax),

Manjistha – Rubia cordifolia

Sarja (Vateria indica)-Rasa and

Sariva – Indian Sarsaparilla – Hemidesmus indicus [the paste is 1/4th in quantity of oil], and water which is 4 times of oil in quantity).

Massage of this oil cures pain in Vatarakta (gout).

Thus, ends the description of Pinda taila. [123]

Dashamoola Ksheera for Parisheka:

दशमूलशृतं क्षीरं सद्यः शूलनिवारणम्| परिषेकोऽनिलप्राये तद्वत् कोष्णेन सर्पिषा||१२४||

Milk is boiled by adding Dasha Mula (bilva – Aegle marmelos, Syonaka – Orchis mascula, Gambhari – Gmelina arborea, Patala – Ficus microcarpa, Ganikarika, Sala Parni, Prishniparni – Uraria picta, Brihati – Solanum indicum, Kantakari – Solanum xanthocarpum and Goksura – Tribulus terrestris).

Affussion with this medicated milk instantaneously cures pain [in Vatarakta or gout]. Similarly, affusion is done with luke warm cow's ghee [for the cure of pain] in Vatarakta or gout caused by the predominance of aggravated Vata.

[124]

Sneha Parisheka:

स्नेहै र्मधुर सिद्धैर्वा चतुर्भिः परिषेचयेत्| स्तम्भाक्षेपक शूलार्त कोष्णैर्दाहे तु शीतलैः||१२५||

Oil, ghee, muscle fat or bone marrow is cooked by adding drugs belonging to sweet or Jivaniya group (Jivaka – Malaxis acuminata, Rishabhaka – Manilkara hexandra, Meda – Polygonatum cirrhifolium, Mahameda, Kakoli – Fritillaria roylei, Masha Parni – Teramnus labialis, Mudga Parni – Phaseolus trilobus, Jivanti – Leptadenia reticulata and Madhuka– Licorice – Glycyrrhiza glabra).

These recipes, when lukewarm are used for affusion if there is

Stabdha – stiffness

Aakshepaka – convulsion and

Shoola – pain in Vatarakta (Gout).

If, however, there is burning sensation, these recipes are cooled, and thereafter, used for affusion. [125]

तद्वद्गव्याविकच्छागैः क्षीरैस्तैल विमिश्रितैः| क्वाथैर्वा जीवनीयानां पञ्चमूलस्य वा भिषक्||१२६||

Oil mixed with the

Milk of cow, sheep or goat or

With the decoction of drugs belonging to Jivaniya group (jivaka, Rishabhaka – Manilkara hexandra, Meda – Polygonatum cirrhifolium, Mahameda, Kakoli – Fritillaria roylei,Ksira Kakoli – Fritillaria roylei,Masha Parni – Teramnus labialis, Mudga Parni – Phaseolus trilobus, Jivanti – Leptadenia reticulata and Madhuka– Licorice – Glycyrrhiza glabra) or

With the decoction of Pancha Mula (Bilva – Aegle marmelos, Syonaka , Gambhari – Gmelina arborea, Patala and Ganikarika) may similarly (lukewarm or cold) be used for affusion in the above mentioned conditions. [126]

Drakshadi Yoga for Seka:

द्राक्षेक्षुरस मद्यानि दधिमस्त्वम्लकाञ्जिकम्| सेकार्थं तण्डुलक्षौद्रशर्कराम्बु च शस्यते||१२७||

Juice of Draksha – Raisin – Vitis vinifera, sugar-cane juice, alcohol, Dadhi Mastu (whey), sour Kanji (gruel), rice water and honey is mixed with water or sugar-solution. These recipes are useful for affusion in Vatarakta (gout). [127]

Kumuda etc for necklace:

कुमुदोत्पल पद्माद्यैर्मणिहारैः सचन्दनैः| शीत तोयानुगैर्दाहे प्रोक्षणं स्पर्शनं हितम्||१२८||

Affusion or touch (external application) of cold water soaked with

Kumuda – Nymphaea alba

Utpala (Nymphaea alba)

Padma, etc,

Necklace of gems and

Chandana – Santalum album is beneficial for curing burning sensation [128]

चन्द्र पादाम्बु संसिक्ते क्षौम पद्मदलच्छदे| शयने पुलिन स्पर्श शीत मारुत वीजिते||१२९||

चन्दनार्द्रस्तनकराः प्रिया नार्यः प्रियंवदाः| स्पर्श शीताः सुख स्पर्शा घ्नन्ति दाहं रुजं क्लमम्||१३०||

The patient should lie on a bed spread over with fine silk cloth and leaves of lotus, sprinkled with water impregnated with the rays of the moon (dew water) and fanned by the cold breezes in the company of women, who speak pleasantly, whose breasts and hands are smeared with the paste of sandalwood and cold and pleasing in touch.

This regimen cures

Daha – burning sensation

Rujam – pain and

Klama – mental fatigue in Vatarakta or gout [129-130]

Raktamokshana and Lepa:
सरागे सरुजे दाहे रक्तं विस्राव्य लेपयेत्| मधुकाश्वत्थ त्वङ्मांसीवीरोदुम्बरशाद्वलैः||१३१||
जलजैर्यवचूर्णैर्वा सयष्ट्याह्वपयोघृतैः| सर्पिषा जीवनीयैर्वा पिष्टैर्लेपोऽर्तिदाहनुत्||१३२||
If Vatarakta is associated with
Sa raga – redness,
Sa ruja -pain and
Daha – burning sensation
Then after:
Visravya – blood-letting,
Lepana (external application) is done with
The paste of
Madhuka – Madhuca longofolia
Asvattha – Ficus religiosa
Tvak – Cinnamonum zeylanica
Mamsi – Nordastachys jatamansi
Vira (Ksira Kakoli – Fritillaria roylei)
Udumbara – Ficus racemosa
Sadvala (Durva (Cynodon dactylon) and
Kamala – Nymphaea alba or
With the paste of Barley-powder mixed with Yastimadhu – Glycyrrhiza glabra, milk and ghee.
The ghee prepared by boiling with the paste of drugs belonging to
Jivaniya group (Jivaka – Malaxis acuminata, Rishabhaka – Manilkara hexandra, Meda – Polygonatum cirrhifolium,
Mahameda – Polygonatum cirrhifolium, Kakoli – Fritillaria roylei, Ksira Kakoloi,Mudga Parni – Phaseolus trilobus,
Masha Parni – Teramnus labialis, Jivanti – Leptadenia reticulata) and
Madhuka – Madhuca longifolia may also be applied
It cures
Daha – burning sensation and
Ruja – pain in Vatarakta or gout. [131-132]

Tiladi Pralepa:
तिलाः प्रियालो मधुकं बिसं मूलं च वेतसात्| आजेन पयसा पिष्टः प्रलेपो दाह रागनुत्||१३३||
These ingredients are made to a paste by triturating with Goat's milk:
Tila
Priyala
Madhuka– Licorice – Glycyrrhiza glabra,
Bisa and
Root of Vetra – Salix caprea
Application of this paste cures
Daha – burning sensation and
Raga – redness in Vatarakta or gout. [133]

Prapaundarikadi Lepa:
प्रपौण्डरीक मञ्जिष्ठा दार्वी मधुक चन्दनैः| सितोपलैरकासक्तुमसूरोशीर पद्मकैः||१३४||
लेपो रुग्दाह वीसर्प राग शोफ निवारणः| पित्तरक्तोत्तरे त्वेते, लेपान् वातोत्तरे शृणु||१३५||
Application of the paste prepared of

Prapaundarika (Nymphaea lotus) – red variety,

Manjistha – Rubia cordifolia,

Daru Haridra

Madhuka– Licorice – Glycyrrhiza glabra,

Chandana (Sandalwood – Santalum album)

Sitopala (sugar of big crystal),

Eraka (Hoggala Grass)

Saktu (roasted corn flour)

Masura

Ushira – Vetiver – Vetiveria zizanioides and

Padmaka – Prunus cerasoides

Cures

Ruja – pain

Daha – burning sensation

Visarpa – erysiples

Raga – redness and

Sopha – swelling.

The above-mentioned recipes (described in verse nos. 128 – ¾ 135] are useful in Vatarakta dominated by aggravated Pitta and Vitiated Rakta (blood). [134- ¾ 135]

Recipes for external Use in Vatarakta Dominated by Vayu

पित्त रक्तोत्तरे त्वेते, लेपान् वातोत्तरे शृणु||१३५||

वातघ्नैः साधितः स्निग्धः स क्षीर मुद्ग पायसः | तिल सर्षप पिण्डैर्वाऽप्युपनाहो रुजापहः||१३६||

Now, listen to the description of lepas (poultices) for Vatarakta caused by the predominance of Vata. The pudding of Mugda (green gram) and milk is prepared by cooking with the decoction of drugs which alleviate Vata, and added with fat (oil or ghee). Application of this pudding as hot poultice (upanaha) cures pain.

Similarly, the application of the bolus of Tila – Sesame (Sesamum indicum) and Sarsapa – Brassica campestris as hot poultice cures pain. [135 ¼- 136]

औदक प्रसहानूप वेशवाराः सुसंस्कृताः| जीवनीयौषधैः स्नेहयुक्ताः स्युरुपनाहने||१३७||

स्तम्भ तोद रुगायाम शोथाङ्ग ग्रह नाशनाः| जीवनीयौषधैः सिद्धा सपयस्का वसाऽपि वा||१३८||

Vesavaras (types of meat preparation) are made of the

Meat of animals belonging to the group of

Audaka (aquatic animals) and

Prasaha (animals and birds who eat by snatching their food) and

Anupa (animals living in marshy land).

Jivaniya group (Jivaka – Malaxis acuminata, Rishabhaka – Manilkara hexandra, Meda – Polygonatum cirrhifolium, Mahameda, Kakoli – Fritillaria roylei, Ksira Kakoli – Fritillaria roylei, Mugda Parni – Phaseolus trilobus, Masha Parni – Teramnus labialis, Jivanti – Leptadenia reticulata and Madhuka– Licorice – Glycyrrhiza glabra) and fat (oil or ghee).

Application of these recipes as hot poultices cures

Stambha – stiffness

Toda – pricking pain

Ruk – ache

Aayama – Stretching

Sotha – oedema and

Anga graha – immobility of limbs.

Muscle fat is cooked by adding drugs belonging to the Jivaniya group, and milk. Use of this recipe as hot poultice cures the aforesaid ailments. [137- 138]

घृतं सहचरान्मूलं जीवन्ती च्छागलं पयः| लेपः पिष्टास्तिलास्तद्वद्भृष्टाः पयसि निर्वृताः||१३९||

Upanaha of these drugs is done by making them into a paste by adding ghee and goat's milk:

Root of Sahacara – Casearia esculanta and

Jivanti – Leptadenia reticulata.

Similarly, seeds of Tila – Sesame (Sesamum indicum) are roasted and immersed in goat's milk. A paste of these seeds is prepared by triturating with the milk (earlier used for immersion).

Application of this paste as hot poultice is also useful for ailments caused by the predominance of aggravated vayu in Vatarakta. [139]

क्षीर पिष्टमुमालेपमेरण्डस्य फलानि च| कुर्याच्छूल निवृत्यर्थं शताह्वामनिलेऽधिके||१४०||

For the cure of pain caused by the predominance of Vata in Vatarakta, the physician should apply the paste of

Uma (Atasi – Linum usitatissimum),

Fruits of Eranda – Ricinus communis or

Satahva prepared by triturating with milk. [140]

समूलाग्रच्छदैरण्डक्वाथे दिव प्रास्थिकं पृथक्| घृतं तैलं वसा मज्जा चानूप मृग पक्षिणाम्||१४१||

कल्कार्थं जीवनीयानि गव्यं क्षीरमथाजकम्| हरिद्रोत्पल कुष्ठैला शताह्वाश्वहनच्छदान्||१४२||

बिल्व मात्रान् पृथक् पुष्पं काकुभं चापि साधयेत्| मधूच्छिष्ट पलान्यष्टौ दद्याच्छीतेऽवतारिते||१४३||

शूलेनैषोर्दिताङ्गानां लेपः सन्धिगतेऽनिले| वातरक्ते च्युते भग्ने खञ्जे कुब्जे च शस्यते||१४४||

Ingredients:

2 Prasthas of each of

Ghrtam – ghee,

Tailam – oil,

Vasa – muscle fat and

Majja – bone marrow of animals and birds inhabiting marshy land and arid zone is cooked by adding the

Decoction of the root and tender leaves (collected from the top of the tree) of

Eranda – Ricinus communis (4 times in quantity of Fat), and

Paste prepared of one Bilva (pala) of each of the drugs belonging to

Jivaniya group (Jivaka – Malaxis acuminata, Rishabhaka – Manilkara hexandra, Meda , Mahameda Kakoli – Fritillaria roylei, Ksira Kakoli – Fritillaria roylei, Mudga Parni – Phaseolus trilobus, Masha Parni – Teramnus labialis, Jivanti – Leptadenia reticulata and Madhuka– Licorice – Glycyrrhiza glabra),

Gavya kshiram – cow-milk

Aja kshiram – goat-milk

Haridra (turmeric – Curcuma longa)

Utpala (Nymphaea alba),

Kushta – Saussurea lappa,

Ela - Elettaria cardamomum Maton)

Satahva,

Leaves of asvahana (Karavira – Nerium indicum) and

Flowers of Kakubha (Arjuna (Terminalia arjuna)

After the medicated fat is cooked, the pot is taken out of the oven, and made to cool down. Thereafter, 8 Palas of Madhucchista (bee's wax) is added, and mixed together.

This medicated fat is applied externally to cure pain in a patient of

Ardita (facial paralysis),

Sandhi gata vata – location of the aggravated Vata in the joints,

Vatarakta (gout),

Khanja (Lameness) and

Kubja (hunch-Back). [141-144]

Abhaynga Lepa Yoga for Vatarakta Dominated by Kapha

शोफ गौरव कण्ड्वाद्यैर्युक्ते त्वस्मिन् कफोत्तरे| मूत्र क्षार सुरापक्वं घृतमभ्यञ्जने हितम्||१४५||

Massage with the medicated ghee prepared by boiling with cow's urine, Ksarodaka (alkaline solution) and alcohol is useful in Vatarakta caused by the predominace of Kapha. And when the ailment is associated with oedema, heaviness, itching etc. [145]

पद्मकं त्वक् समधुकं सारिवा चेति तैर्घृतम्| सिद्धं स मधु शुक्तं स्यात् सेकाभ्यङ्गे कफोत्तरे||१४६||

Ghee is boiled with the paste of

Padmaka – Prunus cerasoides,

Tvak – Cinnamonum zeylanica

Madhuka– Licorice – Glycyrrhiza glabra and

Sariva – Indian Sarsaparilla – Hemidesmus indicus and

Vinegar prepared with honey (Madhusuka).

This medicated ghee is useful for

Seka – affusion and

Abhyanga – massage in Vatarakta caused by the predominance of Kapha. [146]

Parisheka Yoga –

क्षारस्तैलं गवां मूत्रं जलं च कटुकैः शृतम्| परिषेके प्रशंसन्ति वातरक्ते कफोत्तरे||१४७||

Ksara (Alkali preparation), oil, cow's urine or water is boiled by adding drugs having pungent taste. These liquids are useful for affusion in Vatarakta (caused by the predominance of Kapha. [147]

Sarshapadi Lepa:

लेपः सर्षप निम्बार्क हिंस्रा क्षीर तिलैर्हितः| श्रेष्ठः सिद्धः कपित्थत्वग्घृतक्षीरैः ससक्तुभिः||१४८||

Application of the paste of

Sarsapa – Brassica campestris

Nimba – Neem (Azadirachta indica),

Arka – Calotropis gigantea,

Himsra – Nardostachys jatamansi,

Kshira – milk and

Tila – Sesame (Sesamum indicum)

Cures: Vatarakta caused by the predominance of Kapha

Application of the poultice prepared of the bark of

Kapittha,

Ghrta – ghee,

Kshira – milk and

Saktu (roasted corn- flour) is most useful in the treatment of the aforesaid ailment [148]

Poultice – Pralepa for Vatarakta Dominated by Vayu and Kapha:

गृह धूमो वचा कुष्ठं शताह्वा रजनी द्वयम्| प्रलेपः शूलनुद्वातरक्ते वात कफोत्तरे||१४९||

Application of the poultice prepared of

Grha Dhuma (Kitchen-soot),

Vacha (Acorus calamus Linn.),

Kushta – Saussurea lappa,

Satahva,

Haridra (turmeric – Curcuma longa) and

Daru Haridra (Berberis aristata)

Cures: pain in Vatarakta caused by the Predominance of Vata and Kapha [149]

Tagaradi Lepa
तगरं त्वक् शताह्वैला कुष्ठं मुस्तं हरेणुका| दारु व्याघ्रनखं चाम्लपिष्टं वात कफास्रनुत्||१५०||
Application of the poultice prepared by
Tagara – Valerian walichii,
Tvak – Cinnamonum zeylanicum,
Satahva,
Ela (Elettaria cardamomum Maton),
Kushta – Saussurea lappa,
Musta (Cyperus rotundus),
Harenuka
Deva Daru – Cedrus deodara and
Vyaghra Nakha by triturating with sour liquids (kanji etc) cures Vatarakta caused by the predominance of Vayu and Kapha. [150]
madhu shigru adi Seka:
मधु शिग्रोर्हितं तद्वद्बीजं धान्याम्ल संयुतम्|
मुहूर्त लिप्तमम्लैश्च सिञ्चेद्वातकफोत्तरम्||१५१||
      Similarly, paste is prepared of the seeds of sweet variety of Sigru – Moringa oleifera by triturating with Dhanyamla (sour liquid prepared of cereals with husk). It is applied for some time over the affected part, and thereafter, the part is affused with sour liquids (Kanji etc) which is beneficial in Vatarakta dominated by Vata and Kapha. [151]
Recipe for Vatarakta caused by Predominance of all the 3 Doshas

Triphaladi Kalka:
त्रिफला व्योष पत्रैला त्वक्क्षीरी चित्रकं वचाम्| विडङ्गं पिप्पलीमूलं रोमशं वृषक त्वचम्||१५२||
ऋद्धिधं तामलकीं चव्यं समभागानि पेषयेत्| कल्यं लिप्तमयस्पात्रे मध्याह्ने भक्षयेत्ततः||१५३||
वर्जयेद्दधिशुक्तानि क्षारं वैरोधिकानि च| वातास्रे सर्व दोषेऽपि हितं शूलार्दिते परम्||१५४||
Ingredients:
Triphala (Haritaki, Vibhitaki and Amalaki),
Trikatu (Ginger, pepper and long pepper fruit),
Patra – Cinnamomum tamala Nees and Eberum.,
Ela (Elettaria cardamomum) ,
Tvak-Ksheeri(vamsa Locana),
Chitraka – Leadword – Plumbago zeylanica,
Vaca (Acorus calamus Linn.),
Vidanga – Embelia ribes,
Pippali -Mula,
Romasha (Kasisa),
Bark of Vatsaka (Holarrhena antidysenterica Wall.),
Riddhi,
Tamalaki – Phyllanthus niruri and
Cavya – Piper chaba is taken in equal quantities, and made to a paste.
In the morning, this paste is smeared over an iron pot, and the food kept in this pot is taken by the patient during the noon time.
The patient should avoid taking yogurt, Sukta (vinegar), Alkalies and mutually contradictory ingredients of food.
This is an excellent recipe for curing Vatarakta even when caused by the predominance of all the 3 Doshas, and is associated with excruciating pain. [152-154]

Line of Treatment:

बुद्ध्वा स्थान विशेषांश्च दोषाणां च बलाबलम्| चिकित्सितमिदं कुर्यादूहापोह विकल्पवित्||१५५||

The physician well versed in appropriate permutation and combination of therapies should apply the above-mentioned therapeutic measures (for Vatarakta - gout) after determining its location and, relative strength of the Doshas responsible for the causation of the ailment. [155]

कुपिते मार्ग संरोधान्मेदसो वा कफस्य वा| अतिवृद्ध्याऽनिले नादौ शस्तं स्नेहन बृंहणम्||१५६||

व्यायाम शोधनारिष्ट मूत्रपानै विरेचनैः| तक्राभया प्रयोगैश्च क्षपयेत् कफमेदसी||१५७||

बोधवृक्ष कषायं तु प्रपिबेन्मधुना सह| वातरक्तं जयत्याशु त्रिदोषमपि दारुणम्||१५८||

पुराण यवगोधूम सीध्वरिष्ट सुरासवैः| शिलाजतु प्रयोगैश्च गुग्गुलो माक्षिकस्य च||१५९||

Therapy for Vatarakta caused by Occlusion - Because of the obstruction to their course by the aggravated Vata, the Medas and Kapha get provoked in excess in Vata Rata (gout). In such an event, Snehana and Brihmana should not be employed in the beginning. The provoked fat and Kapha is brought to their normal state by exercise, by elimination therapy, by the intake of wine and urine, by Virechana and by the administration of butter-milk as well as Abhaya – Terminalia chebula (Haritaki).

Intake of the decoction of Bodhi tree along with honey instantaneously cures Vatarakta (Gout), even if it is of serious nature being caused by the simultaneous aggravation of all the 3 Doshas.

Inkate of old barley or wheat, Sidhu and Arista types of wine, sura (alcohol) Asava (a type of wine), or Silajatu, Guggulu (Commifora mukul Engl.) and honey also cures Vatarakta (gout). [156-159]

Treatment of Gambheera Vatarakta

गम्भीरे रक्तमाक्रान्तं स्याच्चेत्द्वातवज्जयेत्| पश्चाद्वाते क्रियां कुर्याद्वातरक्त प्रसादनीम्||१६०||

If in the Gambheera (Deep seated) Vatarakta blood is vitiated, then for its cure, in the beginning, Vayu is alleviated, and thereafter, the treatment for the alleviation of Vatarakta is given. [160]

Treatment of Suppurated (Paka) Vatarakta

रक्तपित्तातिवृद्ध्या तु पाकमाशु नियच्छति| भिन्नं स्रवति वा रक्तं विदग्धं पूयमेव वा||१६१||

तयोः क्रिया विधातव्या भेद शोधन रोपणैः| कुर्यादुपद्रवाणां च क्रियां स्वां स्वाच्चिकित्सितात्||१६२||

If, in Vatarakta, Pitta and Rakta are vitiated in excess, then this may lead to suppuration, bursting open of the wound and discharge of putrid blood as well as pus. This condition is treated by incision, purification and therapies for the healing of the wound.

Complications of Vatarakta are treated on the lines prescribed for the respective signs and symptoms. [161-162]

Summary:

तत्र श्लोकाः-

हेतुः स्थानानि मूलं च यस्मात् प्रायेण सन्धिषु| कुप्यति प्राक् च यद्रूपं द्विव विधिस्य च लक्षणम्||१६३||

पृथग्भिन्नस्य लिङ्गं च दोषाधिक्यमुपद्रवाः| साध्यं याप्यमसाध्यं च क्रिया साध्यस्य चाखिला||१६४||

वातरक्तस्य निर्दिष्टा समासव्यासतस्तथा| महर्षिणाऽग्निवेशाय तथैवावस्थिकी क्रिया||१६५||

Maharsi Atreya explained to Agnivesha, in brief as well as in detail, the following topics related to Vatarakta (gout):

Hetu – Etiology

Sthanani – Location of the diseases

Mulam – The base (root) of the disease

Kupyati roga – The reason for which the disease generally gets aggravated in the joints

Rupam – Premonitory signs and symptoms

Signs and symptoms of the 2 varieties of Vatarakta

Signs and symptoms of different types of Vatarakta

Signs and symptoms of the disease caused by the predominance of different Doshas

Complications
Curability, Palliability and incurability of the disease
Detailed treated or curable types of the disease and
Treatment of different stages of the disease. [163-165]

इत्यग्निवेशकृते तन्त्रे चरक प्रतिसंस्कृतेऽप्राप्ते दृढबल सम्पूरिते चिकित्सित स्थाने वात शोणित चिकित्सितं नामैकोनत्रिंशोऽध्यायः||२९||
Thus, ends the 29th chapter of Chikitsa section dealing with the "Treatment of Vatarakta" of Agnivesha's work as redacted by Charaka, and supplemented by Dridhabala.

13

Chikitsasthana Chapter 30 Yoni Vyapat Chikitsitam

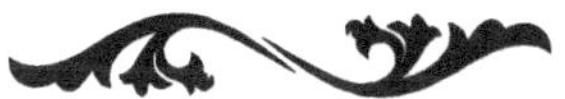

The 30th chapter of Charaka Samhita Chikitsa Sthana is called Yoni Vyapat Chikitsa Adhyaya. It deals with gynecological disorders, seminal disorders and postpartum disorders in women.
Chapter 30

अथातो योनिव्यापच्चिकित्सितं व्याख्यास्यामः||१||
इति ह स्माह भगवानात्रेयः||२||
Now we shall explore the chapter on the "Treatment uterine disorders. Thus said Lord Atreya [1-2]

Prologue:
दिव्य तीर्थौषधिमतश्चित्रधातु शिलावतः| पुण्ये हिमवतः पार्श्वे सुर सिद्धर्षि सेविते||३||
विहरन्तं तपोयोगात्तत्त्व ज्ञानार्थ दर्शिनम्| पुनर्वसुं जितात्मानमग्निवेशोऽनु पृष्टवान्||४||
भगवन्! यदपत्यानां मूलं नार्यः परं नृणाम्| तद्विघातो गदैश्चासां क्रियते योनिमाश्रितैः||५||
तस्मातेषां समुत्पत्तिमुत्पन्नानां च लक्षणम्| सौषधं श्रोतुमिच्छामि प्रजानुग्रहकाम्यया||६||
Punarvasu who has mastered self-control and who knew about truth of this universe by virtue of his penance and meditation was taking a stroll by the slopes of the Himalayas which abounds in celestial and sacred river, medicinal herbs and stones containing varieties of metals of variegated colours, and which is the abode of Gods, Siddhas (higher spiritual persons) and saints.
Agnivesha inquired as below:
"O Lord! Among human beings, women are the root cause of existence. The diseases of the female reproductive system cause many problems. Therefore, please explain the origin, signs, symptoms and treatment of these disorders for the welfare of humanity. [3-6]

Atreya Punarvasu replies as below:
इति शिष्येण पृष्टस्तु प्रोवाचर्षिवरोऽत्रिजः| विंशतिर्व्यापदो योनेर्निर्दिष्टा रोग सङ्ग्रहे||७||
मिथ्याचारेण ताः स्त्रीणां प्रदुष्टेनार्तवेन च| जायन्ते बीजदोषाच्च दैवाच्च शृणु ताः पृथक्||८||
Being thus asked by the disciple, Atreya the foremost of the sages replied, "In Sutrasthana the number of gynaecological disorders (Yonivyapat) is listed as 20.
These 20 uterine ailments are caused by
Mithyachara – wrong regime,
Pradushta Arthava – menstrual morbidities,
Beeja Dosha – defective genes, ovum and
Daiva or Karma.
Now, listen to their description individually (which follows) [7-8]

Vatika Yoni Roga Nidana, Lakshana:

वातलाहारचेष्टाया वातलायाः समीरणः| विवृद्धो योनिमाश्रित्य योनेस्तोदं सवेदनम्||९||

स्तम्भं पिपीलिका सृप्तिमिव कर्कशतां तथा| करोति सुप्तिमायासं वातजांश्चापरान् गदान्||१०||

सा स्यात् सशब्द रुक्फेन तनु रूक्षार्तवाऽनिलात्|

Vatika Yoni Roga causes and symptoms:

If a woman having Vata body type, resorts to Vata increasing food and regimen, it causes Vata increase. The aggravated Vata gets located in the reproductive organs to produce below symptoms –

Stambha – stiffness

Pipilika – a sensation as if ants are crawling

Stambha – numbness

Supti – numbness and such other ailments caused by Vata in that place (reproductive organs).

Because of aggravated Vata, she gets untimely menstrual bleeding which is

Phena – frothy

Tanu – thin and

Ruksha – dry and

Sa syat sa shabda – is associated with sound and pain. [9 – ½ 11]

Paittika Yoni Roga Nidana and Lakshana

व्यापत्कट्वम्ल लवण क्षाराद्यैः पित्तजा भवेत्||११||

दाहपाकज्वरोष्णार्ता नील पीतासितार्तवा| भृशोष्ण कुणप स्रावा योनिः स्यात्पित्तदूषिता||१२||

Paittika Yonivyapat is caused by the intake of Katu (pungent), Amla (sour), Lavana (saline), Kshara (Alkaline) and similar other types of food ingredients as a result of which the woman suffers from

Daha – burning sensation

Paka – suppuration

Jwara – fever and

Ushna – heating sensation.

Her menstrual discharge becomes

Nila, Pita asita artava – blue, yellow or black in colour, and

Bhrsha – in large quantity

Ushna – hot and

Kunapa Gandha – having offensive smell of a dead body [11 ½ – 12]

Kaphaja Yoni Roga Nidana and Lakshana:

कफोऽभिष्यन्दिभिर्वृद्धो योनिं चेद्दूषयेत् स्त्रियाः| स कुर्यात् पिच्छिलां शीतां कण्डुग्रस्ताल्पवेदनाम्||१३||

पाण्डुवर्णा तथा पाण्डु पिच्छिलार्तव वाहिनीम्|

By the intake of Abhisyandi ingredients (which cause obstruction to the channels of circulation, which form a coat on the inner lining of channels), the aggravated Kapha vitiates the reproductive organs of the woman and causes

Picchilam – sliminess

Shitam – cold

Kandu- itching

Vedanam – mild pain and

Pandu varna – pallor of her genital organ.

Pandu picchila artava vahinim – Her menstrual discharge will be pale in colour and slimy. [13- ½ 14]

Sannipatika Yoniroga Nidana Lakshana:

समश्नन्त्या रसान् सर्वान्दूषयित्वा त्रयो मलाः||१४||

योनिं गर्भाशयस्थाः स्वैर्योनिं युञ्जन्ति लक्षणैः| सा भवेद्दाह शूलार्ता श्वेत पिच्छिलवाहिनी||१५||

If the woman indulges in Samashana (intake of wholesome and unwholesome food together), the whole uterus and related organs get vitiated. Following this, the signs and symptoms of all the 3 Doshas – Vata, Pitta and Kapha – as described above are manifested.

She becomes afflicted with

Daha – burning sensation and

Shula – colic pain.

Sveta picchila artava vahini – Her menstrual discharge will be white in colour and slimy. [14 ½ – 15]

Rakta Yoni:

रक्तपित्तकरैर्नार्या रक्तं पित्तेन दूषितम्| अतिप्रवर्तते योन्यां लब्धे गर्भेऽपि सासृजा ||१६||

If the woman resorts to food and regimens which cause Raktapitta (bleeding disorders), then her blood being vitiated by Pitta flows in excess quantity through the genital tract, and the blood- flow does not stop even when the woman becomes pregnant. [16]

Arajaska Yoni Vyapat:

योनिं गर्भाशयस्थं चेत् पित्तं सन्दूषयेदसृक्| साऽरजस्का मता काश्र्य वैवर्ण्य जननी भृशम्||१७||

If Pitta is located in the vaginal tract and Uterus vitiates blood, then there will be no menstruation.

In addition, there will be

Karshya – extreme emaciation and

Vaivarnya – discoloration of the skin.

This ailment of reproductive organs is called Arajaska or amenorrhea. [17]

Acharana Yoniroga :

योन्यामधावनात् कण्डूं जाताः कुर्वन्ति जन्तवः| सा स्यादचरणा कण्डुवा तयाऽतिनरकाङ्क्षिणी||१८||

If the genital tract is not washed properly, then microbes (germs) grow and cause itching. This ailment associated with itching is called Acharana. The woman suffering from this ailment has excessive desire to have sex. [18]

Aticharana Yonivyapat:

पवनोऽतिव्यवायेन शोफ सुप्ति रुजः स्त्रियाः| करोति कुपितो योनौ सा चातिचरणा मता||१९||

Because of excessive sexual intercourse, the aggravated Vata causes

Shopha – swelling

Supti – numbness and

Ruja – pain in the genital tract of the woman.

This ailment is called Aticharana. [19]

Prakcharana Yoniroga

मैथुनादतिबालायाः पृष्ठ कट्यूरु वङ्क्षणम्| रुजन् दूषयते योनिं वायुः प्राक्चरणा हि सा||२०||

If a girl before attaining appropriate age (puberty) indulges in sexual intercourse, the aggravated Vata vitiates reproductive organs and causes pain in back, waist, thighs and groins. This ailment is called Prakcharana. [20]

Upapluta Yoniroga :

गर्भिण्याः श्लेष्मलाभ्यासाच्छर्दिनिःश्वास निग्रहात्| वायुः क्रुद्धः कफं योनिमुपनीय प्रदूषयेत्||२१||

पाण्डुं सतोदमास्रावं श्वेतं स्रवति वा कफम्| कफ वातामयव्याप्ता सा स्याद्योनिरुपप्लुता||२२||

If a pregnant woman indulges in Kapha aggravating food and regimes, and suppresses the manifested natural urge of vomiting and deep breathing, then the Vata in her reproductive organs gets aggravated. This increased Vata carrying Kapha to the genital organs vitiates Kapha. This leads to yellow discharge of mucus and pain. This Vata and kapha aggravated condition is called Upapluta. [21-22]

Paripluta Yoniroga:

पित्तलाया नृसंवासे क्षवथूद्गारधारणात्| पित्त सम्मूर्च्छितो वायुर्योनिं दूषयति स्त्रियाः||२३||

शूना स्पर्शाक्षमा सार्तिर्नीलपीतमसृक् स्रवेत्| श्रोणि वङ्क्षण पृष्ठार्ति ज्वरार्तायाः परिप्लुता||२४||

If a Pitta body type woman suppresses the manifested urge for sneezing and eructation during the sexual intercourse, then the aggravated Vata being afflicted by Pitta vitiates her reproductive organs.

This causes

Shoona – oedema

Sparsha kshama – tenderness and

Sa arti – pain in her genital organ and

Nila pitam asrk – discharge of bluish as well as yellowish blood.

Shroni vankshana prstha arti – She suffers from pain in waist, groin and back, and

Jvara – fever. This ailment is called Paripluta.[23-24]

Udavartini Yoniroga

वेगोदावर्तनाद्योनिमुदावर्तयतेऽनिलः| सा रुगार्ता रजः कृच्छ्रेणोदावृत्तं विमुञ्चति||२५||

आर्तवे सा विमुक्ते तु तत्क्षणं लभते सुखम्| रजसो गमनादूर्ध्वं ज्ञेयोदावर्तिनी बुधैः||२६||

If in a woman the course of the [downward moving] natural urges are reversed and made to move upward, then the aggravated Vata causes upward movement of the reproductive organs. This makes the woman afflicted with pain. She gets painful periods because of the tendency of the discharge to move in the reverse direction. The pain is relieved after discharge of menstrual blood. Because of the tendency of the menstrual flow (Avarta) to move upwards (Urdhva), wise physicians call this ailment as Udavartini. [25- 26]

Karnini Yoni Roga:

अकाले वाहमानाया गर्भेण पिहितोऽनिलः| कर्णिकां जनयेद्योनौ श्लेष्म रक्तेन मूर्च्छितः||२७||

रक्तमार्गावरोधिन्या सा तया कर्णिनी मता|२८|

If the pregnant woman strains prematurely to expel the foetus, then Vata in reproductive organs gets obstructed by the foetus. Being afflicted with Kapha and Rakta (blood), this aggravated Vata gives rise to Karnika (Polyp or nodular growth) in her genital organ. This polyp obstructs the course of blood flow, and the ailment is called Karnini. [27 -1/ 2 28]

Putraghni Yoniroga

रौक्ष्याद्वायुर्यदा गर्भं जातं जातं विनाशयेत्||२८||

दुष्ट शोणितजं नार्याः पुत्रघ्नी नाम सा मता|२९|

When the aggravated Vata, because of its dryness destroys each and every foetus produced from the polluted ovum, the ailment is known as Putraghni. [28 ½ – ½ 28]

Antarmukhi Yoni Roga:

व्यवायमतितृप्ताया भजन्त्यास्त्वन्नपीडितः||२९||

वायुर्मिथ्यास्थिताङ्गाया योनि स्रोतसि संस्थितः| वक्रयत्याननं योन्याः साऽस्थिमांसानिलार्तिभिः||३०||

भृशार्ति मैथुनाशक्ता योनिरन्तर्मुखी मता|३१|

If a woman after a heavy meal enters into sexual intercourse posture, then Vata located in the channels of reproductive organs gets suppressed by food. This aggravated Vata causes distortion of the cervix. As a result, she suffers from pain in the bones and muscles. Because of excruciating pain, sexual act becomes intolerable for her. This ailment of the uterine organ is called Antarmukhi. [29 ½ – ½ 31]

Soochi mukhi Yoniroga

गर्भस्थायाः स्त्रिया रौक्ष्याद्वायु योनिं प्रदूषयन्||३१||

मातृदोषादणुद्वारां कुर्यात् सूचीमुखी तु सा|३२|

If a pregnant woman resorts to wrong regimens, then Vata gets vitiated. Because of dryness of Vata, the genital organ of the female foetus in the womb of the mother becomes narrow in opening (stenosis) [and continues to be so even when the girl is grown up]. This ailment of the uterine organ is called Suchimukhi (needle like or narrow opening of the genital tract). [31 ½ – ½ 32]

Shushka Yoni Roga:

व्यवाय काले रुन्धन्त्या वेगान् प्रकुपितोऽनिलः||३२||

कुर्यादिवण्मूत्रसङ्गार्ति शोषं योनिमुखस्य च|३३|

If during the sexual intercourse, the woman suppresses her natural urges, then the aggravated Vata causes pain, obstruction to the passage of stool and urine, and dryness of the opening of the uterine organ [because of this dryness (Shushka) of the uterine organ (Yoni), the ailment is called Suska Yoni. [32 ½ – 1/ 33]

Vamini Yoni Roga:

षडहात् सप्तरात्राद्वा शुक्रं गर्भाशयं गतम्||३३||

सरुजं नीरुजं वाऽपि या स्रवेत् सा तु वामिनी|३४|

If the semen deposited in the vagina for 6 days or 7 nights is excreted with or without pain, then the ailment is called Vamini. [33 ½ – ½ 34]

Shandi Yoni Roga

बीजदोषातु गर्भस्थ मारुतोपहताशया||३४||

नृद्वेषिण्यस्तनी चैव षण्ढी स्यादनुपक्रमा|३५|

Because of a genetic defect, the Vata in the foetus destroys its developing reproductive organs in the womb of the mother. In later stage of her life, the woman develops aversion for men (sexual intercourse), and her breasts do not grow.

The woman having this ailment is called Shandi, and is incurable. [34 ½ – ½ 35]

Maha Yoni:

विषमं दुःख शय्यायां मैथुनात् कुपितोऽनिलः||३५||

गर्भाशयस्य योन्याश्च मुखं विष्टम्भयेत् स्त्रियाः| असंवृतमुखी सार्ती रूक्ष फेनास्रवाहिनी||३६||

मांसोत्सन्ना महायोनिः पर्व वङ्क्षण शूलिनी|३७|

If the woman sleeps in irregular postures or on an uncomfortable bed during sexual intercourse, then Vata gets aggravated to cause dilatation of the opening of uterus and vagina, since the dilated openings do not get closed, she suffers from pain and discharge of dry and frothy blood from the genital tract. There will be protuberance of the muscles, and she suffers from pricking pain in the joints and groins. [35 ½ – ½ 37]

Complications of Yoniroga :

इत्येतैर्लक्षणैः प्रोक्ता विंशति योनिजा गदाः||३७||

न शुक्रं धारयत्येभिर्दोषैर्योनिरुपद्रुता| तस्मादगर्भं न गृह्णाति स्त्री गच्छत्यामयान् बहून्||३८||

गुल्मार्शःप्रदरादींश्च वातादयैश्चातिपीडनम्|३९|

Thus, 20 Yonirogas are described. When the reproductive organs of the woman are afflicted with these ailments, she becomes incapable of retaining the semen as a result of which she does not conceive.

She becomes liable to many diseases like

Gulma (tumour),

Arsha – piles and

Pradara – menorrhagia because of the excessive affliction by Vata, etc. [37 ½ – ½ 39]

Predominance of Doshas in Yonirogas:
आसां षोडश यास्त्वन्त्या आद्ये द्वे पित्तदोषजे||३९||
परिप्लुता वामिनी च वातपित्तात्मिके मते| कर्णिन्युपप्लुते वातकफाच्छेषास्तु वातजाः||४०||
देहं वातादयस्तासां स्वैर्लिङ्गैः पीडयन्ति हि|४१|

Among the aforesaid [20] uterine diseases, in the last 16 varieties, the first 2, viz.,

Rakta Yoni and Arjaska varieties are caused by the aggravated Pitta,

Paripluta and Vamini varieties are caused by the aggravated Vata and Pitta

Karnini and Upapluta are caused by Vata and Kapha Dosha

And the remaining uterine disorders (viz, Acharana, Aticharana, Prakcharana, Udavartini, Putraghni, Antarmukhi, Suchimukhi, Sushka, Sandhi and Maha Yoni) are caused by aggravated Vata Dosha.

The aggravated Doshas, Viz, Vata etc, afflict the reproductive organs of the patient with their respective signs and symptoms. [39 ½ – ½ 41]

Predominance of Doshas in the 20 varieties of uterine disorders is as follows:

Name of the uterine Disorders – Predominace of Doshas

Vata Dosha dominant Yonivyapat:

Vatika Yoni Roga, Acharana, Aticharana, Prakcharana, Putraghni, Udavartini, Antarmukhi, Suchimukhi,, Shushka, Shandi, Mahayoni,

Pitta Dosha dominant Yoni Roga:

Paittika Yoni Roga, Arajaska, Rakta Yoni

Kaphaja Yoni Roga – Kapha Dosha

Vata and Pitta – Paripluta and Vamini

Vata and Kapha – Upapluta and Karnini

Sannipatika Yoni Roga – Vata Dosha, Pitta & Kapha

Yonivyapat Chikitsa Sutra – line of treatment:
स्नेहन स्वेद बस्त्यादि वातजास्वनिलापहम्||४१||
कारयेद्रक्तपित्तघ्नं शीतं पित्तकृतासु च| श्लेष्मजासु च रूक्षोष्णं कर्म कुर्यादि्वचक्षणः||४२||
सन्निपाते विमिश्रं तु संसृष्टासु च कारयेत्| स्निग्धस्विन्नां तथा योनिं दुःस्थितां स्थापयेत्पुनः||४३||
पाणिना नामयेज्जिह्मां संवृतां वर्धयेत् पुनः| प्रवेशयेन्निःसृतां च विवृतां परिवर्तयेत्||४४||
योनिः स्थानापवृत्ता हि शल्यभूता मता स्त्रियाः| सर्वां व्यापन्न योनिं तु कर्मभिर्वमनादिभिः||४५||
मृदुभिः पञ्चभिर्नारीं स्निग्ध स्विन्नामुपाचरेत्| सर्वतः सुविशुद्धायाः शेषं कर्म विधीयते||४६||

For Vata imbalance uterine disorders, patients are given

Snehana – oleation,

Swedana – sweating treatment (fomentation),

Basti – enema and such other therapies which alleviate Vayu .

For Pittaja Yonirogas – the Patient is given therapies which are cooling and which are curative of Raktapitta (an ailment characterized by bleeding from different parts of the body).

For Kaphaja Yonirogas: physicians should administer therapies which are dry and hot.

If the uterine diseases are caused by the aggravation of 2 or all the 3 Doshas, then the therapies prescribed above are combined and administered. If there is displacement of the uterus, the patient is given oleation and fomentation therapies. The tortuous uterus is pressed by the hand and brought to its normal position. If there is dilatation, after the administration of oleation and fomentation therapies, the passage is constricted.

If the uterus is displaced from its normal position, then it behaves like a foreign body in the woman.

In all the varieties of uterine diseases, after giving Snehana (oleation) and Svedana (fomentation) therapies, Pancha karma (5 elimination and fomentation therapies like emesis etc.,) is administered in a mild form.

When her body is clean of the morbid material, the remaining therapeutic measures (to be described hereafter) are administered. [41 ½ – 46]

Vataja Yonivyapat Chikitsa:

वात व्याधिहरं कर्म वातार्तानां सदा हितम्| औदकानूपजैर्मांसैः क्षीरैः स तिल तण्डुलैः||४७||

सवातघ्नौषधै र्नाडी कुम्भी स्वेदैरुपाचरेत्| अक्तां लवण तैलेन साश्म प्रस्तर सङ्करैः||४८||

स्विन्नां कोष्णाम्बुसिक्ताङ्गी वातघ्नैर्भोजयेद्रसैः|४९|

Treatment of Vatika Yoni Roga:

For the woman suffering from uterine diseases caused by aggravated Vayu, therapeutic measures which are curative of Vatik diseases are always useful.

Her body is smeared with oil mixed with rock- salt and thereafter, Nadi, Kumbhi, Ashma, Prastara and Sankara types of Sweda karmas are administered with the medicines containing meat of aquatic (Audaka) and marshy land-inhabiting animals (Anupa mamsa), milk, de-husked Tila – Sesame and Vayu- alleviating herbs.

After Swedana, she is sprinkled with warm water, and given mamsarasa prepared by boiling with Vayu- Alleviating herbs. [47 ½ – 49]

Bala Ghrita:

बला द्रोण द्वय क्वाथे घृत तैलाढकं पचेत्||४९||

स्थिरा पयस्या जीवन्ती वीर्षभक जीवकैः| श्रावणी पिप्पली मुद्ग पीलु माषाख्यपर्णिभिः||५०||

शर्करा क्षीर काकोली काक नासाभिरेव च| पिष्टैश्चतुर्गुणक्षीरे सिद्धं पेयं यथाबलम्||५१||

वात पित्तकृतान् रोगान् हत्वा गर्भ दधाति तत्|

1 Adhaka each of ghee and oil is cooked by adding 2 Dronas of the decoction of

Bala – Country mallow (root) – Sida cordifolia

Paste of Sthira – Desmodium gangeticum (Shala Parni)

Payasya – Impomoea paniculata

Jivanti – Leptadenia reticulata

Vira(Shatavari – Asparagus racemosus)

Rishabhaka – Manilkara hexandra

Jivaka – Malaxis acuminata

Sravani (morata or Murva – Marsdenia tenacissima)

Mashaparni – Teramnus labialis

Sugar

Ksira Kakoli – Lilium polyphyllum and

Kaka Nasa and

Milk (4 times in quantity of ghee and oil, i.e 8 Adhakas).

This medicated fat is taken in appropriate doses according to the strength of the patient. It cures diseases caused by aggravated Vayu and Pitta, and helps the woman to conceive. [49 ½ – ½ 52]

Kashmaryadi Ghrita

काश्मर्य त्रिफला द्राक्षा कासमर्द परूषकैः||५२||

पुनर्नवादिवरजनी काकनासा सहचरैः| शतावर्या गुडूच्याश्च प्रस्थमक्षसमैर्घृतात्||५३||

साधितं योनि वातघ्नं गर्भदं परमं पिबेत्|

1 Prastha of ghee is cooked by adding [the paste of] 1 Aksha of each of

Kashmarya – Gmelina arborea

Haritaki – Terminalia chebula

Vibhitaka – Terminalia bellerica

Amalaki – Phyllanthus emblica

Draksha – Vitis vinifera
Kasamarda – Cassia occidentalis
Parusaka – Grewia asiatica
Punarnava – Boerhavia diffusa
Haridra – Curcuma longa
Daru Haridra – Berberis aristata
Kaka nasa
Sahacara - Barleria prionitis
Shatavari – Asparagus racemosus and
Guduchi – Tinospora cordifolia.
This medicated ghee is an excellent cure for uterine diseases caused by Vayu. It is also an excellent medicine for the woman to help conceive. [52 ½- ½ 54]

Pippalyadi Yoga
पिप्पली कुञ्चिकाजाजी वृषकं सैन्धवं वचाम्||५४||
यवक्षाराजमोदे च शर्करां चित्रकं तथा| पिष्ट्वा सर्पिषि भृष्टानि पाययेत् प्रसन्नया||५५||
योनि पार्श्वार्ति हृद्रोग गुल्मार्शो विनिवृत्तये|
The paste of
Pippali – Long pepper fruit – Piper longum
Kunchika (Krishna Jeeraka) – Cuminum cyminum
Ajaji (Sveta –Jiraka) – Cuminum cyminum
Vrsaka (Vasaka) – Adhathoda vasika
Saindhava – rock salt
Vacha - Acorus calamus Linn.
Yava Kshara
Ajamoda – Ajowan (fruit) – Trachyspermum roxburghianum
Sugar and
Chitraka – Leadwort – Plumbago zeylanica is sizzled with ghee.
Adjuvant – Prasanna (a type of Alcohol)
Indicated in –
Yoni shoola -Pain in the reproductive organs
Parshva arti – Pain in the sides of the chest
Hrd roga – heart diseases
Gulma – Phantom tumor and
Arsha – piles. [54 ½ – ½ 56]

Vrushakadi Churna:
वृषकं मातुलुङ्गस्य मूलानि मदयन्तिकाम्||५६||
पिबेत् स लवणै मंद्यैः पिप्पली ककुञ्चिके तथा|
The powder of
Vrsaka(Vasa) – Adhatoda vasica
Root of Matulunga – Lemon variety – Citrus decumana / Citrus limon
Madayantika – Lawsonia alba
Pippali – Long pepper fruit – Piper longum and
Kuncika (Krishna Jiraka – Cuminum cyminum) is taken with alcohol added with salt to cure pain in the reproductive organs. [56 ½ – ½ 57]

Rasnadi Dugdha Paka and Guduchyadi Pariseka:

रास्ना श्वदंष्ट्रा वृषकैः पिबेच्छूले शृतं पयः||५७||

गुडूची त्रिफला दन्तीक्वाथैश्च परिषेचयेत्|

Intake of the milk boiled by adding

Rasna (Vanda roxburghi / Pluchea lanceolata),

Svadamstra (goksura) – Tribulus terrerstris and

Vrushaka (vasa) – Adhathoda vasica cures the pain in reproductive organs.

Affusion (Seka) is done over this part with the decoction of

Guduchi – Tinospora cordifolia

Haritaki – Terminalia chebula

Bhibhitaka – Terminalia bellerica

Amalaki – Phyllanthus emblica and

Danti – Baliospermum montanum [57 ½- ½ 58]

Saindhavadi Taila

सैन्धवं तगरं कुष्ठं बृहती देवदारु च||५८||

समांशैः साधितं कल्कैस्तैलं धार्यं रुजापहम्|

Oil is cooked by adding the paste of (quantity to be equal to that of oil)

Saindhava – rock salt

Tagara –Valeriana wallichii

Kushta – Saussurea lappa

Brihati – Solanum indicum and

Devadaru – Cedrus deodara

This medicated oil [Soaked in tampon] is kept inside the vagina which cures local pain. [58 ½ – ½ 59]

Guduchyadi Taila:

गुडूची मालती रास्ना बला मधुक चित्रकैः||५९||

निदिग्धिका देवदारु यूथिकाभिश्च कार्षिकैः| तैलप्रस्थं गवां मूत्रे क्षीरे च द्विगुणे पचेत्||६०||

वातार्तायाः पिचुं दद्याद्योनौ च प्रणयेत्ततः|

1 Prastha of oil is cooked by adding 2 Prasthas of each of Cow's urine and cow's milk and the paste of 1 Karsa of each of

Guduchi – Tinospora cordifolia

Malati – Jasminum grandiflorum

Rasna (Vanda roxburghi / Pluchea lanceolata)

Bala – Sida cordifolia

Madhuka– Licorice – Glycyrrhiza glabra

Chitraka – Plumbago zeylanica

Nidigdhaika –

Devadaru – Cedrus deodara and

Yuthika

A Tampon soaked with this medicated oils is inserted into the vagina and this may be administered in the form of douche for curing uterine diseases caused by Vayu. [59 ½ – ½ 61]

General Treatment for Vatika Yoniroga:

वातार्तानां च योनीनां सेकाभ्यङ्ग पिचु क्रियाः||६१||

(उष्णाः स्निग्धाः प्रकर्तव्यास्तैलानि स्नेहनानि च)|

For the patient suffering from uterine diseases, Seka, massage and pichu- kriya (insertion of tampon soaked in medicated oil in the general tract) is given with recipes which are hot and unctuous. For the purpose of oleation, medicated oils are used. [61 ½ – 1/3 62]

Kalka – medicinal pastes

हिंस्रा कल्कं तु वातार्ता कोष्णमभ्यज्य धारयेत्| पञ्च वल्कस्य पित्तार्ता श्यामादीनां कफातुरा||६२||

The patient suffering from Vatika Yonivyapat is given massage over the genital organs, and thereafter, she should keep a warm paste of Himsra – Nardostachys jatamamsi in vagina.

The patient suffering from Paittika Yoniroga should similarly be given massage, and thereafter, should keep the paste of Pancha Valkala (bark of Nyagrodha – Ficus bengalensis, Udumbara – Ficus racemosa, Asvattha – Ficus religiosa, Parisa – Thespesia populnea and Plaksa – Ficus lacor) in her vagina.

The patient suffering from Kaphaja Yonivyapat should keep the paste of shyama Trivrit, etc., in her vagina (Charaka Vimanasthana 8: 136) similarly after massage. [62 2/3]

Paittika Yoni Vyapat Chikitsa:

पित्तलानां तु योनीनां सेकाभ्यङ्ग पिचु क्रियाः| शीताः पित्तहराः कार्याः स्नेहनार्थं घृतानि च||६३||
(पित्तघ्नौषध सिद्धानि कार्याणि भिषजा तथा)|

General Treatment of Paittika uterine Diseases:

For the patient suffering from Paittika type of uterine diseases, Seka (affusion), Abhyanga (massage) and Pichu-Kriya (insertion of tampon soaked in medicated oil or ghee in the genital tract) is given with the help of recipes which are cooling and alleviators of Pitta. For the purpose of oleation, ghee boiled by adding Pitta alleviating herbs should be used. [63- ½ 64]

Brihat Shatavari Ghrita

शतावरीमूल तुलाश्चतस्रः सम्प्रपीडयेत्||६४||
रसेन क्षीरतुल्येन पचेतेन घृताढकम्| जीवनीयैः शतावर्या मृद्वीकाभिः परूषकैः||६५||
पिष्टैः प्रियालैश्चाक्षांशैर्द्वियष्टिमधुकैर्भिषक्| सिद्धे शीते च मधुनः पिप्पल्याश्च पलाष्टकम्||६६||
सिता दशपलोन्मिश्रल्लिह्यात् पाणितलं ततः| योन्यसृक्शुक्रदोषघ्नं वृष्यं पुंसवनं च तत्||६७||
क्षतं क्षयं रक्तपित्तं कासं श्वासं हलीमकम्| कामलां वातरक्तं च वीसर्प हृच्छिरोग्रहम्||६८||
उन्मादारत्यपस्मारान् वात पित्तात्मकाञ्जयेत्|
इति बृहच्छतावरी घृतम्|

The juice extract of 4 Tulas of the root of Shatavari – Asparagus racemosus and equal amount of milk is boiled with 1 Adhaka of ghee this is cooked by adding the paste of 1 Aksha of each of the drugs belonging to

Jivaniya group (Jivaka – Malaxis acuminata, Rishabhaka Meda Maha meda, Kakoli – Fritillaria roylei, Mudga Parni – Phaseolus trilobus, Masha parni – Teramnus labialis, Jivanti – Leptadenia reticulata and Madhuka– Licorice – Glycyrrhiza glabra)

Shatavari – Asparagus racemosus

Mrdvika – Vitis vinifera

Parusaka

Priyala

Jalaja Yastimadhu – Glycyrrhiza glabra and

Sthalaja Yastimadhu – Glycyrrhiza glabra.

After it is cooked and cooled, 8 Palas of honey, 8 Palas of Pippali – Long pepper fruit – Piper longum (powder) and 10 Palas of Sugar is added to it.

Dosage: 1 Pani Tala (Tola).

Indications:

It cures uterine diseases and morbidities of menstruation and semen. It promotes virility, and helps the woman to get a male progeny.

It also cures

Kshatam – Phthisis

Kshayam – consumption

Rakta Pitta – an ailment characterized by bleeding from different parts of the body)

Kasa – cough

Shvasam – Asthma

Halimaka (a serious type of Jaundice)

Kamala (ordinary Jaundice)

Vata Rakta (gout including other forms of arthritis)

Visarpa – erysipelas

Shiro graham – Stiffness (sluggishness) of the heart and head

Unmada – insanity

Arati (depression and epilepsy caused by Vayu and Pitta).

Apsmara

Thus, ends the description of Brhat Shatavari Ghrita. [64 ½ – ½ 69]

Jeevaneeyadi Ghrita:

एवमेव क्षीर सर्पि जीवनीयोपसाधितम्||६९||

गर्भदं पित्तलानां च योनीनां स्यादिभषग्जितम्|७०|

In the aforesaid manner (i.e by adding the juice of 4 Tulas of the root of Shatavari – Asparagus racemosus), Ksira Sarpi (ghee collected from the cream of milk) is cooked by adding the paste of drugs belonging to Jivaniya group (Jivaka – Malaxis acuminata, Rishabhaka , Meda Maha meda, Kakoli – Fritillaria roylei, Mudga Parni – Phaseolus trilobus, Jivanti – Leptadenia reticulata and Madhuka– Licorice – Glycyrrhiza glabra).

It helps in the conception, and cures uterine diseases caused by aggravated pitta. [69 ½ – ½ 70]

Kaphaja Yoniroga Chikitsa:

योन्यां श्लेष्म प्रदुष्टायां वर्तिः संशोधनी हिता||७०||

वाराहे बहुशः पित्ते भावितैर्लक्तकैः कृता| भावितं पयसार्कस्य यवचूर्णं ससैन्धवम्||७१||

वर्तिः कृता मुहुर्धार्या ततः सेच्या सुखाम्बुना| पिप्पल्या मरिचै र्माषैः शताह्वा कुष्ठ सैन्धवैः||७२||

वर्तिस्तुल्या प्रदेशिन्या धार्या योनि विशोधनी|७३|

For the uterine disorders caused by Kapha, application of wick- bougie in the genital tract for cleansing it is useful. It is to be prepared on a rolled piece of cloth (Laktaka) which is to be impregnated several times with the bile of a wild pig.

The Varti (wick- Bougie) prepared of Barley- flour and rock- salt is impregnated with the latex of Arka – Calotropis gigantea. It is kept in the genital tract for a short period, and thereafter, removed. Then the genital tract is douched with lukewarm water.

A Varti (wick –Bougie) of the shape and size (length and thickness) of the index finger is prepared out of Pippali, Maricha, Masam, Satahva, Kushta – Saussurea lappa and rock- salt, and is inserted in the genital tract which cleanses the reproductive organs. [70 ½ – ½ 73]

Udumbaradi Taila

उदुम्बर शलाटूनां द्रोणमब्द्रोण संयुतम्||७३||

स पञ्चवल्क कुलक मालती निम्ब पल्लवम्| निशां स्थाप्य जले तस्मिंस्तैल प्रस्थं विपाचयेत्||७४||

लाक्षा धव पलाश त्वङ्निर्यासैः शाल्मलेन च| पिष्टैः सिद्धस्य तैलस्य पिचुं योनौ निधापयेत्||७५||

सशर्करैः कषायैश्च शीतैः कुर्वीत सेचनम्| पिच्छिला विवृता कालदुष्टा योनिश्च दारुणा||७६||

सप्ताहाच्छुध्यति क्षिप्रमपत्यं चापि विन्दति|

1 Drona of the Udumbara Shalatu (tender fruit cut into thin slices) of Ficus racemosa

Pancha Valkala (barks of Nyagrodha – Ficus bengalensis, Udumbara – Ficus racemosa, Asvattha – Ficus religiosa, Parisa – Thespesia populnea and Plaksa – Ficus lacor), and

leaves of Kulaka (Patola – Trichosanthes dioica),

Malati – Jasminumgrandifolium and

Nimba – Neem (Azadirachta indica) is kept soaked in 1 Drona of water for the whole night and the next morning, the water is strained out.

With this water, 1 Prastha of oil is cooked by adding the paste of Laksa and the extract of the bark of Dhava – Anogeissus latifolia and Palasha – Butea monosperma and Gum- resin of Salmala – Salmalia malabarica. A tampon (picu) soaked in this medicated oil is kept inserted in the genital tract. Thereafter, the genital tract is douched with the cold decoction of the aforesaid drugs (Udumbara – Ficus religiosa, etc) mixed with Sugar.

This therapy helps in quickly cleaning the genital tract, which is slimy and dilated, and which is afflicted with chronic as well as serious types of uterine diseases within seven days. Thereafter, the woman becomes quickly capable of conception. [73 ½- ½ 77]

Udumbara Ksheera:

उदुम्बरस्य दुग्धेन षट्कृत्वो भावितात्तिलात्||७७||

तैलं क्वाथेन तस्यैव सिद्धं धार्य च पूर्ववत्|

Tila – Sesame is impregnated 6 times with the latex of Udumbara – Ficus racemosa. The oil extracted from these seeds of Tila – sesame is cooked by adding the decoction of Udumbara – Ficus racemosa.

The tampon soaked with this medicated oil is kept inserted into the genital tract in the aforesaid manner [for the cure of uterine diseases]. [77 ½- ½ 78]

Dhatakyadi Taila:

धातक्यामलकीपत्र स्रोतोज मधुकोत्पलैः||७८||

जम्ब्वाम्रमध्य कासीस लोध्र कट्फल तिन्दुकैः| सौराष्ट्रिका दाडिम त्वगुदुम्बर शलाटुभिः||७९||

अक्षमात्रैरजामूत्रे क्षीरे च द्विगुणे पचेत्| तैलप्रस्थं पिचुं दद्याद्योनौ च प्रणयेततः||८०||

कटी पृष्ठ त्रिकाभ्यङ्गं स्नेह बस्तिं च दापयेत्| पिच्छिला स्राविणी योनि विप्लुतोपप्लुता तथा||८१||

उताना चोन्नता शूना सिध्येत् सस्फोट शूलिनी|

Dhataki – Woodfordia fruticosa,

leaves of Amalaki – Phyllanthus emblica/ Emblica officinalis

Srotoja (Srotanjana),

Madhuka– Licorice – Glycyrrhiza glabra

Utpala (Nymphaea alba),

Pulp of the seeds of Jambu – Syzygium cumini and

Amra – mango – Mangifera indica

Kaseesa – Green vitriol

Lodhra - Symplocos racemosa

Katphala – Myrica nagi,

Tinduka

Saurastrika (Tuvari) – Sphatika

bark of Dadima – Pomegranate – Punica granatum and

Udumbara Salatu (tender fruits of Ficus racemosa)

They are ground and made into paste. Goat's urine and milk are taken twice the quantity of the above mentioned paste. 1 Prastha of oil is cooked with all these ingredients.

When the oil is processed and prepared a sterile cloth / wick is dipped in this oil and is inserted into the genital tract (vaginal canal).

Thereafter, massage is done over her lumbar region, back and sacral region, and the patient is given an unctuous type of medicated enema.

This cures the sliminess as well as exudation from the genital tract, uterine diseases like Vipluta, Upapluta, Uttana (Prolapse of Uterus), Unnata (Upward displacement of the uterus) and oedema accompanied with pustular growth as well as pricking pain. [78 ½ – ½ 82]

Dhavana Yoga – Recipe for Douche

करीर धव निम्बार्क वेणु कोशाम्र जाम्बवैः||८२||

जिङ्गिनी वृषमूलानां क्वाथै र्मार्द्वीक सीधुभिः| सशुक्तै र्धावनं मिश्रैर्योन्यास्राव विनाशनम्||८३||

कुर्यात् स तक्र गोमूत्र शुक्तैर्वा त्रिफलारसैः|८४|

Douching of the female genital tract with the decoction of

Karira, Dhava , Nimba – Neem (Azadirachta indica), Arka – Calotropis gigantea, Venu, Koshamra, Jambu

Jingini and root of Vrusha (Vasa) – Adhathoda vasica Mrudvika – Vitis vinfera as well as Sidhu types of wine along with Sukta (vinegar) cures morbid vaginal discharges.

Similarly, douching could be done with butter- milk, cow's urine, sukta (vinegar) or the decoction of triphala [which cures morbid vaginal discharges] [82 ½ – ½ 84]

Pippali Ayoraja Yoga:

पिप्पल्ययोरजःपथ्या प्रयोगा मधुना हिताः||८४||

The portion contains Pippali – Piper longum, powder (Bhasma) of Iron and Haritaki – Terminalia chebula is mixed with honey and given to the patient which is useful in curing Kaphaja Yonivyapats.

Recipes for Enema

श्लेष्मलायां कटु प्रायाः समूत्रा बस्तयो हिताः| पित्ते स मधुर क्षीरा वाते तैलाम्ल संयुताः||८५||

सन्निपात समुत्थायाः कर्म साधारणं हितम्|८६|

In uterine diseases of:

Kaphaja type – enema of recipes containing pungent drugs in general and cow's urine is useful.

Paittika type – enema of recipes containing sweet drugs and milk is useful.

Vatika type – enema of recipes containing oil and sour juice is useful.

Sannipatika type – all the aforesaid therapies mixed together are administered. [85- ½ 86]

Treatment of Rakta Yoni:

रक्तयोन्यामसृग्वर्णैरनुबन्धं समीक्ष्य च||८६||

ततः कुर्याद्यथादोषं रक्तस्थापनमौषधम्| तिल चूर्ण दधि घृतं फाणितं शौकरी वसा||८७||

क्षौद्रेण संयुतं पेयं वातासृग्दर नाशनम्| वराहस्य रसो मेद्यः सकौलत्थोऽनिलाधिके||८८||

शर्करा क्षौद्र यष्ट्याह्व नागरैर्वा युतं दधि| पयस्योत्पल शालूक बिस कालीयकाम्बुदम्||८९||

सपयःशर्करा क्षौद्रं पैत्तिकेऽसृग्दरे पिबेत्|९०|

In Rakta Yoni, the physician should ascertain the association of other Doshas from the colour of the blood, and respective Dosha balancing haemostatic medicines are administered.

Intake of the Yoga containing powder of Tila – Sesame, Yoghurt, ghee, Phanita (Penidium) and pig fat mixed with honey cures Asrugdara (Rakta Yoni) caused by the association of Vayu.

Intake of the soup of fatty meat of pig and Kulattha (horse gram) is useful for curing Rakta Yoni type of uterine diseases caused by the association of Vayu.

Similarly, intake of yoghurt mixed with sugar, honey, Yasti Madhu – Glycyrrhiza glabra and Nagara (ginger) is useful in this condition.

If the rakta yoni (Asrgdara) is caused by the association of Pitta, then the patient should take:

Payasya – Impomoea paniculata (Ksira Vidari (Ipomoea paniculata / Pueraria tuberosa))

Nilotpala – blue lily

Shaluka(Rhizome of lotus),

Bisa (Lotus Stalk),

Kaliyaka - P

   ita Chandana (Sandalwood – Santalum album) or

Ambuda (musta – Cyperus rotundus) mixed with milk, Sugar and honey. [86 ½- ½ 90]

Pushyanuga Churna:

पाठा जम्ब्वाम्रयोर्मध्यं शिलोद्भेदं रसाञ्जनम्||९०||

अम्बष्ठा शाल्मलीश्लेषं समङ्गां वत्सक त्वचम्| बाह्लीकातिविषं बिल्वं मुस्तं लोध्रं स गैरिकम्||९१||

कट्वङ्गं मरिचं शुण्ठीं मृद्वीकां रक्त चन्दनम्| कट्फलं वत्सकानन्ता धातकी मधुकार्जुनम्||९२||

पुष्येणोद्धृत्य तुल्यानि सूक्ष्म चूर्णानि कारयेत्| तानि क्षौद्रेण संयोज्य पिबेत्तण्दुल वारिणा||९३||

अर्शःसु चातिसारेषु रक्तं यच्चोपवेश्यते| दोषागन्तुकृता ये च बालानां तांश्च नाशयेत्||९४||

योनिदोषं रजोदोषं श्वेतं नीलं सपीतकम्| स्त्रीणां श्यावारुणं यच्च प्रसह्य विनिवर्तयेत्||९५||

चूर्णं पुष्यानुगं नाम हितमात्रेयपूजितम्|९६|

इति पुष्यानुग चूर्णम्|

The below mentioned drugs are collected in the Pusya constellation. They are taken in equal quantity and fine powder is prepared of them –

Patha – Cissampelos pariera, seed- Pulp of Jambu , Amra – mango – Mangifera indica, Silodbhava (pasana bheda , Rasanjana (Aqueous extract of Berberis aristata), Ambastha (a type of Patha) – Cissampelos pariera, Resin of Shalmali – Salmalia malabarica, Samanga – Rubia cordifolia, Bark of Vatsaka (Holarrhena antidysenterica Wall.), Bahlika (kunkuma), Ativisa – Aconitum heterophyllum, Bilva – Aegle marmelos, Musta (Cyperus rotundus), Lodhra (Symplocos racemosa), Gairika, Katvanga (aralu) Maricha – Black pepper fruit – piper nigrum,

Sunthi – Zingiber officinale, Mrdvika – Vitis vinfira, Rakta Chandana (Sandalwood – Santalum album), Katphala – Myrica nagi, Vatsaka (Holarrhena antidysenterica Wall.)(fruits), Ananta, Dhataki – Woodfordia fruticosa, Madhuka– Licorice – Glycyrrhiza glabra and Arjuna – Terminalia arjuna.

This powder is mixed with honey, and taken along with rice water (Tandula Vari).

It effectively cures

Arsas (piles) and

Rakta atisara – diarrhoea associated with bleeding, and

Disease of infants caused by Doshas (endogenous) and exogenous factors.

It effectively cures uterine and menstrual disorders associated with white, blue, yellow, brownish, black and pinkish discharges.

This useful recipe called Pusyanuga Churna is held in high esteem by Lord Atreya. Thus, ends the description of Pusyanuga Churna. [90 ½ – ½ 96]

Recipes for Rakta Yoni (Asrugdara)

तण्दुलीयक मूलं तु सक्षौद्रं तण्दुलाम्बुना||९६||

रसाञ्जनं च लाक्षां च छागेन पयसा पिबेत्| पत्रकल्कौ घृते भृष्टौ राजादन कपित्थयोः||९७||

पित्तानिलहरौ, पैते सर्वथैवास्रपित्तजित्| मधुकं त्रिफलां लोध्रं मुस्तं सौराष्ट्रिकां मधु||९८||

मद्यै निम्ब गुडूच्यौ वा कफजेऽसृग्दरे पिबेत्| विरेचनं महातिक्तं पैत्तिकेऽसृग्दरे पिबेत्||९९||

हितं गर्भ परिस्रावे यच्चोक्तं तच्च कारयेत्|१००|

For Asgdara, the following recipes are used:

The paste of the root of Tanduliyaka mixed with honey is taken along with rice water (tandulambu).

Rasanjana and Laksa are taken along with goat's milk.

The paste of the leaves of Rajadana and Kapittha (Feronia limonia) sizzled with ghee. This recipe alleviates pitta and Vayu.

In Paittika type of Asrgdara, the paste of Madhuka – Madhuca longifolia, Haritaki – Terminalia chebula, Bibhitaka

– Terminalia bellerica, Amalaki – Phyllanthus emblica, Lodhra (Symplocos racemosa), Musta (Cyperus rotundus), Saurastrika and honey is taken. It cures Rakta Pitta (an ailment characterized by bleeding from different parts of the body).

In the Kaphaja type of Asrgdara, Nimba and Guduchi is taken along with alcohol.

In Paittika type of Asrgdara, Purgation with Trivrt – Operculina turpethum, etc., is given, and the patient should take Maha Tiktaka Ghrta (Chikitsa 7: 144-150)

Therapeutic measures described for the management of Garbha Srva (threatened abortion) is used (Sarira 8: 24). [96 ½ – ½ 100]

Kashmaryadi Ghrita:

काश्मर्य कुटज क्वाथ सिद्धमुत्तर बस्तिना||१००||

रक्तयोन्यरजस्कानां पुत्रघ्न्याश्च हितं घृतम्|

Ghee cooked with the decoction of Kashmarya and Kutaja –(Holarrhena antidysenterica Wall.) is used for vaginal douche which is beneficial for the treatment of uterine diseases like Rakta Yoni, Arajaska and Putraghni. [100 ½ – ½ 101]

Treatment of Arajaska – amenorrhea:

मृगाजाविवराहासृग्दध्यम्ल फल सर्पिषा ||१०१||

अरजस्का पिबेत् सिद्धं जीवनीयैः पयोऽपि वा|

The woman suffering from Arajaska (amenorrhoea) type of uterine disease should drink the blood of deer, Goat, sheep and pig mixed with Yoghurt, juice of sour fruits and ghee.

She may also take the milk boiled with herbs belonging to Jivaniya Group (Jivaka Rishabhaka , Meda – Polygonatum cirrhifolium, Maha Meda – Polygonatum cirrhifolium, Kakoli – Fritillaria roylei, Ksira kakoli – , Mudga Parni –Teramnus labialis, Mashaparni, Jivanti and Madhuka– Licorice). [101 ½ – ½ 102]

Taila Uttara Basti for Karnini Etc.

कर्णिन्य चरणाशुष्कयोनि प्राक्चरणासु च||१०२||

कफवाते च दातव्यं तैलमुत्तर बस्तिना|

In Karnini, Acharana, Shushka Yoni, Prakcharana and such other diseases caused by Kapha as well as Vayu, the patient is given vaginal douche with the medicated oil prepared by boiling oil with drugs belonging to Jeevaniya group (Jivaka , Rishabhaka , MedaMaha meda,Kakoli – Fritillaria roylei, Ksira Kakoli , Mudga parni – Phaseolus trilobus, Mashaparni –Teramnus labialis, Jivanti – Leptadenia reticulata and Madhuka – Madhuca longifolia). [102 ½- ½ 103]

Treatment of Acharana:

गोपिते मत्स्यपित्ते वा क्षौमं त्रिःसप्तभावितम्||१०३||

मधुना किण्व चूर्ण वा दद्यादचरणापहम्| स्रोतसां शोधनं कण्डू क्लेद शोफहरं च तत्||१०४||

For the cure of Acharana, a piece of silk cloth impregnated for 21 times with cow's bile or fish- bile, and kept inserted into the vaginal tract.

Similarly, for the cure of this ailment, the powder of yeast mixed with honey may be kept inside the genital tract. This cleanses the genital tract, and removes itching, sloughing as well as oedema in the vagina [103 ½ – 104]

Treatment of Prakcharana and Aticharana

वातघ्नैः शतपाकैश्च तैलैः प्रागतिचारिणी| आस्थाप्या चानुवास्या च स्वेद्या चानिलसूदनैः||१०५||

स्नेहद्रव्यैस्तथाऽऽहारैरुपनाहैश्च युक्तितः|

In Prakcharana and Aticharana, the patient is given Asthapana and Anuvasana Basti with the medicated oil cooked for 100 times with Vata balancing medicines. Thereafter, Swedana is appropriately given with fat, food preparations and Upanaha (hot poultice) prepared with drugs which alleviate Vayu. [105 – ½ 106]

Treatment of Vamini:

शताह्वा यवगोधूम किण्व कुष्ठ प्रियङ्गुभिः||१०६||
बलाखुपर्णिकाश्र्याह्वैः संयावो धारणः स्मृतः|

The Samyava (Utkarika or thick gruel) prepared of Shatahva, Barley, wheat, yeast, Kushta – Saussurea lappa, Priyangu (Callicarpa macrophylla), Bala – Sida cordifolia, AkhuParnika and Sryahva (Gandha phiroja) is kept inserted in the genital tract [which helps in the embedment of the embryo in the uterus of the woman suffering from Vamini]. [106 ½ – ½ 107]

Treatment of Vamini and Upapluta

वामिन्युपप्लुतानां च स्नेह स्वेदादिकः क्रमः||१०७||
कार्यस्ततः स्नेह पिचुस्ततः सन्तर्पणं भवेत्|

In Vamini and Upapluta, therapies like Snehana, Swedana etc are given. Thereafter, the tampon (Pichu) soaked with the medicated oil is inserted into the vagina for providing nourishment to the genital tract. [107 ½ – ½ 108]

Treatment of Vipluta

शल्लकी जिङ्गिनी जम्बू धव त्वक्पञ्च वल्कलैः||१०८||
कषायैः साधितः स्नेहपिचुः स्यादि्वप्लुतापहः|

Oil is cooked with the decoction of

Sallaki – Boswellia serrata

Jingini and

the barks of Jambu – Eugenia jambolana

Dhava

Nyagrodha – Ficus bengalensis

Udumbara – Ficus racemosa

Asvattha – Ficus religiosa

Parisa – Thespesia populnea and

Plaksa – Ficus lacor

Tampon soaked with this medicated oil is kept inserted into the gential tract which cures Vipulta Yonivyapat. [108 ½ – ½ 109]

Treatment of Karnini [Kusthadi Varti]

कर्णिन्यां वर्तिका कुष्ठ पिप्पल्यर्काग्र सैन्धवैः||१०९||
बस्त मूत्रकृता धार्या सर्वं च श्लेष्मनुद्धितम्|

Varti (medicated bougie) is prepared with Kushta – Saussurea lappa, Pippali – Piper longum, buds of Arka – Calotropis gigantea and rock salt by triturating with goat's urine.

It is kept inserted into the vagina which cures Karnini type of uterine diseases. All the therapeutic measures prescribed for the treatment of diseases caused by kapha are also beneficial for the cure of this ailment. [109 ½ – ½ 110]

Treatment of Udavarta:

त्रैवृतं स्नेहनं स्वेदो ग्राम्यानूपौदका रसाः||११०||
दशमूल पयो बस्तिश्चोदावर्तानिलार्तिषु| त्रैवृतेनानुवास्या च बस्तिश्चोतरसञ्ज्ञितः||१११||
एतदेव महायोन्यां स्रस्तायां च विधीयते|

In Udavarta Yonivyapat and in Vatika type of Pain, Snehana with Traivrta (ghee, oil and muscle fat), Swedana and Mamsarasa of domesticated (gramya), marshy land (Anupa) inhabiting and aquatic animals (Audaka) are useful. In this disease, enema with Dashamoola ksheerapaka (milk boiled with Dashamoola) is also useful.

The patient is given Anuvasana Basti and Uttarabasti (vaginal douche) with Traivrta (ghee, oil and muscle fat).
The aforesaid therapeutic measures are also to be adopted for the treatment of Maha Yoni and for prolapse of uterus.
[110 ½- ½ 112]

Treatment of Maha Yoni:

वसा ऋक्ष वराहाणां घृतं च मधुरैः शृतम्||११२||
पूरयित्वा महायोनिं बध्नीयात् क्षौम लक्तकैः|

Vasa (muscle fat) of bears and pigs, and ghee are cooked by adding the herbs belonging to the sweet group (Vimanasthana 8/139). This recipe of medicated fat is kept inserted into the vagina of the woman suffering from Maha Yoni Yonivyapat. The vagina should be bandaged with silk cloth. [112 ½ -1/2 113]

Treatment of Prolapse Uterus – Prasruta Yoni Vyapat:

प्रस्रस्तां सर्पिषाऽभ्यज्य क्षीर स्विन्नां प्रवेश्य च||११३||
बध्नीयाद्वेशवारस्य पिण्डेनामूत्रकालतः|

In the case of Prasruta (prolapsed uterus), the uterus is massaged with ghee, fomented with warm milk and inserted into its normal position. Thereafter, the vagina is tied with a pad of Vesavara (a type of meat preparation) till there is the urge for urination. [113 ½ – ½ 114]

Importance of balance of Vata in uterine Diseases

यच्च वात विकाराणां कर्मोक्तं तच्च कारयेत्||११४||
सर्वव्यापत्सु मतिमान्महायोन्यां विशेषतः| नहि वातादृते योनि नारीणां सम्प्रदुष्यति||११५||
शमयित्वा तमन्यस्य कुर्याद्दोषस्य भेषजम्||११६|

In all types of uterine disorders, and especially in the Maha Yoni variety, a wise physician should administer all the therapeutic measures prescribed for the treatment of diseases caused by Vayu.
A woman never suffers from uterine diseases except as a result of affliction by increased Vata Dosha. Therefore, first, the aggravated Vayu is alleviated, and only thereafter, therapies are administered for the alleviation of other Doshas.

Treatment of Leucorrhoea – Pandura Asrugdara:

रोहीतकान्मूलकल्कं पाण्डुरेऽसृग्दरे पिबेत्||११६||
जलेनामलकीबीजं कल्कं वा स सिता मधुम्| मधुनाऽऽमलकाच्चूर्ण रसं वा लेहयेच्च ताम्||११७||
न्यग्रोधत्वक्कषायेण लोध्र कल्कं तथा पिबेत्| आस्रावे क्षौम पट्टं वा भावितं तेन धारयेत्||११८||
प्लक्ष त्वक्चूर्ण पिण्डं वा धारयेन्मधुना कृतम्| योन्या स्नेहाक्तया लोध्र प्रियङ्गु मधुकस्य वा||११९||
धार्या मधुयुता वर्तिः कषायाणां च सर्वशः| स्राव च्छेदार्थमभ्यक्तां धूपयेद्वा घृता प्लुतैः||१२०||
सरला गुग्गुलु यवैः स तैल कटु मत्स्यकैः| कासीसं त्रिफला काङ्क्षी समङ्गाऽऽस्मास्थि धातकी||१२१||
पैच्छिल्ये क्षौद्र संयुक्तश्चूर्णो वैशद्यकारकः| पलाश सर्ज जम्बू त्वक्समङ्गा मोच धातकीः||१२२||
स पिच्छिला परिक्लिन्ना स्तम्भनः कल्क इष्यते| स्तब्धानां कर्कशानां च कार्य मार्दव कारकम्||१२३||
धारयेद्वेशवारं वा पायसं कृशरां तथा| दुर्गन्धानां कषायः स्यात्तौवरः कल्क एव वा||१२४||
चूर्ण वा सर्व गन्धानां पूति गन्धापकर्षणम्| एवं योनिषु शुद्धासु गर्भ विन्दन्ति योषितः||१२५||
अदुष्टे प्राकृते बीजे जीवोपक्रमणे सति|१२६| पञ्चकर्म विशुद्धस्य पुरुषस्यापि चेन्द्रियम्||१२६||
परीक्ष्य वर्णे दोषाणां दुष्टं तद्घ्नैरुपाचरेत्|१२७|

Treatment of Leucorrhoea – Pandura Asrugdara:
For the cure of Pandura Asrugdara (Leucorrhoea) and for its associated ailments, the patient should use following recipes:
Paste of the root of Rohitaka is mixed with sugar, and taken along with water.
Paste of the seeds (Pulp) of Amalaki – Phyllanthus emblica is mixed with sugar and honey, and taken along with water.

The powder or the juice of Amalaki – Phyllanthus emblica is mixed with honey and made into linctus which the patient should use.

In the aforesaid manner, she should take the paste of Lodhra (Symplocos racemosa) along with the decoction of the bark of Nyagodha – Ficus bengalensis.

If there is profuse white discharge from the genital tract, then a piece of silken cloth impregnated with the decoction of the bark of Nyagrodha – Ficus bengalensis is kept inserted in the vagina.

The powder of the bark of Plaksha – Ficus lacor is made to a lump by triturating with honey. This is kept inserted in the vagina after anointing the part with fat.

The powder of Lodhra (Symplocos racemosa), Priyangu (Callicarpa macrophylla) and Madhuka– Licorice – Glycyrrhiza glabra is made into a lump by triturating with honey. This is kept inserted in the vagina after anointing the part with fat.

The varti (medicated bougie) prepared with astringent drugs and honey is kept inserted in the vagina.

For checking the discharge, the vagina is oleated, and thereafter, fumigated by Sarala, Guggulu (Commifora mukul Engl.) And barley mixed with butter, or by bitter fish (saphari) mixed with oil.

If there is sliminess of Vagina, then the powder of Kasisa, Haritaki—Terminalia chebula, Bibhitaka – Terminalia bellerica, Amalaki – Phyllanthus emblica, Kanksi mixed with honey is kept inserted into the genital tract which makes it non- slimy.

If there is sliminess and stickiness of vagina, then the paste of Palasha – Butea monosperma, Sarja (Vateria indica), bark of Jambu – Eugenia jambolana, Samanga – Rubia cordifolia, Moca and Dhataki – Woodfordia fruticosa is kept inserted into the genital tract which is stambhana (Arrests exudation).

In the case of stiffness and roughness of Vagina, softening remedies are used. For this, Vesavara (a type of meat preparation), Payasa (preparation of milk and rice) and Krsara (preparation of Pulses) is kept inserted in the vagina.

If there is foul smell in vagina, the decoction or the paste of Tuvaraka or the powder of Sarva Gandha (group of aromatic drugs) is kept inserted into the genital tract which works as deodorant.

When the gyecic organs get cleansed by the aforesaid measures, the woman becomes capable of conception provided the sperm of her husband and her own ovum are unpolluted, and possessed of natural attributes, and there is entry of the Jiva (soul).

Even if the man is cleansed of his physical morbidities by the administration of Pancha Karma (5 elimination therapies) his semen is examined, and from its colour, the nature of the afflicting Doshas (if any) is ascertained. If any morbidity of Doshas is found, then it is corrected by appropriate therapeutic measures. [116 ½ – ½ 127]

Thus it is said

भवन्ति चात्र-

सलिङ्गा व्यापदो योनेः स निदान चिकित्सिताः||१२७||

उक्ता विस्तरतः सम्यङ्मुनिना तत्त्वदर्शिना|

The great Sage having spiritual insight has explained above in detail the signs, symptoms, etiology and treatment of various types of Yoni Vyapat (uterine disorders). [127 ½ – ½ 128]

Dialogue between disciple and Preceptor

पुनरेवाग्निवेशस्तु पप्रच्छ भिषजां वरम्||१२८||

आत्रेयमुपसङ्गम्य शुक्रदोषास्त्वयाऽनघ!| रोगाध्याये समुद्दिष्टा ह्यष्टौ पुंसामशेषतः||१२९||

तेषां हेतुं भिषक्श्रेष्ठ! दुष्टादुष्टस्य चाकृतिम्| चिकित्सितं च कात्स्न्र्येन क्लैब्यं यच्च चतुर्विधम्||१३०||

उपद्रवेषु योनीनां प्रदरो यश्च कीर्तितः| तेषां निदानं लिङ्गं च चिकित्सां चैव तत्त्वतः||१३१||

समास व्यास भेदेन प्रब्रूहि भिषजांवर!| तस्मै शुश्रूषमाणाय प्रोवाच मुनिपुङ्गवः||१३२||

Again, Agnivesha approached Atreya, the foremost physician and asked, "Oh, Sinless one and foremost among the physicians! In Sutrasthana 19:3, you have stated in brief that there are 8 types of seminal defects. Please explain to us the etiology, signs and symptoms of normal and abnormal semen, and the treatment in their entirety.

Similarly, O foremost Physician! Kindly explain us the etiology, signs and symptoms, and treatment of Klaibya (impotency) which is described to be of 4 types and Pradara (menorrhagia) which is enumerated to be one of the complications of uterine diseases (Shloka 39) appropriately both in brief and in detail".

To the disciple desirous of hearing these details, the Foremost among the physicians (Atreya) replied as follows (to be described in the subsequent verses) [128 ½ -132]

Seminal Defects

Importance of Beeja – semen / sperm

बीजं यस्माद्व्यवाये तु हर्ष योनि समुत्थितम्| शुक्रं पौरुषमित्युक्तं तस्माद्वक्ष्यामि तच्छृणु||१३३||

During sexual intercourse, semen gets ejaculated as a result of excitement. It is the sign of masculinity, the reason for which it is called Bija or seed (the ingredient of procreation) (addressed by Atreya to disciple Agnivesha). [133]

Infertility of Polluted Semen

यथा बीजमकालाम्बु कृमि कीटाग्निदूषितम्| न विरोहति सन्दुष्टं तथा शुक्रं शरीरिणाम्||१३४||

As a seed does not grow when impaired by un-seasonal implantation and when afflicted by water, microbes, insects and fire, similarly the vitiated or polluted semen in human beings does not help in the precreation of an offspring. [134]

Etiology of seminal Pollution – Shukra Dosha Nidana:

अतिव्यवायाद्व्यायामादसात्म्यानां च सेवनात्| अकाले वाऽप्ययोनौ वा मैथुनं न च गच्छतः||१३५||

रूक्ष तिक्त कषायातिलवणाम्लोष्णसेवनात्| नारीणामरसज्ञानां गमनाज्जरया तथा||१३६||

चिन्ता शोकादविस्रम्भाच्छस्त्रक्षाराग्नि विभ्रमात्| भयात्क्रोधादभीचारादव्याधिभिः कर्शितस्य च||१३७||

वेगाघातात् क्षताच्चापि धातूनां सम्प्रदूषणात्| दोषाः पृथक् समस्ता वा प्राप्य रेतोवहाः सिराः||१३८||

शुक्रं सन्दूषयन्त्याशु ...|१३९|

Factors which cause seminal pollution:

Excessive sexual indulgence

Excessive physical exercise

Intake of unwholesome food

Untimely sexual intercourse

Sexual intercourse through tracks other than the female genital organ

Abstinence from sexual rapport during appropriate time

Intake of food which are exceedingly dry, bitter,astringent, saline, sour and hot

Sexual intercourse with women who are not passionate

Old age , worry, grief and lack of confidence [in the sexual partner]

Injury by sharp instruments, alkalies (Ksara) and cauterization (agnikarma)

Fear, anger and application of black magic (Abhicara)

Emaciation by diseases

Suppression of the manifested natural Urges and

Injury to and vitiation of tissue elements

Because of the above mentioned factors, the Doshas individually or jointly get aggravated, and reach the seminal channels instantaneously to vitiate the semen. [135 -1/4 139]

Seminal Morbidities – 8 Shukra Dosha

... तद्वक्ष्यामि विभागशः|

फेनिलं तनु रूक्षं च विवर्णं पूति पिच्छिलम्||१३९||

अन्य धातूप संसृष्टमवसादि तथाऽष्टमम्|

Now the differing types of seminal morbidities will be described by me (Atreya). These are of 8 types as follows:

Phenila (frothy semen), Tanu (thin semen), Ruksa(dry semen), Vivarna (discoloured semen), Puti(semen with putrid smell), Picchila (slimy semen), Anya dhatu-Samsrsta (semen mixed with other tissue elements) and Avasadi (semen sinking to the bottom when placed on water). [139 ¾- ½ 140]

Vataja Shukra Dosha – Seminal Morbidities Caused by Vayu

फेनिलं तनु रूक्षं च कृच्छ्रेणाल्पं च मारुतात्||१४०||
भवत्युपहतं शुक्रं न तद्गर्भाय कल्पते|

When the semen is vitiated by Vayu, it becomes frothy, thin, and dry.
It gets ejaculated with pain, and in small quantities. This type of vitiated semen does not help in conception. [140 ½ – ½ 141]

Seminal defects caused by Pitta

सनीलमथवा पीतमत्युष्णं पूतिगन्धि च||१४१||
दहल्लिङ्गं विनिर्याति शुक्रं पित्तेन दूषितम्|

If the semen is vitiated by Pitta, then it becomes blue or yellow in colour, excessively hot and putrid in smell. It causes burning sensation in the phallus during ejaculation [141 ½ – ½ 142]

Seminal morbidities caused by Kapha

श्लेष्मणा बद्धमार्गं तु भवत्यत्यर्थं पिच्छिलम्||१४२||

If the semen is obstructed by the aggravated kapha, then it becomes exceedingly slimy. [142 ½]

Semen associated with Blood:

स्त्रीणामत्यर्थं गमनादभिघातात् क्षतादपि| शुक्रं प्रवर्तते जन्तोः प्रायेण रुधिरान्वयम्||१४३||

Because of excessive sexual intercourse with women, Injury or ulceration, the semen gets ejaculated generally in association with blood. [143]

Avasadi Shukra:

वेग सन्धारणाच्छुक्रं वायुना विहतं पथि| कृच्छ्रेण याति ग्रथितमवसादि तथाऽऽष्टमम्||१४४||

Because of the suppression of the manifested urge for sex, the semen gets obstructed in its course by the aggravated Vayu, thus making it grathita (Knotty) and Avasadi (which sinks when placed over water). This semen associated with the 8 type of morbidity gets ejaculated with difficulty. [144]

इति दोषाः समाख्याताः शुक्रस्याष्टौ सलक्षणाः|

Thus, the 8 types of semen are described with reference to their signs and symptoms. [1/2 145]

Shuddha Shukra Lakshana: Signs of Pure semen:

स्निग्धं घनं पिच्छिलं च मधुरं चाविदाहि च||१४५||
रेतः शुद्धं विजानीयाच्छ्वेतं स्फटिक सन्निभम्|१४६|

The semen which is
Snigdham(unctuous), Ghanam – dense, Picchilam – slimy, Madhuram – sweet, Vidahi – non-irritating and Sphatika sannibham – white (transparent) like a crystal is to know as pure or normal [145 ½- ½ 146]

Shukradosha Chikitsa Sutra:

वाजीकरणयोगैस्तैरुपयोग सुखै हितैः||१४६||
रक्तपित्तहरै र्योगै र्यॉनिव्यापदिकैस्तथा| दुष्टं यदा भवेच्छुक्रं तदा तत् समुपाचरेत्||१४७||
घृतं च जीवनीयं यच्च्यवनप्राश एव च| गिरिजस्य प्रयोगश्च रेतोदोषानपोहति||१४८||

For the treatment of the vitiated semen, the following measures are taken:
Aphrodisiac recipes which are pleasant to use and beneficial

Therapeutic measures described for the treatment of Rakta Pitta (an ailment characterized by bleeding from different parts of the body- Charaka Chikitsa 4th chapter)

Therapeutic measures described (earlier in this chapter) for the Jivaniya group- Sutra 4: 9)

Chyavana Prasa(Chikitsa 1:1:62-74) and

Shilajatu (Chikitsa 1:3:48- 65)

Vataja Shukra Dosha Chikitsa

वातान्विते हिताः शुक्रे निरूहाः सानुवासनाः|

In Vataja Shukra Dosha, the patient is given Niruha and Anuvasana Basti. [1/2 149]

Treatment of Seminal Morbidities Caused by Pitta:

In the seminal morbidities caused by the aggravated Pitta, the patient is given Abhayamalakiya Rasayana (Chikitsa 1:1: 76- 77) [149 ½]

Treatment of seminal Morbidities caused by Kapha

मागध्यमृतलोहानां त्रिफलाया रसायनम्|

कफोत्थितं शुक्रदोषं हन्याद्भल्लातकस्य च||१५०||

Pippali–Rasayana (Chikitsa 1:3 32-35), Amalaki Rasayana (Chikitsa 1:1: 75), Loha –Rasayana (Chikitsa 1:2: 13) cure Kaphaja Shukradosha. [150]

Treatment of seminal Morbidities Caused by Association of Other Dhatus:

यदन्यधातु संसृष्टं शुक्रं तद्वीक्ष्य युक्तितः| यथादोषं प्रयुञ्जीत दोष धातुभिषग्जितम्||१५१||

If seminal morbidities are caused by the vitiated tissue elements, then after ascertaining their nature and those of the vitiated Doshas, the patient is given appropriate therapeutic measures for the correction of the concerned Doshas and tissue elements. [151]

Treatment of seminal Morbidities in General

सर्पिः पयो रसाः शालि र्यवगोधूम षष्टिकाः| प्रशस्ताः शुक्र दोषेषु बस्ति कर्म विशेषतः||१५२||

इत्यष्टशुक्रदोषाणां मुनिनोक्तं चिकित्सितम्|१५३|

Ghee, milk, meat soup, food ingredients like Shali (rice), barley, wheat and Sastika rice and medicated enema in special are very useful for correcting the treatment of eight types of seminal morbidities. [152 -1/2 153]

IMPOTENCY (KLAIBYA)

Varieties of Impotency:

रेतोदोषोद्भवं क्लैब्यं यस्माच्छुद्ध्यैव सिध्यति||१५३||

ततो वक्ष्यामि ते सम्यगग्निवेश! यथातथम्|१५४|

बीजध्वजोपघाताभ्यां जरया शुक्र सङ्क्षयात्||१५४||

क्लैब्यं सम्पद्यते तस्य शृणु सामान्य लक्षणम्|

Since impotency is caused by the seminal morbidities and it gets corrected by the purification of the semen, now O Agnivesha! I shall appropriately describe [the etiology, signs and treatment of] this disease systematically.

Impotency is of 4 types depending upon its causative factors as follows:

Bijopaghataja Klaibya (impotency caused by seminal diminution)

Dhvajabhangaja Klaibya (impotency caused by non-erectile phallus)

Jaraja Klaibya (impotency caused by old age) and

Shukra Ksayaja Klaibya (impotency caused by excessive loss of semen, i.e by sexual intercourse).

Now listen about their general signs and symptoms [which follows in subsequent verses][153 ½- ½ 155]

Signs and Symptoms of impotency in General

सङ्कल्प प्रवणो नित्यं प्रियां वश्यामपि स्त्रियम्||१५५||
न याति लिङ्ग शैथिल्यात् कदाचिद्यायाति वा यदि| श्वासार्तः स्विन्न गात्रश्च मोघ सङ्कल्प चेष्टितः||१५६||
म्लानशिश्नश्च निर्बीजः स्यादेतत् क्लैब्य लक्षणम्| सामान्य लक्षणं ह्येतद्विस्तरेण प्रवक्ष्यते||१५७||

Even though a man is constantly descrous of sexual intercourse with the partner who is cooperative, he, because of the looseness (absence of erection) of the phallus becomes incapable of performing the sexual act. Even if he rarely attempts sexual act, he gets afflicted with dysponea as well as perspiration in the body, and gets frustrated in his determined effects. His phallus becomes loose (because of the lack of erection), and he does not ejaculate any semen. These are the general signs and symptoms of impotency. Specific signs and symptoms of impotency will, hereafter be, described in detail. [155 ½ – 157]

Etiology and signs of Bijopaghataja Klaibya

शीत रूक्षाल्प सङ्क्लिष्ट विरुद्धाजीर्णभोजनात्| शोक चिन्ता भय त्रासात् स्त्रीणां चात्यर्थ सेवनात्||१५८||
अभिचाराद्विस्रम्भाद्रसादीनां च सङ्क्षयात्| वातादीनां च वैषम्यात्तथैवानशनाच्छ्रमात्||१५९||
नारीणामरसज्ञत्वात् पञ्चकर्मापचारतः| बीजोपघाताद्भवति पाण्डुवर्णः सुदुर्बलः||१६०||
अल्पप्राणोऽल्पहर्षश्च प्रमदासु भवेन्नरः| हृत्पाण्डुरोग तमक कामला श्रम पीडितः||१६१||
छर्द्यतीसार शूलार्तः कास ज्वर निपीडितः| बीजोपघातजं क्लैब्यं ...|१६३|

In Bijopaghataja type (impotency caused by the diminution of semen), the semen gets vitiated and diminished in quantity because of the following:

śīta rūkṣālpa saṅkliṣṭa viruddhā – Intake of cold, dry, scanty, polluted and mutually contradictory ingredients of food.

Ajīrṇabhojanāt- Intake of food before the previous meal is digested

śoka cintā bhaya trāsāt – Grief, anxiety, fear and terror

strīṇāṃ cātyartha sevanāt- Excessive indulgence in sex with woman

Abhicara (affliction by black magic)

Avisrambha (suspicious nature)

rasādīnāṃ ca saṅkṣayāt- Diminution of Rasa (plasma) and other tissue elements

vātādīnāṃ ca vaiṣamyā- Disharmony among Vata and other Doshas

Fasting and farting

nārīṇāmarasajñatvāt – Disliking for women and

pañcakarmāpacārataḥ- Improper administration of PanchaKarma (5 elimination therapies)

Because of the seminal destruction (diminution) as a result of the aforesaid factors, the patient becomes pale in color, very weak and low in vitality. He gets low excitement while meeting female partners, he suffers from - Hrt roga – heart diseases, Pandu roga – anemia, Tamaka shwasa – asthma, Kamala – jaundice, Shrama – physical exhaustion, Chardi – vomiting, Atisara – diarrhoea,, Shoola – colic pain

Kasa- cough and Jwara- fever. [158- 1/3 162]

Etiology of Dhvajabhangaja Klaibya:

... ध्वजभङ्गकृतं शृणु||१६२||
अत्यम्ल लवण क्षार विरुद्धासात्म्यभोजनात्| अत्यम्बुपानादिविषमात् पिष्टान्न गुरु भोजनात्||१६३||
दधि क्षीरानूप मांस सेवनाद्व्याधिकर्षणात्| कन्यानां चैव गमनाद योनि गमनादपि||१६४||
दीर्घरोगां चिरोत्सृष्टां तथैव च रजस्वलाम्| दुर्गन्धां दुष्टयोनिं च तथैव च परिसुताम्||१६५||
ईदृशीं प्रमदां मोहाद्यो गच्छेत् कामहर्षितः| चतुष्पदाभिगमनाच्छेफसश्चाभिघाततः||१६६||
अधावनाद्वा मेढ्रस्य शस्त्र दन्त नख क्षतात्| काष्ठ प्रहार निष्पेषाच्छुकानां चातिसेवनात्||१६७||
रेतसश्च प्रतीघाताद्ध्वजभङ्गः प्रवर्तते|

Hear about the impotency caused by Dhvaja Bhanga (non-erectile phallus) which takes place because of the following factors:

atyamla lavaṇa kṣāra viruddhāsātmyabhojanāt – Intake of excessively sour, saline, alkaline, mutually antagonistic and unwholesome ingredients of food

atyambupānā – Intake of water in excess

Taking meals irregularly

piṣṭānna guru bhojanāt – Intake of pastry and heavy food habitually

dadhi kṣīrānūpa māṃsa sevanādvyādhikarṣaṇāt- Intake of yoghurt, milk and meat of animals inhabiting marshy land

Emaciation because of diseases

kanyānāṃ caiva gamanāda – Cohabitation with young virgin girls

yoni gamanādapi- Sexual intercourse in parts other than vagina

dīrgharogāṃ cirotsṛṣṭāṃ tathaiva ca rajasvalām durgandhāṃ duṣṭayoniṃ ca tathaiva ca parisrutām – Because of excitement and ignorance, sexual intercourse with a woman who is suffering from chronic diseases, in continuation who has shunned sexual relationship for a long time, who is in menstruation, and whose vagina is offensive in smell, afflicted with diseases and has profuse discharge

catuṣpadābhigamanācchephasaścābhighātataḥ- Sexual intercourse with quadruped animals,Trauma to the phallus,not cleaning the phallus properly

adhāvanādvā medhrasya śastra danta nakha kṣatāt- Injury to the phallus by weapons, teeth, nails, beating by a stick or compression

kāṣṭha prahāra niṣpeṣācchūkānāṃ cātisevanāt- Excessive use of Sukas (a type of insect which is applied for the elongation of the phallus) and

retasaśca pratīghātāddhvajabhaṅgaḥ pravartate- Suppression of the urge for seminal ejaculation during sexual intercourse. [¼ 162- 1/3 168]

I shall, hereafter, describe the signs and symptoms caused by Dhvajabhanga (morbidity of the phallus) which are as follows:

śvayathurvedanā medhre rāgaścaivopalakṣyate- Swelling, pain and redness of the phallus

sphoṭāśca tīvrā jāyante liṅgapāko bhavatyapi- Serious types of pustular eruption in and suppression of the phallus

māṃsavṛddhirbhaveccāsya vraṇāḥ kṣipraṃ bhavantyapi- Fleshy growth in the phallus and its quick ulceration

pulākodaka saṅkāśaḥ srāvaḥ śyāvāruṇaprabhaḥ- Exudation which appears like rice water (Pulakodaka) or which is brownish black or pink in color

valayīkurute cāpi kaṭhinaśca parigrahaḥ- Circular and hard indurations below the glans penis

jvarastṛṣṇā bhramo mūrcchā cchardiścāsyopajāyate – Fever, morbid thirst, giddiness, fainting and vomiting

raktaṃ kṛṣṇaṃ sravccāpi nīlamāvila lohitam-Discharge of red, black, blue, turbid and red colored liquid from the urethra

agnineva ca dagdhasya tīvro dāhaḥ savedanaḥ|bastau vṛṣaṇayorvā'pi sīvanyāṃ vaṅkṣaṇeṣu ca – Acute burning sensation as if burnt by fire, and pain in the region of urinary bladder, testicles, perineal suture and groins.

kadācitpicchilo vā'pi pāṇḍuḥ srāvaśca jāyate- Discharge of slimy and pale yellow liquid at times

śvayathurjāyate mandaḥ stimito'lpaparisravaḥ- Mild swelling, numbness and scanty discharge

cirācca pākaṃ vrajati śīghraṃ vā'tha pramucyate- It takes long time to suppurate and may get abated quickly

jāyante krimayaścāpi klidyate pūtigandhi ca- Appearance of maggots in the phallus:

viśīryate maṇiścāsya medhraṃ muṣkāvathāpi ca- Sloughing and foul smell of the phallus and

dhvajabhaṅgakṛtaṃ klaibyamityetat samudāhṛtam- Dropping of the glance penis or of the whole penis or of the testicles

Thus, the impotency caused by Dhwajabhanga (morbidity of the phallus) is explained.

According to some physicians, this type of impotency caused by Dhvajabhanga is of 5 varieties. [168 2/3 – ½ 176]

The 5 varieties of Dhvajabhanga are as follows

(भवन्ति यानि रूपाणि तस्य वक्ष्याम्यतः परम्)।

श्वयथुर्वेदना मेढ्रे रागश्चैवोपलक्ष्यते॥१६८॥

स्फोटाश्च तीव्रा जायन्ते लिङ्गपाको भवत्यपि। मांसवृद्धिर्भवेच्चास्य व्रणाः क्षिप्रं भवन्त्यपि॥१६९॥

पुलाकोदक सङ्काशः स्रावः श्यावारुणप्रभः| वलयीकुरुते चापि कठिनश्च परिग्रहः||१७०||

ज्वरस्तृष्णा भ्रमो मूर्च्छा च्छर्दिश्चास्योपजायते| रक्तं कृष्णं स्रवेच्चापि नीलमाविल लोहितम्||१७१||

अग्निनेव च दग्धस्य तीव्रो दाहः सवेदनः| बस्तौ वृषणयोर्वाऽपि सीवन्यां वङ्क्षणेषु च||१७२||

कदाचित्पिच्छिलो वाऽपि पाण्डुः स्रावश्च जायते| श्वयथुर्जायते मन्दः स्तिमितोऽल्पपरिस्रवः||१७३||

चिराच्च पाकं व्रजति शीघ्रं वाऽथ प्रमुच्यते| जायन्ते क्रिमयश्चापि क्लिद्यते पूतिगन्धि च||१७४||

विशीर्यते मणिश्चास्य मेढ्रं मुष्कावथापि च| ध्वजभङ्गकृतं क्लैब्यमित्येतत् समुदाहृतम्||१७५||

एतं पञ्चविधं केचिद्ध्वजभङ्गं प्रचक्षते|१७६|

Next, I shall explain the signs and symptoms manifested in the dhvajabhanga –

Swelling in the genitals, pain, redness, severe eruptions / blisters which would undergo suppuration, fleshy outgrowths on penis, and quick manifestation of ulcers, manifestation of pulakodaka (whitish fluid) from the ulcers which are blackish or reddish in color

Crookedness of the penis, hardness in penis

Fever, excessive thirst, giddiness, unconsciousness, vomiting,

Discharge of blood having red, black and blue color and is also dirty in appearance from the ulcers / wounds

Severe pain with burning sensation as if burnt by fire – mainly experienced in urinary bladder, scrotum / testes, perineum, and groin

Occasionally pale and sticky discharges can be seen coming from penis,

Swelling of penis sometimes becomes less, coldness is manifested in it and discharges also become less

Sometimes quick and sometimes delayed suppuration,

Worms / parasites develop once the wound / ulcer gets suppurated

The penis will always be in a moist and rotten state and also would emit foul / rotten smell

There is a possibility of the glans, penis and scrotum (testicles) to get decayed / rotten and fall off

These are the signs and symptoms of klaibya caused due to dvajabhanga.

Experts consider dvajabhanga to be of five types.

Jaraja Klaibya:

क्लैब्यं जरा सम्भवं हि प्रवक्ष्याम्यथ तच्छृणु||१७६||

जघन्य मध्य प्रवरं वयस्त्रिविधमुच्यते| अतिप्रवयसां शुक्रं प्रायशः क्षीयते नृणाम्||१७७||

रसादीनां सङ्क्षयाच्च तथैवावृष्यसेवनात्| बलवीर्येन्द्रियाणां च क्रमेणैव परिक्षयात्||१७८||

परिक्षयादायुषश्चाप्यनाहाराच्छ्रमात् क्लमात्| जरासम्भवजं क्लैब्यमित्येतैर्हेतुभिर्नृणाम्||१७९||

जायते तेन सोऽत्यर्थं क्षीणधातुः सुदुर्बलः| विवर्णो दुर्बलो दीनः क्षिप्रं व्याधिमथाश्नुते||१८०||

एतज्जरासम्भवं हि ...|१८१|

Now I shall describe the type of impotency caused by old age which you may hear (addressed by the Preceptor Atreya to the disciple Agnivesha).

Age of a person is divided into 3 parts, viz,

Jaghanya (childhood),

Madhya (adulthood) and

Pravara (old age).

In old age, generally the semen gets diminished.

Impotency takes place in the old age because of the following:

Diminution of tissue elements like Rasa(plasma) etc

Constant use of ingredients which are detrimental to the vitality of a person

Gradual diminution of strength, energy, power of senses and span of life

Inability of take nourishing food and

Physical as well as mental fatigue

Because of the aforesaid factors, the tissue element of the old man becomes diminished and excessively weak. His complexion becomes perverted; he becomes physically and mentally weak; and he succumbs to different types of diseases quickly.

These are the characteristic features of geriatric impotency. [176 ½- ¼ 181]

Kshayaja Type of Impotency

... चतुर्थं क्षयजं शृणु।

अतीव चिन्तनाच्चैव शोकात्क्रोधाद्भयात्तथा॥१८१॥

ईर्ष्योत्कण्ठामदोद्वेगान् सदा विशति यो नरः। कृशो वा सेवते रूक्षमन्नपानं तथौषधम्॥१८२॥

दुर्बल प्रकृतिश्चैव निराहारो भवेद्यदि। असात्म्यभोजनाच्चापि हृदये यो व्यवस्थितः॥१८३॥

रसः प्रधानधातुर्हि क्षीयेताशु ततो नृणाम्। रक्तादयश्च क्षीयन्ते धातवस्तस्य देहिनः॥१८४॥

शुक्रावसानास्तेभ्योऽपि शुक्रं धाम परं मतम्। चेतसो वाऽतिहर्षेण व्यवायं सेवतेऽति यः॥१८५॥

तस्याशु क्षीयते शुक्रं ततः प्राप्नोति सङ्क्षयम्। घोरं व्याधिमवाप्नोति मरणं वा स गच्छति॥१८६॥

शुक्रं तस्मादिवशेषेण रक्ष्यमारोग्यमिच्छता। एवं निदान लिङ्गाभ्यामुक्तं क्लैब्यं चतुर्विधम्॥१८७॥

Now hear about the 4th type of impotency which is caused by the diminution of semen gets diminished because of the following factors:

atīva cintanāccaiva śokātkrodhādbhayāttathā- Constant exposure to worry, grief, anger, fear, envy, anxiety, intoxication and nervousness

kṛśo vā sevate rūkṣamannapānaṃ tathauṣadham- Intake of dry food, drinks and drugs by an emaciated person

durbala prakṛtiścaiva nirāhāro bhavedyadi- Fasting by a person who is weakening nature; and

asātmyabhojanāccāpi – Intake of unwholesome food

By the aforesaid factors, Rasa (plasma) which is the primary tissue element and which is located in the heart gets diminished soon. As a result of this, other tissue elements beginning from Rakta (blood) up to semen get diminished in that person. Among all these tissue elements, semen (Shukra) which is the final product is the most important

If a person because of excessive mental excitement indulges in sexual intercourse in excess, his semen gets diminished soon, and he gets emaciated. He succumbs to serious diseases, and even death.

Therefore, a person desirous of good health should specially preserve his semen.Thus, the etiology and signs as well as symptoms of 4 types of impotency are described. [181 ¾ – 187]

Prognosis:

केचित् क्लैब्ये त्वसाध्ये द्वे ध्वजभङ्गक्षयोद्भवे। वदन्ति शेफसश्छेदाद्वृषणोत्पाटनेन च॥१८८॥

मातापित्रोर्बीजदोषादशुभैश्चाकृतात्मन। गर्भस्थर्य यदा दोषाः प्राप्य रेतोवहाःसिराः॥१८९॥

शोषयन्त्याशु तन्नाशाद्रेतश्चाप्युपहन्यते। तत्र सम्पूर्ण सर्वाङ्गः स भवत्यपुमान् पुमान्॥१९०॥

एते त्वसाध्या व्याख्याताः सन्निपात समुच्छ्रयात्॥१९१।

According to some physicians, impotency caused by Dhwajabhanga (morbidity of Phallus) and Ksaya (diminution of semen) are incurable. In this context, Dhvajabhanga caused by amputation of the phallus and testicles is to be considered as incurable.

The term "Ksaya" in this context of incurability refers to the condition caused due to

- defects or morbidities in sperm and ovum / morbidities during embryonic stage or

- doshas getting aggravated due to the indulgence of a person who doesn't have self control – in inauspicious and unwholesome acts and deeds

The doshas thus afflict the channel carrying sperm (of the fetus), and make it atrophied. Because of this, [in the later part of life] the process of semen formation in the offspring is inhibited. Thus, the man, though having full physical development, becomes emasculated.

Different types of impotencies described before which are caused by the simultaneous vitiation of all the 3 Doshas (sannipata) are also incurable. [188- ½ 191]

Line of treatment of Impotency

चिकित्सितमतस्तूर्ध्वं समास व्यासतः शृणु॥१९१॥

शुक्रदोषेषु निर्दिष्टं भेषजं यन्मयाऽनघ। क्लैब्योपशान्तये कुर्यात् क्षीण क्षतहितं च यत्॥१९२॥
बस्तयः क्षीर सर्पींषि वृष्ययोगाश्च ये मताः। रसायन प्रयोगाश्च सर्वानेतान् प्रयोजयेत्॥१९३॥
समीक्ष्य देह दोषाग्निबलं भेषज कालवित्। व्यवाय हेतुजे क्लैब्ये तथा धातु विपर्ययात्॥१९४॥
दैवव्यपाश्रयं चैव भेषजं चाभिचारजे । समासेनैतदुद्दिष्टं भेषजं क्लैब्य शान्तये॥१९५॥

O! Sinless one (addressed to Agnivesha), hereafter will be described the treatment of impotency in brief as well as in detail which you may hear. These therapies for the cure of impotency, in brief, are as follows:

Remedies described by me (Atreya) for the treatment of seminal morbidities in this chapter

Therapeutic measures described earlier (in the chapter XI) for the treatment of Ksina (Phthisis) and

Medicated enema, medicated milk, medicated ghee aphrodisciac, recipes and rejuvenating recipes.

To the patient suffering from impotency as a result of sexual indulgence (Vyavaya hetuja), and disharmony among the Dhatus (Doshas), the physician well versed in medicaments (Bhesaja) and time (Kala) should administer all the aforesaid therapeutic measures keeping in view the strength of his body, Doshas and Agni (power of digestion and metabolism).

If the impotency is caused by Abhicara (black magic), then such a patient is treated with religious prayers and rituals (Daiva Vyapasrya Chikitsa). Thus, in brief, the remedies for the cure of impotency are described.

PanchaKarma Therapy:

विस्तरेण प्रवक्ष्यामि क्लैब्यानां भेषजं पुनः। सुस्विन्न स्निग्ध गात्रस्य स्नेहयुक्तं विरेचनम्॥१९६॥
अन्नाशनं ततः कुर्यादथवाऽऽस्थापनं पुनः। प्रदद्यान्मतिमान् वैद्यस्ततस्तमनुवासयेत्॥१९७॥
पलाशैरण्डमुस्ताद्यैः पश्चादास्थापयेत्ततः।

Now, the therapeutic measures for the cure of impotency will be described by me (Atreya) in detail.

After giving proper fomentation therapy to the patient whose body is oleated, he is given purgation therapy with a recipe containing fat. This should follow the patient's taking appropriate food (according to prescribed procedure). Thereafter, the wise physician should administer Asthapana type of medicated enema followed by Anuvasana type of enema.

Asthapana type of enema is given again with [the decoction of] the leaves of Palasha – Butea monosperma, Eranda – Ricinus communis, etc., or with Musta (Cyperus rotundus). Etc [196- ½ 198]

Treatment of Bijophataja Type of Impotency:

वाजीकरणयोगाश्च पूर्व ये समुदाहृताः॥१९८॥ भिषजा ते प्रयोज्याः स्युः क्लैब्ये बीजोपघातजे।

Aphrodisiac therapies described earlier may be used by the physician to cure impotency caused by Bijopaghata (Pollution of semen). [198 ½ – ½ 199]

Treatment of Dhvajabhanga Type of Impotency:

ध्वजभङ्गकृतं क्लैब्यं ज्ञात्वा तस्याचरेत् क्रियाम्॥१९९॥
प्रदेहान् परिषेकांश्च कुर्याद्वा रक्तमोक्षणम्। स्नेहपानं च कुर्वीत सस्नेहं च विरेचनम्॥२००॥
अनुवासं ततः कुर्यादथवाऽऽस्थापनं पुनः। व्रणवच्च क्रियाः सर्वास्तत्र कुर्यादिवचक्षणः॥२०१॥

If the impotency is caused by Dhvajabhanga (morbidity of the phallus), then the patient is treated with

Pradeha (application of warm paste of drugs),

Pariseka (affusion with the decoction of drugs),

Rakta Moksana (blood-letting),

Sneha Pana (administration of ghee, etc) and

Vireka (purgation) with a recipe containing fat.

After that, Anuvasana type of medicated enema followed by Asthapana type of medicated enema is administered. The intelligent physician should, thereafter, adopt all the therapeutic measures prescribed for the treatment of wounds. [199 ½- 201]

Treatment of Jaraja and Ksayaja Impotency:

जरा सम्भवजे क्लैब्ये क्षयजे चैव कारयेत्| स्नेह स्वेदोपपन्नस्य सस्नेहं शोधनं हितम्||२०२||

क्षीर सर्पि वृष्य योगा बस्तयश्चैव यापना:| रसायन प्रयोगाश्च तयोर्भेषजमुच्यते||२०३||

विस्तरेणैतदुद्दिष्टं क्लैब्यानां भेषजं मया|२०४|

If the impotency is caused by Jara (old age) and Ksaya (seminal diminution), then the patient should first of all be oleated and fomented. Thereafter, purgation therapy with unctuous ingredients is administered.

These 2 types of impotency are treated with medicated ghee, aphrodisiac recipe, Yapana type of medicated enema (Siddhi 12:16) and rejuvenating recipes (described in Chikitsa 1).

Thus, I (lord Atreya) have explained the treatment of impotency. [202- ½ 204]

PRADARA (MENORRHAGIA)

य: पूर्वमुक्त: प्रदर: शृणु हेत्वादिभिस्तु तम्||२०४||

Now listen (address of the disicple Agnivesha) to the etiology, etc. Of Pradara which has been mentioned earlier (verse no ½ 39) [204 ½]

Etiology, pathogenesis and signs of Pradara

याऽत्यर्थं सेवते नारी लवणाम्लगुरूणि च| कटून्यथ विदाहीनि स्निग्धानि पिशितानि च||२०५||

ग्राम्यौदकानि मेद्यानि कृशरां पायसं दधि | शुक्त मस्तु सुरादीनि भजन्त्या: कुपितोऽनिल:||२०६||

रक्तं प्रमाणमुत्क्रम्य गर्भाशयगता: सिरा:| रजोवहा: समाश्रित्य रक्तमादाय तद्रज:||२०७||

यस्मादिववर्धयत्याशु रसभावादिवमानता| तस्मादसृग्दरं प्राहुरेततन्त्रविशारदा:||२०८||

रज: प्रदीर्यते यस्मात् प्रदरस्तेन स स्मृत:| सामान्यत: समुद्दिष्टं कारणं लिङ्गमेव च||२०९||

If a woman takes excess of saline, sour, heavy , pungent, irritant and unctuous ingredients as food, fatty meat of domesticated and aquatic animals, Krsara (a preparation of rice and pulses), Payasa (a preparation of milk and rice), yoghurt, Vinegar, whey, Sura (a type of alcohol), etc, then the Vayu in her body gets aggravated. This aggravated Vayu causes increases in the quantity of blood, and gets lodged in the channels carrying menstrual fluid which go to the (are connected with) Uterus.

Since by propelling blood of the body to these menstrual fluids it causes increase in menstrual blood immediately because of the liquid nature of the former (blood). This condition is called Asrdagara (menorrhagia) by the experts in this field of specialty (gynaecology)

Since the quantity of menstrual fluid is augmented or expanded, it is called Pradara.

Thus, the etiology and signs of Pradara are explained in general. [205- 209]

Varieties of Pradara

चतुर्विधं व्यासतस्तु वाताद्यै: सन्निपातत:|

अत:परं प्रवक्ष्यामि हेत्वाकृतिभिषग्जितम्||२१०||

Regarding the details of this disease, Pradara is of 4 varieties, viz,

Vatika Pradara

Paittika Pradara

Kaphaja Pradara and

Sannipatika Pradara (the last one caused by the simultaneous aggravation of all 3 Doshas). [210]

Etiology, Pathology and Signs of Vatika Pradara:

रूक्षादिभि: मारुतस्तु रक्तमादाय पूर्ववत्| कुपित: प्रदरं कुर्याल्लक्षणं तस्य मे शृणु||२११||

फेनिलं तनु रूक्षं च श्यावं चारुणमेव च| किंशुकोदक सङ्काशं सरुजं वाऽथ नीरुजम्||२१२||

कटि वङ्क्षण हृत्पार्श्व पृष्ठ श्रोणिषु मारुत:| कुरुते वेदनां तीव्रामेतद्वातात्मकं विदु:||२१३||

Because of the intake of dry, brownish black, Kimshukodaka sankasa (pink or like the juice of Kimsuka (Palasha – Butea monosperma)) which may or may not be associated with pain, and if the aggravated Vayu causes Kati vankshna hrt parshva prstha shroni ruk (excruciating pain in the waist, groins, cardiac region, sides of the chest, back and hips), then this ailment is to be diagnosed as Vatika type of pradara. [211- 213]

Etiology and signs of Paittika Pradara:

अम्लोष्ण लवण क्षारैः पित्तं प्रकुपितं यदा| पूर्ववत् प्रदरं कुर्यात् पैत्तिकं लिङ्गतः शृणु||२१४||

सनीलमथवा पीतमत्युष्णमसितं तथा| नितान्तरक्तं स्रवति मुहुर्मुहुरथार्तिमत्||२१५||

दाह राग तृषा मोह ज्वर भ्रम समायुतम्| असृग्दरं पैत्तिकं स्याच्छ्लैष्मिकं तु प्रवक्ष्यते||२१६||

When the Pitta aggravated by the intake of sour, hot, saline and alkaline ingredients causes Pradara in the aforesaid manner, then it is called Paittika Pradara. Now, listen to its signs and symptoms.

If the menstrual discharge is blue, yellow, excessively hot, black or red, if it flows frequently associated with pain, and if the patient suffers from

Daha – burning sensation

Raga – redness

Trshna – thirst

Moha – unconsiciousness

Jwara – fever and

Bhrama – giddiness then this is to be diagnosed as Paittika type of Asrgdara (pradara) [214- ¾ 216]

Etiology and Signs of Kaphaja Pradara:

गुर्वादिभिर्हेतुभिश्च पूर्ववत् कुपितः कफः| प्रदरं कुरुते तस्य लक्षणं तत्त्वतः शृणु||२१७||

पिच्छिलं पाण्डुवर्णं च गुरु स्निग्धं च शीतलम्| स्रवत्यसृक् श्लेष्मलं च घनं मन्द रुजाकरम्||२१८||

छर्द्यरोचक हृल्लास श्वास कास समन्वितम्|

Hereafter will be described Kaphaja type of Pradara

Kapha, aggravated by the intake of ingredients which are heavy, etc., causes Pradara in the manner stated before. Now, listen to the characteristic features of this type of Pradara.

In this type of Pradara, the menstrual discharge is

Picchilam – slimy

Pandu varnam – pale in color

Guru – heavy

Snigdha – unctuous

Shitalam – cold

Sravat shlesham ya ghanam – mucous or dense;

There is

Manda ruja – dull pain, and the patient suffers from

Chardi – vomiting

Arochaka – anorexia

Hrllasa – nausea

Shvasa – asthma and

Kasa – cough. [216 ¼- ½ 219]

Sannipatika Type of Pradara:

(वक्ष्यते क्षीरदोषाणां सामान्यमिह कारणम्||२१९||

यतदेव त्रिदोषस्य कारणं प्रदरस्य तु)|

त्रिलिङ्ग संयुतं विद्यान्नैकावस्थमसृग्दरम्||२२०||

The factors in general to be described as cases of the morbidity of mother's milk (verse nos. 232- 235) are also the causative factors of Sannipatika type of Pradara.

In these types of Pradara, all the signs and symptoms of aforesaid 3 types of Pradara (Viz., Vatika Pradara, Paittika

Pradara and Kaphaja Pradara) are manifested in complete form. This Sannipatika Pradara is not characterized by the signs and symptoms of only one of them. [219 ½-220]

An associated Ailment:

नारी त्वतिपरिक्लिष्टा यदा प्रक्षीणशोणिता| सर्व हेतु समाचारादतिवृद्धस्तदाऽनिलः||२२१||

रक्तमार्गेण सृजति प्रत्यनीकबलं कफम्| दुर्गन्धं पिच्छिलं पीतं विदग्धं पित्ततेजसा||२२२||

वसां मेदश्च यावद्धि समुपादाय वेगवान्| सृजत्यपत्यमार्गेण सर्पि र्मज्ज वसोपमम्||२२३||

शश्वत् स्रवत्यथास्रावं तृष्णा दाह ज्वरान्विताम्| क्षीणरक्तां दुर्बलां स तामसाध्यां विवर्जयेत्||२२४||

If a woman who is excessively exhausted and who is excessively depleted of blood, resorts to all the aforesaid factors (described in respect of Vatika, Paittika and Kapha) having opposite attributes through the channels of blood, the Kapha being afflicted (lit. Burnt) by the heat of Pitta becomes foul smelling, Slimy and yellow. The aggravated Vayu moving rapidly makes this Kapha (fluid) along with Vasa (muscle fat) and Medas (adipose tissue) to be discharged through the vaginal tract. The fluid, thus discharged, appears like ghee, Majja (bone marrow) and Vasa (muscle fat).

This discharge from the vaginal tract takes place constantly, and the patient suffers from

Trshna – morbid thirst

Daha – burning sensation and

Jwara – fever

Curability: This patient whose blood is depleted and who is very weak is incurable, and the physician should avoid treatment of such a patient. [221-224]

Characteristics of Healthy Menstruation:

मासान्निष्पिच्छ दाहार्ति पञ्चरात्रानुबन्धि च| नैवातिबहु नात्यल्पमार्तवं शुद्धमादिशेत्||२२५||

गुञ्जाफलसवर्णं च पद्मालक्तक सन्निभम् | इन्द्रगोपक सङ्काशमार्तवं शुद्धमादिशेत्||२२६||

The menstruation which appears every month, which is (free from)

Nis pichha – free from sliminess of discharge,

Daha arti – burning sensation and pain,

Pancha ratra anubandhi – which continues for 5 nights and

Na ati bahu na ati alpam – which is neither excessive nor scanty is to be considered as normal.

Gunja phala sa varnam – the menstrual discharge which is of the color of Gunja fruits or

Padma alaktaka sannibham – of lotus or of or of Indra Gopa (trombidium) is considered as unpolluted. [225- 226]

Treatment of Pradara:

योनीनां वातलाद्यानां यदुक्तमिह भेषजम्| चतुर्णां प्रदराणां च तत् सर्वं कारयेद्भिषक्||२२७||

रक्तातिसारिणां यच्च तथा शोणित पित्तिनाम्| रक्तार्शसां च यत् प्रोक्तं भेषजं तच्च कारयेत्||२२८||

The therapeutic measures prescribed before for the treatment of different types of Yoni vyapat (uterine disorders) in this chapter are used by the physician for the treatment of [4 types of] Pradara (menorrhagia).

Similarly, [for the treatment of these 4 types of Pradara], the therapeutic measures prescribed for Raktatisara or diarrhoea associated with bleeding (Chikitsa 19:71- 100), Raktapitta (an ailment characterized by bleeding from different parts of the body – Chikitsa 4) and Rakta arshas or bleeding piles (Chikitsa 14) used. [227-228]

MORBIDITIES OF BREAST MILK

धात्री स्तन स्तन्य सम्पद्युक्ता विस्तरतः पुरा| स्तन्य सञ्जननं चैव स्तन्यस्य च विशोधनम्||२२९||

वातादिदुष्टे लिङ्गं च क्षीणस्य च चिकित्सितम्| तत्सर्वमुक्तं ये त्वष्टौ क्षीरदोषाः प्रकीर्तिताः||२३०||

वातादिष्वेव तान् विद्याच्छास्त्रचक्षुर्भिषक्तमः| त्रिविधास्तु यतः शिष्यास्ततो वक्ष्यामि विस्तरम्||२३१||

Earlier, detailed description has already been pro d on the following topics:

Dhatri Sampat (characristics of a wet nurse)- Sarira 8: 52

Stana Sampat (qualities of well formed breasts) Sarira 8: 52

Stanya –Sampat (qualities of healthy breast milk) Sarira 8: 53-54

Stanya –Samjanana (galactogogue drugs)- Sutra 4: 12 and Sarira 8: 57

Stanya Visodhana (drugs for purification of breast milk) Sutra 4: 12 and Sarira 8 : 56

Signs of breast milk vitiated by Vayu, etc- Sarira 8: 55

Treatment of diminished breast milk- Sutra 4:12 and Sarira 8; 56 and

8 types of morbidities of breast milk – Sutra 19:4:1

The aforesaid 8 morbidities of breast milk are also caused by Vayu, etc. Which an able physician well versed in the scriptures should know.

Disciples are of 3 different types, viz Tikshna / Pravara (Superior more intelligent), Madhya (mediocre intelligence) and Manda (low intelligence). Therefore the comprehension of all (including those disciples who are of low intelligence), details of these 8 types of morbidities of breast milk will be described hereafter. [229-231]

Etiology and Pathogenesis Lactational Morbidities:

अजीर्णासात्म्य विषम विरुद्धात्यर्थभोजनात्| लवणाम्ल कटु क्षार प्रक्लिन्नानां च सेवनात्||२३२||

मनःशरीर सन्तापाद स्वप्नान्निशि चिन्तनात्| प्राप्त वेग प्रतीघाताद प्राप्तोदीरणेन च||२३३||

परमान्नं गुडकृतं कृशरां दधि मन्दकम् | अभिष्यन्दीनि मांसानि ग्राम्यानूपौदकानि च||२३४||

भुक्त्वा भुक्त्वा दिवास्वप्नान्मद्यस्यातिनिषेवणात्| अनायासादभीघातात् क्रोधाच्चातङ्ककर्शनैः||२३५||

दोषाः क्षीरवहाः प्राप्य सिराः स्तन्यं प्रदूष्य च| कुर्युरष्टविधं भूयो दोषतस्तन्निबोध मे||२३६||

In a woman, Doshas get aggravated because of the following:

ajīrṇāsātmya bhojanāt – Intake of food before the previous meal is digested

viṣama viruddhātyartha bhojanāt- Intake of unwholesome, irregular and mutually contradictory food

Atyartha bhojanat – Intake of food in excess quantity

lavaṇāmla kaṭu kṣāra praklinnānāṃ ca sevanāt- Intake of saline, sour, pungent , alkaline and pasty / moist food

manaḥśarīra santāpāda svapnānniśi cintanāt- Affliction with mental as well as physical miseries

Remaining awake at night and worry

Suppression of the manifested natural urges, and forceful excitation of the unmanifested ones.

Sleep during day time after frequent intake of Krsara (a preparation of jaggery, Krsara (a preparation of rice and pulses), Mandaka Dadhi (Yoghrut not fully fermented or matured), ingredients which are Abhisyandi (which cause obstruction to the channels of circulation) and the meat of domesticated, marshy land- inhabiting as well as aquatic animals

Excessive intake of alcohol

Lack of exercise and affliction with trauma and anger and

Excessive emaciation because of chronic diseases.

The Doshas aggravated by the above mentioned factors reaches the Galactic channels to vitiate the breast milk, thus causing 8 types of morbidities [as described in Sutra 19 : 4:1]

Hereafter, the signs of the vitiation of breast milk by different Doshas will be described which you (addressed to Agnivesha) may understand. [232- 236]

Morbidities of Breast milk caused by different Doshas:

वैरस्यं फेनसङ्घातो रौक्ष्यं चेत्यनिलात्मके| पित्ताद्वैवर्ण्य दौर्गन्ध्ये स्नेह पैच्छिल्य गौरवम्||२३७||

कफाद्भवति रूक्षाद्यैरनिलः स्वैः प्रकोपणैः|

If the breast milk is vitiated by Vayu, then it becomes

Vairasyam – distasteful,

Phena sangatam – froathy and

Raukshyam – dry.

Breast milk vitiated by Pitta becomes

Vaivarnya – discolored and

Daurgandhya – foul smelling.

If it is vitiated by Kapha, then the breast milk becomes

sneha – unctuous

paichchilyam – slimy and

Guru – heavy. [237- ¼ 238]

Pathogenesis and signs of Breast milk Vitiated by vayu:

कफाद्भवति रूक्षाद्यैरनिलः स्वैः प्रकोपणैः| क्रुद्धः क्षीराशयं प्राप्य रसं स्तन्यस्य दूषयेत्||२३८||

विरसं वात संसृष्टं कृशी भवति तत् पिबन्| न चास्य स्वदते क्षीरं कृच्छ्रेण च विवर्धते||२३९||

तथैव वायुः कुपितः स्तन्यमन्तर्विलोडयन्| करोति फेन सङ्घातं तत्तु कृच्छ्रात् प्रवर्तते||२४०||

तेन क्षामस्वरो बालो बद्ध विण्मूत्र मारुतः| वातिकं शीर्षरोगं वा पीनसं वाऽधिगच्छति||२४१||

पूर्ववत् कुपितः स्तन्ये स्नेहं शोषयतेऽनिलः| रूक्षं तत् पिबतो रौक्ष्याद्बल ह्रासः प्रजायते||२४२||

By the intake of Vayu provoking ingredients, like those which are dry etc, the Vayu gets aggravated. Having reached the breasts, it afflicts the taste of the breast –milk.

By taking this tasteless milk, the child becomes emaciated. He does not relish this type of milk. And thus, his growth gets impaired. In addition, the aggravated Vayu churns up the milk inside the breast, and makes it a mass of frothy substance. As a result of this, the milk flows out of the breasts with difficulty.

By taking polluted milk, the child becomes weak of voice, and suffers from stasis of stool, urine and flatus. He may also get Vatika type of head- diseases and Pinasa (chronic coryza)

The Vayu aggravated by the aforesaid factors dries up the unctousness (sneha) of the milk, and makes it dry. By taking this milk, the strength of the child gets reduced due to the dryness of the milk. [238 ¾ – 242]

Pathogenesis and signs of Breast –milk vitiated by Pitta

पित्तमुष्णादिभिः क्रुद्धं स्तन्याशयमभिप्लुतम्| करोति स्तन्य वैवर्ण्यं नील पीता सितादिकम्||२४३||

विवर्णगात्रः स्विन्नः स्यात्तृष्णालुर्भिन्नविट् शिशुः| नित्यमुष्णशरीरश्च नाभिनन्दति तं स्तनम्||२४४||

पूर्ववत् कुपिते पित्ते दौर्गन्ध्यं क्षीरमृच्छति| पाण्डुवामयस्तत्पिबतः कामला च भवेच्छिशोः||२४५||

Pitta, aggravated by ingredients which are hot etc., afflicts the breast of a woman. As a result of this, the milk becomes discolored, blue, yellow, black, etc. In the child who takes this milk, there will be

Vivarna gatra – discoloration of the body,

Svinna – perspiration,

Trshna -morbid thirst and

Atisara – diarrhea. His body remains warm constantly, and it dislikes breast feed.

The Pitta aggravated in the aforesaid manner causes foul smell in the breast milk, and the child taking this milk gets afflicted with anemia and Jaundice. [243-245]

Pathogenesis and Signs of Breast milk Vitiated by Kapha:

क्रुद्धो गुर्वादिभिः श्लेष्मा क्षीराशयगतः स्त्रियाः| स्नेहान्वितत्वात्तत्क्षीरमतिस्निग्धं करोति तु||२४६||

छर्दनः कुन्थनस्तेन लालालुर्जायते शिशुः| नित्योपदिग्धैः स्रोतोभि निद्रा क्लम समन्वितः||२४७||

श्वास कास परीतस्तु प्रसेक तमकान्वितः| अभिभूय कफः स्तन्यं पिच्छिलं कुरुते यदा||२४८||

लालालुः शून वक्त्राक्षिर्जडः स्यात्तत् पिबञ्छिशुः| कफः क्षीराशयगतो गुरुत्वात् क्षीर गौरवम्||२४९||

करोति गुरु तत् पीत्वा बालो हृद्रोगमृच्छति| अन्यांश्च विविधात्रोगान्कुर्यात्क्षीर समाश्रितान्||२५०||

Kapha, aggravated by the intake of ingredients which are heavy, etc., afflicts the breast milk of the woman. Because of the unctuous attribute of this aggravated Kapha, the afflicted breast milk becomes excessively unctuous.

The child feeding on this Breastmilk suffers from

Chardanah – vomitting

Kunthanastena – gripping pain and

Lala srava – excessive salivation.

Since the channels in his body remain constantly smeared with this aggravated Kapha, the child constantly feels sleepy and fatigued (inactive).

He suffers from

Svasa (dyspnoea)

Kasa – cough

Lala srava – dribbling of saliva and

Tamaka (Asthma).

Because of the affliction by Kapha, the breast milk becomes slimy. The child feeding on this type of breastmilk suffers from excessive salivation, swelling of the face as well as dullness of the eyes.

When the aggravated Kapha which is heavy in attribute afflicts the breasts, the milk also becomes heavy. The child taking this milk suffers from heart diseases and other different types of diseases caused by the polluted milk. [246-250]

Affliction by other ailments:

क्षीरे वातादिभिर्दुष्टे सम्भवन्ति तदात्मकाः|

When the Breast milk is afflicted with aggravated Vayu, etc., then other diseases specific to these Doshas also afflict the child. [½ 251]

Emetic therapy:

तत्रादौ स्तन्यशुद्ध्यर्थं धात्रीं स्नेहोपपादिताम्||२५१||
संस्वेद्य विधिवद्वैद्यो वमनेनोपपादयेत्|

For the purification of the polluted breast milk, in the beginning the wet nurse (or the mother) is given oleated and fomentation therapies. Thereafter, the physician should appropriately administer emetic therapy to her. [251 ½- ½ 252]

Recipe of Emetic Therapy:

वचा प्रियङ्गु यष्ट्याह्व फलवत्सक सर्षपैः||२५२||
कल्कै निम्ब पटोलानां क्वाथैः सलवणैर्वमेत्|

The patient suffering from the pollution of breastmilk is given emetic therapy with a recipe containing the paste of Vacha (Acorus calamus Linn.). Priyangu (Callicarpa macrophylla), Yastimadhu – Glycyrrhiza glabra, Madana Phala – Randia dumetorum, bark of Kutaja – Connessi (Holarrhena antidysenterica Wall.) and Sarsapa – Brassica campestris, and the decoction of nimbi – Azadirachta indica as well as Patola – Trichosanthes dioica mixed with Salt. [252 ½ – ½ 253]

Purgation Therapy:

सम्यग्वान्तां यथान्यायं कृत संसर्जनां ततः||२५३||
दोष काल बलापेक्षी स्नेहयित्वा विरेचयेत्|

After proper emesis, the patient is given Samsarjana Karma (rehabilitating diet). Thereafter, depending upon the nature of the aggravated Doshas, seasonal nature and strength of the patient, she is given purgation therapy preceded with oleation therapy. [253 ½- ½ 254]

Recipe of Purgation Therapy:

त्रिवृतामभयां वाऽपि त्रिफलारस संयुताम्||२५४||
पाययेन्मधुसंयुक्तामभयां वाऽपि केवलाम्|
(पाययेन्मूत्रसंयुक्तां विरेकार्थं च शास्त्रवित्)||२५५||

The physician proficient in scriptures should administer purgation therapy to the patient with the following recipes: The paste Trivrt – Operculina turpethum or Abhaya – Terminalia chebula mixed the decoction of Triphala or honey or

Only Haritaki – Terminalia chebula mixed with cow's urine [254 ½ – 255]

Food and drinks:
सम्यग्विरिक्तां मतिमान् कृतसंसर्जनां पुनः| ततो दोषावशेषघ्नैरन्नपानैरुपाचरेत् ||२५६||
शालयः षष्टिका वा स्युः श्यामाका भोजने हिताः| प्रियङ्गवः कोरदूषा यवा वेणु यवास्तथा||२५७||
वंश वेत्र कलायाश्च शाकार्थं स्नेह संस्कृताः| मुद्गान् मसूरान् यूषार्थं कुलत्थांश्च प्रकल्पयेत्||२५८||
निम्ब वेत्राग्र कुलक वार्ताकामलकैः शृतान्| स व्योष सैन्धवान् यूषान्दापयेत्स्तन्यशोधनान्||२५९||
शशान् कपिञ्जलानेनान् संस्कृतांश्च प्रदापयेत्|

After proper purgation, a wise physician should again give Samsarjana Karma (rehabilitating diet) to the patient and, thereafter, for the alleviation of the residual Doshas, she is treated with different types of food and drinks [which are as follows]:
Sali and Sastika types of rice, Syamaka , Priyangu (Callicarpa macrophylla), Kodrava , Barley and Venu Yava – Barley (Hordeum vulgare) (seeds of Bamboo) are useful as food;
Bamboo shoots, Vertra and Kalaya sizzeled with fat are given vegetable preparation.
Vegetables soup prepared of Mudga – Vigna radiata, Masura and Kulattha may also be given
Vegetable soups prepared by boiling tender leaves of Nimba – Neem (Azadirachta indica) and Vetra
, Kulaka (Karavellaka), Vartaka and Amalaki, and added with Ginger, black pepper, long pepper and rock- salt may be given for the purification of breast milk and
The meat of Sasa, Kapinijala and Ena may be given after sizzling, to the patient to take. [257- ½ 260]

Recipes for Treatment of Polluted Breast milk in General:
शाङ्र्गेष्टा सप्तपर्ण त्वगश्वगन्धाशृतं जलम्||२६०||
पाययेताथवा स्तन्य शुद्धये रोहिणी शृतम्| अमृता सप्तपर्ण त्वक्क्वाथं चैव सनागरम्||२६१||
किराततिक्तक क्वाथं श्लोकपादेरितान् पिबेत्| त्रीनेतान्स्तन्य शुद्ध्यर्थमिति सामान्य भेषजम्||२६२||
कीर्तितं स्तन्यदोषाणां पृथगन्यं निबोधत|

For the purification of the polluted breast milk, the patient is given the following recipes
Decoction of Sarngesta, bark of Saptaparna – Raulwolfia serpentina, and Ashwagandha – Winter Cherry / Indian ginseng (root) – Withania somnifera
Dccoction of Katukarohini – Picrorhiza kurroa
Decoction of Amrta(Guduchi – Tinospora cordifolia) and the bark of Saptaparna – Raulwolfia serpentina
Decoction of ginger
Decoction of Kirata Tikta – Swertia chirata
Thus, the recipes for the purification of polluted breast milk in general are described. Hereafter, treatment of specific morbidities of the breast milk will be described which may be listed to (addresses to Agnivesha). [260 ½- ½ 263]

Recipes for corrections Distaste of breast milk
पायये दिवरस क्षीरां द्राक्षा मधुक सारिवाः||२६३||
श्लक्ष्ण पिष्टां पयस्यां च समालोड्य सुखाम्बुना| पञ्चकोल कुलत्थैश्च पिष्टैरालेपयेत् स्तनौ||२६४||
शुष्कौ प्रक्षाल्य निर्दुह्यातथा स्तन्यं विशुध्यति|

If there is distaste(bad taste) of the breast milk, then the patient is made to drink the fine paste of Draksha – Raisin – Vitis vinifera, Madhuka– Licorice – Glycyrrhiza glabra, Sariva – Indian sarsaparilla – Hemidesmus indicus and Payasya – Impomoea paniculata mixed with warm water.
The paste of Pancha Kola (Pippali , Pippali –mula, Cavya – Piper chaba, Chitraka – Plumbago zeylanica and Nagara) and Kulatha is applied over the breasts. After it is dried up, the breasts are washed, and the accumulated milk is squeezed out. Thus the breast milk gets purified [and the bad taste of the milk is removed]. [263 ½ – ½ 265]

Treatment of frothy milk:

फेनसङ्घातवत्क्षीरं यस्यास्तां पाययेत् स्त्रियम्||२६५||

पाठा नागर शाङ्गेष्टा मूर्वाः पिष्ट्वा सुखाम्बुना| अञ्जनं नागरं दारु बिल्वमूलं प्रियङ्गवः||२६६||

स्तनयोः पूर्ववत् कार्यं लेपनं क्षीर शोधनम्| किराततिक्तकं शुण्ठीं सामृतां क्वाथयेद्भिषक्||२६७||

तं क्वाथं पाययेद्धात्री स्तन्यदोष निबर्हणम्| स्तनौ चालेपयेत् पिष्टै र्यवगोधूम सर्षपैः||२६८||

If the Breast milk is like thick foam, then the woman is given to drink the paste of Patha – Cissampelos pariera, Nagara – Zingiber officinale, Sarngesta and Murva –Marsedenia tenacissima along with lukewarm water.

In the aforesaid manner, her breast is anointed with the paste of anjana, Nagara – Zingiber officinale, Devadaru (Cedrus deodara), root of bilva – Aegle marmelos and Priyangu (Callicarpa macrophylla) [after the paste is dried up, the breasts are washed and the accumulated milk is squeezed out]. This purifies the polluted breastmilk [and frothiness of the milk is corrected]

The decoction of Kirata tikta – Swertia chirata, Sunthi – Zingiber officinale and Amrta – Tinospora cordifolia is given to the wet nurse to drink which purifies polluted [frothy] milk.

In the aforesaid manner, the breasts are anointed with the paste of barley, wheat and mustard seed. [After the paste is dried up, the breasts are washed, and the accumulated milk is squeezed out. This purifies the polluted (frothy) breast milk]. [265 ½ -268]

Treatment of dry Milk

षड्विरेकाश्रितीयोक्तैरौषधैः स्तन्य शोधनैः| रूक्षक्षीरा पिबेत् क्षीरं तैर्वा सिद्धं घृतं पिबेत्||२६९||

पूर्ववज्जीवकाद्यं च पञ्चमूलं प्रलेपनम्| स्तनयोः संविधातव्यं सुखोष्णं स्तन्य शोधनम्||२७०||

Milk boiled with the drugs described in Sutra 4: 12., for the purification of breast milk, is taken by the woman who has unctuous breast milk.

Ghee cooked with the above mentioned drugs is also useful in this condition (dryness of breast milk).

In the aforesaid manner, the luke-warm paste of Jivaka, etc., (jivaka – Malaxis acuminata, Rishabhaka – Meda , Maha meda, Kakoli – Fritillaria roylei, Ksira Kaloli, Mudga parni, Masa parni, jivanti and Madhuka– Licorice – Glycyrrhiza glabra) or Panchamula (bilva – Aegle marmelos, syonaka, gambari – Gmelina arborea, Patali and Ganikarika) is applied over the breast . After the paste is dried up, it is washed and the accumulated milk is squeezed out. This purifies the [dry] breast milk [269- 270]

Treatment of Discolored Breast –milk:

यष्टीमधुक मृद्वीका पयस्या सिन्धुवारिकाः| शीताम्बुना पिबेत्कल्कं क्षीर वैवर्ण्य नाशनम्||२७१||

द्राक्षा मधुक कल्केन स्तनौ चास्याः प्रलेपयेत्| प्रक्षाल्य वारिणा चैव निर्दुह्यात्तौ पुनः पुनः||२७२||

Intake of the paste of Yastimadhu – Glycyrrhiza glabra, Mrdvika – Vitis vinfera, Payasya – Impomoea paniculata, Ksira Vidari (Ipomoea paniculata / Pueraria tuberosa)) and Sindhuvara (Vitex negundo)(nirgundi) along with cold water corrects the discoloration of the breast milk.

The breasts of the woman having discolored milk are smeared with the paste of Draksha – raisins and Vitis vinifera & Madhuka– Licorice – Glycyrrhiza glabra. After the paste gets dried up, they are washed with water, and [the accumulated milk] is squeezed out repeatedly. This helps in correcting the polluted (discolored) breast milk. [271-272]

Treatment of foul odour in breast milk:

विषाणिकाजशृङ्ग्यौ च त्रिफलां रजनीं वचाम्| पिबेच्छीताम्बुना पिष्ट्वा क्षीर दौर्गन्ध्य नाशिनीम्||२७३||

लिह्याद्वाऽप्यभयाचूर्णं सव्योषं माक्षिक प्लुतम्| क्षीर दौर्गन्ध्य नाशार्थं धात्री पथ्याशिनी तथा||२७४||

सारिवोशीर मञ्जिष्ठा श्लेष्मातक कुचन्दनैः| पत्राम्बु चन्दनोशीरैःस्तनौ चास्याः प्रलेपयेत्||२७५||

Intake of the paste of visanika (mesasrngi), Aja sring, , Haritaki – Terminalia chebula, Bibhitaki – Terminalia bellerica, Amalaki – Phyllanthus emblica, Haridra (turmeric – Curcuma longa) and Vacha (Acorus calamus Linn.) along with cold water cures foul odour of the breast milk.

The wet –nurse should take the powder of Abhaya – Terminalia chebula, Sunthi – Zingiber officinale, Pippali – Long pepper fruit – Piper longum and Maricha – Black pepper fruit – piper nigrum mixed with the honey along with wholesome diet for the removal of foul odour in her breast milk.

The breasts of the woman having foul odour in her milk is anointed with the paste of

Sariva – Indian Sarsaparilla – Hemidesmus indicus,

Ushira – Vetiver – Vetiveria zizanioides,

Manjistha – Rubia cordifolia

Slesmataka,

Kachandana,

Patra – Cinnamomum tamala Nees and Eberum.(tamala Patra – Cinnamomum tamala Nees and Eberum.),

Ambu (Hrivera) – Pavoria odorata

Chandana (Sandalwood – Santalum album) and after the paste is dried up, the breasts are washed with water, and the accumulated milk is squeezed out. [273- 275]

Treatment of unctuousness of Breastmilk:

Shloka & Translation is needed here

The woman having very unctuous breast milk should take the paste of Devadaru (Cedrus deodara), Musta (Cyperus rotundus) and Patha – Cissampelos parriera mixed with rock- salt along with Lukewarm water. By this, the unctuousness of the breast milk gets quickly corrected. [276]

Treatment of Sliminess in Breast –milk:

Shloka and Translation needed

The woman whose breast milk is slimy should drink the decoction prepared with sarngeshta, abhaya – Terminalia chebula, vaca – Acorus calamus or Musta – Cyperus rotundus, Shunti – ginger and Patha - Cissampelos parriera should be ground and given for drinking. These recipes will cleanse the breast milk. Also, Takrarista which is Prescribed for the treatment of piles (Chikitsa 14; 71: 75) shall be administered.

Her breasts are anointed with the paste of Vidari (Ipomoea paniculata / Pueraria tuberosa), Bilva – Aegle marmelos and Madhuka– Licorice – Glycyrrhiza glabra. After the paste gets dried up, the breasts are washed, and the accumulated milk is squeezed out]. [277-278]

Treatment of Heaviness in Breast milk:

त्रायमाणामृता निम्ब पटोल त्रिफलाशृतम्| गुरु क्षीरा पिबेदाशु स्तन्यदोष विशुद्धये||२७९||

पिबेद्वा पिप्पलीमूल चव्य चित्रक नागरम्| बला नागर शाङ्र्गेष्टा मूर्वाभिर्लेपयेत् स्तनौ||२८०||

पृश्निपर्णी पयस्याभ्यां स्तनौ चास्याः प्रलेपयेत्| अष्टावेते क्षीरदोषा हेतु लक्षण भेषजैः||२८१||

निर्दिष्टाः क्षीर दोषोत्थास्तथोक्ताः केचिदामयाः|२८२|

The woman whose breast milk is heavy should take the decoction of

Tryamana – Gentiana kuroo, Amrta – Tinospora cordifolia, Nimba – Neem (Azadirachta indica), Patola – Trichosanthes dioica, Haritaki – Terminalia chebula, Bibhitaka – Terminalia bellerica and

Amalaki – Phyllanthus emblica.

By this her breast milk gets purified (heaviness removed) quickly.

She may also take the decoction of

Pippali Mula – Long pepper fruit – Piper longum-,

Cavya – Piper chaba

Chitraka – Plumbago zeylanica and

Nagara – Zingiber officinale for the removal of heaviness in her breast milk.

Her breasts are anointed with the paste of

Bala – Sida cordifolia,

Nagara – ginger

Sarngesta - Kakamaci and

Murva – Marsedenia tenacissima

After the paste is dried up, her breasts are washed with water, and the accumulated milk is squeezed out. This purifies (removes heaviness of) the breast milk.

Similarly, application of the paste of

Prsni parni – Uraria picta and

Payasya – Impomoea paniculata (Vidari (Pueraria tuberosa)-Kanda) [in the aforesaid manner corrects the heaviness of the breast –milk].

Thus, etiology, signs and treatment of 8 galactic disorders, and some other ailments arising out of the polluted milk are described. [279– ½ 282]

TREATMENT OF PAEDIATRIC DISEASES:

दोष दूष्य मलाश्चैव महतां व्याधयश्च ये||२८२||

त एव सर्वे बालानां मात्रा त्वल्पतरा मता| निवृत्तिर्वमनादीनां मृदुत्वं परतन्त्रताम्||२८३||

वाक्चेष्टयोरसामर्थ्यं वीक्ष्य बालेषु शास्त्रवित्| भेषजं स्वल्पमात्रं तु यथाव्याधि प्रयोजयेत्||२८४||

मधुराणि कषायाणि क्षीरवन्ति मृदूनि च| प्रयोजयेदिभषग्बाले मतिमानप्रमादतः||२८५||

अत्यर्थं स्निग्ध रूक्षोष्णमम्लं कटु विपाकि च| गुरु चौषधपानान्नमेतद्बालेषु गर्हितम्||२८६||

समासात् सर्व रोगाणामेतद्बालेषु भेषजम्| निर्दिष्टं शास्त्र विद्वैद्यः प्रविविच्य प्रयोजयेत्||२८७||

The Doshas, dhatus (tissue elements), Malas (waste products) and the diseases of adults are all present in children. But in the case of the latter, these are only a small quantity and of mild intensity.

The physician well versed in scriptures should avoid the administration of Vamana (emesis) and such other therapies of PanchaKarma to a child., in view of his tenderness, dependency on others and inability to speak as well as act.

The dose of the medicine for children is very small and appropriate to the disease. The wise physician should carefully administer sweet and stringent drugs which are mild. Medicines, diet and drinks which are excessively unctuous, dry, hot, sour, and pungent in Vipaka (the taste that emerges after digestion) and heavy are contraindicated for children.

In brief, these are the guiding principles for administering medicines to children for all their ailments. A physician well versed in scriptures should administer therapies to children after considering all aforesaid aspects. [282 ½ – 287]

Thus it is said:

भवन्ति चात्र-

इति सर्व विकाराणामुक्तमेत चिचिकित्सितम्|

स्थानमेतदिध तन्त्रस्य रहस्यं परमुत्तमम्||२८८||

This Chikitsa Sthana (section of Therapeutics) deals with the therapeutic measures for all the diseases. It constitutes the most significant secret of this treatise (Charaka Samhita). [288]

Portion of treatment supplemented by Drdhabala:

अस्मिन् सप्तदशाध्यायाः कल्पाः सिद्धय एव च| नासाद्यन्तेऽग्निवेशस्य तन्त्रे चरक संस्कृते||२८९||

तानेतान् कापिल बलिः शेषान् दृढबलोऽकरोत्| तन्त्रस्यास्य महार्थस्य पूरणार्थं यथातथम्||२९०||

The 17th chapter of this section (on therapeutics) and the successive 2 sections, viz., Kalpa (section on Pharmacetics) and Siddhi (section on Therapeutic Perfection) are not available in the Agnivesha's Treatise which was redacted by Charaka. Therefore, Drdhabala, the son of kapilabala reconstructed and supplemented them appropriately leading to the completion of this treatise endowed with great objective. [289-290]

Treatment of Unnamed Diseases:

रोगा येऽप्यत्र नोदिदष्टा बहुत्वान्नामरूपतः| तेषामप्येतदेव स्याद्दोषादीन् वीक्ष्य भेषजम्||२९१||

There are several other diseases which are not described in this Section with names and forms. Even such diseases are to be treated on the lines suggested in this Section after examining the Doshas and such other factors involved in their manifestation. [291]

Line of Treatment in General:

दोष दूष्य निदानानां विपरीतं हितं ध्रुवम्| उक्तानुक्तान् गदान् सर्वान् सम्यग्युक्तं नियच्छति||२९२||

Therapies which are opposite to the properties of the Doshas, Dusyas (tissue elements) and etiological factors involved in the causation of the disease are certainly useful to cure it. If appropriately used, such therapeutic measures will cure all the diseases whether they are named or not in the text [292]

Appropriate Use of Therapeutic Measure:

देश काल प्रमाणानां सात्म्यासात्म्यस्य चैव हि| सम्यग्योगोऽन्यथा ह्येषां पथ्यमप्यन्यथा भवेत्||२९३||

Therapeutic measures are appropriately used keeping in view the following:

Desha (location)

Kala (time)

Pramana (Dose)

Satmya (Wholesomeness) and

Asatmya (unwholesomeness)

Otherwise, even a useful therapy (Pathya) may turn out to be harmful (apathya). [293]

Desha (Administration of Drugs Through Particular Channel)

आस्यादामाशयस्थान् हि रोगान् नस्तःशिरोगतान्| गुदात् पक्वाशयस्थांश्च हन्त्याशु दत्तमौषधम्||२९४||

शरीरावयवोत्थेषु विसर्प पिडकादिषु| यथादेशं प्रदेहादि शमनं स्यादिवशेषतः||२९५||

If a drug is administered through the mouth, it works quickly on diseases located in the stomach.

Administration of a drug by inhalation quickly cures diseases of the head.

Administration of a therapy through the anus quickly cures diseases located in the colon.

For the cure of disease located in various parts of the body like Visarpa (erysipelas or Herpes), Pidaka (pimples) etc., application of therapies externally like Pradeha (application of hot poultices), etc, in that particular part afflicted by the disease are useful. [294 -295]

Kala (Time of Administration of Drugs)

दिनातुरौषध व्याधि जीर्ण लिङ्गर्त्ववेक्षणम्| कालं विद्यादिदिनावेक्षः पूर्वाह्णे वमनं यथा||२९६||

रोग्यवेक्षो यथा प्रातर्निरन्नो बलवान् पिबेत्| भेषजं लघु पथ्यान्नैर्युक्तमद्यात्तु दुर्बलः||२९७||

भैषज्य कालो भुक्तादौ मध्ये पश्चान्मुहुर्मुहुः| सामुद्गं भक्त संयुक्तं ग्रास ग्रासान्तरे दश||२९८||

अपाने विगुणे पूर्वं, समाने मध्य भोजनम्| व्याने तु प्रातरशितमुदाने भोजनोत्तरम्||२९९||

वायौ प्राणे प्रदुष्टे तु ग्रास ग्रासान्तरिष्यते| श्वास कास पिपासासु त्ववचार्य मुहुर्मुहुः||३००||

सामुद्गं हिक्किने देयं लघुनाऽन्नेन संयुतम्| सम्भोज्यं त्वौषधं भोज्यैर्विचित्रैररुचौ हितम्||३०१||

ज्वरे पेयाः कषायाश्च क्षीरं सर्पि विरेचनम्| षड्हे षड्हे देयं कालं वीक्ष्यामयस्य च||३०२||

क्षुद्वेग मोक्षौ लघुता विशुद्धि जीर्ण लक्षणम्| तदा भेषजमादेयं स्यादिध दोषवदन्यथा||३०३||

चयादयश्च दोषाणां वर्ज्यं सेव्यं च यत्र यत्| ऋताववेक्ष्यं यत् कर्म पूर्व सर्वमुदाहृतम्||३०४||

(उपक्रमाणां करणं प्रतिषेधे च कारणम्| व्याख्यातमबलानां सविकल्पानामवेक्षणे||३०५||

मुहुर्मुहुश्च रोगाणामवस्थामातुरस्य च| अवेक्षमाणस्तु भिषक् चिकित्सायां न मुह्यति)||३०६||

इत्येवं षड्विधं कालमनवेक्ष्य भिषग्जितम्| प्रयुक्तमहिताय स्यात् सस्यस्याकालवर्षवत्||३०७||

The term"Kala" (time) in the present context has reference to the following:

Dina (different parts of the day)

Atura (nature of the patient)

Ausadha (time of taking medicine)

Vyadhi (nature of the disease)

Jirna Linga (stage of the digestion of food) and

Rtu (nature of the season)

Examples of these aspects of Kala (time) are as follows:

as regards the time with reference to the different parts of the day, the morning is the most suitable time for the administration of emetic therapy

(b) as regards the time with reference to the nature of the patient , a strong person should take medicines in the morning on empty stomach and a weak person should take medicines along with light and wholesome food.

(c) As regards the time (frequency) of taking medicine it is of ten categories as follows:

Bhuktadau or before the meals (i. e once on empty stomach in the morning and once before the night meal)

Bhukta Madhye (during the meal, i.e in the middle of the meal)

(iv-v) Bhukta Pascat (after the meals, i.e in the morning meal and after the evening meal)

(vi)Muhurmuhuh (repeatedly during the day and night)

(vii) Samudga (before as well as after the meal)

(viii) Bhakta Samyukta (mixed with the food)

(ix) Grase (along with each morsel of food)

(x) Grasantare (between two meals)

If the Apana Vayu is vitiated, then the medicine is given before food.

If the Samana Vayu is vitiated, then the medicine is given during the meal.

If Vyana Vayu is vitiated then the medicine is given after the morning meal.

If Udana Vayu is vitiated, then the medicine is given after the meal.

If Prana Vayu is vitiated, then the medicine is given along with each morsel of food or in between morsels of food.

In asthma, cough and morbid thirst, the medicine is given at short intervals frequently.

To the patient suffering from hiccups, medicine is given before and after food adding to the light articles of food.

In anorexia, medicine is mixed with various types of food.

(d) As regards the time with reference to the diseases (Vyadhi), the patient suffering from fever is given peya (thin gruel), Kashaya (decoctions), medicated milk, medicated ghee and purgation therapy consecutively at an interval of 6 days after observing the time (number of the days of suffering) of disease.

(e) Jirna Linga: Appearance of hunger, proper evacuation of stool and urine, lightness of the body and purity [of eructation]- these are the signs of proper digestion. Medicines are given to the patient only thereafter. [This according to Chakrapani, refers to the time of medicine which is administered before food]. Otherwise, the medicine will produce harmful effects.

As regards the time with reference to the nature of seasons , accumulation, etc., of Doshas, the ingredients to be used to avoid such accumulation, etc.., and regimens to be used in different seasons depending upon the condition of Doshas are already described (in Sutra 6).

Administration of therapeutic measures, reasons for prohibiting their use, and examination of the permutation and combination of Doshas in a weak patient are already described.

The physician who very frequently keeps on observing the development of the disease and the conduct of the patient will not commit mistakes in treatment.

Administration of therapeutic measures without careful examination of the 6 conditions of Kala (time) leads to harmful effects as the unseasonal rain damages the crops. [296-307]

Aggravation of Doshas in Different Seasons etc:

व्याधीनामृत्वहोरात्रवयसां भोजनस्य च| विशेषो भिद्यते यस्तु कालावेक्षः स उच्यते||३०८||

वसन्ते श्लेष्मजा रोगाः शरत्काले तु पित्तजाः| वर्षासु वातिकाश्चैव प्रायः प्रादुर्भवन्ति हि||३०९||

निशान्ते दिवसान्ते च वर्षान्ते वातजा गदाः| प्रातः क्षपादौ कफजास्तयोर्मध्ये तु पित्तजाः||३१०||

वयोन्त मध्य प्रथमे वात पित्त कफामयाः| बलवन्तो भवन्त्येव स्वभावाद्वयसो नृणाम्||३११||

जीर्णान्ते वातजा रोगा जीर्यमाणे तु पित्तजाः| श्लेष्मजा भुक्तमात्रे तु लभन्ते प्रायशो बलम्||३१२||

With reference to Kala (time), the specific classification of diseases[on the basis of aggravated Doshas] during different seasons, different parts of the day and night, different ages (parts of the span of life) and different stages of the digestion of food will be described hereafter.

Generally Kaphaja diseases are manifested in the spring, Paittika diseases are manifested [the beginning of] the rainy season.

Vatika diseases get aggravated [the term 'Varsante' here should read as 'Vardhane'] – during the end of the night and the day (afternoon),

Kaphaja diseases get aggravated during the morning and evening; and

Paittika diseases get aggravated during the midday and midnight.

As regards the age, vata gets aggravated during old age, pittaja diseases get aggravated during the middle age and kaphaja diseases get aggravated during the early age (childhood and early adolescence)

As regards the digestion of food - Vata gets aggravated after the digestion of food

Paittika diseases get aggravated during the digestion of food, and

Kaphaja diseases get aggravated immediately after taking food. [308- 312]

III Dose (Quantity) of Medicine:

नाल्पं हन्त्यौषधं व्याधिं यथाऽऽपोऽल्पा महानलम्| दोषवच्चातिमात्रं स्यात्सस्यस्यात्युदकं यथा||३१३||

सम्प्रधार्य बलं तस्मादामयस्यौषधस्य च| नैवातिबहु नात्यल्पं भैषज्यमवचारयेत्||३१४||

As a small amount of water cannot extinguish fire, similarly medicine in small quantities cannot cure a disease. As irrigation with overflood is harmful for the crops, similarly medicine in excessive quantities (dose) is harmful for the patient.

Therefore, after carefully examining the strength of the disease and the medicine, the remedial measures are administered in a quantity (dose) which is neither too large nor too small. [313-314]

IV Satmya (wholesomeness):

औचित्याद्यस्य यत् सात्म्यं देशस्य पुरुषस्य च| अपथ्यमपि नैकान्तात्त्यजंल्लभते सुखम्||३१५||

बाह्लीकाः पह्लवाश्चीनाः शूलीका यवनाः शकाः| मांस गोधूम माध्वीक शस्त्र वैश्वानरोचिताः||३१६||

मत्स्य सात्म्यास्तथा प्राच्याः क्षीर सात्म्याश्च सैन्धवाः| अश्मकावन्तिकानां तु तैलाम्लं सात्म्यमुच्यते||३१७||

कन्दमूल फलं सात्म्यं विद्यान्मलयवासिनाम्| सात्म्यं दक्षिणतः पेया मन्थश्चोत्तरपश्चिमे ||३१८||

मध्यदेशे भवेत् सात्म्यं यवगोधूम गोरसाः| तेषां तत्सात्म्ययुक्तानि भैषजान्यवचारयेत्||३१९||

सात्म्यं ह्याशु बलं धत्ते नातिदोषं च बह्वपि|३२०|

If a non- homologous (Apathya) item [of food and regimen] has become wholesome (Satmya) to a person because of habit (aucitya) or the nature of the place of Habitat (desha), then sudden and total withdrawal of this item (even though it is non- homologous or Apathya) does not give happiness to a person.|

Persons like Bahlikas, Pahlavas, Cinas, Sulikas, Yavanas and Shakas are habituated with meat, wheat, Madhvika (a type of wine), carrying arms and fire [for keeping them warm].

People living in the eastern part (of India) are habituated with taking fish which is wholesome for them.

People of Sindh are habituated with taking milk which is wholesome for them.

For people living in the southern part (of India), intake of Peya (thin gruel) is wholesome.

For the people of northern and western parts (of India), intake of mantha (roasted corn- flour mixed with water) is wholesome.

For the people living in the middle part (of India), intake of barley wheat and milk- products is wholesome.

For the (people living in the aforesaid geographical areas and people of aforesaid ethnic origin), medicines are administered by adding to the food and drinks which are wholesome to them.

The wholesome ingredients promote strength instantaneously. If given in excess, these wholesome items do not produce any harmful effect. [315- ½ 320]

Mistakes committed by Ignoring Desha etc

योगैरेव चिकित्सन् हि देशाद्यज्ञोऽपराध्यति||३२०|| वयो बल शरीरादिभेदा हि बहवो मताः |३२१|

The physician treating a patient simply with recipes without paying any attention to factors like Desha (habitation in different areas), etc, may commit mistakes (may not achieve success). On the basis of age, strength and physical features, physiques are of innumerable types. Accordingly, patients are also innumerable types. [320- ½ 321]

Usefulness of Therapies Generally Considered as Harmful:

तथाऽन्तःसन्धिमार्गाणां दोषाणां गूढचारिणाम्||३२१||

भवेत् कदाचित् कार्याऽपि विरुद्धाभिमता क्रिया| पित्तमन्तर्गतं गूढं स्वेदसेकोपनाहनैः||३२२||

नीयते बहिरुष्णैर्हि तथोष्णं शमयन्ति ते| बाह्यैश्च शीतैः सेकाद्यैरूष्माऽन्तर्याति पीडितः||३२३||

सोऽन्तर्गूढं कफं हन्ति शीतं शीतैस्तथा जयेत्| श्लक्ष्ण पिष्टो घनो लेपश्चन्दनस्यापि दाहकृत्||३२४||

त्वग्गतस्योष्मणो रोधाच्छीतकृच्चान्यथाऽगुरोः| छर्दिघ्नी मक्षिका विष्ठा मक्षिकैव तु वामयेत्||३२५||

द्रव्येषु स्विन्न जग्धेषु चैव तेष्वेव विक्रिया|३२६|

If the morbidities have afflicted the deep- seated organs like those in the Kostha (thoracic and abdominal viscera) and joints, at times, for their cure, therapeutic measures generally considered as contradictory (viruddha) may be useful.

If Pitta is deep-seated and located in the internal pathway (thoracic and abdominal visceras), then by the application of hot fomentation, Seka (affusion) and Upadeha (hot poultices), it comes out to the exterior of the body resulting in the alleviation of Pitta or heat. Thus, heat – producing therapies may cure Pitta which is hot in nature.

By the application of external therapies like Seka (affusion) etc., which are cooling in nature, the external heat is pressed to go inside, and cure the deep- seated Kapha in the internal path way (thoracic and abdominal visceras). Thus, a cooling therapy may cure Kapha which is cold in nature.

Sandal-wood is cooling in nature. But if it is made into a fine paste and applied over the skin in a thick layer, it causes burning sensation (heat production) by obstructing the evaporation of heat from the skin. Similarly, Aguru – Aquallaria agallocha which is hot in potency, [if made to a coarse paste and applied in a thin layer over the skin] produces cooling effects.

Intake of the whole fly causes emesis; but intake of the stool of fly is anti-emetic. Similarly, modification of effects (manifestation of opposite effects) can be observed if an article [of food or drugs] is subjected to physical heat or taken internally [and exposed to the effects of the digestive fire].

Need for proper examination of Desha, etc.

तस्माद्दोषौषधादीनि परीक्ष्य दश तत्त्वतः||३२६||

कुर्याच्चिकित्सितं प्राज्ञो न योगैरेव केवलम्|३२७|

Therefore, a wise physician should carry out treatment after examining the diseases and drugs with reference to 10 items (commentary), and only by recipes [described with reference to the diseases in the classics]. [326 ½ – ½ 327]

Re- occurrence of disease:

निवृत्तोऽपि पुन व्याधिः स्वल्पेनायाति हेतुना||३२७||

क्षीणे मार्गीकृते देहे शेषः सूक्ष्म इवानलः| तस्मात्तमनुबध्नीयात् प्रयोगेणानपायिना||३२८||

सिद्ध्यर्थं प्राक्प्रयुक्तस्य सिद्धस्याप्यौषधस्य तु|३२९|

Even if disease is cured, it may reoccur by minor form of etiological factors because by the earlier disease the body has become already weak., and the channels for the manifestation of the disease have already become vulnerable.This reccurrence takes place like the flaring up of a small quantity of residual fire [after the main fire is extinguished]. Therefore, the body is immured from such recurring attacks of the disease by the continuous use of effective and otherwise harmless drugs which were used before for the treatment of the primary disease. [327 ½ – ½ 329]

Effects of wholesome food and regimens:

Should be replaced with Shlokas - 329 ½- ½ 331

काठिन्यादूनभावाद्वा दोषोऽन्तः कुपितो महान्||३२९||

पथ्यैर्मृद्वल्पतां नीतो मृदुदोषकरो भवेत्|

पथ्यमप्यश्नतस्तस्माद्यो व्याधिरुपजायते||३३०||

ज्ञात्वैवं वृद्धिमभ्यासमथवा तस्य कारयेत्|३३१|

Doshas may get aggravated in 2 different ways, viz.,

Kathinya (with compactness) which occurs internally, and

Punarbhava (with non- compactness) which occurs in gross form.

By wholesome food and regimes, these compact and non-compact Doshas may get softened or reduced in quantity respectively as a result of which the morbid manifestation will be of mild nature. Therefore, if a disease is manifested in spite of the intake of wholesome food, etc., then for its cure, after ascertaining its nature, wholesome food, etc., is increased in quantity or is taken habitually for a long duration.[329 ½- ½ 331]

Management of Aversion for wholesome Items and Linking for Unwholesome Ones:

सातत्यात्स्वाद्वभावाद्वा पथ्यं द्वेष्यत्वमागतम्||३३१||

कल्पना विधिभिस्तैस्तैः प्रियत्वं गमयेत् पुनः| मनसोऽर्थानुकूल्यादिध तुष्टिरूर्जा रुचिर्बलम्||३३२||

सुखोपभोगता च स्याद्व्याधेश्चातो बलक्षयः| लौल्याद्दोषक्षयाद्व्याधेर्वैधर्म्याच्चापि या रुचिः||३३३||

तासु पथ्योपचारः स्याद्योगेनाद्यं विकल्पयेत्|३३४|

Because of constant use and unpalatability, a wholesome regime may [at times] become repulsive. Such wholesome but repulsive regimes may again be made palatable by processing them through different modes of cooking.

Therapeutic measures agreeable to the mind and senses promote

Tusti (mental satisfaction)

Urja(mental strength)

Ruchi (relish)

Bala (strength) and

Sukha Bhogata (non-resistance to the use of therapeutic measures) as a result of which the strength of the disease gets diminished.

If a patient has developed liking for a particular unwholesome ingredient because of Laulya (desire to indulge because of mental perversion), Ksaya (diminution of Doshas) Vyadhi (nature of the disease) and Vyadhi – Vaidharmya (desire to take ingredients which are opposed to the attributes of the disease), then such events are managed by the administration of suitable wholesome regimens, different types of recipes and different food preparations. [331 ½- ½ 334]

To sum up:

तत्र श्लोकाः:-

विंशति व्यापदो योनेर्निदानं लिङ्गमेव च||३३४||

चिकित्सा चापि निर्दिष्टा शिष्याणां हित काम्यया| शुक्र दोषास्तथा चाष्टौ निदानाकृतिभेषजैः||३३५||

क्लैब्यान्युक्तानि चत्वारि चत्वारः प्रदास्तथा| तेषां निदानं लिङ्गं च भैषज्यं चैव कीर्तितम्||३३६||

क्षीर दोषास्तथा चाष्टौ हेतुलिङ्गभिषग्जितैः| रेतसो रजसश्चैव कीर्तितं शुद्धि लक्षणम्||३३७||

उक्तानुक्त चिकित्सा च सम्यग्योगस्तथैव च| देशादि गुणशंसा च कालः षड्विध एव च||३३८||

देशे देशे च यत् सात्म्यं यथा वैद्योऽपराध्यति| चिकित्सा चापि निर्दिष्टा दोषाणां गूढचारिणाम्||३३९||

The topics described in this chapter for the benefits of the disciples are as follows:

Etiology, signs, symptoms and therapeutic measures for the treatment of 20 varieties of genetic diseases (yoni Dosha);

Etiology, signs , symptoms and therapeutic measures for the treatment of 8 types of seminal morbidities (Shukra Dosha)

Etiology, signs , symptoms and therapeutic measures for the treatment of 4 types of impotency (Klaibya)

Etiology, signs , symptoms and therapeutic measures for the treatment of 4 types of menorrhagia (Pradara)

Etiology, signs , symptoms and therapeutic measures for the treatment of 8 types of galactic morbidities (Ksira Dosha)

Signs of pure (natural or normal) semen (Shukra) and Menstrual blood (Rajas)

Treatment of diseases which are described by name and which are not described by name in the text

Appropriate line of treatment for the aforesaid diseases

Highlighting the excellence of the knowledge of the attributes of Desha (Habitat) etc

6 types of times for the administration of therapeutic measures (bhesaja Kala)

Homologation in different countries

Non-achievement of success by the physician because of the ignorance of the aforesaid factors; and

Treatment of deep-seated morbidities. [334 ½- 339]

Interpretations:

यो हि सम्यङ्न जानाति शास्त्रं शास्त्रार्थमेव च| न कुर्यात् स क्रियां चित्रमचक्षुरिव चित्रकृत्||३४०||

A physician who is not well versed in the scriptures and their interpretations should not attempt treatment of diseases as a painter without eyesight should not attempt painting a picture. [340]

Colophon of the Chapter:

इत्यग्निवेशकृते तन्त्रे चरक प्रति संस्कृतेऽप्राप्ते दृढबल सम्पूरिते चिकित्सा स्थाने योनिव्यापच्चिकित्सितं नाम त्रिंशोऽध्याय:||३०||

Thus, ends the 30th chapter on the treatment of uterine diseases [etc] in the Chikitsa section of Agnivesha's work as redacted by Charaka, and supplemented by Dridhabala.

Colophon of the Section: (Sthana)

अग्निवेशकृते तन्त्रे चरक प्रतिसंस्कृते| चिकित्सितमिदं स्थानं षष्ठं परिसमापितम्||३४१||

Thus, ends the 6th section called Chikitsa Sthana (section on Therapeutics) of Agnivesha's work as redacted by Charaka.

End of Chikitsa Sthana

कल्पस्थानम् Kalpa Sthanam

14

Kalpasthana Chapter 1 Madana Kalpam

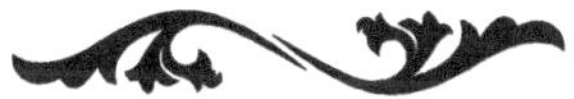

अथातो मदनकल्पं व्याख्यास्यामः||१||

इति ह स्माह भगवानात्रेयः||२||

Now we shall expound the chapter dealing with the "pharmaceutics of madana (randia dumetorum)". Thus, said lord Atreya. [1-2]

Purpose of composing this section

In the previous section on the "treatment of diseases", several recipes for emesis and purgation are prescribed in the context of the treatment of various diseases. In the present chapter on "pharmaceutics", these recipes will be described in detail along with their applicability in the treatment of various diseases. Thus, this is a section on recipes (kalpa).

Needs for describing this section before Siddhi Sthana

Basti (medicated enema), etc. are also described for the treatment of diseases in the previous section i.e., section dealing with treatment of diseases. Therefore, the section dealing with various aspects of this enema therapy (siddhi-sthana) is also required to be described as a part of the treatment of diseases. But while administering Pancha- karma (five specialised elimination therapies) in general emetic (vamana) and purgation (virechana) therapies are to be administered before the administration of basti (medicated enema therapy). Therefore, Kalpa- sthana dealing with these emetics and purgatives is placed before the description of basti therapy. Basti therapy will be described later in the siddhi section.

Purpose of describing emetics before purgatives

Generally, purgation therapy is administered only after the administration of emetic therapy. Therefore, the chapters describing emetic therapy are placed before the before the dealing with the purgative therapy in this section.

Purgation of describing madanaphala in the first chapter:

Among the emetic drugs, madana-phala is the best because it does not produce any adverse effect (vide para no 13). Therefore, the chapter dealing with the recipes containing this drug is placed in the beginning of this section.

Objects of kalpa –sthana

अथ खलु वमनविरेचनार्थ वमनविरेचनद्रव्याणां सुखोपभोगगतमैः सहान्यैर्द्रव्यैर्विविधैः कल्पनार्थं भेदार्थं विभागार्थं चेत्यर्थः , तद्योगानां च क्रियाविधेः सुखोपायस्य सम्यगुपकल्पनार्थं कल्पस्थानमुपदेक्ष्यामोऽग्निवेश!||३||

O, Agnivesha! Hereafter, kalpa-sthana (section on pharmaceutics) will be described by me (refers to preceptor Atreya) for the appropriate processing of the recipes with the following objectives:

Preparation of recipes for emesis and purgation which includes main drugs added with the subsidiary ones of the likes of sura (alcohol), suvira (vinegar) and kovidara having the most useful effects to facilitate emetic and purgative actions along with their varieties and proportions;

Preparation of these recipes appropriately through different pharmaceutical processes to facilitate easy action are explained. [3]

Definition of vamana and Virechana

तत्र दोषहरणमूर्ध्वभागं वमनसञ्ज्ञकम्, अधोभागं विरेचनसञ्ज्ञकम्; उभयं वा शरीरमलविरेचनादि्विरेचनसञ्ज्ञां लभते||४||

Vamana i.e., therapeutic emesis is the process of expelling morbid material through the upward tract (mouth).

Virechana i.e., therapeutic purgation is the process of expelling morbid material through the downward tract (anus). Virechana is the common term used to describe both these therapies / processes since both expel the morbid material from the body. [4]

Mode of action of emetics and purgatives:

तत्रोष्ण-तीक्ष्ण-सूक्ष्म-व्यवायि-विकाशीन्यौषधानि स्ववीर्येण हृदयमुपेत्य धमनीरनुसृत्य स्थूलाणुस्रोतोभ्यः केवलं शरीरगतं दोषसङ्घातमाग्नेयत्वाद् विष्यन्दयन्ति, तैक्ष्णाद् विच्छिन्दन्ति, स विच्छिन्नः परिप्लवन् [१] स्नेहभाविते काये स्नेहाक्तभाजनस्थमिव क्षौद्रमसज्जन्नणुप्रवणभावादामाशयमागम्योदानप्रणुन्नोऽग्निवाय्वात्मकत्वादूर्ध्वभागप्रभावादौषधस्योर्ध्वमुत्क्षिप्यते, सलिलपृथिव्यात्मकत्वादधोभागप्रभावाच्चौषधस्याधः प्रवर्तते, उभयतश्चोभयगुणत्वात्|

इति लक्षणोद्देशः||५||

Drugs used for emesis and purgation are ushna (hot), tikshna (sharp), suksma (subtle), vyavayi (those pervading the entire body before joints) in nature. By the virtue of their own potency these drugs reach the heart, and circulate through the vessels.

Because of their agneya nature (predominance of Agni mahabhuta i.e., fire element), they liquefy the compact (adhered) doshas (morbid material).

They separate the adhered doshas located in the gross and suitable channels of the entire body owing to their tikshna guna i.e., sharpness attribute.

The morbid material, after separation from the channels, moves floating without adhesion in the body which has been subjected to oleation i.e., lubrication therapy, just like the honey kept in a pot smeared with the fat floats without getting adhered to the pot.

Because of its nature to move through subtle channels and to flow (towards the gastro- intestinal) this morbid material reaches the stomach, and gets propelled by udana Vayu.

The morbid material gets expelled through the upward tract (mouth) because of the predominance of Agni and Vayu mahabhutas (fire and air elements) in these emetic drugs and because of their specific action to move upwards.

On the other hand, the purgative drugs owing to the predominance of Prithvi and Jala mahabhutas (earth and water elements), and because of their prabhava i.e., specific actions move downwards to expel the morbid material through the downward tract (anus).

Combination of both these attributes results in the expulsion of the morbid material through both the upward and downward tracts. This is the brief description of the mode of actions of emetic and purgation. [5]

Innumerability of recipes

तत्र फल-जीमूतकेक्ष्वाकु-धामार्गव-कुटज-कृतवेधनानां, श्यामा-त्रिवृच्चतुरङ्गुल-तिल्वक-महावृक्ष-सप्तला-शङ्खिनी-दन्ती-द्रवन्तीनां च, नानाविधदेशकालसम्भवास्वाद-रस-वीर्य-विपाक-प्रभावग्रहणाद् देह-दोष-प्रकृति-वयो-बलाग्नि-भक्ति-सात्म्य-रोगावस्थादीनां नानाप्रभावत्वाच्च , विचित्रगन्ध-वर्ण-रस-स्पर्शानामुपयोगसुखार्थमसङ्ख्येयसंयोगानामपि च सतां द्रव्याणां विकल्पमार्गोपदर्शनार्थ षड्विरेचनयोगशतानि व्याख्यास्यामः||६||

[Emetic drugs, viz] Phala, Jimutaka, Iksvaku, Dhamargava, Kutaja and Krtavedhana, and purgative drugs, viz., Shyama, Trivrt, Chaturangula, Tilvaka, Mahavrksa, Saptala, Sankhini, Danti and Dravanti are of different types depending upon the below mentioned aspects –

desha - habitat, kala - time of their availability, sambhava - origin, ashvada - palatability, rasa - taste,

virya - potency, vipaka - the taste that emerges after digestion and prabhava - specific action

Patients for whom these drugs are to be used are also of different types depending upon the nature of their physique, condition of the doshas, constitution, age, strength, power of digestion and metabolism, liking for a particular type of recipe, wholesomeness, stage of the disease etc. Therefore, in order to cater to the requirement of all these factors the recipes of drugs become innumerable in types. Individual description of the recipes with permutation and combination is impossible. Therefore, by way of illustration, we shall confine our description only to six hundred recipes with multiple smell, colour, taste and touch which are helpful with immediate effects. [6]

Promoting therapeutic efficacy of drugs:

तानि तु द्रव्याणि देश-काल-गुण-भाजन-सम्पद्वीर्यबलाधानात् क्रियासमर्थतमानि भवन्ति॥७॥

These drugs used for emesis and purgation become capable of producing maximum therapeutic effects when their potency is augmented by –

desha-sampat (collecting the plants from the appropriate habitat),

kala- sampat (collecting these plants in the appropriate season),

guna- sampat (collecting plants when these are enriched with excellent attributes) and

bhajana-sampat (strong these plants in appropriate containers) [7]

Varieties of habitat

त्रिविधः खलु देशः- जाङ्गलः, आनूपः, साधारणश्चेति।

तत्र जाङ्गलः पर्याकाशभूयिष्ठः, तरुभिरपि च कदर-खदिरासनाश्वकर्ण-धव-तिनिश-शल्लकी-साल-सोमवल्क-बदरी-तिन्दुकाश्वत्थ-वटामलकीवनगहनः, अनेकशमी-ककुभ-शिंशपाप्रायः, स्थिरशुष्कपवनबलविधूयमानप्रनृत्यत्तरुणविटपः, प्रततमृगतृष्णिकोपगूढतनुखरपरुषसिकताशर्कराबहुलः, लावतित्तिरिचकोरानुचरितभूमिभागः, वातपित्तबहुलः, स्थिरकठिनमनुष्यप्रायो ज्ञेयः, अथानूपो हिन्तालतमालनारिकेलकदलीवनगहनः, सरित्समुद्रपर्यन्तप्रायः, शिशिरपवनबहुलः, वञ्जुलवानीरोपशोभिततीराभिः सरिद्भिरुपगतभूमिभागः, क्षितिधरनिकुञ्जोपशोभितः, मन्दपवनानुवीजितक्षितिरुहगहनः, अनेकवनराजीपुष्पितवनगहनभूमिभागः, स्निग्धतरुप्रतानोपगूढः, हंस-चक्रवाक-बलाका-नन्दीमुख-पुण्डरीक-कादम्ब-मद्गु -भृङ्गराज-शतपत्र-मत्तकोकिलानुनादिततरुविटपः, सुकुमारपुरुषः, पवनकफप्रायो ज्ञेयः; अनयोरेव द्वयोर्देशयोर्विरुद्वनस्पतिवानस्पत्यशकुनिमृगगणयुतः स्थिरसुकुमारबलवर्णसंहननोपपन्नसाधारणगुणयुक्तपुरुषः साधारणो ज्ञेयः॥८॥

Habitats (dcsha) arc of three types, viz jangala (dry forest land), anupa (marshy land) and sadharana (normal land).

1. The jangala- desha (dry forest land) is characterized as follows:

It abounds in open sky

It has deep forests consisting of trees like kadara, khadira, asana, ashva-karna, dhava, tinisa, sallaki, sala, soma-valka, vasari, tinduka, ashvattha, vata and amalaki;

It is mostly surrounded by trees of shami, kakubha and simsapa in large numbers.

The tender branches of these trees dance, being swayed by the force of continuous dry wind;

It abounds in thin, dry and sands as well as gravels which give rise to mirages;

This area is inhabited by lava, tittiri and cakora and the people inhabiting this type of land are dominated by Vayu and pitta and most of them are sturdy and hardy.

2. The anupa- desha (marshy land) is characterized as follows:

It contains deep forests of trees like hintala, tamala, narikela, and kadali;

It is located generally at the banks of rivers and sea;

Mostly cold wind blows here;

This type of land is located in the neighbourhood of rivers whose banks are beautified by plants like vanjula and vanira.

It has mountains covered with beautiful creepers;

The trees in this thick forest weave with the gentle breeze;

The area is surrounded by thick forest with beautiful and blooming trees.

It is covered with tender branches of trees;

The branches of trees located here are echoed with the sound produced by birds like hamsa, cakravaka, balaka, nandi_ mukha, pundarika, kadamba, madgu, bhrngaraja, satapara, and inebriated kokila and

People inhabiting this type of land are of tender body, and generally they are dominated by Vayu and kalpha.

3. The sadhrana- desha(normal land) is characterized as follows:

It has creepers, vanaspati (trees having fruits without apparent flowers), vanaspatya (trees having both fruits and flowers) birds and beasts described above in respects of jangala desha (dry forest land) and anupa desha(marshy land) and;

Persons inhabiting this land are study, tender, endowed with strength, complexion and compactness, as well as other attributes of people inhabiting in the land of general nature. [8]

Appropriate habitat for drug collection

तत्र देशे साधारणे जाङ्गले वा यथाकालं शिशिरातपपवनसलिलसेविते समे शुचौ प्रदक्षिणोदके श्मशान-चैत्य-देवयजनागार-सभा-श्वभ्राराम वल्मीकोषरविरहिते कुशरोहिषास्तीर्णे स्निग्धकृष्णमधुरमृत्तिके सुवर्णवर्णमधुरमृत्तिके वा मृदावफालकृष्टेऽनुपहतेऽन्यैर्बलवत्तरैर्द्रुमैरौषधानि जातानि प्रशस्यन्ते||९||

Medicinal plants, for producing excellent therapeutic effects, are collected from places having the following characteristic features:

These are to be collected from sadharana desha (forests of normal land) or jangala desha (dry land forests)

Plants should have been exposed to seasonal cold, sun, wind and rain appropriately;

Plants should have been grown over plains and clean land surrounded by water reservoirs, rivers etc on the right side;

Plants should not have been grown in a crematorium, caitya (scared tomb), prayer ground, assembly ground, pits, parks, ant-hills and saline soil;

The land should have enormous growth of kusa and rohisa grass;

The soil is unctuous, black in colour and sweet in taste or golden in colour and sweet in taste and

The land should not have been ploughed, and

There should not be other big trees in the vicinity over- shadowing the medicinal plants. [9]

Appropriate time and method of drug collection:

तत्र यानि कालजातान्युपागतसम्पूर्णप्रमाण-रसवीर्य-गन्धानि कालातपाग्निसलिलपवनजन्तुभिरनुपहतगन्ध-वर्ण-रस-स्पर्श-प्रभावाणि प्रत्यग्राण्युदीच्यां दिशि स्थितानि; तेषां शाखापलाशमचिरप्ररूढं वर्षावसन्तयोर्ग्राह्यं, ग्रीष्मे मूलानि शिशिरे वा शीर्णप्ररूढपर्णानां, शरदि त्वक्कन्दक्षीराणि, हेमन्ते साराणि, यथर्तु पुष्पफलमिति; मङ्गलाचारः कल्याणवृत्तः शुचिः शुक्लवासाः सम्पूज्य देवता अश्विनौ गोब्राह्मणांश्च कृतोपवासः प्राङ्मुख उदङ्मुखो वा गृह्णीयात्||१०||

Drugs are collected in the appropriate season when they have attained maturity in respect of their size, taste, potency and smell. Their smell, colour, taste, touch and specific action should have remained unaffected by time (like over maturity), excessive exposure to sun-rays, fire, water and wind, and parasites. They are endowed with all attributes. They are collected from the northern side.

Fresh branches and tender leaves are culled in the rainy season and spring season. Their roots are collected in summer or late winter (Shishira) when the leaves of the trees have ripened and withered out. Their barks, rhizomes and latex are collected in hemanta (early winter), wood including exudates are collected during appropriate seasons [when flowers and fruits appears in the plant].

One should collect the various parts of these plants while facing towards the east or north after performing auspicious rites in a spirit of compassion, while living a pure life, while wearing white dress, after offering prayers to the gods, asvins, cows and brahmins, and while observing fast. [10]

Proper storage:

गृहीत्वा चानुरूपगुणवद्भाजनस्थान्यागारेषु प्रागुदग्द्वारेषु निवातप्रवातैकदेशेषु नित्यपुष्पोपहारबलिकर्मवत्सु, अग्नि-सलिलोपस्वेद-धूम-
रजो-मूषक-चतुष्पदामनभिगमनीयानि स्वच्छन्नानि शिक्येष्वासज्य स्थापयेत्||११||

The collected plant products are kept in appropriate containers well covered with a lid and hung on a swing.
The store-room should have doors facing towards the east or the north. The room is immune to the wind or
storm and there is only one window for ventilation. Flower- offerings and sacrificial rituals are performed in the
store-room every day. It is free from the hazards of fire, water, moisture, smoke, dust, mice and quadrupeds.
[11]

Adjuvants according to doshas

तानि च यथादोषं प्रयुञ्जीत सुरा-सौवीरक-तुषोदक-मैरेय-मेदक-धान्याम्ल -फलाम्ल-दध्यम्लादिभिर्वाते, मृद्वीकामलक [२] -मधु-
मधुक-परूषक-फाणितक्षीरादिभिः पित्ते, श्लेष्मणि तु मधु-मूत्र-कषायादिभिर्भावितान्यालोडितानि च; इत्युद्देशः|
तं विस्तरेण द्रव्य-देह-दोष-सात्म्यादीनि प्रविभज्य व्याख्यास्यामः||१२||

Different adjuvants are required to be used along with these drugs in accordance with the doshas involved in the
causation of the disease.
For treating the diseases caused by Vayu - these drugs are impregnated and mixed with sura, sauviraka, maireyaka,
medaka, dhanyamla, phalamla (juice of sour fruits like pomegranate), dadhyamla (sour yogurt), etc.
For the treatment of diseases caused by pitta, these drugs are to be used by adding mrdvika, amalaka, madhu (honey),
madhuka, parusaka, phanita, milk etc.
For the treatment of diseases caused by kapha, these recipes are to be added with madhu (honey), murta (urine),
kashaya (decoctions of kapha- alleviating drugs), etc.
Thus, the adjuvants are described in brief.
We shall hereafter describe them in detail in relation to different categories of dravya (nature of drug), deha
(requirement of various types of physique), doshas (aggravated to cause the disease) and satmya (homologation).
[12]

Collection, storage and recipes of madana-phala:

वमनद्रव्याणां मदनफलानि श्रेष्ठतमान्याचक्षते, अनपायित्वात्|
तानि वसन्तग्रीष्मयोरन्तरे पुष्याश्वयुग्भ्यां मृगशिरसा वा गृह्णीयान्मैत्रे मुहूर्ते|
यानि पक्वान्यकागान्यहरितानि पाण्डून्यक्रिमीण्यपूतीन्यजन्तुजग्धान्यह्रस्वानि; तानि प्रमृज्य कुशपुटे बद्ध्वा, गोमयेनालिप्य,
यवतु(बु)षमाषशालिकुलत्थमुद्गपलानामन्यतमे निदध्यादष्टरात्रम्|
अत ऊर्ध्वं मृदूभूतानि मधिवष्टगन्धान्युद्धृत्य शोषयेत्|
सुशुष्काणां फलपिप्पलीरुद्धरेत् |तासां घृतदधिमधुपललविमृदितानां पुनः शुष्काणां नवं कलशं सुप्रमृष्टवालुकमरजस्कमाकण्ठं पूरयित्वा
स्वच्छन्नं स्वनुगुप्तं शिक्येष्वासज्य सम्यक् स्थापयेत्||१३||

Fruits of madana are considered to be the best among the emetic drugs because they are free from any adverse side
effects. These fruits are to be collected during the middle of the spring and summer in a maitra muhurta (auspicious
period of the day) when the moon is in the constellation of pushya, asvini or mrgasiras. These fruits are fully
matured, not perforated, not green but yellowish white in colour, not rotten, not infested with parasites and not small
in size. These fruits are cleaned and tied up inside a bundle of barley husk, masha, sali type of paddy, kulattha or
mudga for eight nights.
Afterwards, when they have become soft and are endowed with a desirable smell like that of honey, these fruits are
taken out of the bundle and dried up. When these are well dried up their seeds are taken out. These seeds are rubbed
with ghee, curd, honey and oil-cake, and dried again. These seeds are kept in a new jar cleaned of sand and dust
particles and filled up to its brim. This jar is properly covered with a lid, and after the performance of protective
rituals, is placed in a swing. [13]

Procedure of administering emetic therapy:

अथ च्छर्दनीयमातुरं द्व्यहं त्र्यहं वा स्नेहस्वेदोपपन्नं श्वश्छर्दयितव्यमिति ग्राम्यानूपौदकमांसरस-क्षीर-दधि-माष-तिल-शाकादिभिः समुत्क्लेशितश्लेष्माणं व्युषितं जीर्णाहारं पूर्वाह्णे कृतबलिहोममङ्गलप्रायश्चित्तं निरन्नमनतिस्निग्धं यवाग्वा घृतमात्रां पीतवन्तं, तासां फलपिप्पलीनामन्तर्नखमुष्टिं यावद्वा साधु मन्येत जर्जरीकृत्य यष्टिमधुकषायेण कोविदार-कर्बुदार-नीप-विदुल-बिम्बी-शणपुष्पी-सदापुष्पी-प्रत्यक्पुष्पी-कषायाणामन्यतमेन वा रात्रिमुषितं विमृद्य पूतं मधुसैन्धवयुक्तं सुखोष्णं कृत्वा पूर्णं शरावं मन्त्रेणानेनाभिमन्त्रयेत्-

'ॐ ब्रह्मदक्षाश्विरुद्रेन्द्रभूचन्द्राकार्निलानलाः। ऋषयः सौषधिग्रामा भूतसङ्घाश्च पान्तु ते।

रसायनमिवर्षीणां देवानाममृतं यथा। सुधेवोत्तमनागानां भैषज्यमिदमस्तु ते।

इत्येवमभिमन्त्र्योदङ्मुखं प्राङ्मुखं वाऽऽतुरं पाययेच्छ्लेष्मज्वरगुल्मप्रतिश्यायार्तं विशेषेण पुनः पुनरापितागमनात्, तेन साधु वमति; हीनवेगं तु पिप्पल्यामलक-सर्षप-वचाकल्कलवणोष्णोदकैः पुनः पुनः प्रवर्तयेदापित्तदर्शनात्।

इत्येष सर्वश्छर्दनयोगविधिः।।१४।।

The person is subjected to oleation and fomentation therapies for two or three days prior to the administration of emetic therapy.

During the night before the day of administration of the emetic therapy, he is given the diet consisting of the soup of the meat of gramya (domesticated), anupa (marshy land- inhabiting) and audaka (aquatic) animals, milk, curd, masha, sesame seeds, vegetables, etc, for the excitation of kapha.

On the next morning when the food taken in the previous night is digested, after performing bali (religious sacrifices), homa (sacred ritual of offering oblations of ghee to fire), mangala (auspicious rituals) and prayascitta (rituals for neutralizing effects of possible sinful acts), and when the stomach is empty, the patient who is anati snigdha (has not been given with excessive oleation), is given gruel added with some ghee for intake.

Seeds of madana phala, a fistful in quantity or in a quantity as may be found appropriate, may be crushed, added with the decoction of either yasti-madhu, kovidara (which flowers in the autumn), karbudara (kanchanara which flowers in the spring), nipa (kadamba), vidula (vetasa), bimbi, sanapuspi (ghantarava), sada-puspi (arka- puspika) or pratyakpuspi (ghantarava), sada-puspi (arka puspika) or pratyakpuspi (apamarga), and kept overnight. In the morning, this is obtained, is stirred with hand and filtered. The liquid, thus obtained, is added with honey and rock-salt, made slightly warm, filled up to the brim in a drinking pot, and impregnated with the following mantra. [The mantra has to be recited in its original language for which the script is Romanised below. The translation is furnished thereafter only for the comprehension of its connotations].

Original mantra:

"om brahma- daksasvirudrendra-bhu-candrarkanilanah|

Rsayah sausadhigrama bhutasanghasca pantu te||

Rasayanamivarsinam'devanam amrtam yatha|

Sudhevottamanaganam

Bhisajyam idam astu te||

Translation of the mantra:

May brahma, daksha, the asvins, rudra, indra, the earth, the moon, the sun, the wind, the fire, the sages, all the drugs and all the living beings protect you.

Let the recipe produce effects on you as the rejuvenating recipes have done to the sages, as the ambrosia has done to the gods, and as sudha (a type of ambrosia) has done to the chief of the nagas.

After the recipe has been impregnated with the mantra described above, it is administered to the patient while he is facing towards the east or the north repeatedly. It should be given till the bile comes out along with the vomited material. This is essential, especially for the patients suffering from kaphaja type of fever, gulma, (phantom tumour) and pratishyaya (chronic cold). By this method, emesis takes place properly.

If the urge for vomiting is weak, then this is augmented by the repeated administration of the paste of pippali, amalaka, sarsapa and vacha added with salt and warm water till the bile appears in the vomited material.

This is the method of administering all types of emetic recipes. [14]

Use of honey and rock- salt:

सर्वेषु तु मधुसैन्धवं कफविलयनच्छेदार्थं वमनेषु विदध्यात्।

न चोष्णविरोधो मधुनश्छर्दनयोगयुक्तस्य, अविपक्वप्रत्यागमनाद्दोषनिर्हरणाच्च||१५||

In all the emetic recipes, honey and rock-salt is added in order to facilitate the liquefaction and chedana (separation of adhesion) of kapha. The emetic recipe should always be administered hot. This honey added to hot emetic recipes is not incompatible with heat (i.e., taken after it is added to hot water which generally products toxic reactions) because this honey is thrown out undigested along with vomited material, and helps in the elimination of morbid doshas. [15]

Eight recipes of madana- phala in pill from

फलपिप्पलीनां द्वौ द्वौ भागौ कोविदारादिकषायेण त्रिःसप्तकृत्वः स्रावयेत्, तेन रसेन तृतीयं भागं पिष्ट्वा मात्रां हरीतकीभिर्बिभीतकैरामलैर्वा तुल्यां वर्तयेत्, तासामेकां द्वे वा पूर्वोक्तानां कषायाणामन्यतमस्याञ्जलिमात्रेण विमृद्य बलवच्छ्लेष्मप्रसेकग्रन्थिज्वरोदरारुचिषु पाययेदिति समानं पूर्वेण||१६||

Two (out of three) parts of the seeds of madana phala is added with (six times of) the decoctions of kovidara, etc (including karbudara, nipa, vidula, bimba, sana-puspi, sada-puspi, and pratyak –puspi- these eight drugs are described in para no. 14), and strained twenty-one times. With this liquid, the (remaining) third part of the seeds is triturated and made to paste. From out of this paste, pills of the size of haritaki, bibhitaka or amalaki are prepared. One or two of these pills are given by rubbing with one anjali (approximately 192 ml) of the decoction either of the eight drugs (described above) to a patient suffering from praseka (salivation), granthi (tumour or nodules), jvara (fever), udara (obstinate abdominal diseases including ascites) and aruchi (anorexia).

The remaining procedure as described above (in para no 14) is adopted for these recipes also. [16]

Recipes of madana-phala prepared with milk

फलपिप्पलीक्षीरं, तेन वा क्षीरयवागूमधोभागे रक्तपित्ते हृद्दाहे च; तज्जस्य वा दध्न उत्तरं कफच्छर्दितमकप्रसेकेषु ; तस्य वा पयसः शीतस्य सन्तानिकाञ्जलिं पित्ते प्रकुपिते उरःकण्ठहृदये च तनुकफोपदिग्धे, इति समानं पूर्वेण||१७||

The four recipes of madana phala prepared by boiling with milk are as follows:

According to the procedure prescribed for ksira-paka, the seeds of madana phala are cooked by adding milk.

Gruel is prepared by adding this milk. Both the above-mentioned recipes are useful as emetics for patients suffering from adhoga raktapitta (a disease characterized by bleeding through the downward tracts) and hrd-daha i.e. burning sensation in the cardiac region.

Cream is taken out of the yoghurt prepared of the above-mentioned medicated milk. This is useful in the kaphaja type of chardi (vomiting), tamaka (asthma) and praseka (ptyalism).

The milk described in item no.1 above is cooled, and the cream from this milk is taken out. This cream is administered in the dose of one anjali (192 ml). This is useful when pitta is aggravated, and the chest, throat as well as heart is adhered with a thin layer of kapha.

The rest of the procedure, to be followed in this connection is as described before (in the paragraph no. 14) [17]

Recipe of madana- phala prepared with butter:

फलपिप्पलीशृतक्षीरान्नवनीतमुत्पन्नं फलादिकल्ककषायसिद्धं कफाभिभूताग्निं विशुष्यद्देहं च मात्रया पाययेदिति समानं पूर्वेण||१८||

The butter collected from the milk boiled with the seeds of madana-phala is cooked by adding the paste and decoction of madana-phala, (jimutaka, iksvaka, dhamargava, kutaja and krta- vedhana). This medicated ghee is administered in appropriate doses to a patient suffering from the suppression of Agni (enzymes responsible for digestion) by kapha, and dehydration of the body.

The rest of the procedure to be followed in this connection is as described earlier (in para no. 14). [18]

Recipe of madana-phala for inhalation

फलपिप्पलीनां फलादिकषायेण त्रिःसप्तकृत्वः सुपरिभावितेन पुष्परजःप्रकाशेन चूर्णेन सरसि सञ्जातं बृहत्सरोरुहं सायाह्नेऽवचूर्णयेत्, तद्रात्रिव्युषितं प्रभाते पुनरवचूर्णितमुद्धृत्य हरिद्राकृसरक्षीरयवागूनामन्यतमं सैन्धवगुडफाणितयुक्तमाकण्ठं पीतवन्तमाघ्रापयेत् सुकुमारमुत्क्लिष्टपित्तकफमौषधद्वेषिणमिति समानं पूर्वेण||१९||

Seeds of madana-phala is well impregnated with the decoction of phala, (jumutaka, iksvaku, dhamargava, kutaja and krta-vedhana) for twenty-one times, and made to fine powder resembling the pollens of flowers. In the evening, a big lotus flower growing in a pond is sprinkled with this powder and kept there overnight. In the next morning, the same powder is once again sprinkled over the lotus flower petals and the flower is plucked. This powder (sprinkled on the lotus petals) is given for inhalation to a patient who is of tender nature, in whom pitta and kapha are excited and who has an aversion to taking medicine orally. This inhalation therapy is administered after the patient is fully fed (up to the throat) with haridra, krshara (a type of gruel preparation containing rice and lentils), milk or gruel after adding rock-salt, jiggery and phanita (treacle).

The rest of the process to be followed in this connection is the same as described before (in para no. 14). [19]

Recipes of madana-phala in the form of treacle and powder

फलपिप्पलीनां भल्लातकविधिपरिसुतं स्वरसं पक्त्वा फाणितीभूतमातन्तुलीभावाल्लेहयेत्; आतपशुष्कं वा चूर्णीकृतं जीमूतकादिकषायेण पित्ते कफस्थानगते पाययेदिति समानं पूर्वेण||२०|| फलपिप्पलीचूर्णानि पूर्ववत् फलादीनां षण्णामन्यतमकषायसुतानि वर्तिक्रियाः फलादिकषायोपसर्जनाः पेया इति समानं पूर्वेण||२१||

The juice of madana-phala is extracted according to the procedure already described for extracting the essence of bhallataka (vide cikitsa 1:3:14). It should then be cooked till it is reduced to the consistency of treacle, and till threads appear when a portion of the paste is pulled out. This linctus is taken by the patient.

The seeds of madana-phala are dried in the sun, added with the decoction of jimutaka, etc, made to a powder, and administered to the patient who is suffering from ailments caused by the migration of the morbid pitta to the place (seat) of kapha.

The rest of the procedure to be followed in this connection is as described before (in para no. 14)

Recipes of madana-phala in the form of varti

The decoction of any of the six drugs, viz, madana-phala, jimutaka, iksvaka, dhamargava, kutaja and krtavedhana and made into vartis (enlongated pills). These are to be taken mixed with the decoction of madana–phala etc.,

The rest of the procedure to be followed in this connection is as described before (in para no 14). [21]

Recipes of madana-phala in the form of linctus

फलपिप्पलीनामारग्वध   -वृक्षक-स्वादुकण्टक-पाठा-पाटला-शाङ्र्गेष्टा-मूर्वा-सप्तपर्ण-नक्तमाल-पिचुमर्द-पटोल-सुषवी-गुडूची-सोमवल्क-द्वीपिकानां पिप्पली-पिप्पलीमूल-हस्तिपिप्पली-चित्रक-शृङ्गवेराणां चान्यतमकषायेण सिद्धो लेह इति समानं पूर्वेण||२२||

Seeds of madana-phala is made into linctus by boiling with the decoction of one of the below mentioned –

Aragvadha, Vrksaka (kutaja), Svadukantaka (vikankata), Patha, Patala, Sarngesta (gunja), Murva, Saptaparna, Naktamala, Picumarda, Patola, Susavi (karvellaka), Guduchi, Somavalka, Dvipika, Pippali, Pippalimula, Hastipippali, Chitraka, Srngavera [and to the patient for emesis]

The rest of the procedure to be followed in this connection is as described before (in para no 14). [22]

Preparation of madana-phala in the form of utkarika nd modaka

फलपिप्पलीष्वेला-हरेणुका-शतपुष्पा-कुस्तुम्बुरु-तगर-कुष्ठ-त्वक्-चोरक-मरुबकागुरु-गुग्गुल्वेलवालुक-श्रीवेष्टक-परिपेलव-मांसी-शैलेयक-स्थौणेयक-सरल पारावतपद्यशोकरोहिणीनां विंशतेरन्यतमस्य कषायेण साधितोत्कारिका उत्कारिकाकल्पेन, मोदका वा मोदककल्पेन, यथादोषरोगभक्ति प्रयोज्या इति समानं पूर्वेण||२३||

Seeds of madana-phala are cooked with the decoction of one of the twenty drugs, viz

Ela, Harenuka, Satapuspa, Kustumburu, Tagara, Kustha, Tvak, Coraka, Marubaka, Aguru, Guggulu

Elavaluka, Srivestaka, Paripelava (kaivarta –mustaka), Mamsi, Saileyaka

Sthauneyaka (granthiparnaka), Sarala, Paravata padi and Ashoka-rohini (katurohini)

With the pastes, thus obtained (twenty types each of), utkarika (pancake) and modaka (sweetmeat) is prepared, following the procedure prescribed for utkarika and modaka respectively. These are to be administered in accordance with the aggravated doshas, the nature of the disease, and liking of the patient.

The rest of the procedure to be followed in this connection is as described in para no. 14. [23]

Preparation of madana- phala in the form of saskuli and pupa:

फलपिप्पलीस्वरसकषायपरिभावितानि तिलशालितण्डुलपिष्टानि तत्कषायोपसर्जनानि शष्कुलीकल्पेन वा शष्कुल्यः, पूपकल्पेन वा पूपाः इति समानं पूर्वेण||२४||

एतेनैव च कल्पेन सुमुख-सुरस-कुठेरक-काण्डीर-कालमालक-पर्णासक-क्षवक-फणिज्झक-गृञ्जन-कासमर्द-भृङ्गराजानां पोटेक्षुवालिका-कालङ्कतक-दण्डैरकाणां चान्यतमस्य कषायेण कारयेत्||२५||

The paste of tila and shali-rice are prepared by adding the juice or decoction or the seeds of madana-phala. This paste is further processed by adding the decoction of the seeds of madana-phala. From this paste, saskuli (a type of pancake) and pupa (preparation of sweetmeat) is prepared, and administered to the patient.

The rest of the procedure to be followed in this connection is as described earlier 9 in para no. 14)

[the paste of tila and sali-rice prepared with the juice or decoction of the seeds of madana-phala may be further processed by adding the] decoction of [one of the fifteen drugs, viz,]

Sumukha, Surasa, Kutheraka, Kandira, Kalamala, Parnasaka, Ksavaka, Phanijjhaka, Granjana, Kasamarda, Bhrngaraja, Pota, Iksuvalika, Kalankataka, Dandairaka (gundra or nala) from this paste, saskulis and pupas may be prepared [and administered to the patient following the procedure earlier described in the paragraph no. 14] [24-25]

Preparation of madana-phala in the form of badara-sadava etc.

तथा बदरषाडव-राग-लेह-मोदकोत्कारिका-तर्पण-पानक-मांसरस-यूष-मद्यानां मदनफलान्यन्यतमेनोपसृज्य यथादोषरोगभक्ति दद्यात्; तैः साधु वमतीति||२६||

Seeds of madana-phala may be added to one of the preparations like -

Badara-sadava (name of a sour liquid preparation of jujube fruit), Raga (an appetiser having sour and pungent tastes), Leha (linctus), Modaka (sweet meat), Utkarika (pan-cake), Tarpana (demulcent drink), Panaka (syrup), Mamsa-rasa ((meat-soup), Yusa (vegetable soup), Madya (alcohol) and given to the patient, depending upon the state of the doshas, nature of the disease and likings. By these preparations the patient vomits well. [26]

Synonymous of madana-phala

मदनः करहाटश्च राठः पिण्डीतकः फलम्| श्वसनश्चेति पर्यायैरुच्यते तस्य कल्पना||२७||

The recipes described in the previous paragraphs are those of the drug whose synonyms are: madana, karahata, ratha, pinditaka, phala and svasana.

Contents of the chapter

तत्र श्लोकाः:-

नव योगाः कषायेषु, मात्रास्वष्टौ [१] , पयोघृते| पञ्च, फाणितचूर्णे द्वौ घ्रेये, वर्तिक्रियासु षट्||२८||

विंशतिर्विंशतिर्लेहमोदकोत्कारिकासु च| शष्कुलीपूपयोश्चोक्ता योगाः षोडश षोडश||२९||

दशान्ये षाडवाद्येषु त्रयस्त्रिंशदिदं शतम्| योगानां विधिवद्दिष्टं फलकल्पे महर्षिणा||३०||

To sum up: -

In this chapter the great sage (Atreya) has described 133 recipes prepared with madana phala. They are as follows –

Nine recipes in the form of decoction (vide para no 14)

Eight recipes in the form of matra (pills)

Five recipes in the form of medicated milk and medicated ghee (vide para no 17-18)

One recipe to be used for inhalation (vide para no 19)

Two recipes in the form of treacle and powder; (vide para no 20)

Six recipes in the form of varti (elongated pill) (vide para no 21)

Twenty recipes in the form of linctus (vide para no. 23)

Twenty recipes in the form of utkarika (pan-cake) (vide para n 23)

Twenty recipes in the form of modaka (sweet-meat) (vide para no. 23)

Sixteen recipes of saskuli (a type of pancake) and (vide para no. 24-25)

Sixteen recipes of pupa (a type of sweet-meat) and (vide para no. 24-25)
Ten recipes prepared by adding madana-phala to badara –sadava etc. (vide para no 26)

Colophon

इत्यग्निवेशकृते तन्त्रे चरकप्रतिसंस्कृतेऽप्राप्ते दृढबलसम्पूरिते कल्पस्थाने मदनकल्पो नाम प्रथमोऽध्यायः||१||

Thus, ends the first chapter of the kalpa- section dealing with the "pharmaceutics of madana-phala" of Agnivesha's work as redacted by charaka, and because of its non- availability supplemented by drdhabala.

15

Kalpasthana Chapter 2
Jeemootaka Kalpam

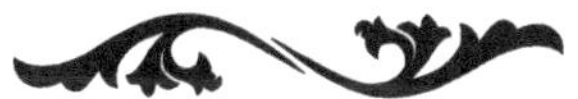

अथातो जीमूतककल्पं व्याख्यास्यामः||१||

इति ह स्माह भगवानात्रेयः||२||

Prologue

Now we shall expound the chapter dealing with the "Pharmaceutics of Jimutaka". Thus, said Lord Atreya. [1-2]

Synonyms of Jimutaka

कल्पं जीमूतकस्येमं फलपुष्पाश्रयं शृणु| गरागरी च वेणी च तथा स्याद्देवताडकः||३||

Now listen [addressed by Atreya to Agnivesha] to the exposition on the pharmaceutics of Jimutaka whose fruits and flowers are used in recipes. The synonyms of Jimutaka are Garagari, Veni and Devatadaka. [3]

Therapeutic Effects of Jimutaka

जीमूतकं त्रिदोषघ्नं यथास्वौषधकल्पितम्| प्रयोक्तव्यं ज्वरश्वासहिक्काद्येष्वामयेषु च||४||

Jimutaka cures all the three doshas when taken with appropriate adjuvants. It is useful in the treatment of fever, asthma, hiccup and such other disorders. [4]

Recipes of Jimutaka Prepared by Boiling with Milk

यथोक्तगुणयुक्तानां देशजानां यथाविधि| पयः पुष्पेऽस्य, निर्वृत्ते फले पेया पयस्कृता||५||

लोमशे क्षीरसन्तानं, दध्युत्तरमलोमशे| शृते पयसि दध्यम्लं जातं हरितपाण्डुके||६||

जीर्णानां च सुशुष्काणां न्यस्तानां भाजने शुचौ| चूर्णस्य पयसा शुक्तिं वातपित्तार्दितः पिबेत्||७||

Jimutaka endowed with all the attributes, growing in appropriate land and collected according to the prescribed procedure as described before [for Madana-Phala in Kalpa 1:9, 10, 14] is used, as followed:

The flower is boiled with milk and this milk is used;

The freshly appeared fruit is boiled with milk and used as gruel;

The fruit with its hairs is boiled with milk; the cream is extracted out of it and is used;

The fruit devoid of hairs is boiled with milk, and curds are prepared from this milk. The cream of this curd is to be used.

The matured fruit which is green and yellowish is boiled with milk. The sour curd prepared out of this milk is to be used; and

The fully matured fruit which is dried should be kept in a clean container.

One Suti (24 gms) of this fruit is made into powder and taken by adding milk to it.

This is useful for a patient who is suffering from ailments caused by Vayu and Pitta. [5-7]

Recipe of Jimutaka Prepared with Alcohol

आसुत्य च सुरामण्डे मृदित्वा प्रसुतं पिबेत्| कफजेऽरोचके कासे पाण्डुरोगे सयक्ष्मणि||८||

The [powder of the] fruit of Jimutaka is soaked in Sura-Manda (supernatant part of alcohol) and kept overnight. Thereafter the recipe is stirred by hand and strained. The liquid thus obtained, is taken by the patient suffering from anorexia caused by Kapha, bronchitis, anemia and tuberculosis. [8]

Recipes of Jimutaka Prepared by Boiling in decoctions:

द्वे चापोथ्याथवा त्रीणि गुडूच्या मधुकस्य वा| कोविदारादिकानां वा निम्बस्य कुटजस्य वा||९||

कषायेष्वासुतं पूत्वा तेनैव विधिना पिबेत्|

Two or three fruits of Jimutaka are boiled in the decoctions of [one of the twelve drugs, viz]

Guduchi, Madhuka, Kovidara, Karbudara, Nipa, Vidula, Bimba, Sana-puspi, Sada-puspi, Pratyak-puspi Nimbi and Kutaja.

Then the liquid is fermented, filtered out and given to the patient according to the procedure prescribed for Madana-Phala (vide Kalpa 1:14) [9 – ½ 10]

Recipes of Jimutaka Perpetrated by Adding Decoctions

अथवाऽऽरग्वधादीनां सप्तानां पूर्ववत् पिबेत्||१०||

एकैकस्य कषायेण पित्तश्लेष्मज्वरार्दितः|११|

Alternatively, the powder of Jimutaka is taken along with the decoctions of

Aragvadha, Vrksaka, Svadu- Kantaka, Patha, Patala, Sarngesta and Murva by the patient suffering from fever caused by aggravated Pitta and Kapha according to the procedure described earlier (vide kalpa 1:14) [10 ½ - ½ 11]

Recipes of Jimutaka prepared in the form of Pills

मात्राः स्युः फलवच्चाष्टौ कोलमात्रास्तु ता मताः||११||

Eight types of pills (Varti) of Jimutaka are to be prepared on the line suggested for Madana- phala (vide Kalpa 1:16). The size of each of these pills is like that of a Kola (jujube fruit). [11 ½]

Recipes of Jimutaka to be used with Juice

जीवकर्षभकेक्षूणां शतावर्या रसेन वा| पित्तश्लेष्मज्वरे दद्याद्वातपित्तज्वरेऽथवा||१२||

The powder of jimutaka is used along with the juice of one of the four drugs, viz.,

Jivaka, Rsabhaka, Ikshu, Shatavari

It is used in the treatment of fever caused either by pitta or Kapha or by Vayu and Pitta. [12]

Recipes of Jimutaka Prepared in the form of Medicated Ghee:

तथा जीमूतकक्षीरात् समुत्पन्नं पचेद्घृतम्| फलादीनां कषायेण श्रेष्ठं तद्वमनं मतम्||१३||

Ghee is prepared from the milk boiled by adding Jimutaka. This ghee is cooked by adding the decoction of Madana-phala, etc., it is an excellent recipe [for emesis] [13]

तत्र श्लोकौ-

षट् क्षीरे मदिरामण्डे एको द्वादश चापरे| सप्त चारग्वधादीनां कषायेऽष्टौ च वर्तिषु||१४||

जीवकादिषु चत्वारो घृतं चैकं प्रकीर्तितम्| कल्पे जीमूतकानां च [२] योगास्त्रिंशन्नवाधिकाः||१५||

To sum up: -

There are thirty-nine recipes of Jimutaka, as follows:

Six recipes prepared by boiling milk with Jimutaka; (vide verse nos 5-7)

One recipe prepared by soaking Jimutaka in alcohol (Vide verse no. 8)

Twelve recipes prepared by boiling with decoctions (vide verse nos. 9 – ½ 11)

Seven recipes to be used along with decoctions (vide verse nos. (10 1/2 - ½ 11)

Eight recipes in the of pills (varti) (vide verse 11 ½)

Four recipes to be used along with the juice of Jivaka, etc; and (vide verse no. 12)
One recipe of medicated ghee (vide verse no 13) [14-15]

Colophon
इत्यग्निवेशकृते तन्त्रे चरकप्रतिसंस्कृतेऽप्राप्ते दृढबलसम्पूरिते कल्पस्थाने जीमूतककल्पो नाम द्वितीयोऽध्यायः||२||
Thus, ends the second chapter of Kalpa-sthana dealing with the "Pharmaceutics of Jimutak "in Agnivesha's work as redacted by Charaka, and because of its non- availability supplemented by Drdhabala.

16
Kalpasthana Chapter 3 Iksvaku Kalpam

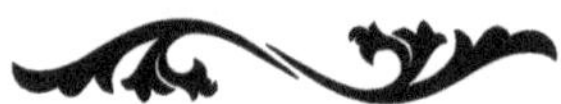

Prologue

अथात इक्ष्वाकुकल्पं व्याख्यास्यामः||१||

इति ह स्माह भगवानात्रेयः||२||

We shall now explore the chapter dealing with the "Pharmaceutics of Iksvaku" Thus, said Lord Atreya. [1-2]

सिद्धं वक्ष्याम्यथेक्ष्वाकुकल्पं येषां प्रशस्यते|३|

I shall [hereafter] explain the effective recipes of Iksvaku, and the types of patients for whom these are very useful. [1/23]

Synonyms

लम्बाऽथ कटुकालाबूस्तुम्बी पिण्डफला तथा||३||

इक्ष्वाकुः फलिनी चैव प्रोच्यते तस्य कल्पना|४|

[Synonyms of iksvaku] are Lamba, Katukalabu, Tumbu, Pindaphala and Phalini. Its recipes will be described [hereafter]. [3 ½ -1/4]

Effects of Iksvaku

कासश्वासविषच्छर्दिज्वरार्ते कफकर्षिते||४||

प्रताम्यति नरे चैव वमनार्थं तदिष्यते|५|

It is useful as emetic for patients suffering from cough, asthma, toxicities, vomiting and fever, for those in whom Kapha has been dried up, for those who are distressed with palpitation. [4 ½- ½ 5]

Recipes of Iksvaku prepared with milk and alcohol

अपुष्पस्य प्रवालानां मुष्टिं प्रादेशसम्मितम्||५||

क्षीरप्रस्थे शृतं दद्यात् पित्तोद्रिक्ते कफज्वरे| पुष्पादिषु च चत्वारः क्षीरे जीमूतके यथा||६||

योगा हरितपाण्डूनां सुरामण्डेन पञ्चमः| फलस्वरसभागं च त्रिगुणक्षीरसाधितम्||७||

उरःस्थिते कफे दद्यात् स्वरभेदे च पीनसे| जीर्णे मध्योद्धृते क्षीरं प्रक्षिपेत्तद्यदा दधि||८||

जातं स्यात् सकफे कासे श्वासे वम्यां च तत् पिबेत्| अजाक्षीरेण बीजानि भावयेत् [२] पाययेत् च||९||

विषगुल्मोदरग्रन्थिगण्डेषु श्लीपदेषु च|

Eight milk preparations and alcoholic preparation of Iksvaku are as follows:

One prastha of milk is boiled by adding one loose fistful of Iksvaku- sprouts which have not yet put forth flowers. This is given to the patient suffering from Kaphaja type of fever associated with aggravated Pitta. (To this recipe four Prasthas of water should also be added while boiling).

As per the description of the recipes of Jimutaka in the earlier chapter (vide Kalpa 2:5-6), four types of milk preparations are to be made out of the flowers, etc, of Iksvaku.

Alcoholic preparation: the matured fruits of Iksvaku which are green and yellowish are kept soaked in Sura-Manda (supernatant part of alcohol) [following the procedure described in Kalpa 2:8]. This constitutes the fifth recipe of flowers and fruits (the earlier four recipes are already described above in item nos. 2-5)

One part of the juice of iksvaku is boiled by adding three parts of milk (and four times of water). This is administered to the patient whose chest is afflicted with aggravated Kapha, and to a person who is suffering from hoarseness of voice and coryza.

The pulp of ripe fruit of Iksvaku is removed. In this shell after removing the pulp, milk is kept until it gets converted into curds. This curd is taken by the patient suffering from cough with phlegm, asthma and vomiting.

Seeds of Iksvaku are impregnated with goat's milk. This milk is given as a potion to a patient suffering from toxicosis, phantom tumour, obstinate abdominal diseases including ascites, nodules), enlargement of thyroid gland and elephantiasis. [5 ½ - ½ 10]

Recipe of Iksvaku to be taken with Whey

मस्तुना वा फलान्मध्यं पाण्डुकुष्ठविषार्दितः||१०||

The pulp of Iksvaku is mixed with whey and taken by the patient suffering from anaemia, obstinate skin diseases including leprosy and toxicities. [10 ½]

Recipe of Iksvaku to be prepared by Boiling with Butter-milk

तेन तक्रं विपक्वं वा सक्षौद्रलवणं पिबेत्|११|

The pulp of Iksvaku boiled by adding butter-milk, and mixed with honey and salt may be taken for emesis. [1/2 11]

Recipe of Iksvaku for inhalation

तुम्ब्या फलरसैः शुष्कैः सपुष्पैरवचूर्णितम्||११||
छर्दयेन्माल्यमाघ्राय गन्धसम्पत्सुखोचितः|१२|

The juice and powder of dried flowers of Iksvaku is sprinkled over a garland. By the very smell of this garland of flowers the patients habituated to pleasant smell will vomit. [11 ½ - ½ 12]

Recipes of Iksvaku with Jaggery etc.

भक्षयेत् फलमध्यं वा गुडेन पललेन च||१२||
इक्ष्वाकुफलतैलं वा सिद्धं वा पूर्ववद्घृतम्|१३|

The pulp of Iksvaku may be taken along with jaggery or oil-cake for emesis.

The medicated oil prepared with the paste of Ikshvaku fruit shall cause vomiting.

The medicated ghee prepared on the lines suggested earlier (in Kalpa 2:13 also caused vomiting. [12 ½ - ½ 13]

Recipes of Iksvaku Used by Increasing Number of Seeds

पञ्चाशद्दशवृद्धानि फलादीनां यथोत्तरम्||१३||
पिबेद्विमृद्य बीजानि कषायेष्वाशतं पृथक्|१४|

The seeds of Iksvaku beginning with fifty in number are gradually increased by tens till the number comes to one hundred. Thus, either 50, 60, 70, 80, 90, or 100 seeds of iksvaku is crushed and added to the decoctions of one of the six plants, (viz, Madana-phala, Jimutaka, Iksvaku, dhamargava, Vatsaka and Krtavedhana) and used for emesis. [13½ -1/2 14]

Recipes of Iksvaku to be used With Decoctions

यष्ट्याह्वकोविदाराद्यैर्मुष्टिमन्तर्नखं पिबेत्||१४||

One closed fist full of the seeds of Iksvaku is taken along with the decoctions (nine) of any one of the below mentioned is used for producing emesis –

Yastimadhu, Kovidara, Karbudara, Nipa, Vidula, Bimbisana-puspi, Sada-puspi, Pratyak- puspi [14 ½]

Recipe of Iksvaku in the form of Pills

कषायैः कोविदाराद्यैर्मात्राश्च फलवत् स्मृताः|१५|

Pills (Matras) are prepared out of Iksvaku by adding the decoctions of any one of Kovidara, {Karbudara, Nipa, Vidula, Bimbi, Sada-Puspi or PratyakPuspi, on the lines suggested for Madana- Phala (vide Kalpa 1: 16) and used for emesis. [1/2 15]

Recipes of Iksvaku in the form of Linctus

बिल्वमूलकषायेण तुम्बीबीजाञ्जलिं पचेत्||१५||

पूतस्यास्य त्रयो भागाश्चतुर्थः [१] फाणितस्य तु| सघृतो बीजभागश्च पिष्टानर्धांशिकांस्तथा [२] ||१६||

महाजालिनिजीमूतकृतवेधनवत्सकान्| तं लेहं साधयेद्दर्व्या घट्टयन्मृदुनाऽग्निना||१७||

यावत् स्यातन्तुमतोये पतितं तु न शीर्यते| तं लिहन्मात्रया लेहं [३] प्रमथ्यां च पिबेदनु||१८||

कल्प एषोऽग्निमन्थादौ चतुष्के पृथगुच्यते|१९|

One Anjali (192 gms) of the seeds of Iksvaku are boiled by adding (eight Anjalis) the decoction of the root of Bilva. It is boiled till the liquid is reduced to one fourth. To three parts of this strained decoction one part of Phanita (treacle or half boiled sugar- cane juice) and one part of ghee are added. To this, half parts each of the paste of Maha-Jakini (pita-Kosataki), Jimutaka, Krtavedhana (jyotsnika) and Vatsaka are added. The linctus is prepared over mild fire and by strewing with the help of a large spoon. This is done till the stuff becomes thick in consistency, and threads appears when a part of it is pulled out, and it does not spread when a part of it is put into water. This linctus is taken in appropriate doses and thereafter, Pramathya (decoction of digestion- stimulant drugs) is used as a post prandial drink.

Similarly, recipes of linctus of Iksvaku seeds can be prepared by adding the decoction of the roots of one of Agnimantha (Shyonaka, Patala and Gambhari) separately. [15 ½ - ½ 19]

Recipe of Iksvaku to be used along with Mantha

शक्तुभिर्वा पिबेन्मन्थं तुम्बीस्वरसभावितैः||१९||

कफजेऽथ ज्वरे कासे कण्ठरोगेष्वरोचके|२०|

Saktu (roasted barley flour) is impregnated with the juice of tumbi (Iksvaku). Patients suffering from Kaphaja type of fever, cough, diseases of the throat and anorexia should take the mantha i.e., thin gruel prepared from this saktu as a potion. [19 ½ - ½ 20]

Recipe of Iksvaku to be taken along with Meat- soup

गुल्मे मेहे प्रसेके च कल्कं मांसरसैः पिबेत्| नरः साधु वमत्येवं न च दौर्बल्यमश्नुते||२०||

The paste of [the seeds of] Iksvaku are taken with meat soup in phantom tumour, obstinate urinary disorders including diabetes and ptyalism. By this, the person gets vomiting easily and does not suffer from weakness. [20 ½]

Contents of Chapter

तत्र श्लोकाः:-

पयस्यष्टौ सुरामण्ड-मस्तु-तक्रेषु च त्रयः| घ्रेयं सपललं तैलं वर्धमानाः फलेषु षट्||२१||

घृतमेकं कषायेषु नवान्ये मधुकादिषु| अष्टौ वर्तिक्रिया लेहाः पञ्च मन्थो रसस्तथा||२२||

योगा इक्ष्वाकुकल्पे ते चत्वारिंशच्च पञ्च च| उक्ता महर्षिणा सम्यक् प्रजानां हितकाम्यया||२३||

To sum up:

In this chapter on the Pharmaceutics of Iksvaku, the great sage, with the healthy well-being of the people in view, has described forty-five recipes of Iksvaku which are as follows:

Eight recipes prepared with milk (vide verse nos. 5- 10)

One recipe with Sura-Manda (supernatant part of Alcohol)

Two recipes one each of whey and buttermilk (vide verse no 10-11)

One recipe for inhalation (vide verse no 11-12)
One recipe to be taken with Palala (oil-cake)
One recipe of medicated oil (vide verse no 13)
Six recipes with increased number of seeds (vide verse no. 13-14)
One recipe of medicated ghee (vide verse no 13)
Nine recipes to be taken along with decoctions of Yastimadhu or other drugs; (vide verse no. 14)
Eight recipes in the form of pills: (vide verse nos 15)
Five recipes of linctus (vide verse nos. 15-19)
One recipe of medicated Saktu; and (vide verse nos 19-20)
One recipe to be taken along with meat-soup (vide verse no. 20) [21-23]

Colophon
इत्यग्निवेशकृते तन्त्रे चरकप्रतिसंस्कृतेऽप्राप्ते दृढबलसम्पूरिते कल्पस्थाने इक्ष्वाकुकल्पो नाम तृतीयोऽध्यायः॥३॥
Thus, ends the third chapter of Kalpa-Sthana dealing with the Pharmaceutic of Iksvaku" in Agnivesha's work as redacted by Charaka, and because of its non- availability supplemented by Drdhabala.

17

Kalpasthana Chapter 4
Dhamargava Kalpam

Prologue

अथातो धामार्गवकल्पं व्याख्यास्यामः||१||

इति ह स्माह भगवानात्रेयः||२||

Now we shall explore the chapter dealing with the "Pharmaceutics of Dhamargava", thus said Lord Atreya. [1-2]

Synonyms of Dhamargava

कर्कोटकी कोठफला महाजालिनिरेव च|

धामार्गवस्य पर्याया राजकोशातकी तथा||३||

The synonyms of dhamargava (pita-Ghosaka) are Karkotaki, Kothaphala,Maha-Jalini and raja-Kostaki.

Therapeutic Effects

गरे गुल्मोदरे कासे वाते श्लेष्माशयस्थिते| कफे च कण्ठवक्रस्थे कफसञ्चयजेषु च||४||

रोगेष्वेषु प्रयोज्यं स्यात् स्थिराश्च गुरवश्च ये|५|

Dhamargava is useful in the treatment of stable and obstinate diseases including toxicities, phantom tumour, and obstinate abdominal diseases including ascites, cough, aliments caused by the localization of aggravated Vayu in the seat of kapha, diseases of throat and mouth and other diseases caused by the accumulation of kapha. [4- ½ 5]

Recipes of Dhamargava to be used with Decoctions

फलं पुष्पं प्रवालं च विधिना तस्य संहरेत्||५||

प्रवालस्वरसं शुष्कं कृत्वा च गुलिकाः पृथक्| कोविदारादिभिः पेयाः कषायैर्मधुकस्य च||६||

The fruits, flowers and tender leaves of Dhamargava are collected according to procedure. The juice of the tender leaves of Dhamargava is dried and made into pills. These pills are to be taken as a potion mixed with the decoction of one of the drugs, viz, Kovidara, (Karbudara, Nipa, Vidula, Bimbi, Sanapuspi, Sadapuspi, Pratyakpuspi) or Yastimadhu. [6]

Recipes of Dhamargava Prepared with milk and Alcohol

पुष्पादिषु पयोयोगाश्चत्वारः पञ्चमी सुरा|

पूर्ववत्...|७|

Four milk preparations and one alcoholic preparations of Dhamargava is made according to the procedure described before (vide Kalpa 2: 5-6) [3/4 7]

Recipe of Dhamargava prepared with decoction

... जीर्णशुष्काणामतः कल्पः प्रवक्ष्यते||७||

मधुकस्य कषायेण बीजकण्ठोद्धृतं फलम्| सगुडं व्युषितं रात्रिं कोविदारादिभिस्तथा||८||
दद्याद्गुल्मोदरार्तेभ्यो ये चाप्यन्ये कफामयाः|९|

Now the recipes prepared of matured and fruits of Dhamargava will be described.

The seeds of Dhamargava are removed from the fruit. The fruit should then be filled up with decoctions of Yastimadhu mixed with jaggery and kept overnight. Similarly, the fruit can be filled up with jaggery mixed with the decoctions of one Kovidara, (Karbudara, Nipa, Vidula, Bimbi, Sanapuspi, Sadapuspi or Pratyakpuspi) and kept overnight. These (nine) decoctions are to be used [for emesis] to patients suffering from phantom tumour, obstinate abdominal diseases and other diseases caused by Kapha. [7 ½ - ½ 9]

Recipe of Dhamargava to be given with food

दद्यादन्नेनसंयुक्तंछर्दिहृद्रोगशान्तये||९||

The powder of Dhamargava is added to food and given for the alleviation of vomiting and cardiac ailments. [9 ½]

Recipe of Dhamargava for Inhalation

चूर्णैर्वाऽप्युत्पलादीनि भावितानि प्रभूतशः| रसक्षीरयवाग्वादितृप्तो घ्रात्वा वमेत् सुखम्||१०||

Flowers of Utpala etc., is impregnated with the powder of Dhamargava for several times. The patient having taken the meat-soup), milk, gruel etc., sumptuously should inhale the smell of this impregnated flower which causes emesis with ease. [10]

Recipes of Dhamargava in Pill-form

चूर्णीकृतस्य वर्तिं वा कृत्वा बदरसम्मिताम्| विनीयाञ्जलिमात्रे तु पिबेद्गोऽश्वशकृद्रसे ||११||
पृषतर्ष्यकुरङ्गाह्वगजोष्ट्राश्वतराविके| श्वदंष्ट्रखरखड्गानां चैवं पेया शकृद्रसे ||१२||

Alternatively, with the powder of Dhamargava, the pill of the size of Kola (jujube – fruit) is prepared. This pill is mixed with one Anjali (192 ml) of the juice of cowdung or horse-dung and taken for emesis. This pill may also be used after mixing with the juice of the drug of Prasta (Bindu- Citra- Harina), Rsya (nilanda), Kuranga (Cancala Gati),Gaja (elephant), Ustra (camel), Advatara (vegasara), Avika (sheep), Svadamstra (Mouse- deer), Khara (ass) and Khadga (rhinoceros) for emesis[11-12]

Recipes of Dhamargava in the form of linctus;

जीवकर्षभकौ वीरामात्मगुप्तां शतावरीम्| काकोलीं श्रावणीं मेदां महामेदां मधूलिकाम्||१३||
एकैकशोऽभिसञ्चूर्ण्य सह धामार्गवेण ते| शर्करामधुसंयुक्ता लेहा हृद्दाहकासिनाम्||१४||
सुखोदकानुपानाः स्युः पित्तोष्मसहिते कफे|१५|

Powders of Jivaka, Rsabhaka, Vira, Atmagupta, Shatavari, Kakoli, Sravani, Meda, Mahameda, Madhulika are prepared separately. Each one of these powders is added with (equal quantity of the powder of Dhamargava, and by adding honey as well as sugar, a linctus is prepared. These (ten emetic recipes) are useful in hrd-daha (burning sensation in the cardiac region) and cough. Tepid water is given as a post-prandial drink if aggravated kapha is associated with Pitta which is hot in nature. [13-1/2 15]

Recipe of Dhamargava in the form of Kalpa

धान्यतुम्बुरुयूषेण कल्कः सर्वविषापहः||१५||

Administration of the paste of Dhamargava along with the decoction of Dhanya and Tumburu [as emetic] cures all forms of toxicities. [15 ½]

Recipes of Dhamargava along with Decoction

जात्याः सौमनसायिन्या रजन्याश्चोरकस्य च| वृश्चीरस्य महाक्षुद्रसहहैमवतस्य च||१६||
बिम्ब्याः पुनर्नवाया वा कासमर्दस्य वा पृथक्| एकं धामार्गवं द्वे वा कषाये परिमृद्य तु||१७||
पूतं मनोविकारेषु पिबेद्वमनमुत्तमम्|१८|

Decoction is prepared out of each of Jati, Saumanasyayini (Yuthika), Rajani (Haridra), coraka, Vrscira (white variety of Punarnava), Maha-Saha (haimavati (Vaca), Bimbi, Punarnava (red variety) and Kasamarda separately. Each of these [eleven] decoctions is added with [the powder of] one or two fruits of Dhamargava, squeezed, and filtered. These are excellent recipes for emesis in physic disorders (Mano Vikara). [16-½ 18]

Recipe of Dhamargava in the form of Medicated Ghee

तच्छृतक्षीरजं सर्पिः साधितं वा फलादिभिः||१८||

Dhamargava is boiled with milk and from this milk ghee is prepared. This ghee is cooked by adding the decoctions of madanaphala etc., [this is useful as emetic]. [18 ½]

Contents of Chapter

तत्र श्लोकौ-

पल्लवे नव चत्वारः क्षीर एकः सुरासवे| कषाये विंशतिः कल्के दश द्वौ च शकृद्रसे||१९||

अन्न एकस्तथा घ्रेये दश लेहास्तथा घृतम्| कल्पे धामार्गवस्योक्ताः षष्टिर्योगा महर्षिणा||२०||

To sum up: -

The great sage has described sixty recipes of Dhamargava as follows:

Nine recipes of tender leaf (vide verse no. 6)

Four recipes prepared by boiling with milk (vide verse no. 7)

One recipe prepared with alcohol (vide verse no. 7)

Twenty recipes prepared with decoctions nine in verse nos 7-9, and eleven in verse nos. 16-18)

One recipe in the form of paste (vide verse no. 15)

Twelve recipes to be used along with the juice of dung's of various animals: (vide verse nos. 11-12)

One recipe to be taken along with food; (vide verse no. 9)

One recipe for inhalation (vide verse no. 10)

Ten recipes in the form of linctus; and (vide verse nos. 13-15)

One recipe of medicated ghee (vide verse no. 18) [19-20]

Colophon

इत्यग्निवेशकृते तन्त्रे चरकप्रतिसंस्कृतेऽप्राप्ते दृढबलसम्पूरिते कल्पस्थाने धामार्गवकल्पो नाम चतुर्थोऽध्यायः||४||

Thus, ends the fourth chapter of Kalpa- Sthana dealing with the "Pharmaceutics of Dhamargava" in Agnivesha's work as a redacted by Charaka., and because of its non- availability supplemented by Drdhabala.

18

Kalpasthana Chapter 5 Vatsaka Kalpam

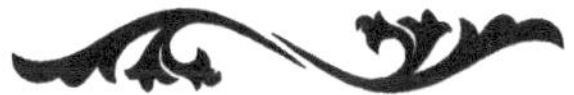

Prologue

अथातो वत्सककल्पं व्याख्यास्यामः||१||

इति ह स्माह भगवानात्रेयः||२||

Now we shall explore the chapter dealing with the "pharmaceutics of Vatsaka. Thus said Lord Atreya" [1-2]

Varieties and symptoms of Vatsaka

अथ वत्सकनामानि भेदं स्त्रीपुंसयोस्तथा| कल्पं चास्य प्रवक्ष्यामि विस्तरेण यथातथम्||३||

वत्सकः कुटजः शक्रो वृक्षको गिरिमल्लिका| बीजानीन्द्रयवास्तस्य तथोच्यन्ते कलिङ्गकाः||४||

बृहत्फलः श्वेतपुष्पः स्निग्धपत्रः पुमान् भवेत्| श्यामा चारुणपुष्पा स्त्री फलवृन्तैस्तथाऽणुभिः ||५||

I shall hereafter describe appropriately the symptoms of Vatsaka, along with the distinctive features of its female and male varieties and its recipes in detail.

Synonyms of Vatsaka are: Kutaja, sarkra, vrksaka and Giri- mallika. Its seeds are called Indrayava and Kalingaka.

The male varieties of Vatsaka have big fruits, white flowers and smooth (unctuous) leaves.

The female variety has bluish black and pink flowers. It has tiny fruits as well as tiny stalks. [3-5]

Therapeutic Effects of Vatsaka

रक्तपित्तकफघ्नस्तु सुकुमारेष्वनत्ययः| हृद्रोगज्वरवातासृग्वीसर्पादिषु शस्यते||६||

Vatsaka cures Raktapitta (an ailment characterized by bleeding from various parts of the body) and Kapha. It is useful for patients suffering from heart diseases, fever, gout and erysipelas. It is free from any adverse effects even if administered to persons of tender (delicate) nature. [6]

Recipes of Vatsaka in the form of decoction

काले फलानि सङ्गृह्या तयोः शुष्काणि निक्षिपेत् | तेषामन्तर्नखं मुष्टिं जर्जरीकृत्य भावयेत् ||७||

मधुकस्य कषायेण कोविदारादिभिस्तथा| निशि स्थितं विमृद्यैतल्लवणक्षौद्रसंयुतम्||८||

पिबेतद्वमनं श्रेष्ठं पित्तश्लेष्मनिबर्हणम्||९|

Fruits of both the varieties of Vatsaka are collected in appropriate time (season), dried and coarsely powdered. A closed fist (quantity as would fit inside a closed fist) of this powder is impregnated by adding the decoction of madhuka, Kovidara, (karbudara, Nipa, Vidula, Bimbi, Sanapuspi or Pratyakpuspi). After keeping soaked for the night, the powder and decoction are stirred [and filtered] after adding salt and honey. This liquid (decoction) is taken as a portion. These are the excellent emetic recipes for the elimination of pitta and kapha. [7- ½ 9]

Recipes of Vatsaka in powder form

अष्टाहं पयसाऽऽर्केण तेषां चूर्णानि भावयेत्||९||

जीवकस्य कषायेण ततः पाणितलं पिबेत्| फलजीमूतकेक्ष्वाकुजीवन्तीनां पृथक् तथा||१०||

सर्षपाणां मधूकानां लवणस्याथवाऽम्बुना|११|

The powder [of the fruits of Vatsaka] should be impregnated in the milky latex of Arka for eight days. One Pani-tala (quantity that fits in the concavity of the hand) of this is taken with the decoction of Jivaka.

Similarly, this powder can be taken separately with the decoctions of Madanaphala, Jimutaka, Iksvaku or Jivanti in 1 karsha quantity. Alternatively 1 karsha of this powder shall be taken mixed with decoction of mustard, juice of flowers of madhuka or with salt water. [9 ½ - 11½]

Recipe of Vatsaka to be taken with Krsara

कृशरेणाथवा युक्तं विदध्याद्वमनं भिषक्||११||

per the above description in the verse no. 7-8] may also be added to Krshara (a preparation of rice and pulses) and administered by the physician [to the patient] for emesis. [11 ½]

Contents of the chapter

तत्र श्लोकः:-

कषायैर्नव चूर्णैश्च पञ्चोक्ताः सलिलैस्त्रयः| एकश्च कृशरायां स्याद्योगास्तेऽष्टादश स्मृताः ||१२||

To sum up:

Eighteen recipes of vatsaka are described in this chapter as follows:

Nine recipes in the form of decoctions (vide verse nos. 7-9)

Five recipes in powder form (vide verse no. 9-10)

Three recipes should be taken along with water; and (vide verse no .11)

One recipe to be taken with Krsara (Vide verse no. 11) [12]

Colophon

इत्यग्निवेशकृते तन्त्रे चरकप्रतिसंस्कृतेऽप्राप्ते दृढबलसम्पूरिते कल्पस्थाने वत्सककल्पो नाम पञ्चमोऽध्यायः||५||

Thus, ends the fifth chapter of Kalpa-sthana dealing with the "Pharmaceutics of Vatsaka" in Agnivesha's work as redacted by Charaka, and because of its non-availability, supplemented by Drdhabala.

19

Kalpasthana Chapter 6 Kruta Vedhana Kalpam

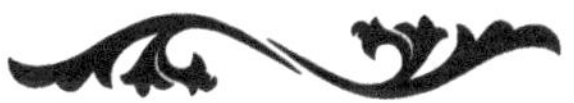

Prologue

अथातः कृतवेधनकल्पं व्याख्यास्यामः॥१॥

इति ह स्माह भगवानात्रेयः॥२॥

Now we shall explore the chapter dealing with the "Pharmaceutics of Krtavedhana". Thus said Lord Atreya [1-2]

Synonyms of Krtavedhana

कृतवेधननामानि कल्पं चास्य निबोधत| क्ष्वेडः कोशातकी चोक्तं मृदङ्गफलमेव च॥३॥

Now listen to the synonyms of Krtavedhana, and its recipes. Its synonyms are Ksveda, Koshataki and Mrdanga Phala. [3]

Attributes and Therapeutic effects of Krta-Vedhana

अत्यर्थकटुतीक्ष्णोष्णं गाढेष्विष्टं गदेषु च| कुष्ठपाण्ड्वामयप्लीहशोफगुल्मगरादिषु॥४॥

It is exceedingly pungent, sharp and hot. It is useful in deep seated diseases, viz, obstinate skin diseases including leprosy, anaemia, splenic disorders, oedema, phantom tumours, toxicosis etc. [4]

Recipes of Krtavedhana prepared with Milk and Alcohol

क्षीरादि कुसुमादीनां सुरा चैतेषु पूर्ववत्॥५|

Preparations of the flower, etc of krtavedhana along with milk and alcohol is made on the lines suggested before and used for emesis. [½ 5]

Recipes of Krtavedhana to be taken along with Decoctions

सुशुष्काणां तु जीर्णानामेकं द्वे वा यथाबलम्॥५॥

कषायैर्मधुकादीनां नवभिः फलवत् पिबेत्|

Depending upon his strength, the patient should take one or two of the ripe fruits of Krtavedhana along with the decoctions of any one of the nine drugs, viz, Madhuka, (Kovidara, Karbudara, Nipa, Vidula, Bimbi, Sanapuspi, Sadapuspi, or Pratyakpuspi). This potion is to be used according to the procedure prescribed for Madanaphala (vide Kalpa 1: 14). [5½ - 6½]

Recipes of Krtavedhana in the form of Linctus

क्वाथयित्वा फलं तस्य पूत्वा लेहं निधापयेत्॥६॥

कृतवेधनकल्कांशं फलाद्यर्धांशसंयुतम् [३] |

The decoction of the fruit of Krtavedhana is prepared and filtered. To this liquid, one part of the paste of Krtavedhana and half part of the paste of Madanaphala etc. is added. This is cooked, made into linctus and used for emesis. [6 ½ -

Recipes of Krtavedhana in the form of Decoction

पृथक् चारग्वधादीनां त्रयोदशभिरासुतम्||७||

The powder of Krtavedhana is macerated with the decoctions of any one of the thirteen drugs, viz, Aragvadha, Vrksaka, Svadukantaka, Patala, Sarngesta, Murva, Saptaparna, Naktamala, Piccumarda, Patola, Susavi and Guduci. These recipes may be used for emesis.] [7 ½]

Recipes of Krtavedhana in slimy form

शाल्मलीमूलचूर्णानां पिच्छाभिर्दशभिस्तथा|८|

Krtavedhana is added with the powders of the roots of one of the drugs viz, Salmali, salalaka, Bhadaraparni, Elaparni, Upodika, uddala, dhanvana, Rajadana, Upacitra and Gopi. Powder of these ten recipes becomes slimy when mixed with water. These ten slimy recipes are used for emesis. [8½]

Recipes of Krtavedhana in the form of Pills:

वर्तिक्रियाः षट् फलवत्, फलादीनां घृतं तथा||८||

On the lines suggested for Madanaphala, six types of vartis (elongated pills) are prepared. In the same manner, medicated ghee should also be prepared. Administration of these pills and the medicated ghee causes emesis. [8 ½]

Recipes of Krtavedhana in the form of Linctus

कोशातकानि पञ्चाशत् कोविदाररसे पचेत्| तं कषायं फलादीनां कल्कैर्लेहं पुनः पचेत्||९||

क्ष्वेडस्य तत्र भागः स्याच्छेषाण्यर्धाशिकानि तु| कषायैः कोविदाराद्यैरेवं तत् कल्पयेत् पृथक्||१०||

Fifty fruits of Krtavedhana are cooked by adding the juice (or decoction) of Kovidara. This is then added with the paste of Madanaphala, (Jimutaka, Iksvaku, Dhamargava, Kutaja or Krtavedhana), cooked again and made into linctus. To the decoction, one part of the paste of Ksveda or Krtavedhana (which is one fourth of the decoction) and half of the paste of each of madana phala, (jimutaka, Iksvaka, Dhamargava and Kutaja) is added before cooking. Similarly, these recipes of linctus are to be prepared separately with the decoctions of –
Kovidara, Karbudara, Nipa, Vidula, Bimbi, Sanapuspi, Sadapuspi, Pratyakpuspi [9-10]

Recipes of Krtavedhana in the form of meat-soup:

कषायेषु फलादीनामानूपं पिशितं पृथक्| कोशातक्या समं पक्त्वा रसं सलवणं पिबेत्||११||

फलादिपिप्पलीतुल्यं तद्वत् क्ष्वेडरसं पिबेत्|१२|

To the decoctions of Madanaphala, Jimutaka, Iksvaku, Dhamargava, Kutaja, Krtavedhana [the powder of] kosataki or Krtavedhana and equal quantities of the meat of aquatic animals are added and cooked. This meat-soup is administered with salt. This will act as an emetic. Similarly, with the decoction of koshataki or Krtavedhana meat of aquatic animals and equal quantity of 9 [the powder of] Madanaphala, Jimutaka, Dhamargava, Kutaja and Krtavedhana [all taken together] is cooked. This meat-soup may also be administered for emesis. [11 ½ - 12]

Recipe of Krtavedhana Prepared by boiling with sugarcane Juice

क्ष्वेडं कासी पिबेत् सिद्धं मिश्रमिक्षुरसेन च||१२||

The powder of Krtavedhana is boiled by adding sugarcane juice and administered [for emesis] to the patient suffering from Kasa (coughing). [12 ½]

Contents of the Chapter:

तत्र श्लोकौ-

क्षीरे द्वौ द्वौ सुरा चैका क्वाथा द्वाविंशतिस्तथा| दश पिच्छा घृतं चैकं षट् च वर्तिक्रियाः शुभाः||१३||

लेहेऽष्टौ सप्त मांसे च योग इक्षुरसेऽपरः| कृतवेधनकल्पेऽस्मिन् षष्टिर्योगाः प्रकीर्तिताः||१४||

To sum up: -

In this chapter describing the Pharmaceutics of Krtavedhana, sixty recipes of this drug are described, as follows:

Four preparations with milk (vide verse no. 5)

One preparation with alcohol; (vide verse no. 5)

Twenty-two preparations in the form of decoction: (vide verse nos. 5-7)

Ten preparations in the form Piccha (slimy form); (vide verse no. 8)

One preparation in the form of medicated ghee, (vide verse no. 8)

Six preparations in the form of Varti (pills); (Vide verse nos. 8)

Eight preparations in the form of linctus; (vide verse nos. 9-10)

Seven preparations of meat-soup and (vide verse nos. 11-12)

One preparation with the juice of sugar-cane (vide verse no. 12) [13-14]

Colophon

इत्यग्निवेशकृते तन्त्रे चरकप्रतिसंस्कृतेऽप्राप्ते दृढबलसम्पूरिते कल्पस्थाने कृतवेधनकल्पो नाम षष्ठोऽध्यायः||६||

Thus ends the sixth chapter dealing with the "Pharmaceutics of Krtavedhana" in the Kalpa section of Agnivesha's work as redacted by Charaka, and because of its non- availability, supplemented by Drdhabala.

20

Kalpasthana Chapter 7 Shyama Trivrt Kalpam

Prologue

अथातः श्यामात्रिवृत्कल्पं व्याख्यास्यामः||१||

इति ह स्माह भगवानात्रेयः||२||

Now we shall explore the chapter dealing with the "Pharmaceutics of Shyama- Trivrt". Thus, said Lord Atreya. [1-2]

Importance of Trivrt as purgative

विरेचने त्रिवृन्मूलं श्रेष्ठमाहुर्मनीषिणः |

तस्याः सञ्ज्ञा गुणाः कर्म भेदः कल्पश्च वक्ष्यते||३||

According to wise physicians, the root of Trivrt is the best among the purgatives. Its synonyms, attributes, actions, varieties and recipes will be described [hereafter]. [3]

Synonyms

त्रिभण्डी त्रिवृता चैव श्यामा कूटरणा तथा|

सर्वानुभूतिः सुवहा शब्दैः पर्यायवाचकैः||४||

The synonyms of Trivrt are Tribhandi, Trivrta, Shyama, Kutarana, sarvanubhuti and Suvaha. [4]

Attributes

कषाया मधुरा रूक्षा विपाके कटुका च सा| कफपित्तप्रशमनी रौक्ष्याच्चानिलकोपनी||५||

सेदानीमौषधैर्युक्ता वातपित्तकफापहैः| कल्पवैशेष्यमासाद्य सर्वरोगहरा भवेत्||६||

Trivrt is astringent and sweet in taste, dry (non-unctuous) and pungent in Vipaka. It alleviates Kapha and Pitta. Because of its non-unctuousness it aggravates Vayu. However, when drugs for the alleviation of Vayu, Pitta and Kapha are added to it in a recipe, it becomes capable of curing all types of diseases (caused by Vayu, Pitta and Kapha). [5-6]

Varieties

मूलं तु द्विविधं तस्याः श्यामं चारुणमेव च| तयोर्मुख्यतरं विद्धि मूलं यदरुणप्रभम्||७||

Trivrt is of 2 types depending on the two types of its roots –

Shyama Trivrt - one having black coloured roots and

Aruna Trivrt - the other one having pink coloured roots

Trivrt having pink coloured root is more useful. [7]

Utility of Pink variety

सुकुमारे शिशौ वृद्धे मृदुकोष्ठे च तच्छुभम्|

It is useful as a purgative for persons having tender / sensitive personality, for children, for old people and for persons having soft bowel movement (mrdu-Kostha) [½ 8]

Utility of Black variety

मोह्येदाशुकारित्वाच्छ्यामा क्षिण्वीत मूर्च्छयेत् ||८||

तैक्ष्ण्यात् कर्षति हृत्कण्ठमाशु दोषं हरत्यपि| शस्यते बहुदोषाणां क्रूरकोष्ठाश्च ये नराः||९||

The black variety of Trivrt, causes unconsciousness, loss of tissue elements and fainting because of its instantaneous action. Because of its sharp action, it causes spasm in the cardiac region and throat. It eliminates the morbid material from the body instantaneously. [Therefore] it is useful for persons having excessively aggravated doshas and hard bowel movement (Krura-Kostha). [8½ - 9]

Method of collection

गुणवत्यां तयोर्भूमौ जातं मूलं समुद्धरेत्| उपोष्य प्रयतः शुक्ले शुक्लवासाः समाहितः||१०||

गम्भीरानुगतं श्लक्ष्णमतिर्यग्विसृतं च यत्| तद्विपाट्योद्धरेद्गर्भं त्वचं शुष्कां निधापयेत्||११||

The root of Trivrt growing in good soil is culled (uprooted) from the earth carefully. This is done in the bright half of the lunar month. It shall be done by a person who has observed fasting, wearing white apparel and has concentration of mind. The roots which have penetrated deep into the earth, which are smooth and which are not spreading side-ways are collected. By splitting these roots, the pith is removed and the bark of the root is collected. After drying, the root bark is stored appropriately. [10-11]

Preparatory Measures:

स्निग्धस्विन्नो विरेच्यस्तु पेयामात्रोषितः सुखम्|१२|

The person who has undergone oleation and fomentation therapies earlier is given Peya (thin gruel) as food in the previous night so that he purges easily [by the administration of purgative, in the next morning). [½ 12]

Recipes of Trivrt to be taken along with sour liquid etc.

अक्षमात्रं तयोः पिण्डं विनीयाम्लेन ना पिबेत्||१२||

गोऽव्यजामहिषीमूत्रसौवीरकतुषोदकैः| प्रसन्नया त्रिफलया शृतया च पृथक् पिबेत्||१३||

One Aksa (12 gms) of paste of either of the two varieties of Trivrt, made into a form of round bolus is mixed with sour drinks (kanjika). This when taken causes purgation. Similarly, the urine of cow, sheep, goat or buffalo, sauviraka (vinegar), Tusodaka (a sour drink prepared of pulses), Prasanna (a type of winc) or the decoction of Triphala is separately used to take Trivrt paste for purgation. [12- ½ - 13]

Recipes of Trivrt in Powder form

एकैकं सैन्धवादीनां द्वादशानां सनागरम्| त्रिवृद्द्विगुणसंयुक्तं चूर्णमुष्णाम्बुना पिबेत्||१४||

Two parts of the powder of the root of Trivrt is mixed with the powder of one part of either of the twelve drugs (types of salt) viz,

Saindhava, Sauvarcala, Kala, Vida , Pakya, Anupa, Kupya, Valukaja, Maulaka, Saka or Audbhida

these recipes are taken along with the powder of Nagara [for purgation] [14]

पिप्पली पिप्पलीमूलं मरिचं गजपिप्पली| सरलः किलिमं हिङ्गु भार्गी तेजोवती तथा||१५||

मुस्तं हैमवती पथ्या चित्रको रजनी वचा| स्वर्णक्षीर्यजमोदा च शृङ्गवेरं च तैः पृथक्||१६||

एकैकार्धांशसंयुक्तं पिबेद्गोमूत्रसंयुतम्|१७|

One part of the powder of the Trivrt root is added with half part of the powder of either of the below mentioned drugs – Pippali, Pippalimula , Maricha, Gajapippali, Sarala , Kilima, Hingu, Bhargi, Tejovati, Musta, Haimavati , Pathya , Chitraka, Rajani (haridra), Vacha, Svarna– Ksiri , Ajamoda, Srngavera

each of these should be taken along with cow's urine for purgation [15- ½ 17]

Recipe of Trivrt added with Madhuka
मधुकार्धांशसंयुक्तं शर्कराम्बुयुतं पिबेत्||१७||

One part of the powder of Trivrt is added with half part of the powder of madhuka. This potion is taken with sugar-water for purgation. [17 ½]

Recipes of Trvrit prepared along with Jivaka etc.
जीवकर्षभकौ मेदां श्रावणीं कर्काटाह्वयाम्|
मुद्गमाषाख्यपर्ण्यौ च महतीं श्रावणीं तथा||१८|| काकोलीं क्षीरकाकोलीमिन्द्रां छिन्नरुहां तथा|

The powder of Trivrt is taken along with the powder of either of the below mentioned drugs –
Jivaka, Rsabhaka, Meda, Sravani or mundi, Karakatasrngi, Mudgaparni, Masaparni, Mahasrvani, Kakoli, Ksirakakoli, Indra or kokilaksa, Chinnaruha, Ksirasukla or ksiravidari or Payasya or arkapuspi [for purgation]
Similarly, the powder of Trvrit is taken along with the powder of yastyahva (Madhuka) [for purgation].
The above mentioned recipes are useful for diseases caused by Vayu or Pitta. Other recipes which are useful for the diseases caused by Kapha and Vayu [will be described later]. [18- ½ 20]

Recipes of Trivrt to be taken along with Milk etc.,
क्षीरशुक्लां पयस्यां च यष्ट्याह्वं विधिना पिबेत्||१९|| वातपित्तहितान्येतान्यन्यानि तु कफानिले|२०|
क्षीरमांसेक्षुकाश्मर्यद्राक्षापीलुरसैः पृथक्||२०|| सर्पिषा वा तयोश्चूर्णमभयार्धांशिकं पिबेत्|२१|

One part of the Trivrt powder and half part of the powder of Haritaki may be taken along with either
Milk, Meat-soup, Juice of sugar-cane , Decoction of Kasmarya, Grape-juice, Juice of Pilu, Ghee [for purgation] [20 ½ - ½ 20]

Recipe of trivrt in the form of Linctus (No.s 1)
लिह्याद्वा मधुसर्पिभर्यां संयुक्तं ससितोपलम्||२१||

[The powder of Trivrt is] added with honey and ghee, [and made into linctus]. Intake of this linctus along with sugar with large crystals [causes purgation]. [21 1/2]

Recipe of trivrt in the form of Linctus (No.2)
अजगन्धा तुगाक्षीरी विदारी शर्करा त्रिवृत्| चूर्णितं क्षौद्रसर्पिभर्यां लीढ्वा साधु विरिच्यते||२२||
सन्निपातज्वरस्तम्भदाहतृष्णादितो नरः|

The powder of Ajagandha (ajamoda), tugaksiri, Vidari, sugar and Trvrt are added with honey as well as ghee. Intake of this linctus is useful as a mild purgative for the patient suffering from fever caused by the aggravation of all the three Doshas, stiffness of the body, burning syndrome and morbid thirst. [22- 1/2 23]

Recipe of Trvrit in the form of Linctus (No.3)
श्यामात्रिवृत्कषायेण कल्केन च सशर्करम्||२३||
साधयेद्विधिवल्लेहं लिह्यात् पाणितलं ततः|

With the decoction and paste of the black Trivrt root, a linctus is prepared according to the prescribed procedure by adding sugar. One Pani tala (12 gms. approx) of this linctus is taken [for purgation] [23 ½- 24½]

Recipe of Trivrt in the form of Linctus (No.4)
सक्षौद्रां शर्करां पक्त्वा कुर्यान्मृद्भाजने नवे||२४|| क्षिपेच्छीते त्रिवृच्चूर्णं त्वक्पत्रमरिचैः सह|
मात्रया लेहयेदेतदीश्वराणां विरेचनम्||२५||

Sugar is boiled with honey in a new earthen pot. After it is cooked and cooled, the powder of Trivrt along with cinnamon bark, cinnamon leaves and black pepper are added. This linctus is taken in appropriate dosse. This is a useful purgative for persons belonging to aristocratic class (rich people) [24 ½ - 25]

Recipe of Trivrt in the form of Linctus (No. 5)

कुडवांशान् रसानिक्षुद्राक्षापीलुपरुषकात्| सितोपलापलं क्षौद्रात् कुडवार्धं च साधयेत्||२६||
तं लेहं योजयेच्छीतं त्रिवृच्चूर्णेन शास्त्रवित्| एतदुत्सन्नपितानामीश्वराणां विरेचनम्||२७||

One Kudava (192 ml. Approx) of the juice of each sugar-cane, grape, Pilu and Parusaka, one Pala (48 gms. approx) of crystalline sugar and half kudava of honey is cooked. After it is cooled, the physician well versed in scriptures shall add to it the powder of Trvrit. This is a good purgative for aristocratic persons having excessively aggravated Pitta. [26-27]

Recipes Prepared with sugar

शर्करामोदकान् वर्तीर्गुलिकामांसपूपकान्|
अनेन विधिना कुर्यात् पैत्तिकानां विरेचनम्||२८||

Following the above-mentioned procedure, recipes of Trvrit are prepared in the form of Sarkara-Modaka (sweet-meat prepared of Sugar), Sarkara-Varti (rolls made of sugar), Sarkara Gulika (pills made of Sugar) and sarkara Mamsa Pupaka (pan-cake of sugar prepared with meat). These recipes are not to be used as purgatives by people suffering from diseases caused by Pitta. [28]

Recipe of Trivrt in the form of Linctus (No. 6)

पिप्पलीं नागरं क्षारं श्यामां त्रिवृतया सह|
लेहयेन्मधुना सार्धं श्लेष्मलानां विरेचनम्||२९||

[The powder of] Trivrt (the variety having pink root) is added with the powders of Pippali, Nagara, Ksara (alkali preparation) and Shyama Trivrt (the variety having black root). To this honey is added. It is given in the form of linctus for purgation to patients suffering from diseases caused by Kapha. [29]

Recipes of Trivrt in the form of Linctus (No.7)

मातुलुङ्गाभयाधात्रीश्रीपर्णीकोलदाडिमात्| सुभृष्टान् स्वरसांस्तैले साधयेतत्र चावपेत्||३०||
सहकारात् कपित्थाच्च मध्यमम्लं च यत् फलम्| पूर्ववद्बहलीभूते त्रिवृच्चूर्णं समावपेत्||३१||
त्वक्पत्रकेशरैलानां चूर्णं मधु च मात्रया| लेहोऽयं कफपूर्णानामीश्वराणां विरेचनम्||३२||

The juices of Matulunga, Abhaya, Dhatri, Sriparni, Kola and Dadima are well sizzled and cooked in oil by adding the pulp of Sahakara (mango), Kapittha and sour fruit (matulunga). When it becomes thick, the powder of the Trivrt root along with the powders of Tvak, Patra, Kesara and ela are added. To this, honey is added and made into linctus. Intake of this linctus in appropriate dose is useful as purgative for aristocratic persons having aggravated Kapha. [30-32]

Recipes of Trivrt in the form of Panaka (Syrup) etc.

पानकानि रसान् यूषान्मोदकान् रागषाडवान्|
अनेन विधिना कुर्यादिवरेकार्थं कफाधिके||३३||

Following the above-mentioned procedure, the recipes [of Trivrt] are prepared in the forms of
Panaka (syrup), Rasa (Meat-soup), Yusha (vegetable soup), Modaka (sweet-meat), Raga-sadava (sour drinks having a pungent taste).
These recipes are to be administered for purgation to a person having aggravated Kapha. [33]

Recipes of Trivrt in the Tarpana (Demulcent Drink)

भृङ्गैलाभ्यां समा नीली तैस्त्रिवृतैश्च शर्करा| चूर्णं फलरसक्षौद्रशक्तुभिस्तर्पणं पिबेत्||३४||
वातपित्तकफोत्थेषु रोगेष्वल्पानलेषु च| नरेषु सुकुमारेषु निरपायं विरेचनम्||३५||

A Tarpana (demulcent drink) is prepared from the powder of one part of bhrnga (Guda-Tvak), one part of ela, two parts of Nili, three parts of Trivrt and seven parts of sugar by adding the juice of Dadima, honey and roasted corn-flour. This is an innocuous purgative for patients suffering from diseases caused by Vayu, Pitta and Kapha, for persons who have less digestive power, and also for persons who have delicate constitution. [34-35]

Recipes of Trivrt in the form of Modaka

शर्करात्रिफलाश्यामात्रिवृत्पिप्पलिमाक्षिकैः| मोदकः सन्निपातोर्ध्वरक्तपित्तज्वरापहः||३६||

A modaka (sweet-meat of large size) is prepared with sugar, Haritaki, Bibhitaka, Amalaki, black variety of Trivrt, Pippali, and honey. Intake of this [purgative recipe] cures Sannipata (diseases caused by the simultaneous aggravation of all the three Doshas), Urdhvaga raktapitta (a disease characterized by bleeding from the upper openings of the body) and fever. [36]

Recipe of Trivrt in the form of Linctus (NO.8)

त्रिवृच्छाणा मतास्तिस्रस्तिस्रश्च त्रिफलात्वचः| विडङ्गपिप्पलीक्षारशाणास्तिस्रश्च चूर्णिताः||३७||

लिह्यात् सर्पिर्मधुभ्यां च मोदकं वा गुडेन तु| भक्षयेन्निष्परीहारमेतच्छोधनमुत्तमम्||३८||

गुल्मं प्लीहोदरं श्वासं हलीमकमरोचकम्| कफवातकृतांश्चान्यान् व्याधीनेतह्यपोहति||३९||

Three Sanas of the powder of Trivrt is added with one Sana of the powder each of Haritaki pulp, Bibhitaka pulp, Amalaki pulp, Vidanga, Pippali and Ksara (alkali preparation). This powder is added with ghee and honey, and made to a linctus or (made to) a Modaka (sweet-meat) with Jaggery. This is an excellent purgative and it does not require any dietetic prohibitions. Intake of this cures phantom tumour, splenomegaly, asthma, chronic jaundice, anorexia and such other diseases caused by the aggravation of Kapha and Vayu. [37-39]

Kalyanaka Guda- recipe of Trivrt in the form of Modaka (No. 2)

विडङ्गपिप्पलीमूलत्रिफलाधान्यचित्रकान्| मरिचेन्द्रयवाजाजीपिप्पलीहस्तिपिप्पली||४०||

लवणान्यजमोदां च चूर्णितं कार्षिकं पृथक्| तिलतैलत्रिवृच्चूर्णभागौ चाष्टपलोन्मितौ||४१||

धात्रीफलरसप्रस्थांस्त्रीन् गुडार्धतुलां तथा| पक्त्वा मृद्वग्निना खादेद्बदरोदुम्बरोपमान्||४२||

गुडान् कृत्वा न चात्र स्यादिविहाराहारयन्त्रणा| मन्दाग्नित्वं ज्वरं मूर्च्छां मूत्रकृच्छ्रमरोचकम्||४३||

अस्वप्नं गात्रशूलं च कासं श्वासं भ्रमं क्षयम्| कुष्ठार्शःकामलामेहगुल्मोदरभगन्दरान्||४४||

ग्रहणीपाण्डुरोगांश्च हन्युः पुंसवनाश्च ते| कल्याणका इति ख्याताः सर्वर्त्वृतुषु यौगिकाः||४५||

इति कल्याणकगुडः|४६|

One Karsa (12 gm. approx) each of Vidanga, Pippalimula, Haritaki, Vibhitaka, Amalaki, Dhanyaka, Chitraka, Maricham, Indrayava, Ajaji, Pippali, Hasti-Pippali (Gaja- Pipplai), Saindhava Lavana, and Ajamoda is made into powders separately and mixed together. To this, powder eight Palas each of Sesame oil and powder of Trivrt are added. The recipe is cooked over mild fire by adding three Prasthas of the juice of amalaki and half tula of jaggery. From out of this paste, pills (Guda) of the size of Badara or Udumbara are made out. While taking this recipe there is no restriction of food and regimen. During the intake of this recipe there is no restriction of food and regimen. Intake of this (purgative) cures mandagni (suppression of the power of digestion), Jvara (fever) ,Murccha (fainting), Mutra-Krcchra (dysuria), Arocaka (anorexia), Asvapna (insomnia), Gatra-Sula (body ache), Kasa (cough), svasa (asthma), Bhrama (giddiness), Ksaya (consumption), Kustha (obstinate skin diseases including leprosy), Arsas (piles), Kamala (Jaundice), Meha (obstinate urinary disorders including diabetes), Gulma (Phantom tumour), Udara (obstinate abdominal disorders including ascites), Bhagandra (anal fistula), grahani (sprue syndrome) and Pandu (anemia). This recipe also helps in procreating a male progency (pumsavana). This recipe is called Kalyanaka (which bestows auspiciousness). It is useful in all the seasons.

Thus ends the description of Kalyanaka-Guda. [40]

Recipe of Trivrt in the form of Modaka (no. 3)

व्योषत्वक्पत्रमुस्तैलाविडङ्गामलकाभयाः समभागा भिषग्दद्यादिद्विगुणं च मुकूलकम्||४६||

त्रिवृतोऽष्टगुणं भागं शर्करायाश्च षड्गुणम्| चूर्णितं गुडिकाः कृत्वा क्षौद्रेण पलसम्मिताः||४७||

भक्षयेत् कल्यमुत्थाय शीतं चानु पिबेज्जलम्| मूत्रकृच्छ्रे ज्वरे वम्यां कासे श्वासे भ्रमे क्षये||४८||तापे पाण्डुवामयेऽल्पेऽग्नौ शस्ता निर्यन्त्रणाशिनः| योगः सर्वविषाणां च मतः श्रेष्ठो विरेचने||४९||

मूत्रजानां च रोगाणां विधिज्ञेनावचारितः।५०।

One part each of Sunthi, Pippali, Maricha, Tvak, Patra, Musta, Ela, Vidanga, Amalaki and Haritaki, two parts of Mukulaka (danti), eight parts of Trivrt and six parts of sugar is made to powder. To this, honey is added and large size pill(s) or Gudika measuring one Pala each is prepared. One such pill is taken in the morning after waking up from the bed. Thereafter cold water is taken. It is an excellent recipe for purgation. When it is administered by an expert (physician) it is useful in treating Mutrakrcchra (Dysuria), Jvara (fever) , vami (vomiting), kasa (cough), Svasa (asthma), Bhrama (giddiness), Ksaya (consumption), tapa (burning syndrome), Pandu (anemia) and useful for all types of poisoning and all types of urinary diseases. While this recipe is taken, no dietetic restriction is necessary. [46- 50½]

Recipe of Trivrt in the form Modaka (No. 4)

पथ्याधात्र्युरूबूकाणां प्रसृतौ द्वौ त्रिवृत्पलम्।।५०।। दश तान्मोदकान् कुर्यादीश्वराणां विरेचनम्।५१।

One Pala (48 gms. approx) of the powders of Trivrt is added with two Prasrtas of the powder of Pathya, Dhatri and Urubuka (castor seed). [This is added with honey in adequate quantity]. From out of this paste, ten large sized pills are prepared. Intake of this pill helps in the purgation of aristocratic persons. [50 ½- 51½]

Recipe of trivrt in the form Modaka (No. 5)

त्रिवृद्धैमवती श्यामा नीलिनी हस्तिपिप्पली।।५१।। समूला पिप्पली मुस्तमजमोदा दुरालभा।
कार्षिकं नागरपलं गुडस्य पलविंशतिम्।।५२।। चूर्णितं मोदकान् कुर्यादुदुम्बरफलोपमान्।
हिङ्गुसौवर्चलव्योषयवानीबिडजीरकैः।।५३।। वचाजगन्धात्रिफलाचव्यचित्रकधान्यकैः।
मोदकान् वेष्टयेच्चूर्णैस्तान् सतुम्बुरुदाडिमैः।।५४।। त्रिकवङ्क्षणहृद्बस्तिकोष्ठार्शःप्लीहशूलिनाम्।
हिक्काकासारुचिश्वासकफोदावर्तिनां शुभाः ।।५५।।

One Karsa of the powder each of Trivrt (the variety having pink root), Haimavati, Shyama, (the variety of Trivrt having black root), Nilini, hastipippali, Pippalimula, Pippali, Musta, Ajamoda and duralabha, one Pala of the powder of Nagara and twenty Palas of Guda (jaggery) are mixed together. From this paste Modakas (large size pills) of the size of Hingu, sauvarcala, Sunthi, Pippali, Maricha, Yavani, Bida, Jiraka, Vacha, Ajagandha, Haritaki, Vibhitaka, Amalaki, Cavya, Chitraka, Dhanyaka, Tumburu and Dadima. These Modakas are very useful for patients suffering from pain in Trika (Lumbo-Sacral region), Vanksana (Pelvic region), Hrt (cardiac region), Basti (region of urinary bladder) and Kostha (colon), Arsas (piles), Pliha (Splenic disorder), Hikka (hiccup), Kasa (cough), Aruchi (Anorexia), Svasa (Asthma) and Kaphaja Udavarta (upward movement of wind in the abdomen caused by aggravated Kapha). [51½ - 55]

Recipe of Trivrt Useful in Rainy season

त्रिवृतां कौटजं बीजं पिप्पलीं विश्वभेषजम्। क्षौद्रद्राक्षारसोपेतं वर्षास्वेतद्विरेचनम्।।५६।।

[The powder of] Trivrt, seeds of Kutaja, Pippali and Visvabhesaja (Sunthi) is mixed with honey and grape-juice. This purgative recipe is useful in the rainy season. [56]

Recipe of Trivrt Useful in autumn

त्रिवृद्दुरालभामुस्तशर्करोदीच्यचन्दनम्। द्राक्षाम्बुना सयष्ट्याह्वसातलं जलदात्यये।।५७।।

The powder of trivrt, Duralabha, Musta, sugar, Udicya, Chandana, Draksha, Yastimadhu and Satala (carma- Kasa) is taken along with grape juice. It is useful in autumn. [57]

Recipe for Trivrt for Winter:

त्रिवृतां चित्रकं पाठामजाजीं सरलं वचाम्। स्वर्णक्षीरीं च हेमन्ते पिष्ट्वा तूष्णाम्बुना पिबेत्।।५८।।

The paste of Trivrt, Chitraka, Patha, Ajaji, Sarala, Vacha and SvaranaKsiri is taken along with hot water. This recipe is useful for purgation in the winter season. [58]

Recipe of trivrt for summer Season:

शर्करा त्रिवृता तुल्या ग्रीष्मकाले विरेचनम्|

The recipe containing sugar and equal quantity of trivrt is useful for purgation during the summer season. [½ 59]

Recipe for Trivrt for all Seasons (No. 1)

त्रिवृत्त्रायन्तिहपुषाः सातलां कटुरोहिणीम् ||५९||

स्वर्णक्षीरीं च सञ्चूर्ण्य गोमूत्रे भावयेत्र्यहम्| एष सर्वर्तुको योगः स्निग्धानां मलदोषहृत्||६०||

Trivrt, Trayanti, Hapusa, Satala, Katurohini and Svarnakshiri is made to powder, and impregnated with cow's urine for three days. This recipe for purgation is useful in all the seasons. It helps in eliminating morbid matter from the body of persons having excessive unctuousness of the body. [59 ½- 60]

Recipe of Trivrt for All Seasons (No. 2)

त्रिवृच्छ्यामा दुरालम्भा वत्सकं हस्तिपिप्पली| नीलिनी त्रिफला मुस्तं कटुका च सुचूर्णितम्||६१||

सर्पिर्मांसरसोष्णाम्बुयुक्तं पाणितलं ततः| पिबेत् सुखतमं ह्येतद्रूक्षाणामपि शस्यते||६२||

Trivrt (having pink root), Shyama (the variety of Trivrt having black root), Duralabha, Vatsaka, Hasti-Pippali, Nilini, Haritaki, Vibhitaka, Amalaki, Musta, and Katuka, are made into fine powder. One Panitala (12 gms, approx) of this recipe is taken along with ghee, meat-soup and hot water. This is an excellent recipe for purgation, and is useful even for persons having excessive dryness of the body. [61-62]

Recipes of Trivrt in the Form of Powder

त्र्यूषणं त्रिफला हिङ्गु कार्षिकं त्रिवृतापलम्| सौवर्चलार्धकर्षं च पलार्धं चाम्लवेतसात्||६३||

तच्चूर्णं शर्करातुल्यं मद्येनाम्लेन वा पिबेत्| गुल्मपार्श्वार्तिनुत्सिद्धं जीर्णे चाद्याद्रसौदनम्||६४||

One Karsa (12 gms. appr) each of sunthi, Pippali, Maricha, Haritaki, Bibhitaka, Amalaki and Hingu, one Pala (48 gms. appr) of Trivrt, half Karsa (6 gms, appr) of Sauvarcala and half Pala (24 Gms Approx) of Amlavetasa are made into powder. It should be taken along with either alcohol or the juice of sour fruits. After the recipe is digested, the patient is given rice with meat-soup to eat. It is an effective recipe for purgation to cure phantom tumour and pain in the sides of the chest. [63- 64]

Recipe of Trivrt in the Form of Tarpana (Demulcent Drink)

त्रिवृतां त्रिफलां दन्तीं सप्तलां व्योषसैन्धवम्| कृत्वा चूर्णं तु सप्ताहं भाव्यमामलकीरसे||६५||

तद्योज्यं तर्पणे यूषे पिशिते रागयुक्तिषु|६६|

Trivrt, haritaki, bibhitaki, Amalaki, Danti, saptala, Sunthi, Pippali, Maricha and Saindhava are made into powder and impregnated with the juice of amalaki – Indian gooseberry - for seven days. This powder is added to Tarpana (demulcent drink), Yusha (vegetable soup), Pisita (meat preparations or meat- soup) and Raga (preparations having pungent taste). [65- ½ 66]

Recipes of Trivrt in the form of medicated Ghee and milk:

तुल्याम्लं त्रिवृताकल्कसिद्धं गुल्महरं घृतम्||६६||श्यामात्रिवृतयोर्मूलं पचेदामलकैः सह|

जले तेन कषायेण पक्त्वा सर्पिः पिबेन्नरः||६७|| श्यामात्रिवृत्कषायेण सिद्धं सर्पिः पिबेत्तथा|

साधितं वा पयस्ताभ्यां सुखं तेन विरिच्यते||६८||

Ghee is boiled with equal quantities of sour juice and the paste of Trivrt. This medicated ghee cures phantom tumour. The root of Shyama (the variety of Trivrt having black root) and Trivrt (the variety having pink root) is cooked with water by adding Amalaki. With this decoction, ghee is cooked [and used for purgation].

Milk is boiled with Shyama (the variety of Trivrt having black root) and Trivrt (the variety having pink root) may similarly be used as a comfortable (painless) purgative. [66 ½ - 68]

Recipe of Trivrt in the form of Alcohol Drink:

त्रिवृन्मुष्टींस्तु सनखानष्टौ द्रोणेऽम्भसः पचेत् [१] |पादशेषं कषायं तं पूतं गुडतुलायुतम्||६९||

स्निग्धे स्थाप्यं घटे क्षौद्रपिप्पलीफलचित्रकैः|प्रलिप्ते मधुना मासं जातं तन्मात्रया पिबेत्||७०||

ग्रहणीपाण्डुरोगघ्नं गुल्मश्वयथुनाशनम्| सुरां वा त्रिवृतायोगकिण्वां तत्क्वाथसंयुताम्||७१||

Eight fistfuls of Trivrt are cooked in one drone of water till one fourth of the liquid remains. The decoction should then be strained out and added with one Tula of Jaggery, honey, pippali, Madanaphala and Chitraka. This is kept in an unctuous jar whose inside wall has been smeared with honey for one month. When well fermented, it is taken in appropriate dose. It cures Grahani (sprue syndrome), Pandu (Anemia), Gulma (Phantom tumour) and Svayathu (Oedema).

The wine made out of the decoction of Trivrt by adding Kinva (yeast) may also be used for purgation. [69-71]

Recipes of Trivrt in the form of kanji (sour Drink)

यवैः श्यामात्रिवृत्क्वाथस्विन्नैः कुल्माषमम्भसा|आसुतं षडहं पल्ले जातं सौवीरकं पिबेत्||७२||

भृष्टान् वा सतुषाञ्छुद्धान् यवांस्तच्चूर्णसंयुतान्|आसुतानम्भसा तद्वत् पिबेज्जातं तुषोदकम्||७३||

Barley is steam boiled with the decoction of Shyama (the variety of Trivrt having black root) and Trivrt (the variety having pink root). This steam boiled barley (Kulmasa) is added with water and made to ferment for six days in a vessel covered with a heap of grains. The Sauviraka (sour drink) thus prepared is used for purgation.

Alternatively, the unhooked and clean grains of barely are roasted. To this, the powder of trivrt is added along with water and made to ferment in the above mentioned manner. When fermented, this Tusodaka (a type of sour drink) is used for purgation. [72-73]

Recipes of Trivrt in the form of Badara etc:

तथा मदनकल्पोक्तान् षाडवादीन् पृथग्दश| त्रिवृच्चूर्णेन संयोज्य विरेकार्थं प्रयोजयेत्||७४||

As described in Kalpa 1:26 with the help of the powder of Trivrt, ten different recipes in the form of Badarasadava, Raga, Leha, Modaka, Utkarika, Tarpana, Panaka , Mamsa-rasa Yusha and Madya are prepared and used for purgation. [74]

Recapitulation

भवतश्चात्र-

त्वक्केशराम्रातकदाडिमैलासितोपलामाक्षिकमातुलुङ्गैः|मद्यैस्तथाऽम्लैश्च मनोनुकूलैर्युक्तानि देयानि विरेचनानि||७५||

शीताम्बुना पीतवतश्च तारय सिञ्चेन्मुखं छर्दिविघातहेतोः|हृदयांश्च मृत्पुष्पफलप्रवालानम्लं च दद्यादुपजिघ्रणार्थम्||७६||

Thus, it is said: -

Purgative recipe is administered along with Tvak (cinnamon), Kesara (Saffron), Amrataka, Dadima (Pomegranate), Ela (cardamom), sitopala (sugar having big crystals), honey, Matulunga, wine and sour drink which are pleasing to the patient.

To prevent the tendency for vomiting after the intake of purgative recipes, the face of the patient is sprinkled with cold water, and he is asked to inhale the smell of the earth, flowers, fruits, tender leaves and sour ingredients, the aroma of which is pleasing to his heart. [75- 76]

Contents of Chapter:

तत्र श्लोकाः-

एकोऽम्लादिभिरष्टौ च दश द्वौ सैन्धवादिभिः| मूत्रेऽष्टादश यष्ट्यां द्वौ जीवकादौ चतुर्दश||७७||

क्षीरादौ सप्त लेहेऽष्टौ चत्वारः सितयाऽपि च| पानकादिषु पञ्चैव षड्रतौ पञ्च मोदकाः||७८||

चत्वारश्च घृते क्षीरे द्वौ चूर्णे तर्पणे तथा| द्वौ मद्ये काञ्जिके द्वौ च दशान्ये षाडवादिषु||७९||

श्यामायास्त्रिवृतायाश्च कल्पेऽस्मिन् समुदाहृतम्|शतं दशोत्तरं सिद्धं योगानां परमर्षिणा||८०||

To sum up: -

In this chapter on the Pharmaceutics of Shyama Trivrt, the great sage has illustrated one hundred and ten recipes of effective purgatives as follows:

Nine recipes prepared with sour juice, etc: (vide verse nos. 12-13)

Twelve recipes prepared with rock-salt etc: (vide verse no. 14)

Eighteen recipes with cow's urine: (vide verse nos. 15-16]

Two recipes prepared by adding Yasti-Madhu: (vide verse nos. 17-19)

Fourteen recipes prepared with Jivaka etc; (vide verse nos 18-20)

Seven recipes prepared with milk etc. (vide verse nos. 20-21)

Eight recipes prepared in the form of linctus (vide verse nos. 21-27, 29- 32, 37-39)

Four recipes prepared with sugar (vide verse no> 28)

Five recipes in the form of syrup etc; (vide verse no. 33)

Six recipes for different seasons; (vide verse nos (56-62)

Five recipes prepared in the form of Modaka; (vide verse nos 36, 40-55)

Four recipes (one) in the form of powder (vide verse nos. 34-35) and the other in the form of Tarpana (vide verse no 69- 71)

Two recipes in the form of Kanji (fermented sour drink) and (vide verse nos. 72-73)

Ten recipes in the form of sadava etc (vide verse no. 74) [77-80]

Colophon

इत्यग्निवेशकृते तन्त्रे चरकप्रतिसंस्कृतेऽप्राप्ते दृढबलसम्पूरिते कल्पस्थाने श्यामात्रिवृत्कल्पो नाम सप्तमोऽध्यायः||७||

Thus, ends the seventh chapter dealing with the "Pharmaceutics of Shyama- Trivrt" in 'Kalpa Sthana' section of Agnivesha's work as redacted by Charaka, and because of its non-availability, supplemented by Drdhabala.

21

Kalpasthana Chapter 8
Chaturangula Kalpam

Prologue

अथातश्चतुरङ्गुलकल्पं व्याख्यास्यामः||१||

इति ह स्माह भगवानात्रेयः||२||

We shall now explore the chapter dealing with the: "Pharmaceutics of Chaturangula ", thus, said Lord Atreya. [1-2]

Synonyms

आरग्वधो राजवृक्षः शम्पाकश्चतुरङ्गुलः|

प्रग्रहः कृतमालश्च कर्णिकारोऽवघातकः||३||

The synonyms of Chaturangula are Aragvadha, Rajavrksa, Sampaka, Chaturangula, Pragraha, Krtamala, Karnikara and Avaghataka.

Therapeutic Utility

ज्वरहृद्रोगवातासृगुदावर्तादिरोगिषु| राजवृक्षोऽधिकं पथ्यो मृदुर्मधुरशीतलः||४||

बाले वृद्धे क्षते क्षीणे सुकुमारे च मानवे| योज्यो मृद्वनपायित्वादिविशेषाच्चतुरङ्गुलः||५||

Because of its mildness, sweet taste and cooling effect, Rajavrksa (Chaturangula) is exceedingly useful (as a purgative) for diseases like fever, cardiac ailments, gout and upward movement of wind in the abdomen. Because of mildness it doesn't produce any complications. Chaturangula is especially suitable as a purgative for children, old people, patients suffering from phthisis and emaciation, and for persons having delicate constitution. [4-5]

Processing of Aragvadha

फलकाले फलं तस्य ग्राह्यं परिणतं च यत्| तेषं गुणवतां भारं सिकतासु निधापयेत्||६||

सप्तरात्रात् समुद्धृत्य शोषयेदातपे भिषक्| ततो मज्जानमुद्धृत्य शुचौ भाण्डे निधापयेत्||७||

During appropriate seasons of fruiting, the matured fruits of Aragvadha (Chaturangula) are collected. These fruits endowed with therapeutic attributes are taken in large quantities and kept covered with sand for seven days. Thereafter, these fruits are taken out of the sand and dried in the sun. The pulp of these fruits is then taken out and stored in a clean jar. [6-7]

Recipes of Aragvadha (Chaturangula) to be taken along with Fruit Juice:

द्राक्षारसयुतं दद्याद्दाहोदावर्तपीडिते| चतुर्वर्षमुखे बाले यावद्द्वादशवार्षिके||८||

चतुरङ्गुलमज्जस्तु प्रसृतं वाऽथवाऽञ्जलिम्|९|

The patient aged between four to twelve years and suffering from daha (burning sensation) as well as udavarta (upward movement of wind in the abdomen) is given one prastha (48 gms. appr) or one anjali (96gms. appr) of the pulp of Aragvadha (Chaturangula) along with grape juice. [8 - ½ 9]

Recipes of Aragvadha (Chaturangula) to be taken along with Sura-Manda etc,

सुरामण्डेन संयुक्तमथवा कोलसीधुनादधिमण्डेन वा युक्तं रसेनामलकस्य वा|

कृत्वा शीतकषायं तं पिबेत् सौवीरकेण वा||१०||

Sita-Kashaya or cold infusion of one Prasrta (48 gms. appr) or one Anjali (96 gms. appr) or pulp of aragvadha may also be given along with the following vehicles:

Sura-Manda (supernatant fluid of Sura type of alcoholic drink)

Kola-Sidhu (a type of wine prepared of Jujube-fruit)

Dadhi-manda (whey)

Juice of Amalaki or

Sauviraka (a type of vinegar) [9 ½ - 10]

Recipes of Aragvadha to be taken with Decoctions

त्रिवृतो वा कषायेण मज्ज्ञः कल्कं तथा पिबेत्|

तथा बिल्वकषायेण लवणक्षौद्रसंयुतम्||११||

Similarly, the pulp of Aragvadha is made into paste and taken along with the decoction of either Trivrt or Bilva by adding salt and honey. [11]

Recipes of Aragvadha prepared in the form of Linctus

कषायेणाथवा तस्य त्रिवृच्चूर्णं गुडान्वितम्| साधयित्वा शनैर्लेहं लेहयेन्मात्रया नरम्||१२||

Linctus is prepared from the decoction of Argavadha added with the powder of Trivrt and Jaggery, by cooking over mild fire. This linctus is taken in appropriate dose [for purgation] [12]

Recipes of Aragvadha Prepared in the form of Medicated Ghee:

चतुरङ्गुलसिद्धाद्वा क्षीराद्यदुदियाद्घृतम्| मज्ज्ञः कल्केन धात्रीणां रसे तत्साधितं पिबेत्||१३||

तदेव दशमूलस्य कुलत्थानां यवस्य च| कषाये साधितं सर्पिः कल्कैः श्यामादिभिः पिबेत्||१४||

Milk is boiled with Aragvadha. From the cream of this medicated milk, ghee is prepared. This ghee is cooked by adding the paste of the pulp of Aragvadha and the juice of Amalaki [this medicated ghee is taken for purgation].

The ghee prepared in the above mentioned manner is cooked by adding the decoction of Dashamula (bilva, Syonaka, Gambhari, Patala, Ganikarika, Salaparni, Prsniparni, Brhti, Kantakari and Gokshura), Kulattha and Yava as well as the paste of nine drugs (viz Syama, Trivrt, Chaturangula , Tilvaka , Mahavrksa, Patala, Sankhini, Danti and Dravanti). [13-14]

Recipe of Aragvadha in the form of Aristha

दन्तीक्वाथेऽञ्जलिं मज्ज्ञः शम्पाकस्य गुडस्य च| दत्वा मासार्धमासस्थमरिष्टं पाययेत् [१] च||१५||

In the decoction of Danti, one Anjali (96 gms, appr) each of the pulp of Sampaka (aragvadha) and Jaggery is added and kept [to ferment] for half a month. The Arista (medicated wine) thus prepared is taken as a potion [for purgation]. [15]

Use of Aragvadha added to Food and Drinks

यस्य यत् पानमन्नं च हृद्यं स्वाद्वथ वा कटु|लवणं वा भवेत्तेन युक्तं दद्यादि्वरेचनम्||१६||

[Aragvadha] is administered as purgative adding to either sweet, pungent or saline food and drinks which are pleasing to the heart of the patient. [16]

Contents of Chapter

तत्र श्लोकाः

द्राक्षारसे सुरासीध्वोर्दध्नि चामलकीरसे| सौवीरके कषाये च त्रिवृतो बिल्वकस्य [१] च||१७||

लेहेऽरिष्टे घृते द्वे च योगा द्वादश कीर्तिताः| चतुरङ्गुलकल्पेऽस्मिन् सुकुमाराः सुखोदयाः||१८||

To sum up:-

In this chapter dealing with the pharmaceutics of Aragvadha, twelve purgative recipes are described for the happiness of persons of delicate nature. These recipes are as follows:

One recipe to be taken along with grape juice (vide verse no. 8)

One recipe each of (1) Sura (alcohol), (2) Sidhu (a type of wine), (3) Dadhi (whey), (4) Juice of Amalaki, (5) Sauvira), (6) decoction of Trivrt and, (7) Decoction of Bilva: (vide Verse nos. 9-11)

One recipe in the form of Linctus (vide verse no. 12)

One recipe in the form of medicated wine: and (vide verse no. 15)

Two recipes in the form of medicated ghee (vide verse nos. 13-14) [17-18]

Colophon

इत्यग्निवेशकृते तन्त्रे चरकप्रतिसंस्कृतेऽप्राप्ते दृढबलसम्पूरिते कल्पस्थाने चतुरङ्गुलकल्पो नामाष्टमोऽध्यायः||८||

Thus, ends the eighth chapter of Kalpa-Sthana dealing with the "Pharmaceutics of Chaturangula" in Agnivesha's work as redacted by Charaka, and because of its non- availability supplemented by Drdhabala.

22

Kalpasthana Chapter 9 Tilvaka Kalpam

Prologue

अथातस्तिल्वककल्पं व्याख्यास्यामः॥१॥

इति ह स्माह भगवानात्रेयः॥२॥

Now we shall explore the chapter dealing with the "Pharmaceutics of Tilvaka". Thus, said Lord Atreya. [1-2]

Synonyms

तिल्वकस्तु मतो लोध्रो बृहत्पत्रस्तिरीटकः।

Tilvaka is known by the synonyms like Lodhra, Brhatpatra and Tiritaka. [½ 3]

Processing of Tilvaka

तस्य मूलत्वचं शुष्कामन्तर्वल्कलवर्जिताम्॥३॥ चूर्णयेतु त्रिधा कृत्वा द्वौ भागौ श्चोतयेत्ततः।

लोध्रस्यैव कषायेण तृतीयं तेन भावयेत्॥४॥ भागं तं दशमूलस्य पुनः क्वाथेन भावयेत्।

शुष्कं चूर्णं पुनः कृत्वा तत ऊर्ध्वं प्रयोजयेत्॥५॥

The dry root-bark of Tilvaka which is free from its inner layer should be pounded. It should be made into three parts. Two parts of this powder is added with water and strained by the process of percolation. With this liquid the third part of the powder of Tilvaka is impregnated with the decoction of Dashamula (Bilva, Shyonaka, Gambhari, Patala, Ganikarika, Shalaparni, Prsniparni, Brhati, Kantakari and Gokshura). This should then be dried and made into a powder again and used [in recipes] [3 ½ -5]

Recipes of Tilvaka with Whey etc.:

दधितक्रसुरामण्डमूत्रैर्बदरसीधुना ।रसेनामलकानां वा ततः पाणितलं पिबेत्॥६॥

One Panitala (12 gms appr) of this powder is taken along with the following vehicles:

Dadhi- Takra (whey)

Sura-manda (supernatant part of alcohol)

Cow's urine

Badara-Sidhu (a type of sour drink prepared of Jujubes) and

Juice of Amalaki [6]

Recipe of Tilvaka in the form of Sauviraka

मेषशृङ्ग्यभयाकृष्णाचित्रकैः सलिले शृते। मरुजान् सुनुयातच्च जातं सौवीरकं यदा॥७॥

भवेदञ्जलिना तस्य लोध्रकल्कं पिबेत् सदा।८।

To the decoction of Meshashringi, Abhaya, Krsna and Chitraka, roasted barley is added and fermented. The paste of Lodhra is mixed with one Anjali (96 ml. appr) of this Sauviraka, and taken as a potion. [7- ½ 8]

Recipe of Tilvaka in the form of Sura
सुरां लोध्रकषायेण जातां पक्षस्थितां पिबेत्||८||
Sura (alcohol drink) prepared of the decoction of Lodhra by keeping (fermenting) it for a fortnight is taken as a potion. [8 ½]

Recipe of Tilvaka in the form of Arista
दन्तीचित्रकयोर्द्रोणे सलिलस्याढकं पृथक्| समुत्क्वाथ्य गुडस्यैकां तुलां लोध्रस्य चाञ्जलिम्||९||
आवपेतत् परं पक्षान्मद्यपानां विरेचनम्|१०|
One Drona each of Danti and Chitraka are added with one Adhaka of water and decoction is prepared. To this decoction, one Tula of Jaggery and one Anjali of the powder of Lodhra is added and allowed to ferment. The Arista (medicated wine) thus prepared by keeping the recipe for a fortnight is an excellent purgative potion for persons habituated to the intake of wine. [9 – ½ 10]

Recipe of Tilvaka Prepared along with Kampillaka.
कम्पिल्ललककषायेण दशकृत्वः सुभाविताम्||१०||
मात्रां कम्पिल्ललकस्यैव कषायेण पुनः पिबेत्|११|
The powder of Tilvaka is well impregnated with the decoction of Kampillaka for ten times. A dose of this recipe should be taken again with the decoction of Kampillaka. [10 ½ - ½ 11]

Recipes of Tilvaka in the form of Linctus
चतुरङ्गुलकल्पेन लेहोऽन्यः कार्य एव च||११|| त्रिफलायाः कषायेण ससर्पिर्मधुफाणितः|
लोध्रचूर्णयुतः सिद्धो लेहः श्रेष्ठो विरेचने||१२|| तिल्वकस्य कषायेण कल्केन च सशर्करः|
सघृतः साधितो लेहः स च श्रेष्ठो विरेचने||१३||
A linctus of Tilvaka is prepared on the line suggested for Chaturangula (vide Kalpa 8:12).
Linctus is prepared by adding the powder of Lodhra, ghee, honey and Phanita (penidium) to the decoction of Triphala (haritaki, Vibhitaka and Amalaki). It is an excellent recipe for purgation.
To the decoction of Tilvaka, its paste, sugar and ghee is added and cooked. This linctus is excellently useful for purgation. [11 ½ - 13]

Recipes of Tilvaka in the form of medicated Ghee:
अष्टाष्टौ त्रिवृतादीनां मुष्टींस्तु सनखान् पृथक्| द्रोणेऽपां साधयेत् पादशेषे प्रस्थं घृतात् पचेत्||१४||
पिष्टैस्तैरेव बिल्वांशैः समूत्रलवणैरथ| ततो मात्रां पिबेत् काले श्रेष्ठमेतद्विरेचनम्||१५||
लोध्रकल्केन मूत्राम्ललवणैश्च पचेद्घृतम्| चतुरङ्गुलकल्पेन सर्पिषी द्वे च साधयेत्||१६||
Eight fistful quantity of each of Shyama, Trivrt (Chaturangula), Mahavrksa, Saptala, Sankhini, Danti and Dravanti) and sixteen fistfuls of Tilvaka Powder is boiled by adding one Drona of water separately till one fourth of the liquid remains. These decoctions should then be mixed together. To this, one Prastha of ghee, one Bilva of the paste each of the nine drugs described above, and one Pala each of cow's urine as well as salt are added. This should then be cooked. It is taken at the appropriate time and in appropriate dose which is an excellent potion for purgation. 'By adding the paste of Lodhra, cow's urine, sour liquid and salt, ghee may also be cooked. In Kalpa 8: 13-14, two recipes of medicated ghee of Chaturangula are described. Following the same procedure, two recipes of medicated ghee containing Tilvaka may also be prepared [and used for purgation]. [14-16]

Contents of Chapter
तत्र श्लोकौ-
पञ्च दध्यादिभिस्त्वेका सुरा सौवीरकेण च| एकोऽरिष्टस्तथा योग एकः कम्पिल्लकेन च||१७||
लेहास्त्रयो घृतेनापि चत्वारः सम्प्रकीर्तिताः| योगास्ते लोध्रमूलानां कल्पे षोडश दर्शिताः||१८||

To sum up: - in this chapter, sixteen recipes of the root of Lodhra are described as follows:

1-5. Five recipes with Dadhi-Takra, Sura-manda, Mutra, Badara-Sidhu and Juice of Amalaki vide verse no. 6)

One recipe of Lodhra in the form of Sura (vide verse no. 8)

One recipe along with Sauviraka (vide verse nos. 7-8)

One recipe in the form of arista (vide verse no. 9)

One recipe of Lodhra to be taken along with Kampillaka (vide verse nos 10-11)

11-13 three recipes of Lodhra prepared in the form of linctus and (vide verse nos. 11-13)-

13-14 four recipes of Lodhra in the form of medicated ghee (vide verse nos. 14-16) [17-18]

Colophon

इत्यग्निवेशकृते तन्त्रे चरकप्रतिसंस्कृतेऽप्राप्ते दृढबलसम्पूरिते कल्पस्थाने तिल्वककल्पो नाम नवमोऽध्यायः ||९||

Thus, ends the ninth chapter of Kalpa- section dealing with the "Pharmaceutics of Tilvaka" in Agnivesha's work as redacted by Charaka, and because of its non- availability, supplemented by Charaka.

23

Kalpasthana Chapter 10 Sudha Kalpam

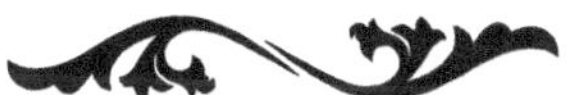

Prologue

अथातः सुधाकल्पं व्याख्यास्यामः||१||

इति ह स्माह भगवानात्रेयः||२|

Now we shall expound the chapter dealing with the "Pharmaceutics of Sudha". Thus said Lord Atreya [1-2]

Effects of Sudha

विरेचनानां सर्वेषां सुधा तीक्ष्णतमा मता| सङ्घातं हि भिनत्त्याशु दोषाणां कष्टविभ्रमा||३||

तस्मान्नैषा मृदौ कोष्ठे प्रयोक्तव्या कदाचन| न दोषनिचये चाल्पे सति मार्गपरिक्रमे [||४||

Among all the purgative drugs, Sudha is the strongest (sharpest) one. It quickly disintegrates the accumulated impurities. Wrong use of these drugs may lead to consequences which are difficult to handle. Therefore, it should never be administered to a person having a soft bowel. It should also not be administered when there is less accumulation of Doshas and when other therapeutic measures are available for correcting the disease. [3-4]

Indications of Sudha:

पाण्डुरोगोदरे गुल्मे कुष्ठे दूषीविषार्दिते| श्वयथौ मधुमेहे च दोषविभ्रान्तचेतसि||५||

रोगैरेवंविधैर्ग्रस्तं ज्ञात्वा सप्राणमातुरम्| प्रयोजयेन्महावृक्षं सम्यक् स ह्यवचारितः||६||

सद्यो हरति दोषाणां महान्तमपि सञ्चयम्|७|

Maha-Vrksa (sudha) is administered to a strong person suffering from anaemia, obstinate abdominal diseases including ascites, phantom tumour, obstinate skin diseases including leprosy, poisoning caused by artificially made toxic ingredients, oedema, obstinate urinary disorders, insanity and such other diseases if properly administered, it quickly eliminates the Doshas even if they are excessively accumulated. [5- ½ 7]

Varieties of Sudha

द्विविधः स मतोऽल्पैश्च बहुभिश्चैव कण्टकैः||७||

सुतीक्ष्णैः कण्टकैरल्पैः प्रवरो बहुकण्टकः|

Sudha is of two types

1. one which has small but numerous thrones,

2. the other type which has less but sharp thorns

The one having numerous thrones (i.e. former) is better than the other (i.e. the latter). [7 ½ - ½ 8]

Synonyms:

स नाम्ना स्नुग्गुडा नन्दा सुधा निस्त्रिंशपत्रकः||८||

Synonyms of Sudha are - Snuk, Guda, Nanda, Sudha and Nistrimsa-Patraka. [8 ½]

Methods of collection

तौ विपाट्याहरेत् क्षीरं शस्त्रेण मतिमान् भिषक्| द्विवर्षं वा त्रिवर्षं वा शिशिरान्ते विशेषतः||९||

He help of a sharp instrument. By doing so they should collect its milky latex. The tree of Sudha is two to three years old, and the milk is collected especially at the end (last part) of the winter. [9]

Recipes of Sudha to be Taken along with Sauviraka etc.,

बिल्वादीनां बृहत्या वा कण्टकार्यास्तथैकशः| कषायेण समांशं तं कृत्वाङ्गारेषु शोषयेत्||१०||

ततः कोलसमां मात्रां पिबेत् सौवीरकेण वा| तुषोदकेन कोलानां रसेनामलकस्य वा||११||

सुरया दधिमण्डेन मातुलुङ्गरसेन वा|१२|

The milk of Sudha is mixed with equal quantities of the decoction of either bilva (Syonaka, Gambhari, Patala and Ganikarika), Kantakari, and dried in a pan kept over charcoal fire. From this paste, pills of the size of Kola are prepared. These pills are taken along with either of the following vehicles:

Sauviraka (sour vinegar)

Tusodaka (sour fermented liquid prepared of husked paddy, etc)

Juice of Kola (Jujube- fruit);

Juice of Amalaki

Sura (alcohol)

Dadhi-Manda (whey) or

Juice of Matulunga [10 – ½ 12]

Recipes of Sudha to be taken with Ghee etc

सातलां काञ्चनक्षीरीं श्यामादीनि कटुत्रिकम् ||१२|| यथोपपत्ति सप्ताहं सुधाक्षीरेण भावयेत्|

कोलमात्रां घृतेनातः पिबेन्मांसरसेन वा|१३||

From amongst Satala, Kancanaksiri, Syama, {Trivrt, Chaturangula, Tilvaka, Mahavrksa, Saptala, Sankhini, Danti, Dravanti], Sunthi, Pippali and Marica, as many as are available are collected. They are made into powder. This powder is impregnated with the latex of Sudha for one week. From this paste, pills of the size of the one Kola are prepared. These pills are taken with either of the following vehicles:

Ghee or

Meat-soup [12 ½- 13]

Recipe of Sudha in the form of Panaka

त्र्यूषणं त्रिफलां दन्तीं चित्रकं त्रिवृतां तथा| स्नुक्क्षीरभावितं सम्यग्विदध्याद्गुडपानकम्||१४||

Sunthi, Pippali,Maricha, Haritaki, Vibhitaka, Amalaki, Danti, Chitraka and Trivrt are impregnated with the milky latex of Snuhi. In the form of syrup prepared with jaggery, [it is administered for purgation]. [14]

Recipes of Sudha to be Used for Inhalation

त्रिवृतारग्वधं दन्तीं शङ्खिनीं सप्तलां समम्|गोमूत्रे रजनीं कृत्वा शोषयेदातपे ततः||१५||

सप्ताहं भावयित्वैवं स्नुक्क्षीरेणापरं पुनः| सप्ताहं भावयेच्छुष्कं ततस्तेनापि भावितम्||१६||

गन्धमाल्यं तदाघ्राय प्रावृत्य पटमेव च|सुखमाशु विरिच्यन्ते मृदुकोष्ठा नराधिपाः||१७||

Trivrt, aragvadha, danti, Sankhini and Saptala are taken in equal quantities and made to a powder. This powder is impregnated and made into a powder. This is impregnated with cow's urine for one night and dried in the sun. This powder should again be impregnated for onc week with the milky latex of Snuhi. Aromatic garlands are sprinkled with this powder and upper garments are impregnated with the water mixed with this powder [of the milky latex]. By the inhalation of this garland or by wearing this upper garment, a person of royal descent or a person who has soft bowel gets purgation easily and quickly. [15-17]

Recipe of Sudha Prepared in the form of Linctus

श्यामात्रिवृत्कषायेण स्नुक्क्षीरघृतफाणितैः|लेहं पक्त्वा विरेकार्थं लेहयेन्मात्रया नरम्||१८||

The decoction of syama-Trivrt is added with the milky latex of snuhi, ghee and Phanita (Penidium), and cooked. This linctus is taken by a person in appropriate doses for the purpose of purgation.

Recipes of Sudha to be taken with Vegetable soup etc.

पाययेतु सुधाक्षीरं यूषैर्मांसरसैर्घृतैः|१९|

The milky latex of Sudha is given as a potion along with vegetables-soup, meat–soup or ghee for purgation. [½ 19]

Recipes of Sudha to be taken with Dried fish or Dried Meat

भावितान्छुष्कमत्स्यान् वा मांसं वा भक्षयेन्नरः||१९||

Dry fish or dry meat is impregnated with the milky latex of Sudha and taken [for purgation]. [19 ½]

Recipes of Sudha in the form of Medicated Ghee and Alcohol

क्षीरेणामलकैः सर्पिश्चतुरङ्गुलवत् पचेत्| सुरां वा कारयेत् क्षीरे घृतं वा पूर्ववत् पचेत्||२०||

Following the procedure described in respect of Chaturangula (vide Kalpha 8: 13), medicated ghee is prepared of the milky latex of Sudha and taken along with [the juice of] Amalaki.

Sura (alcoholic drink) is prepared of the powder of Sunthi, Pippali, Maricha, Vibhitaki, Amalaki, Danti, Citraka and Trivrt impregnated with the milky latex of Snuhi. Medicated ghee may also be prepared with the latex of Snuhi [these recipes may be used for purgation] according to the method prescribed before. [20]

Contents of Chapter

तत्र श्लोकौ-

सौवीरकादिभिः सप्त सर्पिषा च रसेन च| पानकं घ्रेयलेहौ च योगा यूषादिभिस्त्रयः||२१||

द्वौ शुष्कमत्स्यमांसाभ्यां सुरैका द्वे च सर्पिषी| महावृक्षस्य योगास्ते विंशतिः समुदाहृताः||२२||

To sum up:-

In this chapter, twenty recipes of Mahavrksa (sudha) are illustrated as follows:

(1-7). Seven recipes of Sudha to be taken along with Sauviraka etc. (vide verse nos. 10-12)

(8-9). Two recipes of Sudha to be taken along with ghee and meat-soup (vide verse nos. 13)

(10) One recipe in the form of Syrup (vide verse no. 14)

(11) One recipe of Sudha for inhalation (vide verse nos. 15-17)

(12) One recipe of Sudha in the form of linctus (vide verse no. 18)

(13- 15) Three recipes of Sudha to be taken along with vegetable-soup, meat soup and ghee (vide verse no. 19)

(16-17) Two recipes of Sudha to be taken along with dry fish and dry meat (vide verse no. 19)

(18). One recipe of Sudha to be taken in the form of alcoholic drink and (vide verse no. 20)

(19_20) two recipes of Sudha to be prepared in the form of medicated ghee (including alcohol) (vide verse no. 20) [21-22]

Colophon

इत्यग्निवेशकृते तन्त्रे चरकप्रतिसंस्कृतेऽप्राप्ते दृढबलसम्पूरिते कल्पस्थाने सुधाकल्पो नाम दशमोऽध्यायः||१०||

Thus, ends the tenth chapter of Kalpha- Sthana dealing with the "Pharmaceutic of Sudha" in the Agnivesha's work redacted by Charaka, and because of its non- availability, Supplemented by Drdhabala.

24

Kalpasthana Chapter 11 Saptala Sankhini Kalpam

Prologue

अथातः सप्तलाशङ्खिनीकल्पं व्याख्यास्यामः||१|| इति ह स्माह भगवानात्रेयः||२||

Now we shall explore the chapter dealing with the "Pharmaceutics of Saptala and Sankhini". Thus said Lord Atreya [1-2]

Synonyms

सप्तला चर्मसाह्वा च बहुफेनरसा च सा| शङ्खिनी तिक्तला चैव यवतिक्ताऽक्षि(क्ष)पीडकः||३||

Synonyms of Saptala - Saptala, Carmasahva and Bahuphenarasa.
Synonyms of Shankhini - Sankhini, Tiktala, Yavatikta and Aksipidaka are synonymous. [3]

Therapeutic Effects:

ते गुल्मगरहृद्रोगकुष्ठशोफोदरादिषु| विकासितीक्ष्णरूक्षत्वाद्योज्ये श्लेष्माधिकेषु तु||४||

Because of their attributes, viz - tendency to cause looseness of joints, sharpness and un-unctuousness (dryness), these two drugs (saptala & sankhini) are used in the treatment of phantom tumour, poisoning, heart diseases, obstinate skin diseases including leprosy, oedema, obstinate abdominal diseases including ascites and such other conditions caused by aggravated kapha. [4]

Method of Collection

नातिशुष्कं फलं ग्राह्यं शङ्खिन्या निस्तुषीकृतम्| सप्तलायाश्च मूलानि गृहीत्वा भाजने क्षिपेत्||५||

The fruits of Sankhini are collected when these are not very dry and ex-corticated. The roots of Saptala are collected for use. Both of these are preserved in a pot. [5]

Recipes of Saptala and Sankhini to be taken along with Decoctions etc.

अक्षमात्रं तयोः पिण्डं प्रसन्नालवणायुतम्| हृद्रोगे कफवातोत्थे गुल्मे चैव प्रयोजयेत्||६||

प्रियालपीलुकर्कन्धुकोलामातककदादिमैः| द्राक्षापनसखर्जूरबदराम्लपरूषकैः||७||

मैरेये दधिमण्डेऽम्ले सौवीरकतुषोदके| सीधौ चाप्येष कल्पः स्यात् सुखं शीघ्रविरेचनः||८||

One Aksa of the paste of Saptala and Sankhini is added with Prasanna (a type of wine) and salt. This is useful for treating heart diseases caused by Kapha and vayu, and for treating phantom tumours. This recipe is administered with the below mentioned vehicles – Decoction of Priyala, Decoction of Pilu, Decoction of Karkandhu, Decoction of Kola, Juice of Amrataka, Juice of Dadima, Juice of Draksa, Juice of Panasa, Juice of Kharjura, Badaramla (sour preparation of Jujube – fruit), Juice of Parusaka, Maireya (a sour drink), Amla Dadhimanda (sour whey), Sauviraka (Vinegar), Tusodaka (another sour drink prepared of Paddy etc) and, Sidhu (a type of wine)

Intake of these recipes helps in easy and quick purgation. [6-8]

Recipes of Saptala and Sankhini in the form of medicated oil

तैलं विदारिगन्धाद्यैः पयसि क्वथिते पचेत्|सप्तलाशङ्खिनीकल्के त्रिवृच्छ्यामार्धभागिके||९||

दधिमण्डेन सन्नीय सिद्धं तत् पाययेत च|शङ्खिनीचूर्णभागौ द्वौ तिलचूर्णस्य चापरः||१०||

हरीतकीकषायेण तैलं तत्पीडितं पिबेत्| अतसीसर्षपैरण्डकरञ्जष्वेष संविधिः||११||

Milk is boiled by adding drugs belonging to Vidarigandhadi group. Oil is cooked by adding this milk, the paste of Saptala and Sankhini (one part), and Trivrt as well as Syama (half parts). This medicated oil is added to Dadhi-Manda (whey) and administered as a potion [for purgation].

Two parts of the powder of Sankhini is added with one part of the powder of sesame seed, and oil is expressed out of it. This oil is taken along with the decoction of Haritaki [for purgation].

Following the same procedure, oil is expressed from the seeds of Atasi, Sarsapa, Eranda and Karanja, [and taken along with the decoction of Haritaki for Purgation]. [9-11]

Recipes of Saptala and Sankhini in the form of Medicated Ghee etc

शङ्खिनीसप्तलासिद्धात् क्षीराद्यदुदियाद्घृतम्| कल्कभागे तयोरेव त्रिवृच्छ्यामार्धसंयुते||१२||

क्षीरेणालोड्य सम्पक्वं पिबेतच्च विरेचनम्| दन्तीद्रवन्त्योः कल्पोऽयमजशृङ्ग्यजगन्धयोः||१३||

क्षीरिण्या नीलिकायाश्च तथैव च करञ्जयोः| मसूरविदलायाश्च प्रत्यक्पर्ण्यास्तथैव च||१४||

द्विवर्गार्धाशकल्केन तद्वत् साध्यं घृतं पुनः| शङ्खिनीसप्तलाधात्रीकषाये साधयेद्घृतम् [३] ||१५||

त्रिवृत्कल्पेन सर्पिश्च त्रयो लेहाश्च लोध्रवत्| सुराकम्पिल्लयोर्योगः कार्यो लोध्रवदेव च||१६||

From the milk boiled with Sankhini and Saptala, ghee is extracted. This ghee is cooked by adding one part of the paste of Saptala and Sankhini, and half part of the paste of Trivrt as well as Syama. This medicated ghee is mixed with milk and taken as potion [for purgation].

In the place of paste of Trivrt and syama, the above mentioned ghee may also be prepared by adding half part of the paste of the following drugs:

Danti and Dravanti;

Ajasrngi (dugdhika) and Niliki;

Two varieties of Karanja and

Masuravidala (Syamalata) and Pratyakparni (Musikaparni)

Medicated ghee may also be prepared by boiling ghee with the decoction of Sankhini, Saptala and Amalaki.

Medicated ghee of Saptala may be prepared according to the procedure described for the preparation of medicated ghee of Trvrit (vide Kalpha 8: 66-68).

Following the procedure prescribed for Lodhra, these types of Leha or linctus (vide Kalpa (: 11-13), Sura or alcoholic drink (vide Kalpa 9: 8-9) and recipe of Kampillaka (vide Kalpa 9-10-11) may also be prepared of Saptapala and Santhini. [12-16]

Recipes of Saptapala and Sankhiniin the form of Fermented Drink:

दन्तीद्रवन्त्योः कल्पेन सौवीरकतुषोदके| अजगन्धाजशृङ्ग्योश्च तद्वत् स्यातां विरेचने||१७||

According to the procedure described with respect to Danti-Dravanti (vide Kalpa 12: 35), Sauviraka (Vinegar) and Tusodaka (a type of Sour drink prepared of Husked paddy, etc) of Saptala and Sankhini is also prepared.

Similarly, Guda type of wine of Saptala and sankhini may also be prepared by adding Ajagandha and Ajasrngi (on the lines suggested in Kalpa 12: 33)

These [four recipes] are useful for purgation. [17]

Contents of Chapter

तत्र श्लोकौ-

कषाया दश षट् चैव षट् तैलेऽष्टौ च सर्पिषि| पञ्च मद्ये त्रयो लेहा योगः कम्पिल्लके तथा||१८||

सप्तलाशङ्खिनीभ्यां ते त्रिंशदुक्ता नवाधिकाः| योगाः सिद्धाः समस्ताभ्यामेकशोऽपि च ते हिताः||१९||

To sum up:-

In this chapter thirty nine types of effective recipes of Saptala and Sankhini are described as follows:

1-6. sixteen recipes of saptala and Sankhini to be taken along with decoctions Etc. (vide verse nos. 6-8)

17-22. six recipes of Saptala and Sankhini to be prepared in the form of oil (vide verse nos. (9-11)

23-30. eight recipes of Saptala and Sankhini to be prepared in the form of medicated ghee: (vide verse nos. (12-16)

31-35. five recipes of Saptala and Sankhini to be prepared by fermentation and (vide verse no. 16-17)

36—39.Three recipes of Saptala –Sankhini to be prepared in the form of linctus and one recipe of Saptala – Sankhini to be prepared by adding Kampillaka (vide verse no. 16)

For the preparation of the mentioned recipes, either Saptala or Sankhini separately or both of these taken together are to be used. [18-19]

Colophon

इत्यग्निवेशकृते तन्त्रे चरकप्रतिसंस्कृतेऽप्राप्ते दृढबलसम्पूरिते कल्पस्थाने सप्तलाशङ्खिनीकल्पो नामैकादशोऽध्यायः||११||

Thus, ends the eleventh chapter of Kalpa- section dealing with the "Pharmaceutic of Saptala and Sankhini" in Agnivesha's work as redacted by Charaka, and because of its non-availability, supplemented by Drdhabala.

25

Kalpasthana Chapter 12 Danti Dravanti Kalpam

Prologue

अथातो दन्तीद्रवन्तीकल्पं व्याख्यास्यामः||१||

इति ह स्माह भगवानात्रेयः||२||

We shall now explore the chapter dealing with the "Pharmaceutics of Danti and Dravanti". Thus, said Lord Atreya. [1-2]

Synonyms

दन्त्युदुम्बरपर्णी स्यान्निकुम्भोऽथ मुकूलकः| द्रवन्ती नामतश्चित्रा न्यग्रोधी मूषिकाह्वया||३||

(तथा मूषिकपर्णी चाप्युपचित्रा च शम्बरी| प्रत्यक्श्रेणी सुतश्रेणी दन्ती र(च)ण्डा च कीर्तिता [१])|

The synonyms of Danti are: Udumbara, Nikumbha and Mukulaka. Synonyms of Dravanti are: Citra, Nyagrodhi and Musikahvavya. (It is also known as Musika parni, Upacitra, Sambari, Pratyak, Suta-serni, Danti and ra(ca)anda. [3]

Parts to be collected:

तयोर्मूलानि सङ्गृह्य स्थिराणि बहलानि च| हस्तिदन्तप्रकाराणि श्यावताम्राणि बुद्धिमान्||४||

A wise physician should collect the roots of Danti and Dravanti which are strong, thick (having thick root-bark) and resembling an elephant's tusk. The roots of Danti are dark brown. The roots of Dravanti are coppery in colour. [4]

Processing of Danti and Dravanti

पिप्पलीमधुलिप्तानि स्वेदयेन्मृत्कुशान्तरे|

शोषयेदातपेऽग्न्यर्कौ हतो ह्येषां विकाशिताम्||५||

The roots of Danti and Dravanti are smeared with the paste (of the powder) of Pippali and honey, and covered with Kusha. The bundle is smeared with mud and fomented with steam. Thereafter, the roots are taken out and dried in the sun. By the exposure to the heat of the fire and sun the Vikasi attribute (toxic effect which causes looseness of joints) is removed. [5]

Attributes of Danti and Dravanti

तीक्ष्णोष्णान्याशुकारीणि विकाशीनि गुरूणि च| विलाययन्ति दोषौ द्वौ मारुतं कोपयन्ति च||६||

The roots of Danti and Dravanti are tikshna (sharp), ushna (hot), ashukari (producing effects instantaneously), vikasi (causing looseness of joints) and guru (heavy). They cause liquefaction of Kapha and Pitta. These roots on the other hand aggravate Vayu. [6]

Recipes of Danti and Dravanti to be taken with Yoghurt Etc

दधितक्रसुरामण्डैः पिण्डमक्षसमं तयोः| प्रियालकोलबदरपीलुशीधुभिरेव च||७||

पिबेद्गुल्मोदरी दोषैरभिखिन्नश्च यो नरः|

The root of Danti and Dravanti is made into a paste (by triturating with water). One aksa of this paste is given to the patient along with the following vehicles:

Yoghurt

Butter-milk

Sura-manda (supernatant part of alcohol)

Priyala-Sidhu (a type of wine prepared of Priyala);

Kola-Sidhu (another type of wine prepared of Kola fruit)

Badara-Sidhu (another type of the wine prepared of Badara) and

Pilu-Sidhu (another type of wine prepared of Pillu)

These recipes are useful for patients suffering from phantom tumour and obstinate abdominal diseases including ascites. These recipes are also useful for those who are afflicted by severely aggravated morbid doshas. [7 – ½ 8]

Recipes of Danti and Dravanti to be taken with Meat- soup

गोमृगाजरसैः पाण्डुः कृमिकोष्ठी भगन्दरी||८||

[One Aksa of the paste of Danthi and Dravanti] is taken with the soup of the meat of cow, deer or goat, by the patient suffering from anemia), infestation with intestinal parasites and anal fistula. [8 ½]

Recipes of Danti and Dravanti in the form of Medicated Ghee etc

तयोः कल्के कषाये च दशमूलरसायुते| कक्ष्यालजीविसर्पेषु दाहे च विपचेद्घृतम्||९||

तैलं मेहे च गुल्मे च सोदावर्ते कफानिले| चतुःस्नेहं शकृच्छुक्रवातसङ्गानिलार्तिषु||१०||

Ghee is cooked by adding the paste and decoction of Danthi and Dravanti and [equal quantity] of the decoction of Dashamula. This medicated ghee is useful for patients suffering from herpes in the axilla, boils, erysipelas and burning syndrome.

With the above-mentioned ingredients, oil is cooked. This medicated oil is useful in Meha (obstinate urinary disorders), Gulma (phantom tumour) and Udavarta (upward movement of wind in the abdomen) caused by the aggravation of Kapha and vayu.

With the above-mentioned ingredients, Chathur-Sneha (four types of fat, viz, oil, ghee, muscle-fat and bone –marrow) is cooked. This recipe of medicated fat is useful in conditions of obstruction of faeces, semen and flatus, and other diseases caused by aggravated Vayu. [9-10]

Recipes of Danthi and Dravanti in the form of Linctus

रसे दन्त्यजशृङ्गयोश्च गुडक्षौद्रघृतान्वितः| लेहः सिद्धो विरेकार्थे दाहसन्तापमेहनुत् [3] ||११||

वाततर्षे ज्वरे पैत्ते स्यात् स एवाजगन्धया| दन्तीद्रवन्त्योर्मूलानि पचेदामलकीरसे||१२||

त्रींस्तु तस्य कषायस्य भागौ द्वौ फाणितस्य च| तप्ते सर्पिषि तैले वा भर्जयेत्तत्र चावपेत्||१३||

कल्कं दन्तीद्रवन्त्योश्च श्यामादीनां च भागशः| तत्सिद्धं प्राशयेल्लेहं सुखं तेन विरिच्यते||१४||

To the decoction of Danti and Ajasrngi - jaggery, honey and ghee are added and cooked. This recipe of linctus is used for purgation which cures burning syndrome, heating sensation and obstinate urinary disorders.

In the place of Ajasrngi in the above recipe, Ajagandha may be added. And the linctus is prepared. This is useful in morbid thirst caused by Vayu, and fever caused by Pitta.

The root of Danthi and Dravanti is cooked by adding the juice (decoction) of Amalaki. Three parts of this decoction should be added with two parts of Phanita (Penidium) which is sizzled by adding hot ghee or hot oil. To this, one part each of the paste of Danti, Dravanti, Syama (Trivrt), Chaturangula, Tilvaka, Sudha, Saptala and Sankhini] is added and cooked. This linctus is taken as a potion which helps in easy purgation. [11-14]

Second Group of Sixteen Recipes;

रसे च दशमूलस्य तथा बैभीतके रसे| हरीतकीरसे चैव लेहानेवं पचेत् पृथक् ||१५||

तयोर्बिल्वसमं चूर्णं तद्रसेनैव भावितम्| असृष्टे विशि वातोत्थे गुल्मे चाम्लयुतं शुभम्||१६||

पाटयित्वेक्षुकाण्डं वा कल्केनालिप्य चान्तरा| स्वेदयित्वा ततः खादेत् सुखं तेन विरिच्यते||१७||

मूलं दन्तीद्रवन्त्योश्च सह मुद्गैर्विपाचयेत्| लाववर्तीरकाद्यैश्च ते रसाः स्युर्विरेचने||१८||

तयोर्वाऽपि कषायेण यवागूं जाङ्गलं रसम्| माषयूषं च संस्कृत्य दद्यातैश्च विरिच्यते||१९||

1-3. in the recipe of linctus described in the verse no. 12-14, the decoction of Dashamula or Vibhitaki or Haritaki may be used in place of the decoction of Amalaki and three other recipes of linctus may be prepared.

4. One Bilva of the powder of Danti and Dravanti is impregnated with the decoction of Danti and Dravanti. This is taken with the sour juice. This is useful in the retention of feces and in phantom tumour caused by aggravated Vayu.

5. Stem of the sugarcane is split, and its inner surface is smeared with the paste of Danti and Dravanti. Thereafter the sugar-cane is fermented. When this sugarcane is chewed and its juice sucked it causes easy purgation.

6-13. The root of Danti and Dravanti along with Mudga is cooked with the meat- soup of

Lava, Vartiraka, Vartika, Kapinjala, Cakora, Upacakra, Kakubha, Rakta carmaka.

These eight medicated soups are useful for purgation.

4-15. With the decoction of Danti and Dravanti, gruel (yavagu) or the soup of the meat of animals living in arid zones is prepared. These two recipes are sizzled with spices, and administered as a potion for purgations.

16. Similarly, with the decoction of Danti and Dravanti, yavagu (gruel) is prepared by adding the soup of masa. This is sizzled and administered as a potion for purgation. [15-19]

Third Group of Sixteen Recipes

तत्कषायात्रयो भागा द्वौ सितायास्तथैव च| एको गोधूमचूर्णानां कार्या चोत्कारिका शुभा||२०||

मोदको वाऽस्य कल्पेन कार्यस्तच्च विरेचनम्| तयोश्चापि कषायेण मद्यान्यस्योपकल्पयेत्||२१||

दन्तीक्वाथेन चालोड्य दन्तीतैलेन साधितान्| गुडलावणिकान् भक्ष्यान् विविधान् भक्षयेन्नरः||२२||

दन्ती द्रवन्ती मरिचं यवानीमुपकुञ्चिकाम्| नागरं हेमदुग्धां च चित्रकं चेति चूर्णितम्||२३||

सप्ताहं भावयेन्मूत्रे गवां पाणितलं ततः| पिबेद्घृतेन जीर्णे तु विरिक्तश्चापि तर्पणम्||२४||

सर्वरोगहरं मुख्यं सर्वर्त्वृतुषु यौगिकम्|चूर्णं तदनपायित्वाद्बालवृद्धेषु पूजितम्||२५||

दुर्भक्ताजीर्णपार्श्वार्तिगुल्मप्लीहोदरेषु च| गण्डमालासु वाते च पाण्डुरोगे च शस्यते||२६||

पलं चित्रकदन्त्योश्च हरीतक्याश्च विंशतिः| त्रिवृत्पिप्पलिकर्षौ द्वौ गुडस्याष्टपलेन तत्||२७||

विनीय मोदकान् कुर्याद्दशैकं भक्षयेत्ततः| उष्णाम्बु च पिबेच्चानु दशमे दशमेऽह्नि च||२८||

एते निष्परिहाराः स्युः सर्वरोगनिबर्हणाः| ग्रहणीपाण्डुरोगार्शःकण्डूकोठानिलापहाः||२९||

दन्तीद्विपलनिर्यूहो द्राक्षार्धप्रस्थसाधितः | विरेचनं पितासरो पाण्डुरोगे च शस्यते||३०||

दन्तीकल्कं समगुडं शीतवारियुतं पिबेत्| विरेचनं मुख्यतमं कामलाहरमुत्तमम्||३१||

श्यामादन्तीरसे गौडः पिप्पलीफलचित्रकैः| लिप्तेऽरिष्टोऽनिलश्लेष्मप्लीहपाण्डूदरापहः||३२||

तथा दन्तीद्रवन्त्योश्च कषाये साजगन्धयोः| गौडः कार्योऽऽजशृङ्ग्या वा स वै सुखविरेचनः||३३||

तच्चूर्णक्वाथमाषाम्बुकिण्वतोयसमुद्भवा| मदिरा कफगुल्माल्पवह्निपार्श्वकटिग्रहे||३४||

अजगन्धाकषायेण सौवीरकतुषोदके| सुराकम्पिल्लके योगौ लोध्रवच्च तयोः स्मृतौ||३५||

Three parts of the decoctions of Danti and Dravanti are added with two parts of sugar and one part of wheat-flour. With this, Utkarika (pan-cake) is prepared and is useful for purgation.

With the above-mentioned ingredients, Modaka (sweet bolus) may also be prepared and used for purgation.

From the decoction of Danti and Dravanti, wine may be prepared and used for purgation.

Different types of eatables made of jaggery or salt can also be prepared by boiling food ingredients with the decoction or oil of Danti. [These eatables may be used for purgation]

Danti, Dravanti, Marica, Yavani, Upakuncika, Nagara, Hemadugdha, and Citraka are made into powder. This is impregnated with cow's urine for the week. One Pani-Tala of this recipe is given to the patient along with ghee. After the potion is digested and the patient is purged, he is given a demulcent drink. This recipe is immensely useful for all kinds of diseases. It can be administered in all the seasons. Since it has no untoward effects, it can be safely given to children and old persons. It is useful in loss of appetite, indigestion, pain in the sides of the chest, phantom tumour, splenomegaly, cervical lymphadenitis, diseases of Vayu and anemia.

One Pala of Citraka, one Palla of Danti, twenty fruits of haritaki, two karsas of Trivrt and two karsas of Pippali are added with eight palas of jaggery. Out of these ingredients, ten Modakas (sweet boluses) are prepared. One of these modakas is taken along with hot water, and this is repeated every tenth day. No dietetic restriction is necessary while using these modakas. These are useful for curing all diseases, specially spure syndrome, anemia, piles, itching, urticaria and diseases caused by Vayu.

The decoction of two Palas of Danti added with half Prastha of Draksa is a purgative useful in cough caused by Pitta and anemia.

The paste of Danti is added with jaggery in equal quantity and taken as a potion along with cold water. It is an excellent purgation recipe for curing jaundice.

The decoction of syama and Danti is added with jaggery and kept for fermentation in a jar. The inner wall of the jar is smeared with the paste of Pippali, Phala and Citraka. This Arista (mediated wine) is useful for ailments caused by vayu and Kapha, and diseases like splenic disorders, anemia and obstinate abdominal diseases including ascites.

The decoction of Danti, Dravanti and Ajagandha is added with jaggery and made to ferment [this arista is useful for purgation].

In the above recipe, Ajasrngi may be added in the place of Ajagandha. This Arista helps in easy purgation.

The decoction of the powder of Danti and Dravanti is added with the decoction of Masa and made to ferment. Out of this fermented (Kinva) wine, alcohol (Madira) is extracted which is useful in treating phantom tumour caused by Kapha, suppression of the power of digestion and stiffness of the sides of the chest and waist.

14. With the decoction of Danti, Dravanti and Ajagandha, Sauviraka (vinegar) and Tusodaka (a type of sour drink) is prepared on the lines suggested for Lodhra (vide Kalpa9: 7). {these two recipes are useful for purgation].

With the decoction of Danti and Dravanti, sura (alcoholic drink) is prepared on the lines suggested for Lodhra (vide Kalpha9:8: 10). This is useful for purgation.

Danti and Dravanti is added with Kampillaka, and the recipe is prepared on the line suggested for Lodhra (vide Kalpha 9: 10-11). This recipe is useful for purgation]. [20-35]

Contents (up to this Portion) of Chapter:

तत्र श्लोकाः-

(दध्यादिषु त्रयः पञ्च प्रियालाद्यैस्त्रयो रसे| स्नेहेषु वै त्रयो लेह्याः षट् चूर्णे त्वेक एव च||३६||

इक्षावेक्स्तथा मुद्गमांसानां च रसास्त्रयः| यवाग्वादौ त्रयश्चैव उक्त उत्कारिकाविधौ||३७||

एकश्च मोदके मद्ये चैकस्तत्क्वाथतैलके| चूर्णमेकं पुनश्चैको मोदकः पञ्च चासवे||३८||

एकः सौवीरकेऽथैको योगः स्यातु तुषोदके| एका सुरैकः कम्पिल्ले तथा पञ्च घृते स्मृताः)||३९||

दन्तीद्रवन्तीकल्पेऽस्मिन् प्रोक्ताः षोडशकास्त्रयः| नानाविधानां योगानां भक्तिदोषामयान्प्रति||४०||

To sum up:

In this (up to this portion of the chapter) the following recipes of Danti and Dravanti are described:

1-3. three recipes to be prepared with Danthi or yoghurt, etc. (vide verse nos. 7-8)

4-7. four recipes to be prepared with Priyala etc (vide verse nos. 7-8)

8-10. three recipes to be prepared in the form of meat-soup vide verse no. 8)

11-13. There recipes to be prepared in the form of medicated fat (vide verse nos. 9-10)

14-19. six recipes to be prepared with the form of powder (vide verse nos. 11-15)

20. One recipe to be prepared in the form of linctus: (vide verse nos. 16)

21. One recipe to be prepared with sugar-cane (vide verse no. 17)

22-39. eight recipes to be prepared with the soup of Mudga and meat-soups; (Rasastrayah' in the text appears to be an error) (vide verse no. 18)

30-32. three recipes to be prepared in the form of Yavagu etc (vide verse no. 19)

33. One recipe in the form of Utkarika (vide verse no. 20)

34. One recipe in the form of Modaka (sweet bolus) (vide verse no. 21)

35. One recipe in the form of alcoholic drink (vide verse no. 21)

36. One recipe of Etables to be prepared with the decoction and oil of Danti and Dravanti (vide verse no. 22)

37. One recipe in powder form (vide verse no. 23-26)

38. One recipe again in the form of Modaka (vide verse nos. 27-29)

39-44. six recipes in the form of Asava (medicated wine) (vide verse nos. 30-34) ["Panca Casave" appears to be an error]

45. One recipe in the form of Sauviraka (vinegar) (vide verse no. 35)

46. One recipe in the form of Tusodaka (sour drink prepared of husked)

47. One recipe in the form of Sura (alcohol) (vide verse no. 35)

48. One recipe to be prepared along with kampillaka and (vide verse no. 35)

49. Five recipes to be prepared in the form of medicated ghee.

["Panca Ghritha Smrtah"] in the text appears to be an error because such five recipes of medicated ghee are not found in the text. Only three recipes of medicated fat are described in verse nos, 9-10 which are already enumerated in item nos. 11- 13 above.].

Summary of Contents

दन्तीद्रवन्तीकल्पेऽस्मिन् प्रोक्ताः षोडशकास्त्रयः| नानाविधानां योगानां भक्तिदोषामयान्प्रति||४०||

In this dealing with the "Pharamaceutics of Danti and Dravanti", three groups each containing sixteen recipes, have been described to suit the likings of the patient, Doshas aggravated and diseases to be treated. [40]

Summary of Kalpa- section

त्रिशतं पञ्चपञ्चाशद्योगानां वमने स्मृतम्| द्वे शते नवकाः पञ्च योगानां तु विरेचने||४१||

ऊर्ध्वानुलोमभागानामित्युक्तानि शतानि षट्|प्राधान्यतः समाश्रित्य द्रव्याणि दश पञ्च च||४२||

In this Kalpa- section, 355 recipes for emesis and 245 recipes for purgation, thus taken together six hundred in total, are described for the purification of the body (by elimination of Doshas) through upward and downward tracts. These recipes are mainly composed of fifteen drugs. [41-42]

Recapitulation

भवन्ति चात्र-

यदि येन प्रधानेन द्रव्यं समुपसृज्यते| तत्सञ्ज्ञकः स योगो वै भवतीति विनिश्चयः ||४३||

फलादीनां प्रधानानां गुणभूताः सुरादयः| ते हि तान्यनुवर्तन्ते मनुजेन्द्रामिवेतरे||४४||

The recipes are invariably named after the principal (most active) drugs used in their composition.

Alcohol, etc, used along with the principal ingredients like Madanaphala, etc., play a secondary role. Their effects follow the attributes of the principal ingredients used in the recipe as the attendants follow the king. [43- 44]

Similarity or Dissimilarity of Potency:

विरुद्धवीर्यमप्येषां प्रधानानामबाधकम्| अधिकं तुल्यवीर्ये हि क्रियासामर्थ्यमिष्यते ||४५||

Sometimes the drugs of secondary nature have antagonistic potency. Even then they do not contradict the effects of the principal drug. If these drugs of secondary nature are similar in potency as that of the principal drugs, then the recipe becomes all the more effective theoretically. [45]

Need for using drugs of dissimilar potency:

इष्टवर्णरसस्पर्शगन्धार्थं प्रति चामयम्| अतो विरुद्धवीर्याणां प्रयोग इति निश्चितम्||४६||

Drugs of antagonistic potency are added to a recipe in order to impart desirable colour, taste, touch and smell. Such addition also helps to effectively cure diseases. [46]

Needs for impregnation:

भूयश्चैषां बलाधानं कार्यं स्वरसभावनैः| सुभावितं ह्यल्पमपि द्रव्यं स्याद्बहुकर्मकृत्||४७||

स्वरसैस्तुल्यवीर्यैर्वा तस्माद्द्रव्याणि भावयेत्|४८|

In addition to adding to the potency of the recipe, it is necessary to impregnate the ingredients of a recipe with the juice or decoction of other drugs. When properly impregnated, even a small quantity of the drug becomes exceedingly effective. Therefore, ingredients of a recipe are impregnated with the juice or decoction of other ingredients having identical potency. [47- ½ 48]

Modification of effects of recipe:

अल्पस्यापि महार्थत्वं प्रभूतस्याल्पकर्मताम्||४८|| कुर्यात् संयोगविश्लेषकालसंस्कारयुक्तिभिः|४९|

By virtue of appropriate Samyoga (addition of ingredients), Vislesa (elimination of ingredients), Kala (appropriate time of administration) and Samskra (processing) even a small quantity of a drug may produce more powerful effects, and otherwise even a recipe in large quantity may produce very mild effects. [48 ½ - ½ 49]

Innumerability of Recipes:

प्रदेशमात्रमेतावद्द्रष्टव्यमिह षट्शतम्||४९|| स्वबुद्ध्यैवं सहस्राणि कोटीर्वाऽपि प्रकल्पयेत्|

बहुद्रव्यविकल्पत्वाद्योगसङ्ख्या न विद्यते||५०||

Six hundred recipes for emesis and purgation, described in this section, are only a fraction of the total number of such recipes. The physician, according to his own wisdom, may prepare thousands and billions of such recipes because the permutation and combination of ingredients are innumerable. Therefore, there is no limit to these recipes. [49 ½ - 50]

Three Categories of Recipe

तीक्ष्णमध्यमृदूनां तु तेषां शृणुत लक्षणम्|

Recipes for emesis and purgation are of three categories, viz, Tikshna (strong or sharp), Madhya (Moderate) and Mrdu (mild). Their characteristic features will be described which you may listen to (addressed to the disciple Agnivesha). [½ 51]

Characteristics of Tikshna recipe

सुखं क्षिप्रं महावेगमसक्तं यत् प्रवर्तते||५१|| नातिग्लानिकरं पायौ हृदये न च रुक्करम्|

अन्तराशयमक्षिण्वन् कृत्स्नं दोषं निरस्यति||५२|| विरेचनं निरूहो वा तत्तीक्ष्णमिति निर्दिशेत्||५३|

Strong type of recipe for emesis, purgation as well as Niruha type of enema has the following characteristics:

It causes purgation and emesis easily, quickly and with strong force;

The morbid material does not get adhered to the gastrointestinal tract;

It does not cause excessive fatigue of the anal region;

It does not cause pain in the cardiac region;

It does not cause any erosion in the gastro-intestinal tract and

It eliminates the morbid material in its entirety. [51 1/2- ½ 53]

Factors Responsible for Making a Recipe Strong

जलाग्निकीटैरस्पृष्टं देशकालगुणान्वितम्||५३|| ईषन्मात्राधिकैर्युक्तं तुल्यवीर्यैः सुभावितम्|

स्नेहस्वेदोपपन्नस्य तीक्ष्णत्वं याति भेषजम्||५४||

The following factors are responsible for increasing the strength of a recipe:

• the ingredients not being impaired by exposure to water, fire and insects;

• the ingredients being imbibed with the beneficial attributes of the soil and season;

• the recipe should have been administered in a slightly higher dose

• the ingredients being appropriately impregnated with drugs having similar potency and

• the patient having been administered with oleation and fomentation therapies. [53 ½ - 54]

Characteristics of Madhya (Moderate) Type of Recipe

किञ्चिदेभिर्गुणैर्हीनं पूर्वोक्तैर्मात्रया तथा| स्निग्धस्विन्नस्य वा सम्यङ्मध्यं भवति भेषजम्||५५||

Recipes having ingredients which are slightly inferior in the above-mentioned characteristics and administered in a lesser dose to a person who has undergone oleation and fomentation therapies appropriately produce moderate effect. [55]

Characteristics of Recipes having Mrdu (Mild) effect

मन्दवीर्यं विरूक्षस्य हीनमात्रं तु भेषजम्|अतुल्यवीर्यैः संयुक्तं मृदु स्यान्मन्दवेगवत्||५६||

Recipes are categorized as mild (Mrdu) when they cause slow urge of emesis and purgation because of the following:

the ingredients are of low potency

the ingredients are of contradictory potencies

the recipe is administered in small doe and

the recipe is administered to a patient who has un-unctuousness (i.e has not been properly oleated) [56]

Suitability of Different Categories of Recipes for different Types of Patients

अकृत्स्नदोषहरणादशुद्धी ते बलीयसाम्|मध्यावरबलानां तु प्रयोज्ये सिद्धिमिच्छता||५७||

Recipes of moderate and mild categories do not cause purification of a patient with strongly aggravated Doshas as these are too mild to eliminate morbid matter (Doshas) in its entirety.

A physician desirous of professional success should administer such therapies only to patients with moderately or mildly aggravated Doshas. [57]

Selection of Recipes for Different Categories of Diseases:

तीक्ष्णो मध्यो मृदुर्व्याधिः सर्वमध्याल्पलक्षणः| तीक्ष्णादीनि बलावेक्षी भेषजान्येषु योजयेत्||५८||

Strong, moderate and mild diseases are characterised by the manifestation of all the symptoms, manifestation of only some symptoms which are moderate in nature, and manifestation of only few symptoms which are of mild nature respectively. For such strong, moderate and mild diseases, therapies of strong, moderate and mild nature are to be used respectively provided the patient is strong, of moderate strength, or of mild strength. [The patient who is strong is given strong therapy, the one who is of moderate strength is given moderate therapy, and the patient who is of mild strength is given mild therapy. [58]

Repeated use of therapy

देयं त्वनिर्हृते पूर्वं पीते पश्चात् पुनः पुनः| भेषजं वमनार्थीयं प्राय आपितदर्शनात्||५९||

Dosha is not eliminated [completely], then it (same recipe) is administered again (to the patient) till there is the appearance of bile (in the vomited material). [59]

Exceptions to this General Rule

बलत्रैविध्यमालक्ष्य दोषाणामातुरस्य च| पुनः प्रदद्याद्भैषज्यं सर्वशो वा विवर्जयेत्||६०||

After ascertaining three different types of the strength of the Doshas (morbid material) and that of the patient, the recipes (of appropriate category) are administered repeatedly. However, if the patient is weak and the disease is of mild nature, then the therapy may be avoided altogether. [60]

Administration of Another Recipe

निर्हृते वाऽपि जीर्णे वा दोषनिर्हरणे बुधः|भेषजेऽन्यत्प्रयुञ्जीत प्रार्थयन्सिद्धिमुत्तमाम्||६१||

If the recipe administered for elimination of Doshas itself gets eliminated or gets digested (without eliminating the Dosha), then another recipe is administered to the patient by a wise physician desirous of professional success. [61]

Necessity to prevent Digestion of Emetic Recipe

अपक्वं वमनं दोषं पच्यमानं विरेचनम्| निर्हरेद्वमनस्यातः पाकं न प्रतिपालयेत्||६२||

An emetic recipe produces emesis only when it is not digested. A purgative recipe causes purgation during the process of its digestion. Therefore, the physician should not lose any time after the recipe is digested [and administer another recipe immediately] [62]

Digestion of Purgative Recipe

पीते प्रसंसने दोषान्न निर्हत्य जरां गते| वमिते चौषधे धीरः पाययेदौषधं पुनः||६३||

If a purgative recipe itself gets digested or gets eliminated by vomiting without eliminating the Doshas (morbid material), [even] then an intelligent physician should administer the purgative recipe again (on the same day).

Repetition of Therapy for strong and weak Patients

दीप्ताग्निं बहुदोषं तु दृढस्नेहगुणं नरम्| दुःशुद्धं तदहर्भुक्तं श्वोभूते पाययेत् पुनः||६४||

दुर्बलो बहुदोषश्च दोषपाकेन यो नरः| विरिच्यते शनैर्भोज्यैर्भूयस्तमनुसारयेत् [१] ||६५||

If a person who has strong digestion, who has more of aggravated Doshas and whose body is strongly unctuous is not fully cleansed of morbid material, then he may be given food on that day, and on the second day, he is given purgation therapy again.

If a weak patient has aggravated Doshas (morbid material) in large quantity, and his Doshas have developed the tendency to undergo Paka (metabolic transformation) leading to purgation, then only giving him food (which causes downward movement of wind in the colon) will again help in slow purgation. [64-65]

Treatment of Residual Doshas

वमनैश्च विरेकैश्च विशुद्धस्याप्रमाणतः | भोजनान्तरपानाभ्यां दोषशेषं शमं नयेत्||६६||

If a person is not fully cleansed by emesis or purgation then the residual Doshas (morbid material) may be alleviated by the appropriate diet like gruel and anta-pana (decoctions of drugs) which stimulate the power of digestion. [66]

Persons to be given mild recipe

दुर्बलं शोधितं पूर्वमल्पदोषं च मानवम्| अपरिज्ञातकोष्ठं च पाययेतौषधं मृदु||६७||

Persons who are weak, who have undergone the process of purification earlier, who have less aggravated Doshas and whose bowel condition is not known are given purificatory recipes of mild nature. [67]

Preference for Milder recipes

श्रेयो मृद्वसकृत्पीतमल्पबाधं निरत्ययम्| न चातितीक्ष्णं यत् क्षिप्रं जनयेत्प्राणसंशयम्||६८||

Mild recipes give less discomfort and do not involve any risk. Therefore, it is better to take such mild recipes if required even frequently than strong recipes which may cause immediate danger to life. [68]

Essentiality of Purification

दुर्बलोऽपि महादोषो विरेच्यो बहुशोऽल्पशः| मृदुभिर्भेषजैर्दोषा हन्युह्र्येनमनिर्हृताः||६९||

If the Doshas are excessively aggravated then even a weak person is given therapeutic doses administered in small Doses, but very frequently with the ingredients having mild effects. If the Doshas are not eliminated, then these may cause death of the patient. [69]

Emetic effects of Purgative Drugs

यस्योध्वं कफसंसृष्टं पीतं यात्यानुलोमिकम्| वमितं कवलैः शुद्धं लङ्घितं पाययेतु तम्||७०||

A purgative recipe may get mixed up with kapha and move upwards. This may cause vomiting. To such patients, emetic therapy and Kavala (gargling therapy) is administered for the elimination of (lit, purification) kapha. He is made to fast, and thereafter, the purgative potion is given to him. [70]

Management of Complications

विबद्धेऽल्पे चिराद्दोषे स्रवत्युष्णं पिबेज्जलम्| तेनाध्मानं तृषा च्छर्दिर्विबन्धश्चैव शाम्यति||७१||

भेषजं दोषरुद्धं चेन्नोर्ध्वं नाधः प्रवर्तते| सोद्गारं साङ्गशूलं च स्वेदं तत्रावचारयेत्||७२||

If the morbid Doshas get obstructed or get eliminated in small quantities or get eliminated after a long time, then hot water is given to the patient for drinking. [Apart from correcting the above-mentioned defects], it relieves flatulence, morbid thirst, vomiting and constipation.

At times, the medicine gets obstructed by morbid Doshas and moves either upwards or downwards. Such a condition gets associated with eructation and bodyache. In such cases, fomentation therapy is administered. [71-72]

Elimination of Residual Medicaments

सुविरिक्ते तु सोद्गारमाश्वेवौषधमुल्लिखेत्| अतिप्रवर्तनं जीर्णे सुशीतैः स्तम्भयेद्भिषक्||७३||

If a person who has been well purged continues to have eructation, the residual medicament inside the gatro-intestinal tract is eliminated by emesis. If after the digestion of the recipe, there is excess of purgation, then it is stopped by excessively using cooling ingredients. [73]

Delayed action

कदाचिच्छ्लेष्मणा रुद्धं तिष्ठत्युरसि भेषजम्| क्षीणे श्लेष्मणि सायाह्ने रात्रौ वा तत्प्रवर्तते||७४||

At times, the recipe being obstructed by Kapha remains in the chest (oesophagus). It produces its effects when Kapha gets diminished either in the evening or at night. [74]

Repetition of Dose

रूक्षानाहारयोर्जीर्णे विष्टभ्योर्ध्वं गतेऽपि वा| वायुना भेषजे त्वन्यत् सस्नेहलवणं पिबेत्||७५||

If because of un-unctuouness (dryness) or fasting, medicine gets digested or if because of aggravated Vayu, it moves upwards along with flatulence, then another dose of the recipe is given to the patient along with unctuous ingredients and salt. [75]

Use of Pitta-alleviating Medicines

तृष्णामोहभ्रममूर्च्छायाः स्युश्चेज्जीर्यति भेषजे| पित्तघ्नं स्वादु शीतं च भेषजं तत्र शस्यते||७६||

If during the digestion of medicines there is morbid thirst, stupor, giddiness or fainting, then Pitta alleviating medicines which are sweet and cooling are given. [76]

Use of Kapha- alleviating medicines

लालाहृल्लासविष्टम्भलोमहर्षाः कफावृते| भेषजं तत्र तीक्ष्णोष्णं कट्वादि कफनुद्धितम्||७७||

If there is salivation, nausea, intestinal stasis and horripilition because of the medication getting covered up by kapha, then the patient is given Kapha alleviating drugs which are sharp, hot, pungent, etc.

Fasting Therapy:

सुस्निग्धं क्रूरकोष्ठं च लङ्घयेद्विरेचितम्| तेनास्य स्नेहजः श्लेष्मा सङ्गश्चैवोपशाम्यति||७८||

If there is no purgation even after the patient has undergone appropriate oleation therapy because of Krurakostha (constipation/ hard bowel) then the patient is made to fast. As a result of this, his Kapha aggravated by oleation therapy and its adherence to the body gets alleviated. [78]

Digestion of Recipe

रूक्ष-बहुवनिल-क्रूरकोष्ठ-व्यायामशालिनाम् दीप्ताग्नीनां च भैषज्यमविरिच्यैव जीर्यति||७९||

तेभ्यो बस्तिं पुरा दत्त्वा पश्चाद्दद्यादि्विरेचनम्| बस्तिप्रवर्तितं [?] दोषं हरेच्छीघ्रं विरेचनम्||८०||

Because of un-unctuousness (dryness) of the body, aggravation of Vayu, Krura- Kostha (constipation / hard nature of the bowel), habitual exercise and strong power of digestion, a recipe may get digested without causing purgation. To such patient's, medicated enema is given prior to the administration of purgation therapy. By this medicated enema, the morbid Doshas get excited and the recipe of purgation eliminates the morbid Doshas quickly. [79-80]

Persons unsuitable for elimination therapy:

रूक्षाशनाः कर्मनित्या ये नरा दीप्तपावकाः| तेषां दोषाः क्षयं यान्ति कर्मवातातपाग्निभिः ||८१||

विरुद्धाध्यशनाजीर्णदोषानपि सहन्ति ते| स्नेह्यास्ते मारुताद्रक्ष्या नाव्याधौ तान् विशोधयेत् [२] ||८२||

In persons who indulge in non-unctuous (dry) food, who are accustomed to physical exercise and whose power of digestion is very strong, the aggravated Doshas get dismissed by the influence of exercise and exposure to wind, sun as well as fire. They are capable of tolerating the effects of an antagonistic diet, intake of food before the previous meal has been digested and indigestion. Such patients are given oleation therapy, and are protected from the aggravation of Vayu. They are protected from the aggravation of Vayu. They should not be given purgation therapy unless they are affected by a (serious) disease. [81-82]

Unctuous and Ununctuous Type of Purgation

नातिस्निग्धशरीराय दद्यात् स्नेहविरेचनम्|स्नेहोत्क्लिष्टशरीराय रूक्षं दद्यादि्वरेचनम्||८३||

Unctuous type of purgation therapy is not to be given to a person whose body is excessively unctuous. To the person whose whole body is saturated with unctuousness, a non-unctuous type of purgation is given. [83]

Appropriate Administration of Purgation Therapy

एवं ज्ञात्वा विधिं धीरो देशकालप्रमाणवित्| विरेचनं विरेच्येभ्यः प्रयच्छन्नापराध्यति||८४||

A wise physician who is acquainted with the above-mentioned procedure (for the administration of purgation including emetic therapies), and who is well- versed with the nature of the land, seasons and dosage, does not commit errors in the administration of purgation including emetic therapies to persons for whom these therapies are indicated. [84]

Proper administration of therapies

विभ्रंशो विषवद्यस्य सम्यग्योगो यथाऽमृतम्| कालेष्ववश्यं पेयं च तस्माद्यत्नात् प्रयोजयेत्||८५||

Purgation including emetic therapies work like poison if inappropriately administered. If properly administered, these work like ambrosia.

It is essential to administer these therapies at the time of need. Therefore, these therapies are to be administered carefully. [85]

Dosage

द्रव्यप्रमाणं तु यदुक्तमस्मिन्मध्येषु तत् कोष्ठवयोबलेषु| तन्मूलमालम्ब्य भवेदि्वकल्प्यं तेषां विकल्प्योऽभ्यधिकोनभावः||८६||

The dosage of recipes described in this section is with reference to persons having moderate type of Kostha (nature of bowel movement), age and strength. Keeping this standard in view, changes in the dosage could be done either by its increases or decreases. [86]

Table of weights and Measures:

षड् ध्वंशयस्तु मरीचिः स्यात् षण्मरीच्यस्तु सर्षपः|अष्टौ ते सर्षपा रक्तास्तण्डुलश्चापि तद्द्वयम्||८७||

धान्यमाषो भवेदेको धान्यमाषद्वयं यवः| अण्डिका ते तु चत्वारस्ताश्चतस्रस्तु माषकः||८८||

हेमश्च धान्यकश्चोक्तो भवेच्छाणस्तु ते त्रयः| शाणौ द्वौ द्रङ्क्षणं विद्यात् कोलं बदरमेव च||८९||

विद्याद्द्वौ द्रङ्क्षणौ कर्षं सुवर्णं चाक्षमेव च| बिडालपदकं चैव पिचुं पाणितलं तथा||९०||

तिन्दुकं च विजानीयात् कवलग्रहमेव च| द्वे सुवर्णे पलार्धं स्याच्छुक्तिरष्टमिका तथा||९१||

द्वे पलार्धे पलं मुष्टिः प्रकुञ्चोऽथ चतुर्थिका| बिल्वं षोडशिका चाम्रं द्वे पले प्रसृतं विदुः||९२||

अष्टमानं तु विज्ञेयं कुडवौ द्वौ तु मानिका| पलं चतुर्गुणं विद्यादञ्जलिं कुडवं तथा||९३||

चत्वारः कुडवाः प्रस्थश्चतुःप्रस्थमथाढकम्| पात्रं तदेव विज्ञेयं कंसः प्रस्थाष्टकं तथा||९४||

कंसश्चतुर्गुणो द्रोणश्चार्मणं नल्वणं च तत्| स एव कलशः ख्यातो घटमुन्मानमेव च||९५||

द्रोणस्तु द्विगुणः शूर्पो विज्ञेयः कुम्भ एव च| गोणी शूर्पद्वयं विद्यात् खारीं भारं तथैव च||९६||

द्वात्रिंशतं विजानीयाद्वाहं शूर्पाणि बुद्धिमान्| तुलां शतपलं विद्यात् परिमाणविशारदः||९७||

शुष्कद्रव्येष्विदं मानमेवमादि प्रकीर्तितम्|९८|

The tables of weights and measures used in Ayurveda is as follows:

(The basic weight is Dhvamsi which is also called trasarenu. According to some physicians, it is also called Dhuli or a floating dust particle)

6 Dhvamsis make one Marici

6 maricis make one (rakta) Sarapa (lit. red mustard seed);

8 Rakta- Sarasapas make one Tandula (lit grain of rice)

2 Tandulas make one Dhanya- Masa (lit black gram)

2 Dhanya-Masas make one Yava (lit. Grain of Barley)

4 Yavas make one Andika.

4 Andikas make one MAssaka (Masa); [it is equivalent to 1 Gram}; its synonyms are Hema and Dhanyaka

3 Masas make one Sana; (It is equivalent to 3 grams)

2 Sanas make on Dranksana; (it is equivalent to grams); its synonyms are Kola and Badara;

2 Dranksanas make one Karsa (It is equivalent to 12 grams); its synonyms are Suvarna, Aksa, Bidala- Padaka, Picu, Pani-tala, Tinduka and Kavala- Graha

2 Suvarnas (Karsas) make one Palardha, i.e half Pala; its is equivalent to 48 grams); its synonyms are Musti, Prakunca, caturthika, Biva, Sodasika and Amra;

2 palardha make One Pala; (it is equivalent to 48 grams); its synonyms are Musti, Prakunca, Caturthika, Bulva, Sodasika and Amra.

2 Palas make one Prasrta; (it is equivalent to 96 grams); its synonym is Astamana

4 Palas make one Anjali; (it is equivalent to192 grams) its synonym is Kudava

2 Kudavas make one Manika; (it is equivalent to 384 grams);

4 Kuduvas make one Prastha; (it is equivalent to 768 grams)

4 Prasthas make one Adhaka; (it is equivalent to 3.072 kilograms); its synonyms is Patra

2 Adhakas (8 Prasthas) make one Kamsa; (it is equivalent to 6.144 kilograms)

4 kamsas make one Drona; (it is equivalent to 24.576 kilograms); its synonymous are Armana, Nalvana, Kalasa, Ghata and Unmana.

2 Dronas make one Surpa; (it is equivalent to 49. 152 kilograms); its synonym is Kumbha;

2 Supas make one Goni; (It is equivalent to 98. 304 kilograms); its synonyms are Khari and Dhara;

32 surpas make one Vaha; (it is equivalent to 1572. 864 kilograms and

100 palas make one Tula; (it is equivalent to 4.800 kilograms).

The above mentioned and such other weights and measures are applicable to dried articles and food ingredients. [87-½ 98]

Doubling the quantity of Liquids and fresh drugs

द्विगुणं तद्द्रवेष्विष्टं तथा सद्योद्धृतेषु च||९८|| यदिध मानं तुला प्रोक्ता पलं वा तत् प्रयोजयेत्

अनुक्ते परिमाणे तु तुल्यं मानं प्रकीर्तितम्||९९||

Liquids are freshly collected. Herbs are taken in double the prescribed quantity for a recipe.

If, in a recipe, the unit of measurement is described in the form of Tula or Pala, then the drug of the same weight (without any change) is used.

When the weight of the ingredients in a recipe is not specified, then all these ingredients should be taken in equal quantities. [98 ½- 99]

Use of water

द्रवकार्येऽपि चानुक्ते सर्वत्र सलिलं स्मृतम्| यतश्च पादनिर्देशश्चतुर्भागस्ततश्च सः||१००||

Some recipes are prepared by processing with liquids. If the type of liquid is not specified, then invariably water has to be used for the preparation of such recipes.

When the quantity of the ingredients is specified as Pada (lit. foot) then this implies one fourth in quantity of the main ingredients in the recipe. [100]

Proportion of Ingredients in preparation of Medicated Ghee, etc:

जलस्नेहौषधानां तु प्रमाणं यत्र नेरितम् |तत्र स्यादौषधात् स्नेहः स्नेहात्तोयं चतुर्गुणम्||१०१||

If in a recipe of medicated ghee or medicated oil, the quantities of water (liquid), fat (ghee or Oil) and other drugs (to be used in the form of paste) are not specified, then the paste of drugs is one part, the fat (oil or ghee) is four parts and water (including decoction, juice, milk etc) is sixteen parts, i.e. the fat is four times in quantity of the paste, and water, decoction, etc., is four times in quantity of the fat. [101]

Three types of paka (cooking)

स्नेहपाकस्त्रिधा ज्ञेयो मृदुर्मध्यः खरस्तथा| तुल्ये कल्केन निर्यासे भेषजानां मृदुः स्मृतः||१०२||

संयाव इव निर्यासे मध्यो दर्वीं विमुञ्चति| शीर्यमाणे तु निर्यासे वर्तमाने [१] खरस्तथा||१०३||

Medicated ghee or medicated oil is prepared according to three different types of Paka (cooking), Viz., Mrdu-Paka (mild cooking), Madhya –Paka (moderate cooking) and Khara –Paka (hard or strong cooking).

When the liquid fraction of the recipe including the paste takes the consistency of Samyava or Gruel (a preparation of ghee, jaggery and broken pieces of wheat in a bolus form), and when the liquid including the paste slides down from the ladle, then this is called Madhya-Paka or moderate cooking,

If the liquid along with the paste snaps when rolled by fingers, it is called Khara-Paka (strong or hard cooking). [102-103]

Therapeutic effects of Medicated Oil Prepared According to Three Types of Paka:

खरोऽभ्यङ्गे स्मृतः पाको, मृदुर्नस्तःक्रियासु च| मध्यपाकं तु पानार्थे बस्तौ च विनियोजयेत्||१०४||

Medicated oil, etc, prepared according to Khara-paka (strong or hard cooking) are useful for massage. Those prepared according to Mrdu-Paka (mild cooking) are useful for inhalation / errhine therapy. Those prepared according to Madhya-Paka (moderate cooking) are useful for being taken internally as a potion and also for medicated enema. [104]

Two traditions for Weights and Measures

मानं च द्विविधं प्राहुः कालिङ्गं मागधं तथा| कालिङ्गान्मागधं श्रेष्ठमेवं मानविदो विदुः||१०५||

Weights and measures are two different types, viz, Kalinga (those traditionally used in the ancient land of Kalinga – Part of present Orissa) and Magadha (those traditionally used in the ancient land of Magadha - part of present-day Bihar). The latter is better than the former. [105]

Summary of Kalpa section

तत्र श्लोकौ-

कल्पार्थः शोधनं सञ्ज्ञा पृथग्घेतुः प्रवर्तने| देशादीनां फलादीनां गुणा योगशतानि षट्||१०६||

विकल्पहेतुर्नामानि तीक्ष्णमध्याल्पलक्षणम्| विधिश्चावस्थिको मानं स्नेहपाकश्च दर्शितः||१०७||

To sum up; - The topics discussed in the Kalpa section are as follows:

Objects of Pharmaceutical process (vide Kalpa 1:3)

Definition of purificatory procedure (vide Kalpa 1:4)

Raison d' enter of the effects of drugs; (vide Kalpa 1:5)

Characteristics of land etc.; (vide Kalpa 1: 7- 11)

Attributes of Madana-Phala etc. (vide Kalpa 1:12)
Six hundred recipes (vide kalpa 12:41-42)
Purpose of Vikalpa (vide kalpa 1:6)
Synonyms of Drugs (vide Kalpa 1:27; 2:3; 3: 3-4; 4:3; 5: 4; 6:3; 7:4; 8:3; 9:3; 10:8; 11:3; 12:3)
Characteristics of recipes having sharp, moderate and mild actions (vide kalpa 12: 51-56)
Management of different types of morbidities; (vide Kalpa 12-59- 85)
Weights and measures and (vide kalpa 12: 87-99, 105)
Methods of preparing medicated oil and ghee; (vide Kalpa 12: 100-104) {106-107]

Colophon

इत्यग्निवेशकृते तन्त्रे चरकप्रतिसंस्कृतेऽप्राप्ते दृढबलसम्पूरिते कल्पस्थाने दन्तीद्रवन्तीकल्पो नाम द्वादशोऽध्यायः||१२||

Thus, ends the twelfth chapter of kalpa-sthana dealing with the "pharmaceutics of Danti and Dravanti" in Agnivesha's work as redacted by Charaka, and because of its non- availability, supplemented by Drdhabala.

इति चरकसंहितायां सप्तमं कल्पस्थानं सम्पूर्णम्|

Thus, ends the seventh section of Charaka Samhitha called Kalpa- Sthana.

सिद्धिस्थानम् Siddhi Sthanam

26

Siddhisthana Chapter 1 Kalpana Siddhi

Prologue

अथातः कल्पनासिद्धिं व्याख्यास्यामः||१|| इति ह स्माह भगवानात्रेयः||२||

Now we shall expound the chapter dealing with "the Procedure for successful administration of PanchaKarma". Thus, said Lord Atreya. [1-2]

Queries of Agniveshaका कल्पना पञ्चसु कर्मसूक्ता, क्रमश्च कः, किं च कृताकृतेषु|

लिङ्गं तथैवातिकृतेषु, सङ्ख्या का, किङ्गुणः, केषु च कश्च बस्तिः||३||

किं वर्जनीयं प्रतिकर्मकाले, कृते कियान् वा परिहारकालः|

प्रणीयमानश्च न याति केन, केनैति शीघ्रं, सुचिराच्च बस्तिः||४||

साध्या गदाः स्वैः शमनैश्च केचित् कस्मात् प्रयुक्तैर्न शमं व्रजन्ति|

प्रचोदितः शिष्यवरेण सम्यगित्यग्निवेशेन भिषग्वरिष्ठः||५||

पुनर्वसुस्तन्त्रविदाह तस्मै सर्वप्रजानां हितकाम्ययेदम्|६|

Agnivesha, the foremost among the disciplines (of Punarvasu Atreya) puts his queries before his preceptor. They are as follows:

What is the prescribed procedure for the administration of Panchakarma (five specialised therapies)? [The answer will be provided in the verse nos.6 2/4 – 2/4 10]

In which order these five therapies should be administered? [The answer will be provided in verse nos. 10 2/4- 2/4 15]

What are the signs of proper, improper and excessive administration of these therapies? [The answer will be provided in the verse nos. 15 2/4 – 24, 40 2/4 – 2/4 47]

What number of enemas should be given? [The answer will be provided in the verse nos. 25-26 and 47 2/4 – 50]

What are the therapeutic effects of medicated enema (Basti)? [The answer will be provided in the verse nos. 27- 34, 38- 2/4 40]

What type of Basti (medicated enema) is useful for which type of disease? [The answer will be provided in the verse nos. 36-37]

What should be avoided during the course of the treatment? [The answer will be provided in the verse nos. 54 2/4- 2/4 55]

What is the interval between the administrations of different therapies? [The answer will be provided in the verse no. 2/4 54]

What is the reason for the enema not entering into the rectum after having administered? [The answer will be provided in verse no. 55 2/4- 2/4 56]

What makes the recipe of enema to come out earlier than the scheduled time? [The answer will be provided in the verse nos. 56 2/4 – 2/4 57]

What is the cause of delay in the evacuation of the administered recipe of medicated enema? And [the answer will be provided in verse no. 2/4 56]

Why do some diseases though curable do not get cured even when recipes for each are administered? [The answer will be provided in verse nos. 57 2/4- 2/4 59]

In relation to these (above mentioned) questions, Punarvasu, who is the foremost among physicians who is well-versed in scriptures, replied as follows with a view of promoting the welfare of human beings. [3-2/4 6]

Duration of Oleation therapy

त्र्यहावरं सप्तदिनं परं तु स्निग्धो नरः स्वेदयितव्य उक्तः ||६||

नातः परं स्नेहनमादिशन्ति सात्म्यीभवेत् सप्तदिनात् परं तु|७|

To a person who has undergone oleation therapy, the fomentation therapy should be administered. It should be administered continuously for a minimum period of three days, or maximum period of seven days. Oleation therapy is not recommended after the seventh day because by then the person's body gets saturated / accustomed with it. [6 2/4- 2/4 7]

Therapeutic Effects of Oleation Therapy:

स्नेहोऽनिलं हन्ति मृदूकरोति देहं मलानां विनिहन्ति सङ्गम्||७||

Oleation therapy –

alleviates aggravated Vayu,

softens the body and

disintegrates the adhered morbid material [in the channels of oleation] [7 2/4]

Therapeutic effects of Fomentation Therapy:

स्निग्धस्य सूक्ष्मेष्वयनेषु लीनं स्वेदस्तु दोषं नयति द्रवत्वम्|८|

Fomentation liquefies the morbid material adhered even in the fine channels of the body of a person who has undergone oleation therapy. [2/4 8]

Measures for Exciting Morbid material:

ग्राम्यौदकानूपरसैः समांसैरुत्क्लेशनीयः पयसा च वम्यः||८|| रसैस्तथा जाङ्गलजैः सयूषैः स्निग्धैः कफावृद्धिकरैर्विरेच्यः|९|

The person who is to be administered emesis is given milk and meat as well as meat-soup of domesticated animals and animals living in aquatic and wetlands in the form of food for causing excitation of kapha.

The person who is to be given purgation therapy is given soup of the meat of animals inhabiting arid zones and vegetable-soup added with fat to bring about the excitation of Pitta, which also do not cause aggravation of Kapha. [8 2/4 – 2/4 9]

Reasons for emetics and Purgatives Working in Opposite Ways:

श्लेष्मोतरश्छर्दयति ह्यदुःखं विरिच्यते मन्दकफस्तु सम्यक्||९|| अधः कफेऽल्पे वमनं विरेचयेद्विरेचनं वृद्धकफे तथोर्ध्वम्|१०|

A person with excessively aggravated kapha vomits without any difficulty, and the person having less aggravated Kapha purges well. However, if there is less of aggravated kapha, the emetic recipe causes purgation through the downward tract. Similarly, if there is aggravated kapha, the purgative recipe causes emesis through the upward tract. [9 2/4- 2/4 10]

Order of Administering Emetic and purgative Therapies:

स्निग्धाय देयं वमनं यथोक्तं वान्तस्य पेयादिरनुक्रमश्च||१०|| स्निग्धस्य सुस्विन्नतनोर्यथावद्विरेचनं योग्यतमं प्रयोज्यम्|११|

Emetic therapy is administered to a person according to the appropriate procedure (described in Kalpa 1:14) after his body has been subjected to oleation therapy.

After emesis, he is given systematic dietetic regimen (samsarjana-Krama) with Peya (thin gruel), etc.

Thereafter, the person who has undergone oleation and fomentation therapies, is administered the best suited purgation therapy appropriately (ref. Sutra 15:17) 10 2/4 – 2/4 11)

Post- therapeutic Measures (Samsarjana – karma):

पेयां विलेपीमकृतं कृतं च यूषं रसं त्रिद्विर्वरथैकशश्च||११|| क्रमेण सेवेत विशुद्धकायः प्रधानमध्यावरशुद्धिशुद्धः|१२|

After the body is cleansed of the morbidities [by emetic and purgation therapies] the patient is given the below mentioned in the form of food –

Peya (thin gruel),

Vilepi (thick gruel),

Akrta as well as Krta yusa (unseasoned and seconded vegetable juice) and

Artaka as well as Krta-Rasa (unseasoned and seasoned meat-soup)

Each of these dietary items is given for three, two or one meal times to the person whose body is cleansed in accordance with either Pradhana Sudhi (maximum cleansing), Madhya Sudhi (moderate cleansing) or Avara Suddhi (minimum cleaning) respectively. [11 2/4 – 2/4 12]

Effects of Samsarjana- Krama

यथाऽणुरग्निस्तृणगोमयाद्यैः सन्धुक्ष्यमाणो भवति क्रमेण||१२|| महान् स्थिरः सर्वपचस्तथैव शुद्धस्य पेयादिभिरन्तरग्निः|१३|

Just like a small spark of fire gets kindled into a big and stable flame when fed gradually with dry grass, cow-dung cake, etc., the internal fire or the enzymes in the body responsible for digestion and metabolism [which was subdued because of purificatory measures] in a purified person grows to become strong and stable, and becomes capable of digesting all types of food by the [gradual] administration of Peya - thin gruel), etc. dietetic regimen. [12 2/4- 2/4 13]

Characteristics of three Types of Emesis and Purgation

जघन्यमध्यप्रवरे तु वेगाश्चत्वार इष्टा वमने षडष्टौ||१३||

दशैव ते द्विद्विगुणा विरेके प्रस्थस्तथा द्विद्विचतुर्गुणश्च| पित्तान्तमिष्टं वमनं विरेकादर्ध कफान्तं च विरेकमाहुः||१४||

द्विव्रान् सविट्कानपनीय वेगान्मेयं विरेके वमने तु पीतम्|१५|

In emetic therapy - in Jaghanya or Avara sudhi (minimum type of cleansing), Madhya Sudhi (Moderate type of cleansing) and Pravara Sudhi (maximum type of cleansing), the person gets four, six and eight bouts of vomiting respectively.

In purgation therapy - in Jaghanya Sudhi, Madhya Sudhi and Pravara Sudhi, the patient purges for ten, twenty and thirty times respectively. In these three types of Sudhi, the quantity of stool voided by the patient is two, three and four Prasthas respectively.

It is desirable that the emetic therapy should end up with the vomiting of bile. And the vomited material is half of what is described for purgative therapy [by implication, in the Jaghnya Sudhi, Madhya Sudhi and Pravara sudhi, the vomited material is one, and a half, and two Prastha respectively.]

The purgation therapy should end up with the voiding of Kapha (phlegm).

In the case of purgation therapy, the first two or three motions containing faeces should not be taken into account while measuring the quantity of voided material. Similarly, in the case of emetic therapy, the quantity of drugs taken for the therapy is excluded while measuring the vomited material. [13 ½ - 2/4 15]

Signs of appropriately Administered Emetic Therapy

क्रमात् कफः पित्तमथानिलश्च यस्यैति सम्यग्वमितः स इष्टः||१५||

हृत्पार्श्वमूर्धेन्द्रियमार्गशुद्धौ तथा लघुत्वेऽपि च लक्ष्यमाणे|१६|

Below mentioned are the signs of properly administered emetic therapy –

- Expulsion of Kapha (Phlegm), pitta (bile) and Vayu (flatus and wind) in succession,

- Feeling of clarity in heart, sides of the chest, head and channels of circulation,
- Feeling of clarity of the sense organs,
- Feeling of lightness of the body,
- Feeling energetic,
- Promotion of Agni (power of digestion and metabolism),
- Freedom from diseases (caused by Doshas for which the purgation therapy was administered) and
- Expulsion of faeces, Pitta (bile), kapha (phlegm) and Vayu (flatus) in succession (that order)

Signs of Improperly Administered Purgation Therapy:

दुश्छर्दिते स्फोटककोठकण्डूहृत्खाविशुद्धिर्गुरुगात्रतां च||१६||

Improperly administered purgation therapy (i.e., with the recipe of small quantity), gives rise to

sphotaka (postural eruptions),

kotha (urticaria),

kandu (itching),

lack of clarity in the heart as well as

sense organs and heaviness of the body [16 2/4]

Signs of Emetic Therapy Administered in Excess:

तृण्मोहमूर्च्छानिलकोपनिद्राबलादिहानिर्वमनेऽति च स्यात्|१७|

If there is excessive administration of emetic therapy, then the person suffers from –

thirst,

moha (unconsciousness),

murccha (fainting),

aggravation of Vayu,

insomnia,

debility, etc.

Signs of Appropriately Administered Purgation Therapy

स्रोतोविशुद्धीन्द्रियसम्प्रसादौ लघुत्वमूर्जोऽग्निरनामयत्वम्||१७|| प्राप्तिश्च विट्पित्तकफानिलानां सम्यग्विरिक्तस्य भवेत् क्रमेण|१८|

If the purgation therapy is appropriately administered, the following signs are observed –

purity of the channels of circulation,

clarity of the sense organs,

lightness of the body,

feeling energetic,

promotion of Agni (power of digestion and metabolism),

freedom from diseases (caused by Doshas for which the purgation therapy was administered) and expulsion of feces,

pitta (bile), kapha (phlegm) and Vayu (flatus) in succession

Signs of Improperly administered Purgation Therapy:

स्याच्छ्लेष्मपित्तानिलसम्प्रकोपः सादस्तथाऽग्नेर्गुरुता प्रतिश्या||१८||

तन्द्रा तथा च्छर्दिररोचकश्च वातानुलोम्यं न च दुर्विरिक्ते|१९|

Below mentioned are the signs of improperly administered purgation therapy (i.e., with the recipe of small quantity),

excessive aggravation of kapha, Pitta and Vata,

suppression of Agni (power of digestion and metabolism),

heaviness of the body,

coryza,

drowsiness,

vomiting,

anorexia and

absence of downward movement of the flatus [18 2/4- 2/4 19]

Signs of Purgation Therapy Administered in Excess:

कफास्रपित्तक्षयजानिलोत्थाः सुप्त्यङ्गमर्दक्लमवेपनाद्याः||१९||

निद्राबलाभावतमःप्रवेशाः सोन्मादहिक्काश्च विरेचितेऽति|२०|

Below mentioned are the signs of excessive administration of purgation therapy –

ailments caused by the aggravation of vayu as a result of the diminution of kapha, blood as well as Pitta,

numbness,

malaise,

mental fatigue,

tremor, etc.,

insomnia,

debility,

fainting,

insanity and

hiccup [19 2/4- 2/4 20]

Spacing of Therapies

संसृष्टभक्तं नवमेऽहिन सर्पिस्तं पाययेताप्यनुवासयेद्वा||२०||

तैलाक्तगात्राय ततो निरूहं दद्यात्र्यहान्नातिबुभुक्षिताय| प्रस्यागते धन्वरसेन भोज्यः समीक्ष्य वा दोषबलं यथार्हम्||२१||

नरस्ततो निश्यनुवासनार्हो नात्याशितः स्यादनुवासनीयः |२२|

After Samsarjana-Krama (intake of regulated diet), on the ninth day [of emesis], the patient is given a portion of ghee [if purgation therapy is intended to be given subsequently]. [Similarly, on the ninth day of purgation therapy, after Samsajana-Krama, anuvasana, i.e., unctuous enema is given subsequently].

For three days, thereafter, the body of the person is massaged with medicated oil, and then Niruha or evacuative type of medicated enema is given when the person is not very hungry

After the recipe of Niruha (evacuative enema) has come out, the patient is given meat-soup of Jangala type of animals (thosc inhabiting arid forest zone) or any other appropriate diet depending upon the nature of Doshas and the power of agni (enzymes responsible for digestion and metabolism).

Thereafter, when the patient has not taken a heavy meal in the night, Anuvasana or unctuous type of medicated enema is given to him if the patient is fit for such Anuvasana therapy. [20 2/4- 2/4 22]

Time of Anuvasana:

शीते वसन्ते च दिवाऽनुवास्यो रात्रौ शरद्ग्रीष्मघनागमेषु||२२|| तानेव दोषान् परिरक्षता ये स्नेहस्य पाने परिकीर्तिताः प्राक्|२३|

In the winter and spring seasons, Anuvasana or unctuous type of medicated enema is given during the day time; and in autumn, summer as well as rainy season, it is administered during the night time. Care is taken to avoid mistakes as described earlier (vide Sutra 13: 19-21) in respect of the administration of oleation therapy. [22 2/4 – 2/4 23]

Frequency of Anuvasana Therapy

प्रत्यागते चाप्यनुवासनीये दिवा प्रदेयं व्युषिताय भोज्यम्||२३|| सायं च भोज्यं परतो द्व्यहे वा त्र्यहेऽनुवास्योऽहनि पञ्चमे वा [१] |

त्र्यहे त्र्यहे वाऽप्यथ पञ्चमे वा दद्यान्निरूहादनुवासनं च||२४||

After the recipe of Anuvasana has come out of the anal tract, the patient should not take any food at night. During the next day, food is given to him during the day time and in the evening. Thereafter, on the second, third or fifth day, Anuvasana is given. After that, every third- or fifth-days Niruha type of medicated enema is given followed by Anuvasana. [23 2/4- 24]

Number of Anuvasana Basti:

एकं तथा त्रीन् कफजे विकारे पित्तात्मके पञ्चं तु सप्त वाऽपि| वाते नवैकादश वा पुनर्वा बस्तीनयुग्मान् कुशलो विदध्यात्||२५||

In Kaphaja type of diseases the patient is given one or three Bastis (medicated enema). In Paittika type of diseases the patient is given five or seven bastis, and in Vatika type of diseases the patient is given nine or eleven bastis. In this way an expert physician should give Bastis in odd numbers. [25]

Time Gap for Niruha After Purgation and for Purgation After Niruha:

नरो विरिक्तस्तु निरूहदानं विवर्जयेत् सप्तदिनान्यवश्यम्| शुद्धो निरूहेण विरेचनं च तद्ध्यस्य शून्यं विकसेच्छरीरम्||२६||

After purgation, a person should avoid Niruha – Basti, and after niruha basti one should avoid purgation therapy for seven days because it will have injurious effects on the body which is already empty [of nourishing material] by the earlier therapy. [26]

Effects of Niruha-Basti

बस्तिर्वयःस्थापयिता सुखायुर्बलाग्निमेधास्वरवर्णकृच्च| सर्वार्थकारी शिशुवृद्धयूनां निरत्ययः सर्वगदापहश्च||२७||

विट्श्लेष्मपित्तानिलमूत्रकर्षी दाढ्र्यावहः शुक्रबलप्रदश्च| विश्वक्स्थितं दोषचयं निरस्य सर्वान् विकारान् शमयेन्निरूहः||२८||

Niruha –Basti or evacuative type of medicated enema has the following effects:

It prevents aging process of the body;

It promotes happiness, longevity, strength, power of digestion and metabolism, intellect), voice and complexion

It accomplishes all the objects (including mutually contradictory ones like stability or plumpness and emaciation);

It is harmless for infants, old persons and youth;

It helps in curing all diseases

It helps in drawing out faeces, Kapha, Pitta, Vayu and urine;

It promotes sturdiness of the body

It enriches semen and promotes strength and

While eliminating accumulated Doshas (morbid matter) from the entire body, it (Niruha type of enema) alleviates all the diseases. [27-28]

Effects of Anuvasana- Basti:

देहे निरूहेण विशुद्धमार्गे संस्नेहनं वर्णबलप्रदं च| न तैलदानात् परमस्ति किञ्चिद्द्रव्यं विशेषेण समीरणार्ते ||२९||

स्नेहेन रौक्ष्यं लघुतां गुरुत्वादौष्ण्याच्च शैत्यं पवनस्य हत्वा| तैलं ददात्याशु मनःप्रसादं वीर्यं बलं वर्णमथाग्निपुष्टिम् ||३०||

मूले निषिक्तो हि यथा द्रुमः स्यान्नीलच्छदः कोमलपल्लवाग्र्यः| काले महान् पुष्पफलप्रदश्च तथा नरः स्यादनुवासनेन||३१||

The channels of the body get cleansed by Niruha. Administration of Samsnehana or unctuous (anuvasana) type of medicated enema to such a person promotes his complexion and strength. There is no therapy better than the administration of oil (anuvasana-basti) which is especially useful for the patient afflicted with diseases caused by Vayu.

The oil by its unctuousness, heaviness and heating property counteracts the non-unctuousness (dryness), lightness and cooling attributes of Vayu respectively. Because of this, administration of oil (Anuvasana-Basti) instantaneously produces clarity of mind, and promotes energy, strength complexion and Agni (power of digestion and metabolism). Just as a tree irrigated with water at the root produces blue leaves, becomes beautiful with tender leaves, and during the course of time grows to produce flowers and fruits, similarly, a person becomes [young and beautiful with procreative power]by the administration of Anuvasana or unctuous type of medicated enema. [29-31]

Effects of Niruha and Anuvasana in General:

स्तब्धाश्च ये सङ्कुचिताश्च येऽपि ये पङ्गवो येऽपि च भग्नरुग्णाः| येषां च शाखासु चरन्ति वाताः शस्तो विशेषेण हि तेषु बस्तिः||३२||

आध्मापने विग्रथिते पुरीषे शूले च भक्तानभिनन्दने च| एवम्प्रकाराश्च भवन्ति कुक्षौ ये चामयास्तेषु च बस्तिरिष्टः||३३||

याश्च स्त्रियो वातकृतोपसर्गा गर्भं न गृह्णन्ति नृभिः समेताः| क्षीणेन्द्रिया ये च नराः कृशाश्च बस्तिः प्रशस्तः परमं च तेषु||३४||

Basti or medicated enema is especially useful for the following types of persons:

whose limbs have become stiff and contracted;

who are lame

who are afflicted with fractures and dislocations and

whose whole limbs are afflicted by the movement of different types of aggravated vayu

Basti is also useful for the treatment of the following ailments:

Distension of the abdomen by air

Scybalous stool

Colic pain

Disliking for food; and

Such other ailments affecting the pelvic region

Basti is an excellent therapy for women who are afflicted with the complications of Vayu, and who are unable to conceive in spite of mating with their male partners. It is also extremely useful for men having seminal debility and emaciation of the body. [32- 34]

Selection of Basti for Different Type of Patients:

उष्णाभिभूतेषु वदन्ति शीताञ्छीताभिभूतेषु तथा सुखोष्णान्। तत्प्रत्यनीकौषधसम्प्रयुक्तान् सर्वत्र बस्तीन् प्रविभज्य युञ्ज्यात्||३५||

According to experts, [in the administration of Pancha-Karma therapy) cooling basti (medicated enema) is given to the patients suffering from diseases caused by hot ingredients. And lukewarm Basti is given to the patients suffering from diseases caused by cooling ingredients.

In all cases, different types of Basti containing ingredients having attributes opposite to the attributes of the etiological factors of diseases are administered. [35]

Contra –indications for Anuvasana Basti:

न बृंहणीयान् विदधीत बस्तीन् विशोधनीयेषु गदेषु वैद्यः| कुष्ठप्रमेहादिषु मेदुरेषु नरेषु ये चापि विशोधनीयाः||३६||

To the patients needing [depending on type of] elimination therapy, roborant / bulk promoting (Brmhaniya or Anuvasana) type of Basti should not be given. Patients suffering from diseases like Kushta (obstinate skin diseases including leprosy) and Prameha (obstinate urinary diseases including diabetics), and those having adiposity need elimination therapy which is depleting [to such patients, roborant (Brmhaniya) type of Basti should not be given]. [36]

Contra- indication for Niruha-Basti

क्षीणक्षतानां न विशोधनीयान्न शोषिणां नो भृशदुर्बलानाम्| न मूच्छितानां न विशोधितानां येषां च दोषेषु निबद्धमायुः||३७||

Niruha or evacuative type of Basti should not be given to patients suffering from Kstha-Ksina (phthisis), Sosa (consumption), extreme debility and Murccha (fainting), and to those who have already undergone the process of purification, and to those life is dependent upon the holding up of Doshas (morbid matter). [37]

Importance of Basti Therapy:

शाखागताः कोष्ठगताश्च रोगा मर्मोर्ध्वसर्वावयवाङ्गजाश्च|ये सन्ति तेषां न हि कश्चिदन्यो वायोः परं जन्मनि हेतुरस्ति||३८||

विण्मूत्रपित्तादिमलाशयानां विक्षेपसङ्घातकरः स यस्मात्| तस्यातिवृद्धस्य शमाय नान्यद्बस्तिं विना भेषजमस्ति किञ्चित्||३९||

तस्माच्चिकित्सार्धमिति ब्रुवन्ति सर्वां चिकित्सामपि बस्तिमेके|४०|

There is none other than Vayu which is the most important causative factor of diseases in Sakha (peripheral tissue elements), Kostha (Visceras of the Thorax and Abdomen) (the body), Sarvavayava (covering the entire body) and Anga (individual parts of the body).

Vayu is responsible for the separation (Viksepa=Vibhaga) and combination (sanghata=Samyoga) of stool, urine, Pitta, (Kapha), including other excreta and tissue elements (Asaya: normally meaning receptacle, which has been interpreted by Chakrapani as tissue elements]. When vata gets exceedingly aggravated there is no remedy other than

Basti for its alleviation.

Therefore, Basti is considered by physicians to be half of the entire therapeutic measures. Some physicians even go to the extent of suggesting that Basti represents (not half but) the whole of therapeutic measures. [38 – 2/4 40]

Definition of Basti:

नाभिप्रदेशं कटिपार्श्वकुक्षिं गत्वा शकृद्दोषचयं विलोड्य ||४०||संस्नेह्य कायं सपुरीषदोषः सम्यक् सुखेनैति च यः स बस्तिः |४१|

The therapy which while moving in the umbilical region, lumbar region, sides of the chest and pelvic region churns up the stool including all the other morbid matter located there, and appropriately, eliminates them (stool and other morbid material) with ease after nourishing (lit. oleating) the body is called Basti. [40 ½ - 2/4 41]

Signs of Appropriately Administered Niruha-Basti:

प्रसृष्टविण्मूत्रसमीरणत्वं रुच्यग्निवृद्ध्याशयलाघवानि||४१|| रोगोपशान्तिः प्रकृतिस्थता च बलं च तत् स्यात् सुनिरूढलिङ्गम्|४२|

The following signs are manifested if niruha basti is appropriately administered:

Appropriate elimination of stool, urine and flatus

Promotion of appetite and agni (power of digestion and metabolism)

Lightness of the Asaya (lit. Receptacle: tissue elements according to the earlier commentary of Cakrapani)

Alleviation of diseases and

Restoration of natural health and strength. [41 2/4- 2/4 42]

Signs of improperly Administered Niruha Basti

स्यादुक्छिरोहृद्गुदबस्तिलिङ्गे शोफः प्रतिश्यायविकर्तिके च||४२|| हृल्लासिका मारुतमूत्रसङ्गः श्वासो न सम्यक् च निरूहिते स्युः|४३|

If the niruha or evacuative type of medicated enema is inappropriately administered (i.e., administered in a smaller dose), then this gives rise to the following signs and symptoms:

Pain in the head, cardiac region, anal region, urinary bladder and oedema of penis, coryza, gripping pain and nausea,

Retention of flatus and urine and

Dyspnoea [42 2/4- 2/4 43]

Signs and symptoms of Niruha Basti excessively administered

लिङ्गं यदेवातिविरेचितस्य भवेत्तदेवातिनिरूहितस्य||४३||

The signs and symptoms of Niruha Basti or evacuative type of medicated enema when used in excess quantity are the same as those caused by the excessive administration of purgation therapy (vide verse no 19 2/4- 2/4 20.

Signs and symptoms of properly administered Anuvasana Basti:

प्रत्येत्यसक्तं सशकृच्च तैलं रक्तादिबुद्धीन्द्रियसम्प्रसादः |स्वप्नानुवृत्तिर्लघुता बलं च सृष्टाश्च वेगाः स्वनुवासिते स्युः||४४||

Proper administration of Anuvasana Basti or unctuous type of medicated enema gives rise to the signs and symptoms as follows:

Return of the recipe containing oil, etc., with faecal matter without any obstruction;

Purity of the tissues, viz, blood, etc.

Clarity of intellect and senses

Good and continuous sleep;

Lightness and strength in the body; and

Proper manifestation of natural urges without any obstruction [44]

Signs and symptoms of improperly administered anuvasana basti

अधःशरीरोदरबाहुपृष्ठपार्श्वेषु रुग्रूक्षखरं च गात्रम् |

ग्रहश्च विण्मूत्रसमीरणानामसम्यगेतान्यनुवासितस्य ||४५||

Improper administration of Anuvasana Basti or unctuous type of medicated enema gives rise to signs and symptoms as follows:

Pain in the lower part of the body, abdomen, arms, back and sides of the chest;

Non-unctuousness (dryness) and roughness of the body; and

Obstruction in the passage of stool, urine and flatus [45]

Signs and Symptoms of excessively administered anuvasana basti:

हृल्लासमोहक्लमसादमूर्च्छाविकर्तिका चात्यनुवासितस्य|४६|

Excessive administration of Anuvasana – Basti or unctuous type of medicated enema gives rise to nausea, unconsciousness, mental fatigue, exhaustion, fainting and gripping pain . [2/4 46]

Duration of retaining anuvasana basti:

यस्येह यामाननुवर्तते त्रीन् स्नेहो नरः स्यात् स विशुद्धदेहः||४६||

आश्वागतेऽन्यस्तु पुनर्विधेयः स्नेहो न संस्नेहयति ह्यतिष्ठन्|४७|

If the unctuous material administered for Anuvasana Basti is retained for three Yamas then the body of the person gets cleansed of morbid material. If it comes out quickly (before nine hours) then another Anuvasana Basti or unctuous type of medicated enema is administered. If the unctuous material is not appropriately retained (in the rectum) then an appropriate unctuous effect is not produced in the body of the person. [46 2/4 – 2/4 47]

Different Types of Basti Therapy:

त्रिंशन्मताः कर्म नु बस्तयो हि कालस्ततोऽर्धन ततश्च योगः||४७||

सान्वासना द्वादश वै निरूहाः प्राक् स्नेह एकः परतश्च पञ्च| काले त्रयोऽन्ते पुरतस्तथैकः स्नेहा निरूहान्तरिताश्च षट् स्युः||४८||

योगे निरूहास्त्रय एव देयाः स्नेहाश्च पञ्चैव परादिमध्याः|४९|

In Karma(n) type, thirty Bastis or enema are administered. In the Kala type of Basti therapy, the number of enema is half of the former [as explained in the commentary is sixteen in number, and not fifteen]. In the yoga type of Basti therapy, the number of enema to be given is half of the former [eight according to Chakrapani].

In **Karma-Basti**, twelve Anuvasanas (unctuous type of enema) and twelve Niruhas (Evacuative type of enema) are administered, one alternating with the other. Before this, one Anuvasana Basti in the beginning, and at the end, five Anuvasana Bastis are administered for the purpose of oleation. [Thus, in total, thirty Bastis are to be given in respect of Karma (n) type]

In **Kala basti**, six Anuvasanas and six Niruhas are given, one alternating with the other. Before this, in the beginning, one anuvasana is given for the purpose of oleation. [Thus, in total, sixteen bastis are to be given in Kala Type].

In **Yoga basti**, three Niruhas are to be given in the beginning, in the middle and at the end, five anuvasana bastis are to be given. [Thus, in this type, eight bastis in total are to be given]. [47 2/ 4- 2/4 49]

Number of anuvasana basti for oleation:

त्रीन् पञ्च वाऽऽहुश्चतुरोऽथ षड्वा वातादिकानामनुवासनीयान् [१] ||४९||

स्नेहान् प्रदायाशु भिषग्विदध्यात् स्रोतोविशुद्यर्थमतो निरूहान्|५०|

Some hold the view that after giving three, five, four or six Anuvasana bastis for the purpose of oleation, to patients suffering from diseases caused by Vayu (Pitta and kalpha) the physician should thereafter, administer Niruha Basti for the cleansing of the [obstructed] Srotas or channels of circulation. [49 2/4- 2/4 50]

Shiro virecana or errhine Therapy:

विशुद्धदेहस्य ततः क्रमेण स्निग्धं तलस्वेदितमुत्तमाङ्गम्||५०||

विरेचयेत्त्रिद्विरथैकशो वा बलं समीक्ष्य त्रिविधं मलानाम्|

When the body of the patient is cleansed, his head is consecutively anointed and fomented with the help of the palm. After ascertaining the strength of the three types of Doshas, he is given errhine therapy, once, twice or thrice. [50 2/ 4 – 2/4 51]

Signs and Symptoms of appropriately administered therapy:

उरःशिरोलाघवमिन्द्रियाच्छ्यं स्रोतोविशुद्धिश्च भवेद्विशुद्धे||५१||

Appropriately administered siro-virecana (errhine) therapy gives rise to lightening of the chest and head, clarity of the senses and cleansing of the srotas (channels of circulation). [51 2/4]

Signs and symptoms of inappropriately administered errhine therapy

गलोपलेपः शिरसो गुरुत्वं निष्ठीवनं चाप्यथ दुर्विरिक्ते|

Inappropriate administration of errhine therapy gives rise to adhesion of sticky material in the throat, heaviness of the head and ptyalism. [2/4 52]

Signs and symptoms of excessively administered Errhine therapy:

शिरोक्षिशङ्खश्रवणार्तितोदावत्यर्थशुद्धे तिमिरं च पश्येत्||५२||

Excessive administration of errhine therapy gives rise to cutting and aching pain in head, eyes temples and ears, and fainting. [52 2/4]

Management of conditions arising out of excessive and inappropriate administration of Errhine therapy:

स्यात्तर्पणं तत्र मृदु द्रवं च स्निग्धस्य तीक्ष्णं तु पुनर्न योगे|५३|

For the management of conditions arising out of excessively administered errhine therapy, the patient is given demulcent drinks and medications which are soft and liquid in nature.

For the management of conditions arising out of inappropriate administration of errhine therapy, the patient is given oleation therapy, and thereafter, sharp type of errhine therapy is given to the patient. [2/4 53]

Utility of Pancha-Karma Therapy:

इत्यातुरस्वस्थसुखः प्रयोगो बलायुषोर्वृद्धिकृदामयघ्नः||५३||

Pancha-Karma (five purificatory therapies) described above bestow happiness to both the patients and healthy persons by promoting their strength and longevity, and also by curing their diseases. [53 2/4]

Interval period between two courses of therapy

कालस्तु बस्त्यादिषु याति यावांस्तावान् भवेद्दि्वः परिहारकालः|५४|

The interval between two courses of Basti (including emetic, purgation and errhine therapies) is double the period for which these therapies were originally administered. [2/4 54]

Prohibitions during Panchakarma Therapies

अत्यासनस्थानवचांसि यानं स्वप्नं दिवा मैथुनवेगरोधान्||५४|| शीतोपचारातपशोकरोषांस्त्यजेदकालाहितभोजनं च|५५|

While undergoing panchakarma therapies, the patient should avoid the following:

Excessive sitting, standing, speaking and riding (over vehicles and horses)

Sleep during day time

Sexual intercourse

Suppression of the manifested natural urges

Cooling regimens

Exposure to hot Sun

Grief and anger and

Intake of urinary and unwholesome food

Factors inhibiting recipes of basti to enter and come out smoothly:

बद्धे प्रणीते विषमं च नेत्रे मार्गे तथाऽर्शःकफविड्विबद्धे ||५५||

न याति बस्तिर्न सुखं निरेति दोषावृतोऽल्पो यदि वाऽल्पवीर्यः|५६|

The recipe of Basti does not reach its destination because of the following:

If the nozzle is clogged or inserted obliquely; and

If the rectal passage is blocked by piles, mucus or hard stool

The recipe after enema does not come out with ease because of the following:

if the path in the enema is obstructed by Doshas

If the recipe of enema is less in quantity and

If the recipe is of low potency [55 2/4- 2/4 56]

Factors Responsible for Quicker Elimination of enema

प्राप्ते तु वर्चोनिलमूत्रवेगे वातेऽतिवृद्धेऽल्पबले गुदे वा||५६|| अत्युष्णतीक्ष्णश्च मृदौ च कोष्ठे प्रणीतमात्रः पुनरेति बस्तिः|५७|

The recipes of enema come out though the anus immediately after it is administered because of the following:

If there is sudden urge for voiding faeces, flatus or urine;

If there is excessive aggravation of vayu,

If there is lack of strength in the anal muscles to retain the recipe

If the recipe contains ingredients which are excessively hot and sharp and

If the person has lax bowel (mrdu kostha) [56 2/4- 2/4 57]

Incapability of Basti to Cure of curable Disease:

मेदःकफाभ्यामनिलो निरुद्धः शूलाङ्गसुप्तिश्वयथून् करोति||५७|| स्नेहं तु युञ्जन्नबुधस्तु तस्मै संवर्धयत्येव हि तान् विकारान्|

रोगास्तथाऽन्येऽप्यवितर्क्यमाणाः परस्परेणावगृहीतमार्गाः||५८|| सन्दूषिता धातुभिरेव चान्यैः स्वैर्भैषजैर्नोपशमं व्रजन्ति|५९|

If the Vayu gets occluded by Medas (fat) and Kapha), then it gives rise to colic pain, numbness of the body and oedema. When an ignorant physician administers Sneha (unctuous recipe in order to alleviate these ailments) then they actually get aggravated. Similarly, they produce other diseases which cannot even be imagined and which probably are difficult to cure. Apart from this, they vitiate blood and other tissues and cause many diseases which are incurable in spite of being administered with good and logical treatments. [57 2/4- 2/4 59]

Reasons for Failure in treatment

सर्वं च रोगप्रशमाय कर्म हीनातिमात्रं विपरीतकालम्||५९|| मिथ्योपचाराच्च न तं विकारं शान्तिं नयेत् पथ्यमपि प्रयुक्तम्|६०|

All therapeutic measures administered to alleviate a disease even though wholesome and skilfully given fail to cure it, if they are used in lesser or excessive doses or at the wrong time or in the wrong manner. Therefore, the diseases get cured only when medicines are administered in the proper dose and proper time by wise and experienced physicians. [59 2/4 – 2/4 60]

तत्र श्लोकः:- प्रश्नानिमान् द्वादश पञ्चकर्माण्युद्दिश्य सिद्धाविह कल्पनायाम्||६०||

प्रजाहितार्थं भगवान् महार्थान् सम्यग्जगादर्षिवरोऽत्रिपुत्रः||६१||

To sum up: - Lord Atreya, the foremost among the sages described the successful administration of Panchakarma (five purificatory therapies) for the wellbeing of the people in the form of answer to the twelve queries (described in verse nos. 3-5) [60 2/4- 61]

इत्यग्निवेशकृते तन्त्रे चरकप्रतिसंस्कृतेऽप्राप्ते दृढबलसम्पूरिते सिद्धिस्थाने कल्पनासिद्धिर्नाम प्रथमोऽध्यायः||१||

Thus, ends the first chapter of the siddhi section called "Kalpana- Sidhhi successful administration of therapeutic measures)" in the text of Agnivesha which was redacted by Charaka, and because of its non-availability, supplemented by Drdhabala.

27

Siddhisthana Chapter 2 Pancha Karmiya Siddhi

Prologue

अथातः पञ्चकर्मीयां सिद्धिं व्याख्यास्यामः||१||

इति ह स्माह भगवानात्रेयः||२||

We shall now expound the chapter dealing with the "Indications and contra-Indications for Successful administration of Panchakarma Therapy'. Thus, said Lord Atreya [1-2]

Dialogue

येषां यस्मात् पञ्चकर्माण्यग्निवेश न कारयेत्| येषां च कारयेतानि तत् सर्वं सम्प्रवक्ष्यते||३||

O! Agnivesa, we shall now describe all the topics relating to the type of patients for whom Panchakarma therapies are contra indicated, reasons for which these are contraindicated, and for which type of patients these therapies are indicated. [3]

Persons for whom all Panchakarma therapies are prohibited

चण्डः साहसिको भीरुः कृतघ्नो व्यग्र एव च|सद्राजभिषजां द्वेष्टा तद्दिद्वष्टः शोकपीडितः||४||

यादृच्छिको मुमूर्षुश्च विहीनः करणैश्च यः| वै री वैद्यविदग्धश्च श्रद्धाहीनः सुशङ्कितः||५||

भिषजामविधेयश्च नोपक्रम्या भिषग्विदा| एतानुपचरन् वैद्यो बहून् दोषानवाप्नुयात्||६||

एभ्योऽन्ये समुपक्रम्या नराः सर्वैरुपक्रमैः|अवस्थां प्रविभज्यैषां वर्ज्यं कार्यं च वक्ष्यते||७||

The wise physician should not give Panchakarma therapies to the following types of patients –

Those who are forceful, rash, cowardly, ungrateful and fickle minded;

Those who hate good persons, kings and physicians, and in turn hated by them,

Those who are afflicted by grief

Those who does not believe in God (Yadrcchika = Nastika);

Those who are in the terminal stage of the disease, and are destined to die

Those who are unable to arrange the essential items (Karana) for the treatment;

Those who are inimical to the physician

One who is an imposter and considers himself to be a physician

One who is skeptical; and

Those not having faith in the physician

Those who do not carry out the instructions given by the physician

The physician who administers Panchakarma therapy to the above-mentioned types of patients invites many difficulties upon himself.

Persons other than those mentioned above should be treated with all the different types of Panchakarma therapies.

Hereafter, we shall explain the indications and contraindications of each of the different types of Panchakarma therapies. [4-7]

Contraindications of Emetic Therapies:

अवम्यास्तावत्- क्षतक्षीणातिस्थूलातिकृशबालवृद्धदुर्बलश्रान्तपिपासित क्षुधितकर्मभाराध्वहतोपवासमैथुनाध्ययनव्यायामचिन्ता-
प्रसक्तक्षामगर्भिणी सुकुमारसंवृतकोष्ठदुश्छर्दनोर्ध्वरक्तपित्तप्रसक्तच्छर्दिरूर्ध्ववातास्थापितानुवासित हृद्रोगोदावर्तमूत्राघात-
प्लीहगुल्मोदरराष्ठीलास्वरोपघाततिमिरशिरशङ्खकर्णाक्षिशूलार्ताः||८||

Emetic therapy is contra- indicated for the following:

The patient suffering from Ksata (phthisis)

The patient who is Ksina (suffering from consumption), Ati-sthula (excessively obese), atikrsa (excessively emaciated), Bala (infant), Vrddha (old) and Durbala (weak)

One who is sranta (fatigue), Pipasita (thirsty) and Ksudhita (hungry);

One who is broken down because of hard work, carrying heavy weight and long walks;

Those who have become weak by excessive fasting, sexual indulgence, study, exercise and worry,

Pregnant woman

One having tender health

One whose gastrointestinal tract is occluded by Vayu and

Those who does not respond easily to emetic therapy;

One suffering from aliments characterized by bleeding from upward tract;

One who is suffering from incessant vomiting

Those suffering from upward movement of Vayu or wind;

Those who have taken evacuative type of medicated enema and

Those who have taken unctuous type of medicated enema

One suffering from heart-diseases

One suffering from mis-peristalsis

One suffering from suppression of urination, splenic disorder, Phantom tumour), obstinate abdominal diseases including ascites, enlarged prostate, choked voice and cataract; and

One suffering from pain in the head, temporal region, ears and eyes [8]

Complications caused by emetic therapy administered in contraindicated Conditions

तत्र क्षतस्य भूयः क्षणनाद्रक्तातिप्रवृतिः स्यात्, क्षीणातिस्थूलकृशबालवृद्धदुर्बलानामौषधबलासहत्वात् प्राणोपरोधः,
श्रान्तपिपासितक्षुधितानां च तद्वत्, कर्मभाराध्वहतोपवासमैथुनाध्ययनव्यायामचिन्ताप्रसक्तक्षामाणां
रौक्ष्याद्वातरक्तच्छेदक्षतभयं स्यात्, गर्भिण्या गर्भव्यापदामगर्भभ्रंशाच्चदारुणा रोगप्राप्तिः, सुकुमारस्य हृदयापकर्षणादूर्ध्वमधो वा
रुधिरातिप्रवृतिः, संवृतकोष्ठदुश्छर्दनयोरतिमात्रप्रवाहणाद्दोषाः समुत्क्लिष्टा अन्तःकोष्ठे जनयन्त्यन्तर्विसर्प स्तम्भं जाड्यं वैचित्र्यं मरणं
वा, ऊर्ध्वगरक्तपित्तिन उदानमुत्क्षिप्य प्राणान् हरेद्रक्तं चातिप्रवर्तयेत्, प्रसक्तच्छर्देस्तद्वत्, ऊर्ध्ववातास्थापितानुवासितानामूर्ध्व
वातातिप्रवृतिः, हृद्रोगिणोहृदयोपरोधः, उदावर्तिनो घोरतर उदावर्तः स्याच्छीघ्रतरहन्ता, मूत्राघातादिभिरार्तानां तीव्रतरशूलप्रादुर्भावः,
तिमिरार्तानां तिमिरातिवृद्दिः, शिरःशूलादिषु शूलातिवृद्दिः; तस्मादेते न वम्याः|
सर्वेष्वपि तु खल्वेतेषु विषगरविरुद्धाजीर्णाभ्यवहारामकृतेष्वप्रतिषिद्धं शीघ्रतरकारित्वादेषामिति ||९||

Sl No Emetic therapy given to Effect

1 a person suffering from Ksata (Phthsis) it further aggravates the injury [to the lungs], and causes excessively haemoptysis

2 to a person who is Ksina (suffering from consumption),

Ati-Sthula (excessively obese),

ati-Krsa (excessively emaciated),

Bala (infant),

Vrddha (old) and

Durbala (weak), this endangers their life because such patients are incapable of tolerating the effects of drugs which are used for emesis

3 to a person who is fatigued, thirsty and hungry similar effect is produced (as explained above)

4 to a person who is broken down by doing hard work, carrying excessive weight and long wayfaring, and is weakened by incessant fasting, sexual indulgence, study, exercise and worry, because of excessive dryness caused by these, the vayu in his body gets aggravated, he may get haemorrhage or injury to his lungs

5 to a pregnant woman this may give rise to complications of pregnancy and occurrence of serious diseases because of the abortion of immature foetus

6 person having tender health because of the strain in his heart, this may give rise to haemorrhage through the upward and downward tracts

7 a person whose gastro–intestinal tract is occluded or who does not respond to emetic therapy easily, excessive bouts of urges for vomiting leading to the excitation of Doshas causing internal erysipelas, stiffness, numbness, mental perversion or death

8 to a person suffering from Urdhvaga- Rakta-Pitta (a diseases characterize by bleeding from the upward tracts) it provokes Udana-vayu leading to death or excessive bleeding

9 a person who is already suffering from incessant vomiting similar effects (as mentioned above)

10 a person suffering from Urdhva-Vata (upward movement of the wind), and who has already taken Asthapana or anuvasana types of medicated enema, this causes upward movement of the wind in excess

11 a person suffering from heart-diseases it leads to cardiac arrest

12 person suffering from Udavarta (mis-peristalsis) this leads to severe mis-peristalsis which is serious nature, and which results in quicker death of the patient

13 patients suffering from Mutraghata (Suppression of urination) etc, leads to the manifestation of colic pain of more acute nature

14 a patient suffering from Timira (cataract) leads to excessive increase of this ailment

15 a patient suffering from headache.etc, leads to the excessive aggravation of pain

Therefore, emetic therapy is contraindicated for the above types of patients. However, administration of emetic therapy is not prohibited even in the above mentioned (contraindicated) ailments if the person is suffering from Visa (ailments caused by natural poisons), Gara (ailments caused by artificially prepared poisons), Viruddhahara (ailments caused by the intake of mutually contradictory ingredients), Ajirna Abhyavahara (intake of foods which cause indigestion) and Ama (ailments caused by the product of improper digestion and metabolism), because these ailments produce their effects instantaneously. [9]

Indications of Emetic Therapy

शेषास्तु वम्याः; विशेषतस्तु पीनसकुष्ठनवज्वरराजयक्ष्मकासश्वासगलग्रहगलगण्डश्लीपदमेहमन्दाग्निविरुद्धाजीर्णान्न विसूचिकालसकविषगरपीतदष्टदिग्धविद्धाधःशोणितपित्तप्रसेक (दुर्नाम) हल्लासारोचकाविपाकापच्यपस्मारोन्मादातिसारशोफपाण्डुरोगमुखपाकदुष्टस्तन्यादयः श्लेष्मव्याधयो विशेषेण महारोगाध्यायोक्ताश्च; एतेषु हि वमनं प्रधानतममित्युक्तं केदारसेतुभेदे शाल्याद्यशोषदोषविनाशवत्||१०||

Emetic therapy is indicated for the remaining aliments especially for –

Pinasa (Coryza), Kustha (skin diseases), Nava Jvara (freshly occurring fever), Rajayaksma (tuberculosis), Kasa (cough), Svasa (Asthma), Galagraha (spasm in the throat), Galaganda (Enlargement of thyroid gland), Slipada (elephantiasis), Meha, Mandagni (suppression of the power of digestion), Viruddhanna (ailments caused by the intake of mutually contradictory food ingredients), Ajirnaanna (ailments caused by indigestion of food), Visucika (cholera), Alasaka (flatulence / tympanitis), Visa-Pita (ailments caused by the intake of artificially prepared poisons), Visa-Dasta (poisonous bites), Visa-digdha-Vidddha (ailments caused by injury with weapons smeared with poisons material), Adhah-sonitapitta (an ailment characterized by bleeding from downward tracts), Praseka (Ptyalism), Durnama (piles), Hrllasa (nausea), Arocaka (anorexia), Avipaka (indigestion), Apaci (cervical adenitis), Apasmara (epilepsy), Unmada (insanity), Atisara (diarrhoea), Sopha (Oedema), Pandu-roga (anemia), Mukha-Paka (stomatitis), Dusta-stanya (polluted breast-milk), etc

The emetic therapy is especially useful for diseases caused by Kapha which are described in Sutra 2): 17.

In all the above-mentioned conditions, emesis is the best therapy. As paddy, etc., in a field full of water are likely to get spoiled, but an outlet made through its wall to take out water saves the crop, similarly, emetic therapy cures diseases caused by aggravated kapha by eliminating these Doshas from the body. [1)]

Contra-indications of Purgation Therapy

अविरेच्यास्तु सुभगक्षतगुदमुक्तनालाधोभागरक्तपित्तिविलङ्घितदुर्बलेन्द्रियाल्पाग्निनिरूढकामादिव्यग्राजीर्णिनवज्वरि-
मदात्ययिताध्मातशल्यार्दिताभिहतातिस्निग्धरूक्षदारुणकोष्ठाः क्षतादयश्च गर्भिण्यन्ताः॥११॥

Purgation therapy is contra-indicated for the following:

Subhaga (persons having tender health / delicate nature), Ksata-Guda (persons having anal injury), Mukta-Nala (prolapse rectum), Adhobhaga rakthapitta (an ailment characterized by bleeding through downward tracts), Vilanghita (person who is on fasting), Durbalalendriya (person having weak sensory and motor organs), Alpagni (person having less power of digestion), Nirudha (person who has undergone evacuative type of enema therapy), Kamadi vyagra manasa (person whose mind is agitated by passion etc), Ajirni (Person suffering indigestion), Madatyayita (person suffering from alcoholism), Adhmata (person suffering from abdominal distension), Salyardita (person afflicted with foreign bodies), Abhihata (person with bodily injury), Ati-snigdha (person who is over-unctuous), Ati-Ruksa (person is excessively un-unctuous), Daruna-Kostha (person having hard bowel) and Other persons having ailments beginning from Ksata (phthisis) and ending with Garbhini (pregnancy) as described in Paragraph no. 8[11]

Adverse effects of purgation therapy administered in contra-indicated conditions

तत्र सुभगस्य सुकुमारोक्तो दोषः स्यात्, क्षतगुदस्य क्षते गुदे प्राणोपरोधकरीं रुजां जनयेत्, मुक्तनालमतिप्रवृत्त्या हन्यात्, अधोभागरक्तपित्तिनं तद्वत्, विलङ्घितदुर्बलेन्द्रियाल्पाग्निनिरूढा औषधवेगं न सहेरन्, कामादिव्यग्रमनसो न प्रवर्तते कृच्छ्रेण वा प्रवर्तमानमयोगदोषान् कुर्यात्, अजीर्णिन आमदोषः स्यात्, नवज्वरिणोऽविपक्वान् दोषान् न निर्हरेद् वातमेव च कोपयेत्, मदात्ययितस्य मद्यक्षीणे देहे वायुः प्राणोपरोधं कुर्यात्, आध्मातस्याधमतो वा पुरीषकोष्ठे निचितो वायुर्विसर्पन् सहसाऽऽनाहं तीव्रतरं मरणं वा जनयेत्, शल्यार्दिताभिहतयोः क्षते वायुराश्रितो जीवितं हिंस्यात्, अतिस्निग्धस्यातियोगभयं भवेत्, रूक्षस्य वायुरुग्रप्रग्रहं कुर्यात्, दारुणकोष्ठस्य विरेचनोद्धता दोषा हृच्छूलपर्वभेदानाहाङ्गमर्दच्छर्दिमूर्च्छाक्लमाञ्जनयित्वा प्राणान् हन्युः, क्षतादीनां गर्भिण्यन्तानां छर्दनोक्तो दोषः स्यात्; तस्मादेते न विरेच्याः॥१२॥

If purgation therapy is given to a person in Subhaga (persons having tender health), then he will suffer from the same disorders as described for emetic therapy administered to sukumara (person having tender health) in para no. 9ra

When administered to persons having anal injury it causes ulcers in the anal / rectum region which further causes severe and intolerable pain causing threat to life.

If purgation medicine is given to those having prolapse of rectum there will be excessive defecation which leads to death.

When administered to those having bleeding through downward passages, purgative medicine causes excessive bleeding leading to death.

When purgation medicine is administered to people who have fasted, those having weak sense organs, those having less digestion power and those who have undergone evacuative enema, they cannot tolerate the intensity of medicine i.e., they would suffer from severe purgation.

If purgation recipes are administered to those whose mind is agitated with passion etc the medicine would not produce purgation or the purges (motions) happen with difficulty which in turn causes complications which would be caused by deficit administration of purgation medicine.

When purgation is administered to those having indigestion it causes ama dosha.

When purgation medicine is administered to those who are suffering from alcoholism, the vayu gets severely aggravated in the body which has been emaciated and depleted causes threat to life (can cause death)

When purgation is administered to those suffering from abdominal distension, the vayu accumulated in the colon wanders throughout the gut in all directions and causes severe flatulence or death.

When purgation is administered to those who are afflicted by foreign bodies, the vayu accumulated in the site of foreign body will cause death.

When purgation is administered to those who are over unctuous it may cause atiyoga i.e., symptoms of excessive administration of purgation therapy (symptoms of excessive purgation).

When purgation is administered in people who have excessive dryness of the body, the vayu gets aggravated and causes gripping pain in the body parts

When administered to people having hard bowel, purgation medicine causes severe aggravation of doshas which in turn cause pain in heart, pain in the small joints of the fingers, flatulence, pain in body parts, vomiting, fainting (unconsciousness), fatigue etc which can lead to death.

When purgation medicine is given to a patient who is having ailments beginning from phthisis and ending with pregnancy it will cause the same complications which are mentioned in the context of giving emesis therapy in the same cases.

Therefore, purgation therapy is contra- indicated in the above-mentioned cases. [12]

Indications of purgation Therapy:

शेषास्तु विरेच्याः; विशेषतस्तु
कुष्ठज्वरमेहोर्ध्वरक्तपित्तभगन्दरोदरार्शोब्रध्नप्लीहगुल्मार्बुदगलगण्डग्रन्थिविसूचिकालसकमूत्राघातक्रिमिकोष्ठविसर्प-
पाण्डुरोगशिरःपार्श्वशूलोदावर्तनेत्रास्यदाहहृद्रोगव्यङ्ग्नीलिकानेत्रनासिकास्यस्रवणहलीमकश्वासकासकामला-
पच्यपस्मारोन्मादवातरक्तयोनिरेतोदोषतैमिर्यारोचकाविपाकच्छर्दिश्वयथूदरविस्फोटकादयः पित्तव्याधयो विशेषेण महारोगाध्यायोक्ताश्च;
एतेषु हि विरेचनं प्रधानतममित्युक्तमग्न्युपशमेऽग्निगृहवत्||१३||

In all the other conditions (other than the above), purgation therapy is indicated.

Especially it is indicated for the patients suffering from –

Kustha (skin diseases), Jvara (fever),

Meha, Urdhvaga- Raktapitta (bleeding from the upward tracts), Bhagandara (fistula- in-ano), Udara (obstinate abdominal diseases including ascites), Arsas (piles), Bradhna (inguinal swelling), Pliha (splenic disorders), Gulma (phantom tumour), Arbuda (tumour), Gala-Ganda (thyroid enlargement), Granthi (lymphadenitis), Visucika (choleric diarrhoea), Alasaka (intestinal torpor), Mutraghata (suppression of urination), Krimi-Kostha (parasitic infestation of intestines), Visarpa (erysipelas), Pandu-roga (anaemia), Sirah-sula (headache), Parsva-Sula (pain in the sides of the chest), Udavarta (upward movement of wind in the abdomen),

Netra-daha (burning sensation in the eyes), Asya-Daha (burning sensation in mouth / face),

Hrd-roga (heart diseases), Vyanga (freckles), Nilika (bluish black moles), Netra –Sravana (excessive discharge from eyes), Nasika-sravana (excessive discharge from the nose), Asya-srvana (excessive salivation), Halimaka (a serious type of Jaundice), Svasa (asthma), Kasa (cough), Kamala (jaundice),

Apaci (cervical adenitis), Apasmaara (epilepsy), Unmada (insanity), Vata-Rakta (gout), Yoni-dosa (gynaecological disorders), Reto-Doshas (seminal morbidities), Timira (cataract), Arocaka (anorexia),

Udara (obstinate abdominal disorders including ascites; this appears to be a repetition), Visphotajka (pustular eruptions) etc.

Purgation therapy is also especially useful for Paittika type of diseases described in Sutra 2):14.

For the above-mentioned ailments, purgation therapy is the foremost remedy.

As the extinguisher of fire normalizes Agni-Grha (a house on fire), similarly, purgation therapy, by eliminating aggravated Pitta, cures all the above-mentioned diseases. [13]

Prohibition of Niruha Basti:

अनास्थाप्यास्तु अजीर्ण्यतिस्निग्धपीतस्नेहोत्क्लिष्टदोषाल्पाग्नियानक्लान्तातिदुर्बल
क्षुत्तृष्णाश्रमार्तातिकृशभुक्तभक्तपीतोदकवमितविरिक्तकृतनस्तः कर्मकुद्धभीतमत्तमूर्च्छितप्रसक्तच्छर्दिनिष्ठीविकाश्वास
कासहिक्काबद्धच्छिद्रोदकोदराध्मानालसकविसूचिकामप्रजातामातिसार- मधुमेहकुष्ठार्ताः||१४||

Administration of asthapana or Niruha (evacuation type of medicated enema) is prohibited for the following:

Person who is suffering from Ajirna (indigestion),

Person who is administered with excessive oleation or the one to whom oleation has just been administered
Persons in whom Doshas are excited (Utklista-Dosa) and those suffering from mandagni (suppression of the power of digestion);
To a person fatigued due to excessive riding of vehicle
Persons who are excessively weak, excessively hungry, excessively thirsty and excessively tired due to indulgence in hard (strenuous) work,
Excessively emaciated persons
Persons who have just taken the meal and has just consumed water
Persons who have just taken emetic therapy and those who have just undergone purgation therapy or those who have just taken inhalation therapy
Persons who are angry and fearful
Persons who are intoxicated and those who have fainted
Those suffering from incessant vomiting, ptyalism, asthma, cough and hiccup;
Those suffering from intestinal obstruction, intestinal perforation, ascites associated with meteorism
Those suffering from intestinal torpor, cholera, miscarriage and first stage of diarrhoea and
Those suffering from diabetes mellitus, all pramehas or skin diseases. [14]

Adverse Effects of Niruha Basti administered in contraindicated conditions
तत्राजीर्ण्यतिस्निग्धपीतस्नेहानां दूष्योदरं मूर्च्छाश्वयथुर्वा स्यात्, उत्क्लिष्टदोषमन्दाग्न्योररोचकस्तीव्रः, यानक्लान्तस्य क्षोभव्यापन्नो बस्तिराशु देहं शोषयेत्, अतिदुर्बलक्षुत्तृष्णाश्रमार्तानां पूर्वोक्तोदोषः स्यात्, अतिकृशस्य कार्श्यं पुनर्जनयेत्, भुक्तभक्तपीतोदकयोरुत्क्लिश्योर्ध्वमधो वावायुर्बस्तिमुत्क्षिप्य क्षिप्रं घोरान् विकारान्जनयेत्, वमितविरिक्तयोस्तु रूक्षं शरीरं निरूहः क्षतं क्षार इव दहेत्, कृतनस्तःकर्मणो विभ्रंशं भृशसंरुद्धस्रोतसः कुर्यात्, क्रुद्धभीतयोर्बस्तिरूर्ध्वमुपप्लवेत्, मत्तमूर्च्छितयो र्भृशं विचलितायां सञ्ज्ञायां चित्तोपघाताद् व्यापत् स्यात्, प्रसक्तच्छर्दिनिष्ठीविकाश्वासकासहिक्कार्तानामूर्ध्वीभूतो वायुरूर्ध्वं बस्तिं नयेत्, बद्धच्छिद्रोदकोदराध्मानार्तानां भृशतरमाध्याप्य बस्तिः प्राणान् हिंस्यात्, अलसकविसूचिकामप्रजातामातिसारिणामामकृतो दोषः स्यात्, मधुमेहकुष्ठिनोर्व्याधेः पुनर्वृद्धिः; तस्मादेते नास्थाप्याः||१५||
Administration of Niruha basti in contra-indicated conditions produces adverse effects as follows:
Sl No Niruha Basti (decoction enema) therapy given to Effect
1 person suffering from indigestion, administered with excessive oleation, who has just taken oleation therapy
Dusyodara - obstinate abdominal diseases caused by the aggravation of all the three Doshas, fainting or oedema
2 person having excited Doshas or
person suffering from the suppression of the power of digestion, severe type of anorexia
3 person fatigued due to excessive riding of vehicles,
causes excessive agitation leading to instantaneous emaciation of the body
4 person who is excessively weak and who is suffering from hunger and fatigue, causes the same disorders as described before
5 person who has just taken his meal or water,
causes excitement of vayu as a result of which the recipe of enema is pushed upwards or downwards leading to the causation of serious ailments instantaneously
6 person who has taken his meal or water,
causes excitement of vayu as a result of which the recipe of enema is pushed upwards or downwards leading to the causation of serious ailments instantaneously
7 person who has already taken emetic or purgation therapy,
administration of Niruha basti burns his dehydrated (dry) body as if it is ulcerated by the application of alkalis
8 person who has taken inhalation therapy, Niruha basti causes impairment of senses, and further obstruction of the channels of circulations
9 person who is angry or fearful,

agitation in the upper part of the body

10 intoxicated and fainted persons

causes further agitation in the consciousness leading to the complications because of mental damage

11 persons suffering from incessant vomiting, ptyalism, asthma, cough or hiccup, Niruha basti causes the aggravated vayu in the upper part of the body to draw the recipe of enema upwards

12 person suffering from intestinal obstruction, intestinal perforation or ascites, which are associated with abdominal distension, Niruha basti further increases the intestinal distension and may lead to the death of the patient

13 person suffering from intestinal obstruction, intestinal torpor, cholera, abortion or amatisara (first stage of diarrhoea), Niruha- Basti causes ailments due to ama (product of improper digestion and metabolism)

14 person suffering from Madhu-meha and Kustha (skin diseases), administration of Niruha-Bsti further aggravates these ailments

Therefore, Niruha basti is prohibited for the above-mentioned type of patients. [15]

Indications of Niruha –Basti:

शेषास्त्वास्थाप्या:; विशेषतस्तु
सर्वाङ्गैकाङ्गकुक्षिरोगवातवर्चोमूत्रशुक्रसङ्गबलवर्णमांसरेतःक्षयदोषाध्मानाङ्गसुप्तिक्रिमिकोष्ठोदावर्तशुद्धातिसार-
पर्वभेदाभितापप्लीहगुल्मशूलहृद्रोगभगन्दरोन्मादज्वरब्रध्नशिरःकर्णशूलहृदयपार्श्वपृष्ठकटीग्रहवेपनाक्षेपकगौरवातिलाघव-
रजःक्षयार्तविषमाग्निस्फिग्जानुजङ्घोरुगुल्फपार्ष्णिप्रपदयोनिबाह्वङ्गुलिस्तनान्तदन्तनखपर्वास्थिशूल-
शोषस्तम्भान्त्रकूजपरिकर्तिकाल्पाल्पसशब्दोग्रगन्धोत्थानादयो वातव्याधयो विशेषेण महारोगाध्यायोक्ताश्च; एतेष्वास्थापनं
प्रधानतममित्युक्तं वनस्पतिमूलच्छेदवत्||१६||

In all the other conditions Niruha basti (evacuative type of medicated enema) is indicated. It is especially useful in treating the below mentioned conditions –

Sarvanga-Roga (paralysis of the whole body), Ekanga- Roga (paralysis of one of the limbs), Kuksi-Roga (diseases of pelvic region), Vata-Sanga (retention of flatus), Varcah-Sanga (retention of stool), Mutra-Sanga (retention of urine), Sukra-Sanga (retention of semen), Bala-Ksaya (diminution of strength), Varna Ksaya (diminution of complexion), Mamsa-Dosa (morbidity of muscle tissue), Reto-Dosa (morbidity of semen), Adhmana - bloating, gaseous distension of abdomen (meteorism), Anga- Supti (numbness of limbs), Krimi Kostha (worm infestation / parasitic infestation of the intestine), Udavarta (upward movement of the wind in the abdomen), Suddhatisara (diarrhoea without the association of ama - a product of indigestion and altered metabolism), Parva- bheda (joint pain, pain in the interphalangeal joints), Abhitapa (feeling of burning sensation), Pliha (splenic disorder), Gulma - tumours of the abdomen (phantom tumour), Sula (colic pain), Hrd-roga (heart diseases), Bhagandara (anal fistula), Unmada - Schizophrenia (Insanity), Jvara - fever (fever), Bradhna – prolapsed rectum (inguinal swellings),

Sirah- Sula (headache), Karna-Sula (earache), Hrdaya- Graha (cardiac spasm), Parsva graha (stiffness in the sides of the chest), Prstha graha (stiffness of the back), Kati- graham (stiffness of the lumbar region), Vepathu (tremor), Aksepaka- Arti (convulsions), Gaurava- Arti (excessive heaviness of the body), Atilaghava- arti (excessive lightness of the body), Rajah Ksaya (amenorrhoea), Visamagni (irregular power of digestion), Sphik sula sosa stambha – stiffness, pain, atrophy and stiffness of the buttocks, Janu Sula Sosa Stambha - pain, atrophy and stiffness of knee-joints, Jangha Sula Sosa Stambha – pain, atrophy and stiffness of the thighs, Gulpha Sula Sosa Stambha - pain, atrophy and stiffness of ankles, Parsni Sula Sosa stambha - pain, atrophy and stiffness of heels, Prapada Sula Sosa stambha - pain, atrophy and stiffness of feet, Yoni sula sosa stambha - pain, atrophy and stiffness of female reproductive organs, Bahu sula sosa stambha - pain, atrophy and stiffness of arms, Anguli Sula Sosa Stambha - pain, atrophy and stiffness of fingers, Stananta Sula sosa stambha - pain, atrophy and stiffness at the end of the breasts or nipples, Danta sula Sosa stambha - pain, atrophy and stiffness of teeth, Nakha Sula sosa stambha - pain, atrophy and stiffness of nails, Parva Sula sosa stambha - pain, atrophy and stiffness of bones, Antra-Kujana (intestinal gurgling), Parikartika (sawing pain in the abdomen), Alpalpa-utthana (voiding stools in small quantities, frequently), Sasabdotthana (voiding stools with noise), Ugra-Gandha-utthana (voiding of foul-smelling stool) and such other ailments Niruha- basti is especially useful in Vatika diseases described in Sutra 2):11

For the above-mentioned ailments, Niruha basti is the foremost medication. As a tree gets destroyed by cutting its roots, similarly the above-mentioned diseases get cured by the administration of Niruha basti. [16]

Contra- indications of anuvasana –Basti:

य एवानास्थाप्यास्त एवाननुवास्याः स्युः; विशेषतस्त्वभुक्तभक्तनवज्वरपाण्डुरोगकामलाप्रमेहार्शः प्रतिश्यायारोचकमन्दाग्निदुर्बलप्लीहकफोदरोरुस्तम्भवर्चोभेद विषगरपीतपित्तकफाभिष्यन्दगुरु कोष्ठश्लीपदगलगण्डापचिक्रिमिकोष्ठिनः ||१७||

Anuvasana Basti is prohibited in all the conditions for which Niruha basti is contra- indicated. It is especially contraindicated in the following conditions:

Abhukta- Bhakta (a person who has not taken food) and

The persons suffering from -

Nava-Jvara - fever (freshly occurring fever / acute fever),

Pandu Roga (anaemia),

Kamala - Jaundice, Liver diseases, Prameha – Urinary tract disorders, diabetes and

Arsas (piles),

Pratisyaya (coryza)

Arocaka (anorexia),

Mandagni – low digestion strength (suppression of the power of digestion), Daurbalya (weakness),

Plihodara (splenic disorders),

Kaphodara - Kapha type of Ascites (obstinate abdominal ailments caused by aggravated Kapha),

Uru-Stambha - stiffness / spasticity of thighs,

Varco-Bheda (ingestion of natural poison),

Pittabhisyanda (conjunctivitis caused by aggravated pitta),

Kaphabhisyanda (conjunctivitis caused by aggravated Kapha),

Guru Kostha (hard bowel),

Slipada (elephantiasis),

Galaganda (enlargement of thyroid gland),

Apaci (cervical adenitis) and

Krimi Kostha (intestinal parasites) [17]

Adverse Effects of anuvasana basti in contraindicated conditions

तत्राभुक्तभक्तस्यानावृतमार्गत्वादूर्ध्वमतिवर्तते स्नेहः, नवज्वरपाण्डुरोगकामलाप्रमेहिणां दोषानुत्क्लिश्योदरञ्जनयेत्, अर्शसस्यार्शांस्यभिष्यन्दयाध्मानं कुर्यात्, अरोचकार्तस्यान्नगृद्धिं पुनर्हन्यात्, मन्दाग्निदुर्बलयोर्मन्दतरमग्निं कुर्यात्, प्रतिश्यायप्लीहादिमतां भृशमुत्क्लिष्टदोषाणां भूय एव दोषं वर्धयेत्; तस्मादेते नानुवास्याः||१८||

Administration of Anuvasana Basti in contraindicated conditions produces adverse effects as follows:

Sl No Anuvasana Basti (unctuous enema) therapy given to Effect

1 person who has not taken any food, Anuvasana Basti spreads upwards due to the absence of any obstruction in the alimentary tract

2 person suffering from

Nava-Jvara (fever of recent origin), anaemia,

Jaundice, and

Prameha – Urinary tract disorders, diabetes, causes excitation of Doshas leading to the manifestation of Udara - ascites, enlargement of the abdomen (obstinate abdominal diseases including ascites)

3 person suffering from piles, administration of Anuvasana Basti produces stickiness in the piles leading to Adhmana - bloating, gaseous distension of abdomen (abdominal distension)

4 person suffering from anorexia,

administration of Anuvasana Basti further impairs the desire for food

5 person suffering from

mandagni - low digestion strength (suppression of the power of digestion) and debility, administration of Anuvasana-basti further reduces the power of digestion

6 person suffering from coryza, splenic disorder (and such other ailments described in the no. 7 of the para-17 above), then the administration of Anuvasana Basti causes excessive aggravation of the already aggravated Doshas

So Anuvasana Basti must not be administered to the above category of patients.

Indications of Anuvasana Basti

य एवास्थाप्यास्त एवानुवास्याः; विशेषतस्तु रूक्षतीक्ष्णाग्नयः केवलवातरोगार्ताश्च; एतेषु ह्यनुवासनं प्रधानतममित्युक्तं मूले दुमप्रसेकवत्||१९||

Anuvasana –Basti is indicated in the very conditions for which Niruha- Basti is indicated (vide para no. 16). It is especially indicated for –

the person having un-unctuousness (dryness),

Tiksnagni (sharp power of digestion) and

Kevala- Vata-Roga (diseases caused by Vayu alone, i.e., not associated with Ama - A product of indigestion and altered metabolism),

In these conditions, Anuvasana Basti is the foremost therapy.

As sprinkling of water at the root prevents withering out of the tree. Similarly, administration of Anuvasana – basti cures diseases in the body of the person. [19]

Contraindications of inhalation therapy

अशिरोविरेचनार्हास्तु अजीर्णिभुक्तभक्तपीतस्नेहमद्यतोयपातुकामाः स्नातशिराः स्नातुकामः क्षुत्तृष्णाश्रमार्तमत्तमूर्च्छितशस्त्रदण्डहतव्यवायव्यायामपानक्लान्तनवज्वरशोकाभितप्तविरिक्तानुवासितगर्भिणीनवप्रतिश्यायार्ताः, अनृतौ दुर्दिने चेति||२०|

Shiro- virecana (inhalation therapy) is prohibited for the following:

The person who has indigestion or to a person who has already taken food

The person who has already taken oleation therapy

The person who has taken alcohol or water

The person who has taken head-bath or who desires to take bath

The person who is hungry and thirty

The person who is suffering from fatigue, intoxication or fainting;

The person afflicted by injury with a weapon or a stick;

The person who is fatigued because of sexual intercourse, physical exercise or intake of alcohol:

The person afflicted with freshly occurring fever and grief;

The person who has taken purgation therapy or Anuvasana –Basti;

A pregnant woman;

The person who is suffering from freshly occurring coryza; and

In inappropriate season or on a cloudy day

Adverse effects of Inhalation Therapy in Prohibited Conditions:

तत्राजीर्णिभुक्तभक्तयोर्दोषं ऊर्ध्ववहानि स्रोतांस्यावृत्य कासश्वासच्छर्दिप्रतिश्यायाञ्जनयेत्, पीतस्नेहमद्यतोयपातुकामानां कृते च पिबतां मुखनासास्रावाक्ष्युपदेहतिमिरशिरोरोगाञ्जनयेत्, स्नातशिरसः कृते च स्नानाच्छिरसः प्रतिश्यायं, क्षुधार्तस्य वातप्रकोपं, तृष्णार्तस्य पुनस्तृष्णाभिवृद्धिं मुखशोषं च, श्रमार्तमत्तमूर्च्छितानामास्थापनोक्तं दोषं जनयेत्, शस्त्रदण्डहतयोस्तीव्रतरां रुजं जनयेत्, व्यवायव्यायामपानक्लान्तानां शिरःस्कन्धनेत्रोरःपीडनं, नवज्वरशोकाभितप्तयोरूष्मा नेत्रनाडीरनुसृत्य तिमिरं ज्वरवृद्धिं च कुर्यात्, विरिक्तस्य वायुरिन्द्रियोपघातं कुर्यात्, अनुवासितस्य कफः शिरोगुरुत्वकण्डूक्रिमिदोषाञ्जनयेत्, गर्भिण्या गर्भं स्तम्भयेत् स काणः कुणिः पक्षहतः पीठसर्पी वा जायते, नवप्रतिश्यायार्तस्य स्रोतांसि व्यापादयेत्, अनृतौ दुर्दिने च शीतदोषान् पूतिनस्यं शिरोरोगं च जनयेत्; तस्मादेते न

शिरोविरेचनार्हाः||२१||

Administration of inhalation therapy in contra-indicated conditions gives rise to adverse effects as follows:

Sl No Shiro Virechana – nasal medication therapy given to Effect

1 person suffering from indigestion or he who has already taken food, causes occlusion of the channels of circulation moving upwards causing therapy cough, asthma, vomiting and coryza

2 person who has already taken oleation therapy or he who desires to take oleation therapy, alcohol or water or if he takes water after the therapy, gives rise to ptyalism, discharge from the nose, stickiness of eyes, cataract and head diseases

3 person who has taken head-bath or takes head-bath after the therapy, gives rise to coryza

4 a hungry person aggravates vayu

5 a thirsty person intensifies thirst, and causes dryness of the mouth

6 a person afflicted with fatigue, intoxication or fainting

produces the same adverse effects as mentioned in respect of Niruha- Basti

7 a person injured by weapon or beaten by a stick produces excruciating pain

8 a person fatigued because of sexual indulgence, physical work or taking alcohol (even after a day) causes pain in the head, shoulders, eyes and chest

9 a person suffering from Nava-Jvara (fever of recent origin) and grief, causes the heat to spread into the channels of the eyes resulting in Timira (cataract) and further aggravation of the fever

10 a person who has already taken the purgation therapy

the Vayu in his body gets aggravated leading to the injury to his sense organs

11 a person who has already taken Anuvasana Basti

kapha in his body gets aggravated leading to heaviness of head, itching and parasitic infestation

12 a pregnant woman,

the growth of the foetus gets arrested, and she gives birth to and offspring who may be Kana (blind by one eye), Kuni (with deformity of upper limbs), Paksahata (hemiplegic) or Pitha-Sarpi (with deformity of the lower limbs)

13 a person who is suffering from nava pratisyaya (freshly occurring coryza), may cause morbidity of the channels of circulation

14 on a cloudy day or during inappropriate seasons may cause ailments due to cold, Puti- nasya (putrefied rhinitis) and Shiro-Roga (head –diseases)

Therefore, in the above-mentioned conditions inhalation therapy is prohibited. [21]

Indications of inhalation Therapy

शेषास्त्वर्हाः, विशेषतस्तु शिरोदन्तमन्यास्तम्भगलहनुग्रहपीनसगलशुण्डिकाशालूकशुक्रतिमिरवर्त्मरोगव्यङ्गो
पजिह्विकार्धावभेदकग्रीवास्कन्धांसास्यनासिकाकर्णाक्षिमूर्धकपालशिरोरोगार्दितापतन्त्रकापतानकगलगण्ड-
दन्तशूलहर्षचालाक्षिराज्यर्बुदस्वरभेदवाग्ग्रहगद्गदक्रथनादय   ऊर्ध्वजत्रुगताश्चवातादिविकाराः   परिपक्वाश्च;   एतेषु   शिरोविरेचनं
प्रधानतममित्युक्तं, तद्ध्युत्तमाङ्गमनुप्रविश्य मुञ्जादीषिकामिवासक्तां केवलं विकारकरं दोषमपकर्षति||२२||

Inhalation therapy is indicated for the remaining ailments. It is especially useful in the below mentioned conditions –

Shiro-stambha (stiffness of the head),

Danta-Stambha (Stiffness of teeth),

Manya-stambha (torticollis),

Gala-Graha (spasm of the teeth),

Hanu-Graha (lock-jaw),

Pinasa (chronic coryza),

Gala-Sundika (tonsillitis),

Gala-Saluka (tumour in the throat),

Sukra (corneal ulcer),

Timira (cataract),

Vartma-Roga (diseases of eye-lids),

Vyanga (freckles),

Upa-Jihvika (Uvulitis),

Ardhavabhedaka (hemicrania),

Griva-roga (diseases of the neck),

Skandha-roga (diseases of the shoulders),

Amsa-roga (diseases of the scapula),

Asya-roga (diseases of the mouth),

Nasika-roga (diseases of the nose),

Karna-Roga (diseases of the ears),

Aksi roga (diseases of the eyes),

Murdha-Roga (diseases of the head),

Kapala-roga (diseases of the cranium),

Shiro-roga (diseases of the head),

Ardita (facial paralysis),

Apatantraka (convulsions with unconsciousness),

Apatanaka (convulsions with consciousness),

Galaganda (goitre),

Danta-Sula (toothache),

Danta-harsa (tingling of teeth),

Danta-cala (looseness of teeth)

Aksi-Raji (conjunctivitis),

Arbuda (tumour),

Svarabheda (hoarseness of the voice),

Vag-graham (loss of speech),

Gad-Gada (spasmodic speech),

Krathana (stammering) etc

and diseases of the head and neck which are caused by aggravated Vayu and which are fully matured (free from Ama-Dosa).

For the treatment of the above-mentioned maladies inhalation therapy is the foremost remedy. The recipe administered through inhalation therapy enters into the head (cerebrum), and draws out exclusively the morbid matter as the pith (Isika) is taken out after removing the fibrous coating of Munja (a type of Grass) adhered to it. [22]

Seasonal Propriety of Inhalation Therapy:

प्रावृट्शरद्वसन्तेतरेष्वात्ययिकेषु रोगेषु नावनं कुर्यात् कृत्रिमगुणोपधानात्; ग्रीष्मे पूर्वाह्णे, शीते मध्याह्ने, वर्षास्वदुर्दिने चेति॥२३॥

In the case of an emergency, inhalation therapy can be given even in the seasons other than Pravrt (first part of the rainy season), sarat (autumn) and Vasanta (spring) by artificially creating the congenial environment. In the summer, inhalation therapy should be given in the morning. In the winter, it should be given during the mid-day. In the rainy season it should be given when the sky is free from clouds. [23]

Contents of chapter and Epilogue:

तत्र श्लोकाः-

इति पञ्चविधं कर्म विस्तरेण निदर्शितम्|येभ्यो यन्न हितं यस्मात् कर्म येभ्यश्च यदिधतम्॥२४॥

न चैकान्तेन निर्दिष्टेऽप्यर्थेऽभिनिविशेद्बुधः| स्वयमप्यत्र वैद्येन तर्क्यं बुद्धिमता भवेत्॥२५॥

उत्पद्येत हि साऽवस्था देशकालबलं प्रति| यस्यां कार्यमकार्यं स्यात् कर्म कार्यं च वर्जितम्||२६||

छर्दिर्हृद्रोगगुल्मानां वमनं स्वे चिकित्सिते| अवस्थां प्राप्य निर्दिष्टं कुष्ठिनां बस्तिकर्म च||२७||

तस्मात् सत्यपि निर्देशे कुर्यादूह्य स्वयं धिया| विना तर्केण या सिद्धिर्यदृच्छासिद्धिरेव सा||२८||

To sum up: -

Thus, five elimination therapies taken together called Pancha-karma is explained above in detail with reference to their following aspects;

Contra-indications of these therapies for different categories of diseases.

The reasons for which these therapies are contraindicated and

the ailments for which these therapies are indicted.

A wise physician should not make a judgement exclusively on the suggestions made above in this chapter. He should use his own discretions and reasoning in arriving at the correct judgement.

Due to the nature of the habitat, time and strength of the patient, situations may arise because of which the therapy indicated for an ailment becomes ineffective, and a prohibited therapy may become useful.

In the chapters dealing with the treatment of Chardi (vomiting), Hrd-Roga (heart –diseases) and Gulma (phantom tumour), emetic therapy [though normally prohibited] is prescribed in certain stages of these diseases. Similarly, Basti or enema therapy is prescribed in the chapter dealing with the treatment of Kusthaa (thought is generally prohibited] depending upon the stage of this disease.

Therefore, despite the directions laid down in this chapter, the physician should determine the correct therapy for an ailment by the use of his own discretion. The success achieved without the exercise of the power of reasoning (tarka) is nothing but only the success per chance. [24-28]

इत्यग्निवेशकृते तन्त्रे चरकप्रतिसंस्कृतेऽप्राप्ते दृढबलसम्पूरिते सिद्धिस्थाने पञ्चकर्मीयसिद्धिर्नाम द्विवतीयोऽध्यायः||२||

Thus, ends the second chapter of siddhi- section dealing with "the Perfect administration of Pancha- karma" in Agnivesha's work as redacted by Charaka, and because of its non-availability, supplemented by Drdhabala.

28

Siddhisthana Chapter 3 Basti Sutriya Siddhi

Prologue

अथातो बस्तिसूत्रीयां सिद्धिं व्याख्यास्यामः||१||

इति ह स्माह भगवानात्रेयः||२||

We shall now explore the chapter dealing with the "Achievement of Perfection in the Treatment through (the Knowledge of) the principles of basti (medicated enema)". Thus said Lord Atreya [1-2]

Dialogue

कृतक्षणं शैलवरस्य रम्ये स्थितं धनेशायतनस्य पार्श्वे|महर्षिसङ्घैर्वृतमग्निवेशः पुनर्वसुं प्राञ्जलिरन्वपृच्छत्||३||

बस्तिर्नरेभ्यः किमपेक्ष्य दत्तः स्यात् सिद्धिमान् किम्मयमस्य नेत्रम्| कीदृक्प्रमाणाकृति किङ्गुणं च केभ्यश्च किंयोनिगुणश्च बस्तिः||४||

निरूहकल्पः प्रणिधानमात्रा स्नेहस्य का वा शयने विधिः कः| के बस्तयः केषु हिता इतीदं श्रुत्वोत्तरं प्राह वचो महर्षिः||५||

When Punarvasu, after completing his daily rituals, was leisurely sitting in the beautiful valley of the Himalayas, being surrounded by a group of saints, close to the abode of Kubera (the god of wealth), Agnivesha with folded hands enquired about the following topics:

Which factors should be kept in view (mind) for the successful administration of basti therapy? [to be explained in the verse no.]

Which material is used to prepare the nozzle for giving enema? explained in verse no. 7]

What is the size, shape and quantities of enema receptacles? [explained in the verse nos. 8-2/4 10]

What is the source material to be used in the preparation of the enema receptacle for different persons, and what are its attributes? [explained in verse nos. 10 2/4 -2/4 12]

What are the recipes of niruha- Basti? [explained in the verse nos. 12 2/4 – 2/4 31]

What is the Dosage of Niruha- basti? [explained in the verse nos. 31 2/4- 2/4 33]

What is the Dosage of Anuvasana- Basti? [explained in the chapter no. IV]

In which position, the patient should lie down during the administration of Basti? [explained in the verse nos. 33 2/4- 2/4 34]

What are the recipes of Basti, and for which type of patients these are useful? [explained in the verse nos. 35 2/4-70]

After hearing these queries, the Great Sage replied as follows. [elaborated in subsequent verses and the next chapter]. [3-5]

Factors to be kept in view for successful administration of Niruha

समीक्ष्य दोषौषधदेशकालसात्म्याग्निसत्त्वादिवयोबलानि| बस्तिः प्रयुक्तो नियतं गुणाय स्यात् सर्वकर्माणि च सिद्धिमन्ति||६||

To achieve success in the administration and to obtain the desired therapeutic effects, Basti is administered keeping in view the factors like nature of the Doshas, Medicines, habitat, season, homologation, Agni (power of digestion and metabolism), Sattva (psychic condition), etc., age and strength of the patient. [6]

Material for Enema- Nozzle

सुवर्णरूप्यत्रपुतामरीतिकांस्यास्थिशस्त्रद्रुमवेणुदन्तैः नलैर्विषाणैर्मणिभिश्च तैस्तैर्नेत्राणि कार्याणि सु(त्रि)कर्णिकानि ||७||

The enema-nozzle is made of gold, silver, tin, copper, brass, bronze, bone, iron, wood, bamboo-reed, ivory, pipe, horn or gems. It is fitted with well-polished rings (which are three in number). [7]

Size and shape of Nozzle

षड्द्वादशाष्टाङ्गुलसम्मितानि षड्विंशतिद्वादशवर्षजानाम्| स्युर्मुद्गकर्कन्धुसतीनवाहिच्छिद्राणि वर्त्याऽपिहितानि चैव||८||

यथावयोऽङ्गुष्ठकनिष्ठिकाभ्यां मूलाग्रयोः स्युः परिणाहवन्ति| ऋजूनि गोपुच्छसमाकृतीनि श्लक्ष्णानि च स्युर्गुडिकामुखानि||९||

स्यात् कर्णिकैकाऽग्रचतुर्थभागे मूलाश्रिते बस्तिनिबन्धने द्वे|१०|

For the patients of the six, twenty and twelve years, the length of the nozzle is six, twelve and eight Angulas (one angula or finger's breadth = ¾th of an inch), respectively.

The calibre of the hole inside the nozzle is such as to allow the passage of a seed of Mudga (green Gram), Karkandhu (small variety of Jujube) and satina (pea) respectively. This hole is crooked with a Varti (elongated plug).

The circumference of the nozzle at the base and top is the same as that of the thumb and little finger respectively of the patient of that age (i.e., six, twenty and twelve years old).

It is straight and tapering like the tail of a cow. The mouth (opening at the top) of the nozzle is smooth and globular. One ring (Karnika) is fixed at the level of one fourth from the top, and two other rings are fixed at the base in order to facilitate tying the mouth of the bladder (basti) around the nozzle. [8 – 2/4 10]

Source of Enema- receptacle (Basti) and Its Attributes

जारद्गवो माहिषहारिणौ वा स्याच्छौकरो बस्तिरजस्य वाऽपि||१०|| दृढस्तनुर्नष्टसिरो विगन्धः कषायरक्तः सुमृदुः सुशुद्धः|

नृणां वयो वीक्ष्य यथानुरूपं नेत्रेषु योज्यस्तु सुबद्धसूत्रः||११||

The enema- receptacle is prepared on the bladder of old ox, buffalo, deer, pig or goat. It is firm, thin, and free from vessels and without any foul odour. It is tanned with astringent drugs by which it becomes red in odour. It is very soft and very clean. Keeping in view the age of the patient, the Basti (enema- receptacle or bladder) of appropriate capacity is selected, and it is tied securely to the nozzle of appropriate size with the help of strings. [10 2/4- 11]

In case of Non-availability of Bladder

बस्तेरलाभे प्लवजो गलो वा स्यादङ्कपादः सुघनः पटो वा|१२|

If bladder is not available then the sac in the throat of a pelican (Plava) or a sac prepared of either the skin of a bat or a thick cloth is used as enema- receptacle. [2/4 12]

Auspicious Time for Administration of Basti Therapy

आस्थापनाईं पुरुषं विधिज्ञः समीक्ष्य पुण्येऽहनि शुक्लपक्षे||१२||

प्रशस्तनक्षत्रमुहूर्तयोगे जीर्णान्नमेकाग्रमुपक्रमेत |१३|

The physician well-versed in the method of administering Basti (medicated enema) should give therapy to a suitable patient (for whom Basti therapy is indicated) after he has digested his meal, and has concentration of the mind. It is given on an auspicious day in the Sukla-Paksa (bright fortnight of lunar month) having a propitious Naksatra (constellation), Muhurta (period of the day) and Yoga (Planatory conjunction). [12 2/4 – 2/4 13]

Method of Administering Basti

बलां गुडूचीं त्रिफलां सरास्नां द्वे पञ्चमूले च पलोन्मितानि||१३|| अष्टौ फलान्यर्धतुलां च मांसाच्छागात् पचेदप्सु चतुर्थशेषम्|

पूतं यवानीफलबिल्वकुष्ठवचाशताह्वाघनपिप्पलीनाम्||१४|| कल्कैर्गुडक्षौद्रघृतैः सतैलैर्युतं सुखोष्णैस्तु पिचुप्रमाणैः|गुडात् पलं दिवप्रसृतां तु

मात्रां स्नेहस्य युक्त्या मधु सैन्धवं च||१५|| प्रक्षिप्य बस्तौ मथितं खजेन सुबद्धमुच्छ्वास्य च निर्वलीकम्|

अङ्गुष्ठमध्येन मुखं पिधाय नेत्राग्रसंस्थामपनीय वर्तिम्||१६|| तैलाक्तगात्रं कृतमूत्रविट्कं नातिक्षुधार्तं शयने मनुष्यम्|

समेऽथवेषन्नतशीर्षके वा नात्युच्छ्रिते स्वास्तरणोपपन्ने||१७|| सव्येन पार्श्वेन सुखं शयानं कृत्वर्जुदेहं स्वभुजोपधानम्|
सङ्कोच्य सव्येतरदस्य सक्थि वामं प्रसार्य प्रणयेततस्तम्||१८|| स्निग्धे गुदे नेत्रचतुर्थभागं स्निग्धं शनैरृज्वन पृष्ठवंशम्|
अकम्पनावेपनलाघवादीन् पाण्योर्गुणांश्चापि विदर्शयंस्तम्||१९||प्रपीड्य चैकग्रहणेन दत्तं नेत्रं शनैरेव ततोऽपकर्षेत्|२०|

One Pala each of Bala, Guduchi, Haritaki, Vibhitaka, Amalaki, Rasna, Bilva, Syonaka, Gambhari, Patala, Ganikarika, Salaparni, Prsniparni, Brhati, Kantakari and Goksura, eight fruits of madana and half Tula (200 Tolas) of Goat meat should be added with water, and boiled till one fourth of water remains. Then the decoction is collected by filtration. To this decoction, one Picu (12 g) each of the paste of Yavani, Madana phala, Bilva, Kustha, Vaca, Satahva, Ghana and Pippali, one Pala of Jaggery, two Prastas each of ghee and oil, and appropriate quantities of honey and rock salt should be added. The recipe should then be stirred with a stirrer (Khaja), and kept inside the basti (enema receptacle) should then be tied to the base of the nozzle, the air inside the bladder is taken out, and the bladder is made free from wrinkles. Thereafter, Varti (elongated plug) at the mouth (of the nozzle) is removed, and the opening (in the mouth) is covered with the middle part of the thumb.

The patient whose body is anointed with oil, who has passed urine and stool, and who is not very hungry is made to sleep over a well spread, and not very high bed which is uniform in level or which is slightly low in level at the head-side.

The patient should sleep comfortably on his left side. He should keep his body straight, and use his flooded left hand as a pillow. He should then flex his right leg, keeping the left leg straight (fully extended).

The anus of the patient is lubricated, and the lubricated nozzle is inserted into it up to one fourth part from the top slowly and straight following the position of the vertebral column.

The physician should not shake or tremble his hand, and quickly compress the bladder (enema – receptacle) so that the recipe goes inside at one stretch. Thereafter, he should remove the nozzle slowly. [13 2/4 – 2/4 20]

Improper Administration of basti

तिर्यक् प्रणीते तु न याति धारा गुदे व्रणः स्याच्चलिते तु नेत्रे||२०|| दत्तः शनैर्नाशयमेति बस्तिः कण्ठं प्रधावत्यतिपीडितश्च|
शीतस्त्वतिस्तम्भकरो विदाहं मूच्छां च कुर्यादतिमात्रमुष्णः||२१|| स्निग्धोऽतिजाड्यं पवनं तु रूक्षस्तन्वल्पमात्रालवणस्त्वयोगम्|
करोति मात्राभ्यधिकोऽतियोगं क्षामं तु सान्द्रः सुचिरेण चैति||२२|| दाहातिसारौ लवणोऽति कुर्यात्तस्मात् सुयुक्तं सममेव दद्यात्|२३|

If the nozzle is obliquely inserted, then the fluid will not flow into the rectum. If the nozzle is shifted from one place to the other, then this may cause anal ulcer. If the bladder is compressed slowly, then the enema-fluid may not reach the colon. If the bladder (Basti) is strongly compressed, then the fluid may rush very fast [in the alimentary tract] even up to the throat.

Sl No Nature of Enema Fluid Effect of enema

1 very cold stiffness [of the body]

2 very hot burning sensation and fainting

3 very unctuous numbness [of the body]

4 very un-unctuous aggravation of Vayu

5 very thin or added with less quantity of salt or administered in large quantity it may cause Ati-Yoga (over – action)

6 vicid (thick) then it may cause emaciation (weakness) of the patient and it moves in the colon very slowly

7 contains salt in excess it may cause burning sensation and diarrhoea

Therefore, Basti should be properly and uniformly administered. [20 2/4 – 2/4 23]

Order of adding ingredients of different categories

पूर्वं हि दद्यान्मधु सैन्धवं तु स्नेहं विनिर्मथ्यं ततोऽनु कल्कम्||२३||
विमथ्य संयोज्य पुनर्द्रवैस्तं बस्तौ निदध्यान्मथितं खजेन|२४|

In the beginning, honey and rock-salt is added to the fat (ghee and oil) and stirred. Thereafter, the paste of drugs is added and stirred again. To this, the liquid (decoction) is added and stirred further with the help of a stirrer. This recipe should thereafter, be placed in the Basti (enema – receptacle). [23 2/4- 2/4 24]

Posture of Body during Enema

वामाश्रये हि ग्रहणीगुदे च तत् पार्श्वसंस्थस्य सुखोपलब्धिः||२४||

लीयन्त एव वलयश्च तस्मात् सव्यं शयानोऽर्हति बस्तिदानम्|२५|

As the Grahani (organ of assimilation, i.e duodenum and upper part of the small intestine) and rectum are located in the left side of the body, administration of Basti (enema) while the patient is lying in his left side would bestow pleasant benefits. The patient laying in his left side keeps the sphincters (valayas) submerged [into the surrounding musculature]. Therefore, Basti is given when the patient is lying in his left side. [24 2/4 – 2/4 25]

Management of Complications:

विड्वातवेगो यदि चार्धदत्ते निष्कृष्य मुक्ते प्रणयेदशेषम् ||२५||

उत्तानदेहश्च कृतोपधानः स्याद्वीर्यमाप्नोति तथाऽस्य देहम्|२६|

While administering enema, if in the middle, the patient gets an urge to void feces or flatus, then the nozzle is taken out, and after the patient has voided stool or flatus, the remaining enema- fluid is injected. The patient should thereafter, be made to lie down on his back with a pillow below his head. By doing so, his body gets invigorated with the effect of enema. [25 2/4 – 2/4 26]

Effect of Three Enemas

एकोऽपकर्षत्यनिलं स्वमार्गात् पित्तं द्विृतीयस्तु कफं तृतीयः||२६||

The first enema helps in the elimination of Vata, the second enema helps in the elimination of pitta, and the third enema helps in the elimination of Kapha from their own channels. [26 2/4]

Post- therapeutic measures

प्रत्यागते कोष्णजलावसिक्तः शाल्यन्नमद्यातनुना रसेन| जीर्णे तु सायं लघु चाल्पमात्रं भुक्तोऽनुवास्यः परिबृंहणार्थम्|२७||

निरूहपादांशसमेन तैलेनाम्लानिलघ्नौषधसाधितेन| दत्वा स्फिचौ पाणितलेन हन्यात् स्नेहस्य शीघ्रागमरक्षणार्थम्|२८||

ईषच्च पादाङ्गुलियुग्ममाञ्छेदुतानदेहस्य तलौ प्रमृज्यात्| स्नेहेन पार्ष्ण्यङ्गुलिपिण्डिकाश्च ये चास्य गात्रावयवा रुगार्ताः||२९||

तांश्चावमद्गीत सुखं ततश्च निद्रामुपासीत कृतोपधानः|३०|

After the enema-fluid has returned, the patient is sprinkled with tepid water, and thereafter, given the diet containing Sali rice along with thin meat soup.

In the evening, after the previous meal is digested, the patient is given light food in small quantities.

Thereafter, Anuvasana- Basti (unctuous enema) is given to the patient for all round nourishment of his body.

For anuvasana basti, medicated oil cooked by adding sour and vayu-alleviating drugs should be used. This oil is one-fourth in quantity of the fluid used for

Niruha-Basti. After the administration of oil, the buttocks of the patient are tapped (pressed) with the palms to prevent early return of reciepe (medicated oil) from the anus.

The patient should lie on the bed in supine position, and the toe joints of both of his legs are pulled gently. The soles of his feet are massaged with oil. His heels, toes, calf regions and such other parts which are painful should also be massaged with oil. Thereafter, the patient should sleep comfortably by keeping his head over a pillow (and he should not do any other work) [27- 2/4 30]

Proportion of Ingredients in Basti – recipe:

भागाः कषायस्य तु पञ्च, पित्ते स्नेहस्य षष्ठः प्रकृतौ स्थिते च||३०||

वाते विवृद्धे तु चतुर्थभागो, मात्रा निरूहेषु कफेऽष्टभागः|३१|

In the recipe of Niruha-Basti (total quantity: twelve Prasrutas or 24 Palas) the decoction is five parts (five Prasritas or ten Palas). If this is intended to be given to a patient suffering from Paittika diseases or to a healthy person, then the quantity of Sneha (fat) is one sixth of the total quantity (i.e two Prasritas or four Palas). For Vaittika diseases, the quantity of Sneha (fat) is one-fourth of the total quantity (i.e three Prasritas or six Palas). For Kaphaja diseases, the quantity of Sneha is 1/8 th of the total quantity (i.e 1 ½ Prastas or three palas). [30 2/4- 2/4 31]

Dose of Niruha-Basti for Different Age- groups

निरूहमात्रा प्रसृताधमाद्ये वर्षे ततोऽर्धप्रसृताभिवृद्धिः||३१|| आद्वादशात् स्यात् प्रसृताभिवृद्धिरष्टादशाद् द्वादशतः परं स्युः|
आसप्ततेस्तदिवहितं प्रमाणमतः परं षोडशविद्विधेयम्||३२|| निरूहमात्रा प्रसृतप्रमाणा बाले च वृद्धे च मृदुर्विशेषः|३३|

For thc one-year-old, the dose of niruha- recipe is half Prasrta (one Pala). Thereafter, for each year of age, the dose is increased by half Prasrta up to twelve years. [For the patient of twelve years old, the dose of Niruha recipe should, therefore, be six Prasritas].

After twelve years of age, the dose of Niruha is increased by one Prasrta for each (of age) till eighteenth year of age. [For the patient of eighteen years old the dose of Niruha should therefore be twelve Prasthas, which is the maximum dose]. This dose of Niruha is prescribed up to the age of seventy. After seventy years of age, the dose of Niruha should be similar to that of a patient of sixteen years old [i.e ten Prasritas]

Thus, the dose of Niruha is described for patients of different age groups in terms of Prasrta.

For infants and old people, the ingredients of enema recipe are specifically mild in nature. [31 2/4- 2/4 33]

Bed to be used after Therapy

नात्युच्छ्रितं नाप्यतिनीचपादं सपादपीठं शयनं प्रशस्तम्||३३||
प्रधानमृद्वास्तरणोपपन्नं प्राक्शीर्षकं शुक्लपटोत्तरीयम्|३४|

After the administration of the therapy is over, the patient should lie down on a bed which is neither too high nor with too low pedestal. This bed should have a foot-rest, and is spread with an adequately big and soft mattress. The patient should lie with his head towards the east, and cover himself with white linen. [33 2/4- 2/4 34]

Diet to be given after Therapy

भोज्यं पुनर्व्याधिमवेक्ष्य तद्वत् प्रकल्पयेद्यूषपयोरसाद्यैः||३४||
सर्वेषु विद्यादिवधिमेतमाद्यं वक्ष्यामि बस्तीनत उत्तरीयान्|३५|

The diet of the patient [after the therapy] is determined on the basis of the nature of his disease. It should consist of vegetables – soup, milk, meat-soup, etc. This is the primary and general principle to be followed in all the conditions. Hereafter, the recipes for the Niruha-Basti will be described. [34 2/4- 2/4 35]

Recipe of Niruha (first Recipe)

द्विपञ्चमूलस्य रसोऽम्लयुक्तः सच्छागमांसस्य सपूर्वपेष्यः||३५||
त्रिस्नेहयुक्तः प्रवरो निरूहः सर्वानिलव्याधिहरः प्रदिष्टः|

The recipe containing decoction of Dvi Panchamoola (Dashamoola) is added with sour juice, soup of goat-meat, the paste of drugs described earlier in the verse no. 13 (viz, Bala, Guduchi, Haritaki, Vibhitaka, Amalaki, Rasna, Bilva, Syonaka, Gambhari, Patala, Ganikarika, Salaparni, Prsniparni, Brhati, Kantakari and Goksura), and three types of fat (ghee, oil and muscle- fat) is excellent for Niruha Basti to be given for curing all the diseases caused by aggravation of Vayu. [35 2/4 – 2/4 3]

Second Recipe of Niruha

स्थिरादिवर्गस्य बलापटोलत्रायन्तिकैरण्डयवैर्युतस्य||३६||
प्रस्थो रसाच्छागरसार्धयुक्तः साध्यः पुनः प्रस्थसमस्तु यावत् प्रियङ्गुकृष्णाघनकल्कयुक्तः सतैलसर्पिर्मधुसैन्धवश्च||३७||
स्याद्दीपनो मांसबलप्रदश्च चक्षुर्बलं चापि ददाति बस्तिः |

One Prastha of the decoction of drugs belonging to Sthiradi – group (sthira or Vidarigandha, Prsniparni, Brhati, Kantakari, Eranda, Kakoli, Chandana, Usira, Ela and Madhuka- vide Sutra 4: 170 Bala, Patola, Trayantika, Eranda (it is a repetition) and Yava, and half a Prastha of the liquid remains. To this, the paste of Priyangu, Krsna and Ghana, oil, ghee, honey and rocksalt is added, and used for enema. It stimulates the power of digestion, provides strength to the muscle tissue and even promotes the strength of the eyes (eye- sight). [36 2/4 – 2/4 38]

Third Recipe of Niruha Eranda-Basti

एरण्डमूलं त्रिपलं पलाशा ह्रस्वानि मूलानि च यानि पञ्च||३८||

रास्नाश्वगन्धातिबलागुडूची पुनर्नवारग्वधदेवदारु| भागाः पलांशा मदनाष्टयुक्ता जलद्विकंसे क्वथितेऽष्टशेषे||३९||

पेष्याः शताह्वा हपुषा प्रियङ्गुः सपिप्पलीकं मधुकं बला च| रसाञ्जनं वत्सकबीजमुस्तं भागाक्षमात्रं लवणांशयुक्तम्||४०||

समाक्षिकस्तैलयुतः समूत्रो बस्तिर्नृणां दीपनलेखनीयः| जङ्घोरुपादत्रिकपृष्ठशूलं कफावृतिं मारुतनिग्रहं च||४१||

विण्मूत्रवातग्रहणं सशूलमाध्मानतामश्मरिशर्करे च| आनाहमर्शोग्रहणीप्रदोषानेरण्डबस्तिः शमयेत् प्रयुक्तः||४२||

Three Palas of the root of Eranda, one Pala each of the Pastes of Palasha (Sati), Salaparni, Prsniparni, Brhati, Kantakari, Goksura, Rasna, Asvagandha, Atibala, Guduchi, Punarnava, Aragvadha and Devadaru and the paste of eight seeds of Madana is added with two Kamsas (512 Tolas) of water and boiled till one-eighth of the liquid remains. To this decoction, the paste of one Aksa or Tola each of Sarahva, Hapusa, Priyangu, Pippali, Madhuka, Bala, Rasanjana, seeds of Vatsaka and Musta along with appropriate quantity of rock-salt, honey, oil and cow's urine is added. Administration of this recipe as enema is dipaniya (stimulant of the power of digestion) and Lekhaniya (which scraps out the morbid matter from the body). Administration of the Eranda-Basti cures pain in the calf region, thighs, feet, lumbar region and back, Kaphavrti (occlusion of vayu by kapha), Maruta Nigraha (immobility of Vata), obstruction to the voiding of stool, urine and flatus associated with pain, Adhmanata (tymphanites), Asmari (stone in the urinary tract), Sarkara (Gravel in urine), Anaha (constipation), Arsas (piles) and Grahani Dosha (Sprue syndrome) . [38 2/4 – 42]

Fourth Recipe of niruha

चतुष्पले तैलघृतस्य भृष्टाच्छागाच्छतार्धौ दधिदाडिमाम्लः| रसः सपेष्यो बलमांसवर्णरेतोग्निदश्चान्ध्यशिरोर्तिशस्तः ||४३||

Fifty Palas of the soup of goat-meat should be sizzled with four Palas of ghee and oil, made sour by adding Dadhi (yogurt) and Dadima, and added with the paste (of bala, etc. described earlier in verse no. 13)

Use of this recipe for enema promotes strength, muscles, complexion, semen and agni (power of digestion as well as metabolism), and cures blindness as well as headache. [43]

Fifth recipe of Niruha

जलद्विकंसेऽष्टपलं पलाशात् पक्त्वा रसोऽर्धाढकमात्रशेषः| कल्कैर्वचामागधिकापलाभ्यां युक्तः शताह्वादिवपलेन चापि||४४||

ससैन्धवः क्षौद्रयुतः सतैलो देयो निरूहो बलवर्णकारी| आनाहपार्श्वामययोनिदोषान् गुल्मानुदावर्तरुजं च हन्यात्||४५||

Eight Palas of Palasha is added with two Kamsas (128 Palas) of water, and boiled till the liquid is reduced to half Adhaka (32 Palas). To this decoction, the paste of one Pala each of Vaca and magadhika, and two Palas of Satahva along with rock- salt, honey and oil are added. This recipe is used for Niruha.

It promotes strength and complex. It cures (Constipation), parsvamaya (pain in the sides of the chest), Yoni-Dosha (gynecic diseases), Gulma (phantom tumour) and Udavarta (upward movement of wind in the abdomen). [45]

Six Recipe of Niruha

यष्ट्याह्वयस्याष्टपलेन सिद्धं पयः शताह्वाफलपिप्पलीभिः| युक्तं ससर्पिर्मधु वातरक्तवैस्वर्यवीसर्पहितो निरूहः||४६||

Milk boiled by adding eight palas of Yastimadhu is mixed with [the paste] of satahva, Phala (Madanaphala) and Pippali, ghee and honey. Administration of this recipe in the form of Niruha- Basti cures Vatarakta (gout), vaisvarya (hoarseness of voice) and Visarpa (erysipelas). [46]

Seventh recipe of Niruha

यष्ट्याह्वलोध्राभयचन्दनैश्च शृतं पयोऽग्र्यं कमलोत्पलैश्च| सशर्करं क्षौद्रयुतं सुशीतं पित्तामयान् हन्ति सजीवनीयम्||४७||

The milk boiled with Yastimadhu, Lodhra, Abhaya (Usira), Chandana, Kamala and Utpala is added with sugar as well as honey, and cooled. To this, the [paste] of drugs belonging to Jivaniya- group (Jivika, Rsabhaka, Meda, Maha-meda, Kakoli, Ksirakakoli, Mudgaparni, Masaparni, Jivanti and Madhuka: vide Sutra 4:9) is added.

Niruha –basti administered with this recipe cures diseases caused by aggravated Pitta. [47]

Eighth recipe of Niruha:

द्विकार्षिकाश्चन्दनपद्मकर्धियष्ट्याह्वरास्नावृषसारिवाश्च| सलोध्रमञ्जिष्ठमथाप्यनन्ताबलास्थिरादितृणपञ्चमूलम्||४८||

तोये समुत्क्वाथ्य रसेन तेन शृतं पयोऽर्धाढकमम्बुहीनम्| जीवन्तिमेदर्धिशतावरीभिर्वीरादिवकाकोलिकशेरुकाभिः||४९||

सितोपलाजीवकपद्मरेणु प्रपौण्डरीकैः कमलोत्पलैश्च| लोध्रात्मगुप्तामधुकैर्विदारीमुञ्जातकैः केशरचन्दनैश्च||५०||

पिष्टैर्घृतक्षौद्रयुतैर्निरूहं ससैन्धवं शीतलमेव दद्यात्| प्रत्यागते धन्वरसेन शालीन् क्षीरेण वाऽद्यात् परिषिक्तगात्रः||५१||

दाहातिसारप्रदरास्रपित्तहृत्पाण्डुरोगान् विषमज्वरं च| सगुल्ममूत्रग्रहकामलादीन् सर्वामयान् पित्तकृतान्निहन्ति||५२||

Two Karsas (tolas) each of Chandana, Padmaka, Rddhi, Yastimadhu, Rasna, Vrsa, Sariva, Lodhra, Manjistha, Ananta (Utpala-Sariva), Bala, Vidarigandha, Prsniparni, Brhati, Kantakarika, Eranda, Kakoli, Chandana, Usira, Ela, Madhuka (vide Sutra 4:17), Sali, Kasa, Darbha and Iksu (vide Cikista 1:1:44) is boiled by adding water.

To this decoction, half Adhaka (72 Palas) of milk is added and boiled till the moisture / water content of the liquid gets evaporated, i.e only 72 Palas of milk remains. Thereafter, to this milk, the paste of Jivanti, Meda, Rddhi, Satavari, Vira, Kakoli, Ksirakakoli, Kaseruka, Sitopala (crystal sugar), Jivaka, anthers of lotus, Prapanudarika, Kamala, Utpala, Lodhra, Atmagupta, Madhuka, Vidari, Munjataka, Kesara and Chandana along with ghee, honey and small quantity of rock-salt is added. This recipe, when cold, is given as Niruha basti.

After the return of enema fluid, the patient's body is sprinkled with water, and he is given Sali type of rice either with meat of animals inhabiting arid zone (jangala-mamsa) or milk.

This type of enema cures Daha (burning sensation), Atisara (diarrhoea), Pradara (menorrhagia), Raktapitta (an ailment characterised by bleeding from different parts of the body), Hrdroga (heart- diseases), Pandu Roga (anemia), Visama-Jvara (irregular fever), Gulma (phantom tumour), Mutra-Graha (anuria), Kamala (jaundice) etc. and all the other diseases caused by aggravated Pitta. [48-52]

Ninth recipe of Niruha

द्राक्षादिकाश्मर्यमधूकसेव्यैः ससारिवाचन्दनशीतपाक्यैः| पयः शृतं श्रावणिमुद्गपर्णीतुगात्मगुप्तामधुयष्टिकल्कैः||५३||

गोधूमचूर्णैश्च तथाऽक्षमात्रैः सक्षौद्रसर्पिर्मधुयष्टितैलैः| पथ्याविदारीक्षुरसैर्गुडेन बस्तिं युतं पित्तहरं विदध्यात्||५४||

हृन्नाभिपार्श्वोत्तमदेहदाहे दाहेऽन्तरस्थे च सकृच्छ्रमूत्रे| क्षीणे क्षते रेतसि चापि नष्टे पैत्तेऽतिसारे च नृणां प्रशस्तः||५५||

Milk boiled with Draksa (and such other sweet ingredients), Kashmarya, Madhuka, Sevya, Sariva, Chandana and Sitapaki (Sitali) is added with the paste of one Karsa (tola) each of Sravani, Mudgaparni, Tugaksiri, Atmagupta and Madhuyasti as well as with one Aksa of wheat-flour. To this, honey, ghee, Madhuyasti, oil, haritaki, vidari, sugarcane juice and jaggery is added and given as Basti (medicated enema). This alleviates aggravated Pitta. It is an excellent remedy for the patients suffering from burning sensation in the cardiac region, umbilicus, sides of the chest, head and the interior part of the body, Mutra-Krcchra (Dysuria), Ksina (consumption), Ksata (phthisis), loss of semen and Paittika type of Diarrhoea. [53- 55]

Tenth recipe of Niruha:

कोषातकारग्वधदेवदारुशाङ्र्गेष्टमूर्वाकुटजार्कपाठाः |पक्त्वा कुलत्थान् बृहतीं च तोये रसस्य तस्य प्रसृता दश स्युः||५६||

तान् सर्षपैलामदनैः सकुष्ठैरक्षप्रमाणैः प्रसृतैश्च युक्तान्| फलाह्वतैलस्य समाक्षिकस्य क्षारस्य तैलस्य च सार्षपस्य||५७||

दद्यान्निरूहं कफरोगिणे ज्ञो मन्दाग्नये चाप्यशनिद्विषे च|

Ten Prasritas (one Prasrta = two palas) of decoction is prepared by boiling kosataka, Aragvadha, devadaru, Sarngesta (Gunja), Murva, Kutaja, Arka, Patha, Kulattha and brhati with water. To this, the paste of one Aksa each of Sarsapa, Ela, Madana and Kustha, and one Prasta each of Madana-Phala, oil, honey, Ksara (Alkali preparation) and mustard oil, honey, Ksara (alkali preparation) and mustard oil is added. An expert physician should use this recipe as niruha-basti for the patients suffering from diseases caused by aggravated kapha, Mandagni (suppression of the power of digestion) and asana Dvesa (aversion to food). [56- 2/4 58]

Eleventh recipe of Niruha

पटोलपथ्यामरदारुभिर्वा सपिप्पलीकैः क्वथितैर्जलेऽग्नौ||५८||

Alternatively, water is boiled over fire by adding Patola, Pathya, Devadaru and Pippali. [With this decoction, enema is given according to the procedure described for the tenth recipe.] [58 2/4]

Twelfth recipe of Niruha

द्विपञ्चमूले त्रिफलां सबिल्वां फलानि गोमूत्रयुतः कषायः| कलिङ्गपाठाफलमुस्तकल्कः ससैन्धवः क्षारयुतः सतैलः||५९||

निरूहमुख्यः कफजान् विकारान् सपाण्डुरोगालसकामदोषान्|

हन्यात्तथा मारुतमूत्रसङ्गं बस्तेस्तथाऽऽटोपमथापि घोरम्||६०||

To the decoction of Dvi Panchamula (Dashamoola), Triphala, Bilva (fruit) and Madana phala and Musta prepared by adding cow's urine, the paste of Kalinga, Patha, Madana phala is added. This recipe is mixed with rock-salt, Ksara (Yava-Ksara: and alkali preparation) and oil, and used for Niruha basti. It is excellent for curing diseases caused by aggravated kapha, Pandu-roga (anaemia), Alasaka (intestinal topor), ailments caused by Ama (product of improper digestion and metabolism), obstruction to the improper digestion and metabolism), obstruction to the voiding of flatus as well as urine, and serious types of bladder distension. [59-60]

Thirteenth recipe of Niruha

रास्नामृतैरण्डविडङ्गदार्वीसप्तच्छदोशीरसुराह्वनिम्बैः| शम्पाकभूनिम्बपटोलपाठातिक्ताखुपर्णीदशमूलमुस्तैः||६१||

त्रायन्तिकाशिग्रुफलत्रिकैश्च क्वाथः सपिण्डीतकतोयमूत्रः| यष्ट्याह्वकृष्णाफलिनीशताह्वारसाञ्जनश्वेतवचाविडङ्गैः||६२||

कलिङ्गपाठाम्बुदसैन्धवैश्च कल्कैः ससर्पिर्मधुतैलमिश्रः| अयं निरूहः क्रिमिकुष्ठमेहब्रध्नोदराजीर्णकफातुरेभ्यः||६३||

रूक्षौषधैरप्यपतर्पितेभ्य एतेषु रोगेष्वपि सत्सु दत्तः| निहत्य वातं ज्वलनं प्रदीप्य विजित्य रोगांश्च बलं करोति||६४||

To the decoction of Rasna, Amrta, Eranda, Vidanga, Daruharidra, Saptacchada, Usira, Surahva, Nimba, Sampaka, Bhunimba, Patola, Patha, Tikta, Akhuparni, Dashamoola, Musta, Trayantika, Sigru, Haritaki, Vibhitaka, Amalaki, the decoction of Pinditaka (madana phala) and Mutra (cow's urine) is added. To this liquid, the paste of madhuyasti, krsna (pippali), Phalini, satahva, Rasanjana, Sveta vaca, Vidanga, Kalinga, Patha, Ambuda (musta) and rock-salt along with ghee, honey and oil is added.

Administration of this recipe for Niruha basti cures Krmi (intestinal parasites), Kustha (skin diseases), meha (obstinate urinary disorders including diabetes), bradhna (inguinal swelling), udara (obstinate abdominal diseases including ascites), Ajirna (indigestion) and diseases caused by Kapha. Administration of this Niruha Basti to the aforesaid patients, who are emaciated because of the use of un-unctuous medicines alleviates Vayu, stimulates Agni (power of digestion and metabolism), cures diseases and promotes strength. [61-64]

Recipc of niruha for combined Doshas

पुनर्नवैरण्डवृषाश्मभेदवृश्चीरभूतीकबलापलाशाः | द्विपञ्चमूलं च पलांशिकानि क्षुण्णानि धौतानि फलानि [२] चाष्टौ||६५||

बिल्वं यवान् कोलकुलत्थधान्यफलानि चैव प्रसृतोन्मितानि|पयोजलद्व्याढकवच्छृतं तत् क्षीरावशेषं सितवस्त्रपूतम्||६६||

वचाशताह्वामरदारुकुष्ठयष्ट्याह्वसिद्धार्थकपिप्पलीनाम् | कल्कैर्यवान्या मदनैश्च युक्तं नात्युष्णशीतं गुडसैन्धवाक्तम्||६७||

क्षौद्रस्य तैलस्य च सर्पिषश्च तथैव युक्तं प्रसृतैस्त्रिभिश्च | दद्यान्निरूहं विधिना विविज्ञः स सर्वसंसर्गकृतामयघ्नः||६८||

One Pala each of Punarnava (red variety), eranda vrksa (Vasaka) Asmabheda (Pasana- Bheda), Vrscira (sveta or white variety of Punarnava), Bhutika, bala, Palasha, bilva, syonaka, gambhari, patala, Ganikarika, Salaparni, Prsniparni, Brhati, Kantakari and Goksura and eight fruits of madana-phala is cut into pieces and washed. To this, one Prashta (two Palas) each of Bilva, Yava, Kola, Kulattha, Dhanyaka and madana phala, and two adhakas each of milk and water is added and boiled till the milk i.e., two adhakas of the liquid remains. The milk should then be filtered out through a white cloth. To this milk, the paste of Vaca, satahva, Devadaru, Kustha, Yastimadhu, Siddharthaka, Pippali, yavani and Madana phala is added. When lukewarm, jaggery, rock-salt, one prasrta each of honey, oil and ghee is added to this recipe, and administered as Niruha basti appropriately by a physician well versed in this field. It cures all the diseases caused by samsarga (combination of aggravated Doshas). [65-68]

Number of Bastis for Different Doshas

स्निग्धोष्ण एकः पवने समांसो द्वौ स्वादुशीतौ पयसा च पित्ते| त्रयः समूत्राः कटुकोष्णतीक्ष्णाः कफे निरूहा न परं विधेयाः||६९||

Patients suffering from Vatika diseases are given one Niruha Basti which is unctuous and warm, and which contains meat-soup. For the patients suffering from Paittika diseases, two Niruha bastis which are sweet and cold, and which contain milk is given. Patients suffering from Kaphaja diseases are given three Niruha Bastis which contain cow's urine and which are pungent, hot as well as sharp.

Niruha Basti should not be given in excess of these specified numbers. [69]

Regimen after Niruha –basti

रसेन वाते प्रतिभोजनं स्यात् क्षीरेण पित्ते तु कफे च यूषैः| तथाऽनुवास्येषु च बिल्वतैलं स्याज्जीवनीयं फलसाधितं च||७०||

After the administration of Niuha basti, the patient suffering from vatika diseases is given meat-soup; the patient suffering from Paittika diseases is given milk and the patient suffering from kaphaja diseases is given vegetable soup as a diet.

After the administration of niruha-basti (evacuative type of medicated enema), those requiring Anuvasana-basti (unctuous type of medicated enema) are given this enema containing Bilva Taila (if the diseases are caused by Vayu), Jivaniya taila (if the disease is caused by Pitta) or Madhu Phala Taila (if the disease is caused by Kapha). [70]

इतीदमुक्तं निखिलं यथावद्बस्तिप्रदानस्य विधानमग्र्यम्| योऽधीत्य विद्वानिह बस्तिकर्म करोति लोके लभते स सिद्धिम्||७१||

Thus, the foremost methods of the administration of basti are fully described. The wise physician, who, after studying this, practises Basti (medicated enema) therapy, achieves success in this world. [71]

इत्यग्निवेशकृते तन्त्रे चरकप्रतिसंस्कृतेऽप्राप्ते दृढबलसम्पूरिते सिद्धिस्थाने बस्तिसूत्रीयसिद्धिर्नाम तृतीयोऽध्यायः||३||

Thus, ends the third chapter describing "thePrinciples of Basti" in the text composed by Agnivesha, redacted by Charaka, and because of its non- availability, Supplemented by Drdhabala.

29

Siddhisthana Chapter 4 Sneha Vyapat Siddhi

Prologue

अथातः स्नेहव्यापत्सिद्धिं व्याख्यास्यामः||१||

इति ह स्माह भगवानात्रेयः||२||

We shall now explore the chapter dealing with "the management of complications arising from the Administration of Anuvasana Basti (unctuous enema)". Thus, said Lord Atreya [1-2]

Details of Topics to be Discussed

स्नेहबस्तीन्निबोधेमान् वातपित्तकफापहान्|

मिथ्याप्रणिहितानां च व्यापदः सचिकित्सिताः||३||

Now listen! [Addressed to Agnivesha by the preceptor Atreya] to the description of the following topics:

Recipes for Sneha or Anuvasana Basti (unctuous enema) for the treatment of diseases caused by Vayu, Pitta and Kapha

Complications arising from their wrongful administration and

Treatment of these complications [3]

Anuvasana Rccipe for Vayu (Bilva Taila)

दशमूलं बलां रास्नामश्वगन्धां पुनर्नवाम्| गुडूच्येरण्डभूतीकभार्गीवृषकरोहिषम्||४||

शतावरी सहचरं काकनासां पलांशिकम् | यवमाषातसीकोलकुलत्थान् प्रसृतोन्मितान्||५||

चतुर्द्रोणेऽम्भसः पक्त्वा द्रोणशेषेण तेन च| तैलाढकं समक्षीरं जीवनीयैः पलोन्मितैः||६||

अनुवासनमेतद्धि सर्ववातविकारनुत्|

One Pala each of Bilva, Syonaka, Gambhari, Patala, Ganikarika, Salaparni, Prsniparni, Brhati, Kantakarika, Gokshura, Bala, Rasna, Asvagandha, Punarnava, Guduchi, Eranda, Bhutika(Yavani) Bhargi, Vrsaka (Vasa), Rohisa, Shatavari, Sahacara as well as Kakanasa (Vayasi Phala), and one Prasrta (two Palas) each of Yava, Atasi, Kola as well as Kulattha is added with four Dronas (one Drona= 256 Palas) of water, and cooked till one Drona of the liquid remains. To this decoction, one Adhaka (64 Palas) each of oil and milk, and the paste of one Pala each of Jivaka, Rsabhaka, Meda, Mahameda, Kakoli, Ksirakakoli, Mudgaparni, Mashaparni, Jivanti and Madhuka are added. Anuvasana Basti (unctuous enema) with this recipe cures all the diseases caused by vayu. [4 – ½ 7]

Other Anuvasana Recipes for vayu:

आनूपानां वसा तद्वज्जीवनीयोपसाधिता||७||

शताह्वायवबिल्वाम्लैः सिद्धं तैलं समीरणे|

सैन्धवेनाग्नितप्तेन तप्तं चानिलनुद्धृतम्||८||

Anuvasana Basti prepared of vasa (muscle fat) of animals inhabiting marshy land, boiled with drugs belonging to Jivaniya group (Jivaka, Rsabhaka, Meda, Mahameda, Kakoli, Ksirakakoli, Mudgaparni, Mashaparni, Jivanti and Madhuka), similarly cures Vatika diseases.

Anuvasana Basti with the oil cooked by Satahva, Yava, Bilva and sour juice is also useful in vatika diseases.

Anuvasana Basti with ghee which has been heated by the immersion of hot rock-salt cures diseases caused by Vayu. [7 ½ - 8]

Recipe of Anuvasana Basti for Pitta (Jivaniya –Yamaka)

जीवन्तीं मदनं मेदां श्रावणीं मधुकं बलाम्। शताह्वर्षभकौ कृष्णां काकनासां शतावरीम्||९||

स्वगुप्तां क्षीरकाकोलीं कर्कटाख्यां शटीं वचाम्। पिष्ट्वा तैलं घृतं क्षीरे साधयेतच्चतुर्गुणे||१०||

बृंहणं वातपित्तघ्नं बलशुक्राग्निवर्धनम्। मूत्रेतोरजोदोषान् हरेतदनुवासनम्||११||

Ghee and oil taken together may be cooked by adding four times of milk along with the paste of Jivanti, Madana Phala, Meda, Sravani, Madhuka, Bala, Satahva, Rsabhaka, Krsna (Pippali), Karkanasa, Shatavari, Svagupta (Atmagupta), Ksirakakoli, Karkatakhya (Karkata Srngi), Sati and Vaca. Anuvasana Basti with this recipe is nourishing, alleviator of Vayu and Pitta, promoter of strength, semen and Agni (power of digestion including metabolism) and curative of urinary, seminal and menstrual morbidities. [9-11]

Another Anuvasana Recipe for Pitta

लाभतश्चन्दनाद्यैश्च पिष्टैः क्षीरचतुर्गुणम्। तैलपादं घृतं सिद्धं पित्तघ्नमनुवासनम्||१२||

Ghee cooked with four times of milk, one fourth in quantity of oil, and the paste of drugs belonging to Chandanadi group whichever are available, is used for anuvasana basti which alleviates Pitta. [12]

Anuvasana Recipe for Kapha

सैन्धवं मदनं कुष्ठं शताह्वां निचुलं वचाम्। ह्रीवेरं मधुकं भार्गीं देवदारु सकट्फलम्||१३||

नागरं पुष्करं मेदां चविकां चित्रकं शटीम्। विडङ्गातिविषे श्यामां हरेणुं नीलिनीं स्थिराम्||१४||

बिल्वाजमोदे कृष्णां च दन्तीं रास्नां च पेषयेत्। साध्यमेरण्डजं तैलं तैलं वा कफरोगनुत्||१५||

वृध्नोदावर्तगुल्मार्शःप्लीहमेहाढ्यमारुतान्। आनाहमश्मरी चैव हन्यातदनुवासनात्||१६||

Castor oil, sesame oil is cooked by adding the paste of Saindhava (rock-salt), Madana, Kustha, Satahva, Nicula, Vaca, Hrivera, Madhuka, Bhargi, Devadaru, Katphala, Nagara, Puskara, Meda, Cavika, Chitraka, Sati, Vidanga, Ativisa, Syama, Hraenu, Nilini, Sthira, Bilva, Ajamoda, Krsna, Danti and Rasna. Anuvasana Basti with this medicated oil cures the below mentioned diseases –

Kaphaja diseases,

Bradhna (inguinal enlargement),

Udavarta (upward movement of wind in the abdomen),

Gulma (phantom tumour),

Arshas (piles),

Plihan (splenic disorders),

Meha (obstinate urinary diseases including diabetes),

Adhya-vata (a joint disease), Anaha (tympanites) and

Asmari (calculus) [13-16]

Another Anuvasana recipe for kapha (Madana- Taila)

मदनैर्वाऽम्लसंयुक्तैर्बिल्वाद्येन गणेन वा। तैलं कफहरैर्वाऽपि कफघ्नं कल्पयेदिभषक्||१७||

Oil cooked with Madana Phala by adding sour liquid (vinegar etc.) or by adding (the decoction as well as paste of) Bilva, Syonaka, Gambhari, Patala, Ganikarika, Salaparni, Prsniparni, Brhati, Kantakari and Gokshura, or by adding Kapha alleviating drugs may be used for Anuvasana Basti for the alleviation of kapha. [17]

Recipe for Anuvasana Basti

विडङ्गैरण्डरजनीपटोलत्रिफलामृताः| जातीप्रवालनिर्गुण्डीदशमूलाखुपर्णिकाः||१८||
निम्बपाठासहचरशम्पाककरवीरकाः| एषां क्वाथेन विपचेतैलमेभिश्च कल्कितैः||१९||
फलबिल्वत्रिवृत्कृष्णारास्नाभूनिम्बदारुभिः| सप्तपर्णवचोशीरदार्वीकुष्ठकलिङ्गकैः||२०||
लतागौरीशताह्वाग्निशटीचोरकपौष्करैः | तत् कुष्ठानि क्रिमीन् मेहानर्शांसि ग्रहणीगदम्||२१||
क्लीबतां विषमाग्नित्वं मलं दोषत्रयं तथा| प्रयुक्तं प्रणुदत्याशु पानाभ्यङ्गानुवासनैः||२२||

Oil is cooked by adding the decoction of Vidanga, Eranda, Rajani, Patola, Haritaki, Amalaki, Amrta, tender leaves of Jati, Nirgundi, Bilva, syonaka, Gambhari, Patala, ganikarika, Salaparni, Prsniparni, Brhati, Kantakari, Gokshura, Akhuparni, Nimbi, Patha, Sahacara, Sampaka, and Karavira and the paste of Madana phala, Bilva, Trivrt, Krsna, Rasna, Kalinga, Lata (manjistha), Gauri (haridra), Satahva, Agni, Sati, Coraka and Puskara-mula.

Administration of this medicated oil as potion, for massage or for Anuvasana Basti immediately cures –

Kustha (skin diseases),

Krimi (parasitic infestation),

Meha (obstinate urinary disorders including diabetes),

Arshas (piles),

Grahani (sprue),

Klibata (impotency),

Visamagni (irregular digestion),

Mala (production of morbid matter in excess) and

diseases caused by all the three Doshas [18-22]

Effects of Anuvasana Basti in General

व्याधिव्यायामकर्माध्वक्षीणाबलनिरोजसाम्| क्षीणशुक्रस्य चातीव स्नेहवस्तिर्बलप्रदः||२३||
पादजङ्घोरुपृष्ठांसकटीनां स्थिरतां पराम्| जनयेदप्रजानां च प्रजां स्त्रीणां तथा नृणाम्||२४||

Sneha or Anuvasana Basti [administered with the above mentioned medicated oils] promotes excessive strength of persons who are emaciated and debilitated because of long suffering from diseases, excessive exercise, hard labour, walking long distance, loss of Ojas (vital essence) and diminution of semen. It causes excellent stability of feet, calves, thighs, back, shoulder and lumbar region. It helps in the procreation of off springs by the sterile men and women. [23-24]

Conditions Leading to Complications

वातपित्तकफात्यन्नपुरीषैरावृतस्य च| अभुक्ते च प्रणीतस्य स्नेहबस्तेः षडापदः||२५||

Improper administration of Anuvasana Basti may give rise to complications in following six conditions:

Occlusion of the enema-fluid by vayu

Occlusion of the enema-fluid by Pitta

Occlusion of the enema-fluid by kapha

Occlusion of the enema-fluid by food, taken in excess

Occlusion of enema- fluid by faeces; and

Administration of enema on empty stomach [25]

Factors responsible for occlusion of enema-fluid

शीतोऽल्पो वाऽधिके वाते पित्तेऽत्युष्णः कफे मृदुः| अतिभुक्ते गुर्वर्चःसञ्चयेऽल्पबलस्तथा||२६||
दत्तस्तैरावृतः स्नेहो न यात्यभिभवादपि [१] |अभुक्तेऽनावृतत्वाच्च यात्यूर्ध्वं तस्य लक्षणम्||२७||

The Sneha (unctuous fluid of anuvasana basti) being occluded does not reach its destination because of the following:

If cold recipe is used in small quantity for unctuous enema when vayu is aggravated;

If excessively hot recipes are used for unctuous enema when Pitta is aggravated;

If mild recipe is used for unctuous enema when Kapha is aggravated;

If heavy recipe is used for unctuous enema when the patient has consumed food in excess quantity

If a recipe of mild nature is used for unctuous enema when there is accumulation of stool; and

If the recipe is afflicted because of excessively aggravated Doshas

If the patient has not taken food before the administration of unctuous enema the enema recipe reaches upwards much above the desired level because of the absence of any obstruction.

Hereafter, the signs of different impediments will be described. [26-27]

Signs of impediments by Vayu

अङ्गमर्दज्वराध्मानशीतस्तम्भोरुपीडनैः पार्श्वरुग्वेष्टनैर्विद्यात् स्नेहं वातावृतं भिषक्||२८||

The physician should ascertain the obstruction of the unctuous fluid by Vayu from the signs and symptoms like malaise, fever, adhmana (flatulence), sita (feeling of cold), stambha (stiffness), uru pidana (pain in the thighs), Parsvaruk (pain in the sides of the chest) and Parsva vestana (cramps in the sides of the chest). [28]

Treatment of Vata Impediment

स्निग्धाम्ललवणोष्णैस्तं रास्नापीतद्रुतैलिकैः |सौवीरकसुराकोलकुलत्थ्ययवसाधितैः||२९||

निरूहैर्निर्हरेत् सम्यक् समूत्रैः पाञ्चमूलिकैः| ताभ्यामेव च तैलाभ्यां सायं भुक्तेऽनुवासयेत्||३०||

The occlusion [of the enema-fluid by Vata] is removed by the administration of Niruha-Basti with the recipes of Rasnadi Taila and Pitadru Taila having the characteristic features as follows:

those which are added with unctuous, sour, saline and hot ingredients

those which are prepared by adding sauviraka (vinegar), Sura (alcohol), Kola Kulattha and Yava and

those which are mixed with cow's urine, and the decoction of Bilva, Syonaka, Gambhari, Patala and Ganikarika.

After the evening meals, the patient is given anuvasana basti with the above mentioned Rasna Taila and Pitadru Taila. [29-30]

Signs and treatment of Pitta Impediments

दाहरागतृषामोहतमकज्वरदूषणैः| विद्यात् पित्तावृतं स्वादुतिक्तैस्तं बस्तिभिर्हरेत्||३१||

The occlusion [of the unctuous enema-fluid] by Pitta can be confirmed by the presence / manifestation of burning sensation, redness, morbid thirst, unconsciousness, tamaka (entering into darkness) and fever.

This occlusion can be removed by the administration of enema containing sweet and bitter ingredients. [31]

Signs of kapha Impediments

तन्द्राशीतज्वरालस्यप्रसेकारुचिगौरवैः| सम्मूच्छाग्लानिभिर्विद्याच्छ्लेष्मणा स्नेहमावृतम्||३२||

The occlusion of the unctuous enema fluid by Kapha can be ascertained from the affliction of the patient by drowsiness, cold fever, indolence, salivation, anorexia, heaviness, fainting and depression (Glani). [32]

Treatment of Kapha Impediments

कषायकटुतीक्ष्णोष्णैः सुरामूत्रोपसाधितैः|फलतैलयुतैः साम्लैर्बस्तिभिस्तं विनिर्हरेत्||३३||

The occlusion (of the unctuous fluid by Kapha) can be removed by the administration of Basti prepared by alcohol and cow's urine by adding Madana Phala Taila, as well as astringent, Pungent, sharp hot and sour ingredients. [33]

Signs of impediments by Intake of Food in Excess

छर्दिमूच्छारुचिग्लानिशूलनिद्राङ्गमर्दनैः|आमलिङ्गैः सदाहैस्तं विद्यादत्यशनावृतम्||३४||

The occlusion (of the unctuous fluid) by the intake of food in excess can be ascertained from the afflictions of the patient by vomiting, fainting, anorexia, depression, colic pain, excessive sleep, malaise, signs of Ama (caused by the product of improper digestion and metabolism) and burning sensation. [34]

Treatment of Impediments Caused by Intake of food in Excess

कटूनां लवणानां च क्वाथैश्चूर्णैश्च पाचनम्| विरेको मृदुरत्रामविहिता च क्रिया हिता||३५||

For the type of occlusion (of unctuous fluid by the intake of food in excess), Pacana (metabolic transformation of the undigested products) with pungent and saline decoctions as well as powders, mild purgation and therapies prescribed for correcting Ama (product of improper digestion and metabolism) are useful. [35]

Signs and Treatment of Impediments by Stool

विण्मूत्रानिलसङ्गार्तिगुरुत्वाध्मानहृद्ग्रहैः| स्नेहं विडावृतं ज्ञात्वा स्नेहस्वेदैः सवर्तिभिः||३६||
श्यामाबिल्वादिसिद्धैश्च निरूहैः सानुवासनैः| निर्हरेद्विधिना सम्यग्गुदावर्तहरेण च||३७||

The occlusion (of the unctuous enema-fluid) by stool can be ascertained from the afflictions of the patient by the obstruction to the passage of stool, urine and flatus, pain heaviness, flatulence and cardiac spasm.

Such a patient is treated by oleation, fomentation and Phala Varti (medicated suppository) therapies with Syama, Bilva, etc., Niruha Basti followed by Anuvasana Basti is given appropriately for the removal of obstruction. The treatment of Udavarta (an ailment characterized by upward movement of wind) too shall be considered. [36-37]

Ailments caused by Administration of Basti Empty Stomach and Their treatment

अभुक्ते शून्यपायौ वा वेगात् स्नेहोऽतिपीडितः|धावत्यूर्ध्वं ततः कण्ठादूर्ध्वेभ्यः खेभ्य एत्यपि||३८||
मूत्रश्यामात्रिवृत्सिद्धो यवकोलकुलत्थवान्|तत्सिद्धतैल इष्टोऽत्र निरूहः सानुवासनः||३९||
कण्ठादागच्छतः स्तम्भकण्ठग्रहविरेचनैः|छर्दिघ्नीभिः क्रियाभिश्च तस्य कार्य निवर्तनम्||४०||

If the Anuvasana Basti is given on an empty stomach or on an emptied bowel or if the enema-fluid is injected with great force it goes up speedily, and comes out from the throat or through the orifices in the upper part of the body.

In this condition, oil cooked with cow's urine, Syama Trivrt, Yava, Kola and Kulattha is used for giving Niruha and anuvasana types of medicated enema.

If the enema-fluid starts coming out of the throat, then the patient is given Stambhana therapies (like fanning and sprinkling with cold water); pressure is applied over his throat [to prevent further upward movement of the enema-fluid], and he is given purgative and anti-emetic therapies. [38-40]

Non- elimination of Enema-fluid

यस्य नोपद्रवं कुर्यात् स्नेहबस्तिरनिःसृतः| सर्वेऽल्पो वाऽऽवृतो रौक्ष्यादुपेक्ष्यः स विजानता||४१||

If because of un-unctuousness, the unctuous enema fluid, being obstructed, does not get eliminated totally or partially, but the condition is not associated with complications, then an expert physician should leave the patient alone (i.e., he should not try to bring out the fluid by therapies) [41]

Diet after Anuvasana Basti

युक्तस्नेहं द्रवोष्णं च लघुपथ्योपसेवनम्| भुक्तवान् मात्रया भोज्यमनुवास्यस्त्र्यहात्त्र्यहात्||४२||

After appropriate administration of Anuvasana Basti, the patient is given liquid, hot, light and wholesome food. After the intake of this food in appropriate quantity, the patient may repeatedly be given Anuvasana Basti every third day. [42]

Hot water

धान्यनागरसिद्धं हि तोयं दद्यादिवचक्षणः| व्युषिताय निशां कल्यमुष्णं वा केवलं जलम्||४३||
स्नेहाजीर्णं जरयति श्लेष्माणं तद्भिनत्ति च| मारुतस्यानुलोम्यं च कुर्यादुष्णोदकं नृणाम्||४४||
वमने च विरेके च निरूहे सानुवासने| तस्मादुष्णोदकं देयं वातश्लेष्मोपशान्तये||४५||

In the next morning, after the night, the expert physician should be given water boiled with Dhanyaka and Nagara (Sunthi) or simple warm water.

This warm water helps the patient in the digestion of undigested fat and it disintegrates Kapha. Therefore, after emesis, purgation, Niruha and Anuvasana therapies, warm water is to be given to the patient for the alleviation of Vayu and Kapha. [43-45]

Frequency of Anuvasana Basti

रूक्षनित्यस्तु दीप्ताग्निनर्व्यायामी मारुतामयी| वङ्क्षणश्रोण्युदावृत्तवाताश्चार्हा दिने दिने||४६||

एषां चाशु जरां स्नेहो यात्यम्बु सिकतास्विव| अतोऽन्येषां त्र्यहात्प्रायः स्नेहं पचति पावकः||४७||

Anuvasana Basti can be given every day in the below mentioned conditions / persons –

Persons who are habituated to taking un-unctuous food,

Those who have strong Agni (power of digestion and metabolism),

Those who perform physical exercise,

Those who are afflicted with Vatika diseases,

Those whose pelvic region and hip region are afflicted with Vata, and

Those who are suffering from Udavarta – bloating (upward movement of Vayu)

As the water falling over sand gets absorbed immediately, similarly the fat given to these patients gets immediately digested.

In the case of others, the Agni (digestive enzymes) generally digests Sneha (fat) in three days. [46-47]

Prohibition of Uncooked fat

न त्वामं प्रणयेत् स्नेहं स ह्यभिष्यन्दयेद्गुदम्| सावशेषं च कुर्वीत वायुः शेषे हि तिष्ठति||४८||

Uncooked fat is not used for Anuvasana Basti as it produces stuffiness (Abhisyanda) in the rectum.

Some portion of the fat (enema- liquid) is allowed to remain in Basti (bladder -which is used as receptacle of enema-fluid) because it contains air. [48]

Prohibition of fat after Anuvasana

न चैव गुदकण्ठाभ्यां दद्यात् स्नेहमनन्तरम्| उभयस्मात् समं गच्छन् वातमग्निं च दूषयेत्||४९||

After the administration of anuvasana Basti, fat should not be given through the anus or mouth, because the fat coming from both the sides (upper and lower) simultaneously vitiates Vayu and Agni (enzymes responsible for digestion). [49]

Prohibition of Exclusive administration of Niruha and Anuvasana

स्नेहबस्तिं निरूहं वा नैकमेवातिशीलयेत्| उत्क्लेशाग्निवधौ स्नेहान्निरूहात् पवनाद्भयम्||५०||

तस्मान्निरूढः संस्नेह्यो निरूह्यश्चानुवासितः| स्नेहशोधनयुक्त्यैवं बस्तिकर्म त्रिदोषनुत्||५१||

Either Niruha or Anuvasana should not be taken in excess (without interruption by the other). Excessive administration of Anuvasana [exclusively] gives rise to Utklesa (excitement of Kapha and Pitta) and suppression of the power of digestion. Excessive administration of Niruha [exclusively] leads to the risk of Vayu getting aggravated. Therefore, after Niruha-Basti, the patient is given Anuvasana Basti, and after Anuvasana Basti, Niruha Basti is given. Thus, by giving anuvasna and Niruha appropriately (one after the other), this Basti therapy cures the diseases caused by all the three Doshas. [50-51]

Matra-Basti

कर्मव्यायामभाराध्वया(पा)नस्त्रीकर्षितेषु च| दुर्बले वातभग्ने च मात्राबस्तिः सदा मतः||५२||

यथेष्टाहारचेष्टस्य सर्वकालं निरत्ययः| ह्रस्वायाः स्नेहमात्राया मात्राबस्तिः समो भवेत्||५३||

बल्यं सुखोपचर्यं च सुखं सृष्टपुरीषकृत्| स्नेहमात्राविधानं हि बृंहणं वातरोगनुत्||५४||

Matra Basti is always useful for persons emaciated by Karma (playing with ball, etc.), Vyayama (practicing archery etc.), carrying heavy load, long way-faring, riding vehicles or indulging in sexual intercourse with women and for persons who are weak and who are afflicted with Vatika diseases.

While taking Matra basti, a person can take any food, and may do any work as he likes. It can be safely administered in all the seasons.

The dose of Matra Basti is equal to the minimum quantity in which Anuvasana Basti is prescribed to be administered.

This Matra Basti which is a form of Anuvasana basti promotes strength and can be administered easily. It helps in easy voiding (elimination) of stool. It causes nourishment, and cures diseases caused by aggravated Vayu. [52-54]

Epilogue

तत्र श्लोकौ-

वातादीनां शमायोक्ताः प्रवराः स्नेहबस्तयः| तेषां चाज्ञप्रयुक्तानां व्यापदः सचिकित्सिताः||५५||

प्राग्भोज्यं स्नेहबस्तेर्यद् ध्रुवं येऽहास्त्र्यहाच्च ये स्नेहबस्तिविधिश्चोक्तो मात्राबस्तिविधिस्तथा||५६||

To sum up:

In this chapter, the topics described are as follows:

1. foremost recipes of Anuvasana Basti for the alleviation (elimination) of aggravated Vayu etc., (vide verse nos. 4-24)

2. complications arising out of their administration by ignorant persons, and treatment of these complications (vide verse nos. 25-41)

3. diet to be given before the administration of Anuvasana Basti (vide verse nos. 42-45)

4. persons for whom anuvasana basti is indicated to be taken every day and for whom it is indicated on every third day; (vide verse nos, 46-47)

5. the method of administration Anuvasana Basti and (vide verse nos. 48-51)

6. the methods of administering Matra Basti (vide verse nos. 52-54)

इत्यग्निवेशकृते तन्त्रे चरकप्रतिसंस्कृतेऽप्राप्ते दृढबलसम्पूरिते सिद्धिस्थाने स्नेहव्यापत्सिद्धिर्नाम चतुर्थोऽध्यायः||४||

Thus ends the fourth chapter in Siddhi-Sthana dealing with "the successful treatment of complications arising out of unctuous enema" in the text composed by Agnivesha, redacted by Caraka and because of its Non-availability, supplemented by Drdhabala.

Siddhisthana Chapter 5 Netrabasti Vyapat Siddhi

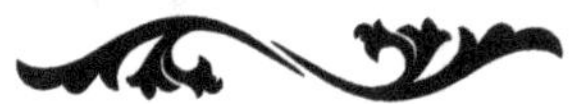

Prologue

अथातो नेत्रबस्तिव्यापत्सिदि्धं व्याख्यास्यामः||१||

इति ह स्माह भगवानात्रेयः||२||

We shall now explore the chapter on "Complications Arising out of the Use of a defective nozzle, and its receptacle (including the Technique of Administration) and their Successful Treatment". Thus said Lord Atreya [1-2]

Topics to be discussed

अथ नेत्राणि बस्तींश्च शृणु वर्ज्यानि कर्मसु| नेत्रस्याज्ञप्रणीतस्य व्यापदः सचिकित्सिताः||३||

Now listen to the description of the following topics:

Types of nnozzles (Netras) and their receptacles (basti) which are not to be used for the administration of enema

Complications arising out of their use

Complications arising out of the mishandling of the nozzles (including enema receptacle) by an inexperienced physician; and

Treatment of these complications [3]

Inappropriate Nozzles and Complications arising out of their Use

ह्रस्वं दीर्घं तनु स्थूलं जीर्णं शिथिलबन्धनम्| पार्श्वच्छिद्रं तथा वक्रमष्टौ नेत्राणि वर्जयेत्||४||

अप्राप्त्यतिगतिक्षोभकर्षणक्षणनस्रवाः| गुदपीडा गतिर्जिह्मा तेषां दोषा यथाक्रमम्||५||

The eight types of nozzles (Netras) which are not to be used for the administration of enema, and complications arising out of their use are as follows:

Characteristics of Nozzles Complications Arising out of their use

1 Hrasva (smaller in size) Aprapti (enema-fluid not reaching its destination)

2 Dirgha (longer in size) Atigati (enema- fluid penetrating far above)

3 Tanu (thinner in shape) Ksobha (irritation caused by the instability of the nozzle in the rectum)

4 Sthula (thicker in shape) Karsana (burning the wall of the rectum)

5 Jirna (worn out) Ksanana (causing injury to the rectum)

6 Sithila- bandhana (loose fixation) Srava (leaking out of the enema- fluid)

7 Parsva chidra (having holes in the side) Guda-Pida (causing pain in the rectum)

8 Vakra (curved) Jihma-gati (tortuous passage of the fluid) [4-5]

Inappropriate Bastis and Complications arising out of their Use

विषममांसलच्छिन्नस्थूलजालिकवातलाः|स्निग्धः क्लिन्नश्च तानष्टौ बस्तीन् कर्मसु वर्जयेत्||६||

गतिवैषम्यविस्रत्वस्रावदौर्ग्राह्यनिस्रवाः|फेनिलच्युत्यधार्यत्वं बस्तेः स्युर्बस्तिदोषतः||७||

The types of Bastis (bladders used as receptacles) which are not to be the administration of enema, and the complications arising out of their use are as follows:

Characteristic of Bladder Complications arising out of their use

01 Visama (irregular in shape) Gati- Vaisamya (irregular flow of enema-fluid)

02 Mamsala (fleshy) Visratva (making the enema-fluid smell fleshy)

03 Chinna (torn) Srava (leaking of the fluid)

04 Sthula (thick) Daurgrahya (difficulty in handling)

05 Jalika (net-work of small perforations) Nisrava (exudation of enema-fluid from the receptacle)

06 Vatala (having air bubbles inside) Phenila (frothiness of fluid)

07 Ati-snigdha (excessively unctuous) Cyuti (slipping away off the receptacle)

08 Klinna (Putrefied) Adharyatva (inability to hold the receptacle) [6-7]

Defective Techniques Employed by Physicians

सवातातिद्रुतोत्क्षिप्ततिर्यगुल्लुप्तकम्पिताः| अतिबाह्यगमन्दातिवेगदोषाः प्रणेतृतः||८||

The defective techniques employed by the (ignorant) physician for administering Basti are as follows:

Sa-vata (pushing the enema fluid along with air)

Ati druta (pushing the enema-fluid too rapidly)

Utksipta (injecting the enema-fluid too high)

Tiryak (injecting the enema-fluid obliquely)

Ullupta (pushing the enema-fluid again after interruption);

Kampita (shaking the nozzle while injecting the enema-fluid)

Atiga (excessive insertion of the nozzle)

Bahyaga (wrong pushing so that instead of entering the anal canal, the enema-fluid flows outside) and

Manda vega (compressing the receptacle too slowly so that the enema-fluid does not reach the colon)

Ati vega (compressing the receptacle too forcibly as a result of which the enema fluid rapidly enters and reaches the distant part of the alimentary canal) [8]

Complications arising out of anucchvasa etc and their treatment

अनुच्छ्वास्य च बद्धे वा दते निःशेष एव वा| प्रविश्य कुपितो वायुः शूलतोदकरो भवेत्||९||

तत्राभ्यङ्गो गुदे स्वेदो वातघ्नान्यशनानि च|१०|

If the enema receptacle is tied to the nozzle without taking out the air from the bladder, or if the entire amount of fluid is rushed into the rectum without leaving any residue in the bladder (basti), then the Vayu (air) entering into the rectum causes colic pain and piercing pain.

In such a condition, massage and fomentation should be given over the anus, and the patient should be given Vayu-alleviating food. [9 ½ 10]

Complications Arising out of Rapid insertion of Nozzle, etc, and Their Treatment

द्रुतं प्रणीते निष्कृष्टे सहसोत्क्षिप्त एव वा||१०|| स्यात् कटीगुदजङ्घार्तिबस्तिस्तम्भोरुवेदनाः |

भोजनं तत्र वातघ्नं स्नेहाः स्वेदाः सबस्तयः||११||

If the nozzle is inserted rapidly, if it is taken out hurriedly, and if it is pushed very high, then there will be pain in the lumbar region, anus and calf region; stiffness of the bladder, and pain in the thigh. In such cases, the patient should be given Vata alleviating food, oleation, fomentation and enema therapy. [1/ 2 10- 11]

Complications caused by oblique insertion of nozzle etc., and their treatment

तिर्यग्वल्यावृतद्वारे बद्धे वाऽपि न गच्छति| नेत्रे तद्द्रजु निष्कृष्य संशोध्य च प्रवेशयेत्||१२||

If the enema nozzle is inserted obliquely, if the passage is obstructed by the anal sphincters, and if there is blockage because of the (fibres in the) recipe itself, then the fluid will not flow into the rectum.

In this case, the nozzle should be taken out, (the passage of the nozzle should be) cleaned, and the nozzle should be inserted again straight. [12]

Complications arising from Interrupted administration of Basti and their treatment

पीड्यमानेऽन्तरा मुक्ते गुदे प्रतिहतोऽनिलः| उरःशिरोर्तिमूर्वश्च सदनं जनयेद्बली||१३||
बस्तिः स्यात्तत्र बिल्वादिफलश्यामादिमूत्रवान्|

If the enema- receptacle is compressed again after an interruption, then the aggravated vayu being obstructed in the rectum causes pain in the chest, head, and prostration of the thighs.

In such conditions, the recipe prepared of Bilvadi (Dashamula), Phaladi and Shyamadi groups of drugs mixed with cow's urine should be given as enema. [13 – ½ 14]

Complication caused by shaking of Nozzle during administration of basti and their treatment.

स्याद्दाहो दवथुः शोफः कम्पनाभिहते गुदे||१४|| कषायमधुराः शीताः सेकास्तत्र सबस्तयः|१५|

If the anus gets injured because of the shaking of the nozzle, then there will be burning sensation, sneezing and oedema. In such conditions, the patient should be given astringent, sweet and cold effusion along with enema. [14 ½ - ½ 15]

Complications caused by excessive penetration of nozzle and their treatment

अतिमात्रप्रणीतेन नेत्रेण क्षणनाद्वलेः||१५|| स्यात् सार्ति दाहनिस्तोदगुदवर्चःप्रवर्तनम्|
तत्र सर्पिः पिचुः क्षीरं पिच्छाबस्तिश्च शस्यते||१६||

If the nozzle is excessively penetrated (or inserted repeatedly), then it causes injury to the anal sphincters leading to pain, burning sensation, pricking pain, prolapsed of the anus and discharge of faecal matter.

In such conditions, Sarpi-pichu (pack of ghee- soaked cotton- pad) should be applied over the anus. Milk and Piccha Basti (mucilaginous enema) are useful in this condition. [15 ½ - 16]

Effects of slow enema, and their management

न भावयति मन्दस्तु बाह्यस्त्वाशु निवर्तते| स्नेहस्तत्र पुनः सम्यक् प्रणेयः सिद्धिमिच्छता||१७||

If the receptacle is inadequately compressed then the enema fluid does not reach its destination, and comes out quickly. In such a condition, Anuvasana- Basti should be administered appropriately again by the physician desirous of success of treatment. [17]

Effects of forceful administration of enema, and their treatment

अतिप्रपीडितः कोष्ठे तिष्ठत्यायाति वा गलम्| तत्र बस्तिर्विरेकश्च गलपीडादि कर्म च||१८||

If the enema-fluid is injected with excess force, then the fluid is either retained in the gastro-intestinal tract, or stomach goes up to reach the throat.

In such case, the patient should be given enema and purgation (if the fluid gets retained in the alimentary tract) or Gala-Pida (application of pressure on the throat) etc. (if the fluid tends to come up from the throat) [18]

तत्र श्लोकः- नेत्रबस्तिप्रणेतृणां दोषानेतान् सभेषजान्| वेति यस्तेन मतिमान् बस्तिकर्माणि कारयेत्||१९||

To sum up: - The physician, who is conversant with the defects of Netra (nozzle) and basti (receptacle of enema), the effects of wrongful techniques applied by the administrator, and treatment of the complications arising out of these factors, should administer basti therapy and only that person gains success.

इत्यग्निवेशकृते तन्त्रे चरकप्रतिसंस्कृतेऽप्राप्ते दृढबलसम्पूरिते सिद्धिस्थाने नेत्रबस्तिव्यापत्सिद्धिर्नाम पञ्चमोऽध्यायः||५||

Thus, ends the fifth chapter of Siddhi-Sthana dealing with "The Success in treatment of Complications Caused by the Use of Improper Nozzle and Receptacle" of Agnivesha's work as redacted by Charaka, and Because of its non-availability, supplemented by Drdhabala.

31

Siddhisthana Chapter 6 Vamana Virechana Vyapat Siddhi

अथातो वमनविरेचनव्यापत्सिद्धिं व्याख्यास्यामः|

इति ह स्माह भगवानात्रेयः||२||

Now we shall explore the chapter on "the successful treatment of complications arising out of wrongly administered emetic and purgative therapies". Thus said Lord Atreya [1-2]

Topics to be discussed in the chapter:

अथ शोधनयोः सम्यग्विधिमूर्ध्वानुलोमयोः| असम्यक्कृतयोश्चैव दोषान् वक्ष्यामि सौषधान्||३||

Now the topics to be described in this chapter are as follows:

Appropriate methods for the administration of the upward and downward purificatory therapies (emesis and purgation);

Complications arising out of the improper administration of these therapies and

Treatment of these complications [3]

Suitable seasons

अत्युष्णवर्षशीता हि ग्रीष्मवर्षाहिमागमाः| तदन्तरे प्रावृडाद्यास्तेषां साधारणास्त्रयः||४||

प्रावृट् शुन्निनभौ ज्ञेयौ शरदूर्जसहौ पुनः| तपस्यश्च मधुश्चैव वसन्तः शोधनं प्रति||५||

एतानृतून् विकल्प्यैवं दद्यात् संशोधनं भिषक्| स्वस्थवृत्तमभिप्रेत्य व्याधौ व्याधिवशेन तु||६||

Greeshma (summer), Varsha (rainy season) and Himagama or Hemanta (winter) are characterised by excessive heat, rain and cold respectively. The three intervening seasons, viz., Pravrt (the period between rainy season and winter) and Vasanta or spring (the period between winter and summer)] are of general nature.

The months composing the three seasons of general nature are as follows:

Pravrt (approx, June- August) is composed of Suci or Aasada (June- July) and Nabha or Sravana (july- August); Sarat or autumn (approx October- December) is composed of urja or Kartika (October – November) and Saha or Margasira (November- December) and Vasanta or spring (February- April) is composed of Tapasya or Phalguna (February- March) and Madhu or Caitra (March- April).

The above mentioned three seasons are suitable for the administration of elimination therapies.

After determining the exact months consisting of the above-mentioned seasons, the physician should give appropriate elimination therapies to a healthy person. However, for a patient, the appropriateness of the time (season) is determined on the basis of the nature of the diseases. [4-6]

Administration of Oleation and Fomentation in Intervals

कर्मणां वमनादीनामन्तरेष्वन्तरेषु च| स्नेहस्वेदौ प्रयुञ्जीत स्नेहं चान्ते प्रयोजयेत्||७||

During the interval between two therapies, viz., emesis, etc., the patient is given oleation and fomentation therapies, and at the end of such therapy, oleation therapy should again be given. [7]

Prohibition of Excessive Oleation

विसर्पपिडकाशोफकामलापाण्डुरोगिणः|अभिघातविषार्तांश्च नातिस्निग्धान् विरेचयेत्||८||

Purgation therapy is to be given to the patient suffering from Visarpa (Erysipelas), Pidaka (pimples), Sopha (oedema), Kamala (Jaundice), Pandu (anaemia), injury and poisoning only when the patient is not excessively oleated. [8]

Nature of Purgation Recipe

नातिस्निग्धशरीराय दद्यात् स्नेहविरेचनम्| स्नेहोत्क्लिष्टशरीराय रूक्षं दद्यादि्वरेचनम्||९||

Unctuous recipe for purgation should not be given to a patient whose body is excessively oleated. If the unctuous element in the body of the patient is excited, then he is given a purgation therapy recipe which is dry in nature. [9]

Conditions responsible for Appropriate Effect

स्नेहस्वेदोपपन्नेन जीर्णे मात्रावदौषधम्| एकाग्रमनसा पीतं सम्यग्योगाय कल्पते||१०||

Factors responsible for appropriate effect (Samyag Yoga) [of the purgation therapy] are the following;
The patient should have taken oleation and fomentation therapies; [to be further explained in the verse nos. [11-13]
The purgation therapy is given only after the previous meal is digested [to be further explained in verse nos. 14]
The purgation therapy is given in appropriate dose; [to be further explained in verse nos. [15-16] and
The patient should take the therapy with concentration of mind. [To be further explained in verse no. Q7] [10]

Need for Oleation and Fomentation Therapies:

स्निग्धात् पात्रादृयथा तोयमयत्नेन प्रणुद्यते| कफादयः प्रणुद्यन्ते स्निग्धाद्देहात्तथौषधैः||११||

आर्द्रे काष्ठं यथा वह्निर्विष्यन्दयति सर्वतः| तथा स्निग्धस्य वै दोषान् स्वेदो विष्यन्दयेत् स्थिरान्||१२||

क्लिष्टं वासो यथोत्क्लेश्य मलः संशोध्यतेऽम्भसा| स्नेहस्वेदैस्तथोत्क्लेश्य शोध्यते शोधनैर्मलः ||१३||

Kapha, etc. morbid doshas can be taken out easily by therapies from the body of the patient who is oleated just like the water can be taken out easily from a pot smeared with oil.
The fomentation therapy helps the stable (adhered) Doshas in an oleated person to get eliminated completely just like the fire makes the liquid content of a piece of wet wood to ooze out in all the directions.
The Malas (morbid and Adhered Doshas) become detached by the application of oleation and fomentation therapies, and elimination therapy just like the dirt adhered to a piece of dirty cloth gets detached [by the application of heat or hot steam and alkaline] which can be washed out easily by rinsing with water. [11-13]

Digestion of food

अजीर्णे वर्धते ग्लानिर्विबन्धश्चापि जायते| पीतं संशोधनं चैव विपरीतं प्रवर्तते||१४||

If elimination therapies are administered before the previous meal is digested, then it gives rise to the following complications:
glani (depression)
vibandha (constipation) and
the therapy works in the opposite way (i.e., the emetic therapy causes purgation and the purgative therapy causes emesis) [14]

Appropriate Dose

अल्पमात्रं महावेगं बहुदोषहरं सुखम्| लघुपाकं सुखास्वादं प्रीणनं व्याधिनाशनम्||१५||

अविकारि च व्यापत्तौ नातिग्लानिकरं च यत्| गन्धवर्णरसोपेतं विद्यान्मात्रावदौषधम्||१६||

Appropriate dose of the recipe for elimination therapies is characterised as follows:
It should be small in quantity, but quick in action

It should be able to eliminate morbid Doshas in large quantity but easily

It should be light for digestion, palatable, pleasing and curative of the concerned diseases

It should not cause serious complications

It should not cause depression/fatigue in excess and

It should possess agreeable smell, colour and taste [15-16]

Concentration of mind

विधूय मानसान् दोषान् कामादीनशुभोदयान् | एकाग्रमनसा पीतं सम्यग्योगाय कल्पते||१७||

Passion etc. are inauspicious impurities of the mind. If a person whose mind is cleansed of these impurities, and whose mind is concentrated on the therapy, takes recipes for the elimination of morbid matter, then appropriate effects (Samyag- Yoga) of the therapy are produced. [17]

Preparatory Measures

नरः श्वो वमनं पाता भुञ्जीत कफवर्धनम्| सुजरं द्रवभूयिष्ठं, लघ्वशीतं विरेचनम्||१८||

उत्क्लिष्टाल्पकफत्वेन क्षिप्रं दोषाः स्रवन्ति हि|१९|

The person scheduled to take the emetic therapy the next day should eat a Kapha aggravating diet which is easy for digestion and which is mostly of liquid nature (in the night of the previous day). The person scheduled to take purgation therapy the next day should take a diet which is light and hot.

Because of the aforesaid diet, the Kapha gets excited or aggravated (in the patient who is to be given emesis the next morning). In the case of the patient who is to be given purgation therapy in the next morning, intake of the above mentioned light and hot diet during the previous night causes reduction of kapha. As a result of this [the emesis and purgation therapies] helps in the elimination of Doshas quickly. [18- ½ 19]

Signs of Appropriate purification

पीतौषधस्य तु भिषक् शुद्धिलिङ्गानि लक्षयेत्||१९|| ऊर्ध्वं कफानुगे पित्ते विट्पित्तेऽनुकफे त्वधः|

हृतदोषं वदेत् कार्श्यदौर्बल्ये चेत् सलाघवे||२०||

After the therapy is administered, the physician should keep observing the appearance of signs of appropriate purification which are as follows:

• In the case of emesis, the bile appears after the elimination of kapha;

• In the case of purgation, Kapha appears after the voiding of stool and bile

• After the therapies (both emesis and purgation) the body becomes emaciated, weak and light

Appearance of the above signs indicates appropriate elimination of the (morbid) Doshas). [19 ½ - 20]

Measures to remove Residual Drugs

वामयेत्तु ततः शेषमौषधं न त्वलाघवे| स्तैमित्येऽनिलसङ्गे च निरुद्गारेऽपि वामयेत्||२१||

आलाघवात्ननुत्वाच्च कफस्यापत् परं भवेत्|२२|

The patient is given emetic therapy to remove the residual drugs (provided all the signs of appropriate administration of elimination therapy are observed). But if only lightness of the body is not observed (in spite of the presence of the remaining signs), then emesis should not be given.

If there is Staimitya (a feeling as if the body is covered with a wet skin) and occlusion of Vata, the emetic therapy is administered, even if there is no eructation, till there is lightness of the body and thinness of Kapha. Giving emesis thereafter leads to serious consequences. [21- ½ 22]

After-care

वमिते वर्धते वह्निः शमं दोषा व्रजन्ति हि||२२|| वमितं लङ्घयेत् सम्यग्जीर्णलिङ्गान्यलक्षयन्|

तानि दृष्ट्वा तु पेयादिक्रमं कुर्यान्न लङ्घनम्||२३||

Emesis promotes the Agni (power of digestion) [after some time], and alleviates Doshas. After emesis, the patient should keep fasting till the appearance of the signs of proper digestion of the medicines. After having observed these signs, the patient is given a regulated diet in the form of Peya (thin gruel), etc. and he should not be made to keep fast any more. [22 ½ -23]

Need for regulated Diet

संशोधनाभ्यां शुद्धस्य हृतदोषस्यदेहिनः| यात्यग्निर्मन्दतां तस्मात् क्रमं पेयादिमाचरेत्||२४||

[Immediately] after purification of the body, and elimination of Doshas from the body by emetic and purgative therapies, the Agni (power of digestion and metabolism) in a person gets subdued. Therefore, for him, a controlled diet in the form of Peya (thin gruel), etc., is recommended. [24]

Dietetic Regimen

कफपित्ते विशुद्धेऽल्पं मद्यपे वातपैत्तिके| तर्पणादिक्रमं कुर्यात् पेयाऽभिष्यन्दयेदि्ध तान्||२५||

If Kapha and Pitta are cleansed partially because of Alpa Yoga or less effect (of emetic and purgative therapies), if the patient is addicted to alcohol, and if he suffers from Vatika or Paittika diseases, then he is given the regulated diet in the form of Tarpana – Nourishing, calming or demulcent drinks, etc., because Peya (thin gruel), etc. produces Abhisyandi effect (i.e., obstruction to the channels of circulation) in such cases. [25]

Signs of Drug- Digestion

अनुलोमोऽनिलः स्वास्थ्यं क्षुत्तृष्णोर्जो मनस्विता| लघुत्वमिन्द्रियोद्गारशुद्धिर्जीर्णौषधाकृतिः||२६||

Signs of complete digestion of drugs used in the recipe are as follows:

Downward movement of the wind in the intestine

A sense of well- being

Proper hunger and thirst

Feeling of energy (promotion of strength) and self confidence

Lightness of the body

Clarity (excellence in the functioning) of sense; and

Purity of eructation (without the smell of drugs)

Signs of residual Drugs

क्लमो दाहोऽङ्गसदनं भ्रमो मूर्च्छा शिरोरुजा| अरतिर्बलहानिश्च सावशेषौषधाकृतिः||२७||

If the drugs of the recipe are not fully digested, and a part remains undigested, then this gives rise to the following signs: Klama (mental fatigue), Burning sensation, Prostration of limbs, Giddiness, Fainting, Headache, Disliking for everything around and, Diminution of strength.

Characteristics of Drugs Producing Undesirable effects

अकालेऽल्पातिमात्रं च पुराणं न च भावितम्| असम्यक्संस्कृतं चैव व्यापद्येतौषधं द्रुतम्||२८||

Drugs of the following nature, if used in the recipes for elimination therapies, produce adverse effects quickly:

Unseasonal and untimely collected

Administration in less or excess dose

Storage for a longer period after collection

Used without proper impregnation and

Improperly processed [28]

Adverse effects and their causative factors

आध्मानं परिकर्तिश्च स्रावो हृद्गात्रयोर्ग्रहः| जीवादानं सविभ्रंशः स्तम्भः सोपद्रवः क्लमः||२९||

अयोगादतियोगाच्च दशैता व्यापदो मताः| प्रेष्यभैषज्यवैद्यानां वैगुण्यादातुरस्य च||३०||

Emetic and purgative therapies may produce ten adverse effects (vyapat) as follows:

Adhmana or Flatulence (caused by Ayoga or under action of the recipe)

Parikartika or gripping pain (caused by Atiyoga or over action of the recipe)

Srava or excessive discharge (caused by Ayoga)

Hrdgraha or stiffness in the cardiac region (caused by Ayoga)

Gatragraha or stiffness of the body (caused by Ayoga)

Jivadana or bleeding (caused by Atiyoga)

Vibhramsa, i.e. Guda-Bhramsa or Prolapsed rectum

Sanjna-Bhramsa or mental perversion (caused by atiyoga) and others like itching (caused by Ayoga):

Stambha or rigidity

Upadrava or complications (caused by Ayoga) and

Klama or mental fatigue (caused by Ayoga)

The above mentioned adverse effects arise out of the Ayoga (under action) and Ati Yoga (over action) of the recipe because of the following.

Presya Vaigunya (defect in the attendant)

Bhaisajya Vaigunya (defect in the recipe)

Vaidya Vaigunya (defect in the physician) and

Atura Vaigunya (defect in the patient) [29-30]

Different types of Actions of Elimination therapies

योगः सम्यक्प्रवृत्तिः स्यादतियोगोऽतिवर्तनम्| अयोगः प्रातिलोम्येन न चाल्पं वा प्रवर्तनम्||३१||

Emesis and purgation therapies act in three different ways as follows:

Yoga or appropriate action resulting in proper elimination of Doshas

Atiyoga or over action which causes excessive elimination of Doshas and

Ayoga or under action which causes action of the drug in the reverse order, non-elimination of Doshas, or their elimination in less quantity. [31]

Movement in reverse direction

श्लेष्मोत्क्लिष्टेन दुर्गन्धमहृद्यमति वा बहु| विरेचनमजीर्णे च पीतमूर्ध्वं प्रवर्तते||३२||

क्षुधार्तमृदुकोष्ठाभ्यां स्वल्पोत्क्लिष्टकफेन वा| तीक्ष्णं पीतं स्थितं क्षुब्धं वमनं स्यादि्वरेचनम्||३३||

प्रातिलोम्येन दोषाणां हरगाते हरकृत्स्नशः| अयोगसञ्ज्ञे, कृच्छ्रेण याति दोषो नवाऽल्पशः||३४||

Intake of purgation therapy by a person with excited (aggravated) Kapha may produce action in reverse direction (i.e., it may cause emesis) because of the following factors:

Foul odour of the recipe

Non-palatability of the recipe

Larger quantity of the recipe and

Intake of the recipe before the previous meal has been digested

Similarly, emetic may produce purgation because of the following factors

Affliction of the patient with hunger

Lax bowel

Less excitement of kapha

Tikshna (sharp) nature of the drug

Sthita or stagnation of the recipe and

Kshubdham or agitating nature of the recipe

If the emetic and purgative therapies produce action in the reverse order, then they become incapable of eliminating the morbid matter entirely. Thus, these conditions are called Ayoga ((inappropriate or under action). In these conditions, the morbid Doshas get eliminated with difficulty or they do not get eliminated at all or they get eliminated only in small quantities. [32-34]

Indigestion of recipe

पीतौषधो न शुद्धश्चेज्जीर्णे तस्मिन् पुनः पिबेत्| औषधं न त्वजीर्णेऽन्यद्भयं स्यादतियोगतः||३५||

If the medicine taken for emesis and purgation does not produce the appropriate cleansing effects, then after its digestion, the therapy is administered again (on the same day). Before the digestion of the earlier recipe, the therapy should not be administered. Repetition of the therapy may lead to AtiYoga (excessive action). [35]

Repetition of Therapy

कोष्ठस्य गुरुतां ज्ञात्वा लघुत्वं बलमेव च| अयोगे मृदु वा दद्यादौषधं तीक्ष्णमेव वा||३६||

If there is Ayoga (under action), then after ascertaining the nature of the bowel (hard or soft bowel) and the strength, the patient is given [repeated dose] of the medicine which is either Mrdu (mild) or Tikshna (Sharp or strong) in nature. [36]

Avoiding Repeat- dose

वमनं न तु दुश्छर्दे दुष्कोष्ठं न विरेचनम्| पाययेतौषधं भूयो हन्यात् पीतं पुनर्हि तौ||३७||

If the patient is a bad subject (not an ideal candidate) for emesis, then a second emetic dose should not be given. Similarly, a second purgative dose should not be given if the patient has a hard bowel. Repeat doses of emesis and purgation to these two categories of patients may lead to their death. [37]

Causes and Complications of Ayoga

अस्निग्धास्विन्नदेहस्य रूक्षस्यानवमौषधम्| दोषानुत्क्लिश्य निर्हर्तुमशक्तं जनयेद्गदान्||३८||

विभ्रंशं श्वयथुं हिक्कां तमसो दर्शनं भृशम् | पिण्डिकोद्वेष्टनं कण्डूमूर्वोः सादं विवर्णताम्||३९||

If the patient is not oleated and fomented, if there is dryness in his body and the ingredients of the recipe have become old (stored for a long time as a result of which their potency has been diminished), then in such a situation the therapy becomes incapable of (completely) eliminating the morbid Doshas in spite of having caused their excitation. This gives rise to ailments like Vibhramsa (action in reverse direction), oedema, hiccup, excessive fainting, and cramps in the calf region, itching, asthenia of the thighs and discoloration of the skin. [38-39]

Another type of Ayoga and its management

स्निग्धस्विन्नस्य चात्यल्पं दीप्ताग्नेर्जीर्णमौषधम्| शीतैर्वा स्तब्धमामे वा दोषानुत्क्लिश्य नाहरेत्||४०||

तानेव जनयेद्रोगानयोगः सर्व एव सः| विज्ञाय मतिमांस्तत्र यथोक्तां कारयेत् क्रियाम्||४१||

Even in a person who is properly oleated and fomented, the Doshas which are already excited do not get eliminated because of the following factors:
• If the recipe is administered in a very small dose
• If the patient has strong power of digestion as a result of which the recipe administered in small dose itself gets digested (without producing its effects)
• If the recipe has become ineffective because of cold ingredients and
• If the recipe is taken when the body of the patient is afflicted with Ama (product of improper digestion and metabolism)

In the above-mentioned conditions, all the complications (like Vibhramsa-Vide verse nos. 38-39 above) are manifested. All the conditions are the result of Ayoga (under action of the purificatory recipe). Having determined this condition, a wise physician should treat them on the suggested lines (vide verse nos. 35-42) [40-41]

Treatment of Ayoga

तं तैललवणाभ्यक्तं स्विन्नं प्रस्तरसङ्करैः|पाययेत पुनर्जीर्णे समूत्रैर्वा निरुहयेत्||४२||

निरूढं च रसैर्धान्वैर्भोजयित्वाऽनुवासयेत्| फलमागधिकादारुसिद्धतैलेन मात्रया||४३||

स्निग्धं वातहरैः स्नेहैः पुनस्तीक्ष्णेन शोधयेत्| न चातितीक्ष्णेन ततो ह्यतियोगस्तु जायते||४४||

After digestion of the previously administered recipe, the patient is given massage with oil mixed with salt, and fomented with Prastara and Sankara type of fomentation therapies (vide sutra 14:41 & 42). Thereafter, he is given another dose of the purificatory recipe or may be given Niruha type of enema mixed with cow's urine.

After Niruha Basti, the patient is given food along with the soup of the meat of animals living in arid zones. Thereafter, Anuvasana Basti is given to him with the medicated oil prepared by boiling with Phala (madana phala), Magadhika (pippali) and Daru (Devadaru) in appropriate doses.

Thereafter, he is oleated with medicated fat prepared by cooking with Vata alleviating drugs, and then purificatory therapy with recipe containing sharp ingredients is given again. The ingredients should not be exceedingly sharp because that may result in Ati Yoga (over action). [42-44]

Signs and treatment of Ati-Yoga

अतितीक्ष्णं क्षुधार्तस्य मृदुकोष्ठस्य भेषजम्| हृत्वाऽऽशु विट्पित्तकफान् धातून्निस्रावयेद्द्रवान्||४५||

बलस्वरक्षयं दाहं कण्ठशोषं भ्रमं तृषाम्| कुर्याच्च मधुरैस्तत्र शेषमौषधमुल्लिखेत्||४६||

वमने तु विरेकः स्यादि्वरेके वमनं पुनः | परिषेकावगाहाद्यैः सुशीतैः स्तम्भयेच्च तत्||४७||

कषायमधुरैः शीतैरन्नपानौषधैस्तथा| रक्तपित्तातिसारघ्नैर्दाहज्वरहरैरपि||४८||

Exceedingly sharp medicated enema given to a patient who is hungry, and who has soft bowel quickly eliminates not only stool, Pitta (bile) and kapha (phlegm), but also the liquid elements (tissues) of the body.

As a result of this loss of strength and voice, burning sensation, dryness of the throat, giddiness and morbid thirst are manifested.

In such a condition, the residual drugs are eliminated with ingredients belonging to the group of sweet drugs (madhura-gana).

In case of Ati Yoga (over-action) of emetic therapy, the patient is given purgation therapy, and in case of atiyoga (over action) of purgation therapy he is given emesis.

The urge for vomiting and purgation in excess because of over-action may be arrested by the following:

Exceedingly cold Pariseka (sprinkling of water), Avagaha (bath) etc. measures,

Intake of food, drinks and medications which are cooling, astringent as well as sweet in taste and

Therapies which are curative of Rakta-Pitta (an ailment characterised by bleeding from different parts of the body), Atisara (diarrhoea), Daha (burning sensation) and Jvara (fever). [45-48]

Recipes for treatment of over-action of Purgation Therapies

अञ्जनं चन्दनोशीरमज्जासृक्शर्करोदकम्| लाजचूर्णैः पिबेन्मन्थमतियोगहरं परम्||४९||

शुङ्गाभिर्वा वटादीनां सिद्धां पेयां समाक्षिकाम्| वर्चःसाङ्ग्राहिकैः सिद्धं क्षीरं भोज्यं च दापयेत्||५०||

जाङ्गलैर्वा रसैर्भोज्यं पिच्छाबस्तिश्च शस्यते| मधुरैरनुवास्यश्च सिद्धेन क्षीरसर्पिषा||५१||

The patient (suffering from the complications of over action of emetic and purgative therapies) should take the following recipes:

Mantha (demulcent drink) prepared with Anjana (daruharidra), Candana, Usira, bone marrow, blood, sugar and water along with the powder of the roasted paddy. This is an excellent recipe for curing over action of elimination therapies.

Peya (thin gruel) prepared of the Sunga (still root) of Vata, etc. (nyagroda, Udumbara, Asvattha and Kapitana), mixed with honey.

Milk and food articles prepared by boiling with drugs which are Varcas Sangrahika or intestinal astringents (vide Sutra 4:5: 15).

Food along with the soup of the meat of animals inhabiting arid zone,

Piccha Basti (mucilaginous medicated enema);

Anuvasana Basti or unctuous enema of Ksira Sarpis belonging to Madhura varga (group of drugs having sweet taste) [49-51]

Treatment of over-action of emetic Therapy

वमनस्यातियोगे तु शीताम्बुपरिषेचितः| पिबेत् कफहरैर्मन्थं सघृतक्षौद्रशर्करम्||५२||

सोद्गारायां भृशं वम्यां मूर्च्छायां धान्यमुस्तयोः| समधूकाञ्जनं चूर्णं लेहयेन्मधुसंयुतम्||५३||

वमतोऽन्तःप्रविष्टायां जिह्वायां कवलग्रहाः| स्निग्धाम्ललवणैर्हृद्यैर्यूषक्षीररसैर्हिताः||५४||

फलान्यम्लानि खादेयुस्तस्य चान्येऽग्रतो नराः| निःसृतां तु तिलद्राक्षाकल्कलिप्तां प्रवेशयेत्||५५||

वाग्ग्रहानिलरोगेषु घृतमांसोपसाधिताम्| यवागूं तनुकां दद्यात् स्नेहस्वेदौ च बुद्धिमान्||५६||

If there is ati-Yoga (over action) of the emetic therapy, then the patient is sprinkled with cold water. He is given Mantha (demulcent drink) prepared of kapha alleviating ingredients and added with ghee, honey and sugar.

In the case of excessive vomiting associated with eructation or fainting, the patient is given to lick, the powder of Dhanya, Musta, Madhuka and Anjana (solid extract of Daru- haridra) mixed with honey.

While vomiting, if the tongue gets drawn inside, then Kavala- Graha (recipe used for rinsing the mouth) with the vegetable-soup, milk or meat-soup prepared by adding unctuous, sour, saline and palatable ingredients is given. Another person may eat sour fruits in front of the patient (to cause salivation of the patient which helps the indrawn tongue to come to its normal position).

If the tongue is protruded out, then it is smeared with the paste of til and Draksa, and pushed back to its normal position.

If there is Vak Graha (obstruction in speech) or other disorders caused by Vata, then a wise physician should give thin gruel prepared with ghee and meat for the patient to eat. In addition, the patient may be given with oleation and fomentation therapies. [52-56]

Need for Regulated diet

वमितश्च विरिक्तश्च मन्दाग्निश्च विलङ्घितः| अग्निप्राणविवृद्ध्यर्थं क्रमं पेयादिकं भजेत् ||५७||

A person who has Mandagni (suppressed power of digestion and metabolism) and who was fasting because of emetic and purgative therapies is given regulated diet in the form of Peya (thin gruel), etc. for the promotion of his Agni and Prana (Vitality) [57]

Etiology, signs and Treatment of Adhmana

बहुदोषस्य रूक्षस्य हीनाग्नेरल्पमौषधम्| सोदावर्तस्य चोत्क्लिशय दोषान्मार्गान्निरुध्य च||५८||

भृशमाध्मापयेन्नाभिं पृष्ठपार्श्वशिरोरुजम्| श्वासविण्मूत्रवातानां सङ्गं कुर्याच्च दारुणम्||५९||

अभ्यङ्गस्वेदवर्त्यादि सनिरूहानुवासनम्| उदावर्तहरं सर्वं कर्माध्मातस्य शस्यते||६०||

If medicines for purifications are administered in a small dose to a patient who is afflicted with excess of morbid Doshas, whose body is dry, who has less of Agni (power of digestion), and who is suffering from Udavarta (upward movement of wind), the medicines while exciting Doshas may cause obstruction to the channels. This causes frequent Adhmana (distension) in the umbilical region, pain in the back, side of the chest as well as head, and serious obstruction to the passage of breath, stool, urine and flatus.

For the treatment of these complications, the patient is given Abhyanga (massage), Svedana (fomentation), Varti (medicated suppository), Svedana (fomentation) Varti (medicated suppository), etc., along with Niruha (evacuative) and Anuvasana (unctuous) types of enema. All the therapies prescribed for the treatment of Udavarta (vide Chikitsa 26: 11-31) are useful for the treatment of the present ailment i.e adhmana (flatulence). [58-60]

Etiology, signs and treatment of Parikartika

स्निग्धेन गुरुकोष्ठेन सामे बलवदौषधम्|क्षामेण मृदुकोष्ठेन श्रान्तेनाल्पबलेन वा||६१||

पीतं गत्वा गुदं साममाशु दोषं निरस्य च|तीव्रशूलां सपिच्छास्रां करोति परिकर्तिकाम्||६२||

लङ्घनं पाचनं सामे रूक्षोष्णं लघुभोजनम्|बृंहणीयो विधिः सर्वः क्षामस्य मधुरस्तथा||६३||

If a person who is oleated, who has costive bowel and who is afflicted with Ama (product of improper digestion and metabolism), or if a person who is weak, who has lax bowel, who is fatigued and who has taken a quick acting medicine for purification, then the recipe reaches the rectum to cause excruciating sawing kind of pain accompanied with slimy and bloody discharge.

In this condition associated with Ama, the patient should keep fasting; take Pachana (digestive stimulants) and food which is dry, hot and light for digestion.

If the patient is weak, then all the nourishing therapies and recipes containing drugs having sweet taste are taken. [61- 63]

Recipes for Parikartika

आमे जीर्णेऽनुबन्धश्चेत् क्षाराम्लं लघु शस्यते| पुष्पकासीसमिश्रं वा क्षारेण लवणेन वा||६४||

सदाडिमरसं सर्पिः पिबेद्वातेऽधिके सति| दध्यम्लं भोजने पाने संयुक्तं दाडिमत्वचा||६५||

देवदारुतिलानां वा कल्कमुष्णाम्बुना पिबेत्| अश्वत्थोदुम्बरप्लक्षकदम्बैर्वा शृतं पयः||६६||

कषायमधुरं शीतं पिच्छाबस्तिमथापि वा| यष्टीमधुकसिद्धं वा स्नेहबस्तिं प्रदापयेत्||६७||

If Parikartika (sawing pain) continues even after the Ama (product of improper digestion and metabolism) gets cooked, intake of alkaline, light to digest and sour foods are beneficial.

If there is predominance of Vata (aggravated), the below mentioned recipes are useful:

Ghee along with pomegranate-juice added with Puspa-kasisa or alkalies or salt

Food and drinks containing sour curd mixed with the skin of the pomegranate;

Paste of Devadaru and Tila should be given for drinking mixed in hot water.

Milk boiled and processed with Ashwattha, Udumbara, Plaksha and Kadamba should be given for drinking.

Cold enemas prepared with astringent and sweet tasting herbs or Pichcha Basti type of enema shall be administered.

Anuvasana Basti with oil/ghee prepared with paste and decoction of Yashtimadhu. [64-67]

Etiology, signs and treatment of Parisrava

अल्पं तु बहुदोषस्य दोषमुत्क्लिश्य भेषजम्| अल्पाल्पं स्रावयेत् कण्डूं शोफं कुष्ठानि गौरवम्||६८||

कुर्याच्चाग्निबलोत्क्लेशस्तैमित्यारुचिपाण्डुताः| परिस्रावः स, तं दोषं शमयेद्वामयेदपि||६९||

स्नेहितं वा पुनस्तीक्ष्णं पाययेत् विरेचनम्| शुद्धे चूर्णासवारिष्टान् संस्कृतांश्च प्रदापयेत्||७०||

Purificatory recipe given in a small dose to a person having excessively aggravated Doshas causes excitation of the morbid material and eliminates them frequently in small quantities, this gives rise to itching, oedema, Kustha (skin diseases), heaviness of the body, diminution of the power of Agni (digestion) and strength, Staimitya (a feeling as if the body has been covered with a wet leather), anorexia and anaemia. This condition is called Parisrava.

This morbidity may be corrected either by alleviation therapy (if there is less of morbid matter) or by emesis (if the morbid material is present in large quantities).

After oleation, the patient may be given with strong purgation therapy again. After purgation, the patient is given recipes of powders, Asavas and Aristas processed with appropriate ingredients (as described in the treatment of Arsas or piles and Grahani or spure syndrome (vide Chikitsa 14, 15). [68-70]

Etiology, signs and treatment of Hrdayopasarana

पीतौषधस्य वेगानां निग्रहान्मारुतादयः| कुपिता हृदयं गत्वा घोरं कुर्वन्ति हृद्ग्रहम्||७१||

स हिक्काकासपार्श्वार्तिदैन्यलालाक्षिविभ्रमैः| जिह्वां खादति निःसञ्ज्ञो दन्तान् किटिकिटापयन्||७२||

न गच्छेदिवभ्रमं तत्र वामयेदाशु तं भिषक्| मधुरैः पित्तमूर्च्छार्तं कटुभिः कफमूर्च्छितम्||७३||

पाचनीयैस्ततश्चास्य दोषशेषं विपाचयेत्| कायाग्निं च बलं चास्य क्रमेणोत्थापयेत्ततः ||७४||

पवनेनातिवमतो हृदयं यस्य पीड्यते| तस्मै स्निग्धाम्ललवणं दद्यात् पित्तकफेऽन्यथा||७५||

Because of the suppression of the manifested natural urges in a person who has taken purificatory recipes, Vata, etc., get aggravated. Pertaining to the heart, these aggravated Doshas give rise to serious ailments like Hrd-Graha (cardiac spasm).

The patient afflicted with these conditions suffers from hiccup, cough, and pain in the sides of the chest, prostration, ptyalism and agitation of the eyes. He bites his tongue, becomes unconscious and gnashes his teeth.

The physician should not commit a mistake. If the patient faints because of aggravated pitta he should immediately administer emetic therapy with sweet ingredients.

If the patient faints because of aggravated Kapha, then the emetic therapy is given with pungent ingredients, thereafter, the residual Doshas are digested by the administration of digestive stimulants after which his Kayagni (digestive power) and strength are restored gradually.

Because of vomiting in excess, if the heart is afflicted by aggravated Vata, then the patient is given unctuous, sour and saline drugs, if this is caused by Pitta or Kapha, then drugs having opposite attributes (like dryness and bitter as well as pungent tastes) are given. [71-75]

Etiology, Signs and Treatment of Anga-Graha

पीतौषधस्य वेगानां निग्रहेण कफेन वा| रुद्धोऽति वा विशुद्धस्य गृह्णात्यङ्गानि मारुतः||७६||

स्तम्भवेपथुनिस्तोदसादोद्वेष्टनमन्थनैः| तत्र वातहरं सर्वं स्नेहस्वेदादि कारयेत् [2] ||७७||

If a person who has taken purificatory therapy, suppresses his manifested natural urges, or if the Vata in his body gets occluded by Kapha, or if the purification is done in excess, then the aggravated Vata causes spasm in different parts of the body of the patient. This produces Stambha (stiffness), Vepathu (trembling), Nistodu (pain), Sada (prostration), Udvestana (spasm) and Manthana (twisting)

For these ailments, all the Vata alleviating therapies like oleation and fomentation are administered. [76-77]

Etiology, signs and Treatment of Jivadana (Bleeding)

अतितीक्ष्णं मृदौ कोष्ठे लघुदोषस्य भेषजम्| दोषान् हृत्वा विनिर्मथ्य जीवं हरति शोणितम्||७८||

तेनान्नं मिश्रितं दद्याद्वायसाय शुनेऽपि वा| भुङ्क्ते तच्चेद्वदेज्जीवं न भुङ्क्ते पित्तमादिशेत्||७९||

शुक्लं वा भावितं वस्त्रमावानं कोष्णवारिणा| प्रक्षालितं विवर्णं स्यात् पित्ते शुद्धं तु शोणिते||८०||

तृष्णामूर्च्छामदार्तस्य कुर्यादामरणात् क्रियाम्| तस्य पित्तहरीं सर्वामतियोगे च या हिता ||८१||

मृगगोमहिषाजानां सद्यस्कं जीवतामसृक्| पिबेज्जीवाभिसन्धानं जीवं तद्ध्याशु गच्छति ||८२||

तदेव दर्भमृदितं रक्तं बस्तिं प्रदापयेत्| श्यामाकाश्मर्यबदरीदूर्वाशिरैः शृतं पयः||८३||

घृतमण्डाञ्जनयुतं शीतं बस्तिं प्रदापयेत्| पिच्छाबस्तिं सुशीतं वा घृतमण्डानुवासनम्||८४||

If a strong purificatory recipe is given to a person who has a laxed bowel, and who has less of morbid Doshas, then after eliminating the morbid Doshas, the recipe causes churning (of the intestine) which results in bleeding.

This (fluid) is mixed with food and given to crows and dogs to eat. If they eat it then it is to be considered as Jiva-Rakta (live or pure blood), and if it is not eaten by them, it should be considered as raktapitta i.e., polluted blood.

A piece of white cloth is impregnated with this fluid and then dried. When washed with lukewarm water, if the piece of cloth becomes/remains discoloured, then the bleeding is to be treated as caused by Raktapitta, and if it becomes absolutely clean, then this is to be treated as Jiva-Rakta (live or pure blood).

If the patient having bleeding suffers from morbid thirst, fainting and intoxication, then the physician should treat him till the last moment of his life. All the therapies which are meant for the alleviation of Pitta, and which are useful for the management of over-action of purificatory therapies (as described in the verse no. 47) are given to him.

He is given to drink the fresh blood of a living deer, cow, buffalo or goat which is life-supporting because it immediately gets transformed into the live-blood. This blood [of animals] may be mixed with the powder of Darbha and used for Basti (medicated enema).

The milk cooked by adding Syama (Priyangu), Kasmarya, Badari, Durva, and Usira is mixed with Ghrta-Manda (supernatant part of ghee) and Anjana (solid extract of daruharidra), and cooled. This may be administered as medicated enema). He may be given very cold Piccha-Basti (mucilaginous enema) or Anuvasana-Basti (unctuous enema) prepared of Ghrta-manda. [78-84]

Etiology, Signs and Treatment of Vibhramsa

गुदं भ्रष्टं कषायैश्च स्तम्भयित्वा प्रवेशयेत्| साम गान्धर्वशब्दांश्च सञ्ज्ञानाशेऽस्य कारयेत्||८५||

यदा विरेचनं पीतं विदन्तमवतिष्ठते| वमनं भेषजान्तं वा दोषानुत्क्लिश्य नावहेत्||८६||

तदा कुर्वन्ति कण्डुवादीन् दोषाः प्रकुपिता गदान्| स विभ्रंशो मतस्तत्र स्यादयथाव्याधि भेषजम्||८७||

If there is prolapse of the rectum (Guda-Bhramsa), it is made stiff by applying astringent drugs, and pushed back into its own location.

If there is unconsciousness (Sanjna-Bhramsa), then the patient is consoled and he is entertained with soothing music. If the intake of purgative recipe stops action after the elimination of stool and doesn't expel morbid pitta and kapha, if the intake of emetic recipe stops action after the elimination of emetic medicine without removing the morbid kapha and pitta, then the aggravated Doshas give rise to ailments like Kandu (itching) etc. This is called Vibhramsa (wrong action) these ailments are to be appropriately treated according to their nature. [85-87]

Etiology, Signs and Treatment of Stambha

पीतं स्निग्धेन सस्नेहं तद्दोषैर्मार्दवाद्वृतम्| न वाहयति दोषांस्तु स्वस्थानात् स्तम्भयेच्च्युतान्||८८||

वातसङ्गगुदस्तम्भशूलैः क्षरति चाल्पशः| तीक्ष्णं बस्तिं विरेकं वा सोऽर्हो लङ्घितपाचितः||८९||

Unctuous type of purificatory recipe taken by an oleated person gets occluded by Doshas because of its mild nature. It becomes incapable of expelling the Doshas. The Doshas displaced from their locations thus get obstructed. This causes obstruction to flatus, stiffness in the anal region and pain in anal region associated with expulsion of faeces (morbid doshas) in smaller quantities. Such a patient is treated by strong enema or purgation after Langhana (fasting therapy) and Pachana (carminative therapy). [88-89]

Etiology, signs and Treatment of Upadravas

रूक्षं विरेचनं पीतं रूक्षेणाल्पबलेन वा|मारुतं कोपयित्वाऽऽशु कुर्याद्धोरानुपद्रवान्||९०||

स्तम्भशूलानि घोराणि सर्वगात्रेषु मुह्यतः|स्नेहस्वेदादिकस्तत्र कार्यो वातहरो विधिः||९१||

Intake of dry type of purgation therapy by a person whose body is dry and who is weak aggravates Vata immediately to cause serious type of complications like serious type of Stambha (stiffness) and colic pain all over the body of the patient who gradually loses consciousness.

In such cases, oleation, fomentation and such other therapies for alleviation of Vata are administered. [90-91]

Etiology, Signs and Treatment of Klama

स्निग्धस्य मृदुकोष्ठस्य मृदूत्क्लिश्यौषधं कफम्| पित्तं वातं च संरुध्य सतन्द्रागौरवं क्लमम्||९२||

दौर्बल्यं चाङ्गसादं च कुर्यादाशु तदुल्लिखेत्| लङ्घनं पाचनं चात्र स्निग्धं तीक्ष्णं च शोधनम्||९३||

Mild purificatory recipe administered to an oleated person having lax bowel excites Kalpha and Pitta because of which the Vata gets obstructed leading to the manifestation of klama (mental fatigue) associated with drowsiness and heaviness. This causes weakness and prostration of limbs.

Such a patient is administered emetic therapy quickly. Langhana (fasting) and Pachana (carminative drugs) are given to the patient followed by purificatory therapy containing unctuous and sharp drugs. [92-93]

Epilogue

तत्र श्लोकौ-

इत्येता व्यापदः प्रोक्ताः सरूपाः सचिकित्सिताः| वमनस्य विरेकस्य कृतस्याकुशलैर्नृणाम् ||९४||

एता विज्ञाय मतिमानवस्थाश्चैव तत्त्वतः| दद्यात् संशोधनं सम्यगारोग्यार्थी नृणां सदा||९५||

To sum up: - The complications along with signs, symptoms and treatment arising out of the administration of emetic and purgative therapies by the unskilled physician are described in this chapter. A wise physician having correct knowledge of these states (complications) should appropriately administer purifictory therapies (free from complications) with the objective of providing good health to the people. [94-95]

इत्यग्निवेशकृते तन्त्रे चरकप्रतिसंस्कृतेऽप्राप्ते दृढबलसम्पूरिते सिद्धिस्थाने वमनविरेचनव्यापत्सिद्धिर्नाम षष्ठोऽध्यायः||६||

Thus, end the sixth chapter of siddhi-Sthana dealing with "successful treatment of Complications of emetic and Purgation Therapies" in Agnivesha's work as redacted by Charaka, and because of its non- availability, supplemented by Drdhabala.

32

Siddhisthana Chapter 7 Basti Vyapat Siddhi

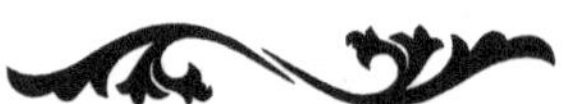

Prologue

अथातो बस्तिव्यापत्सिद्धिं व्याख्यास्यामः||१||

इति ह स्माह भगवानात्रेयः||२||

Now we shall explore the "Successful Treatment of Complications of Basti therapy'. Thus said Lord Atreya [1-2]

Dialogue and topics to be discussed

धीधैर्यौदार्यगाम्भीर्यक्षमादमतपोनिधिम्| पुनर्वसुं शिष्यगणः पप्रच्छ विनयान्वितः||३||

काः कति व्यापदो बस्तेः किंसमुत्थानलक्षणाः| का चिकित्सा इति प्रश्नाञ्छ्रुत्वा तानब्रवीद्गुरुः||४||

Punarvasu, the veritable stone-house of wisdom, fortitude, large-heartedness, profundity, forgiveness, self control and penance was asked with humility by the group of disciples about the following topics:

Which complications arise out of the administration of basti?

What is the number of these complications?

What are their causes?

What are their signs and symptoms? And

What is the treatment of these complications?

Having heard these questions, the teacher said as follows [to be discussed in the subsequent verses]. [3-4]

Complications, Their Number and Etiology in General

नातियोगौ क्लमाध्माने हिक्का हृत्प्राप्तिरूर्ध्वता| प्रवाहिका शिरोङ्गार्तिः परिकर्तः परिस्रवः||५||

द्वादश व्यापदो बस्तेरसम्यग्योगसम्भवाः| आसामेकैकशो रूपं चिकित्सां च निबोधत||६||

Twelve complications arising out of the improper administration (Asamyak Yoga) of Basti or enema are as follows: Ayoga (under action or absence of any action), Ati-yoga (over-action), Klama (mental fatigue), Adhmana (flatulence), Hikka (hiccup), Hrt-Prapti (cardiac disorders), Urdhvata (excessive upward movement), Pravahika (gripping pain), Siro-arti (headache), Anga-arti (body ache), Parikartika (sawing pain) and, Parisrava (excessive discharge)

Signs (including aetiology) and treatment of each one of them will be described thereafter which you may hear (addressed to Agnivesha) [5-6]

Etiology, signs and Treatment of Ayoga:

गुरुकोष्ठेऽनिलप्राये रूक्षे वातोल्बणेऽपि वा| शीतोऽल्पलवणस्नेहद्रवमात्रो घनोऽपि वा||७||

बस्तिः सङ्क्षोभ्य तं दोषं दुर्बलत्वादनिर्हरन्| करोति गुरुकोष्ठत्वं वातमूत्रशकृद्ग्रहम्||८||

नाभिबस्तिरुजं दाहं हृल्लेपं श्वयथुं गुदे| कण्डूगण्डानि वैवर्ण्यमरुचिं वह्निमार्दवम्||९||

तत्रोष्णायाः प्रमथ्यायाः पानं स्वेदाः पृथग्विधाः| फलवर्त्योऽथवा कालं ज्ञात्वा शस्तं विरेचनम्||१०||

• 434 •

बिल्वमूलत्रिवृद्दारुयवकोलकुलत्थवान्| सुरादिमूत्रवान् बस्तिः सप्राक्पेष्यस्तमानयेत्||११||

The enema, while exciting the morbid matter does not help in their elimination because of its weak actions as a result of the following:

• If the patient is of costive bowel;

• If the colon of the patient is dominated by vata

• If the body of the patient is un-unctuous

• If there is aggravation of vata in the body

• If the enema recipe is cold

• If the recipe of enema c ontains less of salt, unctuous material and liquid

• If the enema recipe is dense

• If the enema recipe is of small dose and

As a result of these factors, the patient suffers from the following;

• Heaviness in the gastro-intestinal tract

• Retention of flatus, urine and stool

• Pain in the umbilical region and urinary bladder

• Burning sensation

• A feeling as if the heart is adhered with/enveloped by sticky material)

• Oedema in the rectum

• Itching and abscesses

• Discoloration of the skin

• Anorexia and

• Suppression of the power of digestion

The above-mentioned ailments can be treated with the following therapies and measures:

• Intake of hot Pramathya (warm digestive decoctions which are described in the treatment of diarrhoea- vide Chikitsa 19:20-21)

• Administration of different types of fomentation therapy

• Administration of Phala-Varti (medicated suppository)

• Administration of purgation therapy in appropriate time and

• Administration of enema recipe prepared of the root of Bilva, Trivrt, Devadaru, Yava, Kola, Kulattha, Sura etc., (Sauviraka, Tusodaka, etc.) and cow's urine by adding the paste of drugs described earlier, (viz, Bala etc., described in Siddhi 3:13) [7-11]

Etiology, signs and Treatment of Ati-Yoga

स्निग्धस्विन्नेऽतितीक्ष्णोष्णो मृदुकोष्ठेऽतियुज्यते|तस्य लिङ्गं चिकित्सा च शोधनाभ्यां समा भवेत्||१२||

पृश्निपर्णी स्थिरां पद्मं काश्मर्यं मधुकं बलाम्| पिष्ट्वा द्राक्षां मधूकं च क्षीरे तण्डुलधावने||१३||

द्राक्षायाः पक्वलोष्टस्य प्रसादे मधुकस्य च| विनीय सघृतं बस्तिं दद्याद्दाहेऽतियोगजे [२] ||१४||

Ati-Yoga (over-action) is caused by the administration of excessively sharp and hot recipes as enema to a person who is oleated and fomented, and who has a lax bowel. The signs and treatment are similar to those prescribed for the treatment of atiyoga (over action) of emetic and purgative therapies.

The recipe for Basti is prepared by adding the paste of Prsniparni, Sthira, Padma, Kasmarya, Madhuka, Bala, Draksa and Madhuka to milk, Tandulodaka (rice-water) and sita-Kasaya (cold infusion) of Draksa, baked earth and Madhuka. This basti when administered with ghee cures Daha (burning sensation) caused by Ati-Yoga (over action) of Niruha. [12-14]

Etiology, signs and Treatment of Klama

आमशेषे निरूहेण मृदुना दोष ईरितः|मार्गं रुणद्धि वातस्य हन्त्यग्निं मूर्च्छयत्यपि||१५||

क्लमं विदाहं हृच्छूलं मोहवेष्टनगौरवम्|कुर्यात् स्वेदैर्विरूक्षैस्तं पाचनैश्चाप्युपाचरेत्||१६||

पिप्पलीकतृणोशीरदारुमूर्वाशृतं जलम्|पिबेत् सौवर्चलोन्मिश्रं दीपनं हृद्विशोधनम्||१७||
वचानागरशटयेला दधिमण्डेन मूच्छिताः|पेयाः प्रसन्नया वा स्युररिष्टेनासवेन वा||१८||
दारु त्रिकटुकं पथ्यां पलाशं चित्रकं शटीम्|पिष्ट्वा कुष्ठं च मूत्रेण पिबेत् क्षारांश्च दीपनान्||१९||
बस्तिमस्य विदध्याच्च समूत्रं दाशमूलिकम्|समूत्रमथवा व्यक्तलवणं माधुतैलिकम्||२०||

If a mild recipe is used for NiruhaBasti, when there is residual Ama (product of improper digestion) in the gastrointestinal tract, then the Doshas (Pitta and Kapha along with Ama) excited by enema obstruct the channel of vata that causes perversion and suppression of the power of digestion, further aggravation of vata, mental fatigue, burning sensation, cardiac pain, stupefaction, cramps and heaviness.

Such a patient is treated by fomentation with un-unctuous ingredients, and Pachana (carminatives).

The patient should drink water boiled with Pippali, kattrna, Usira, Devadaru and Murva by adding sauvarcala salt which stimulates the power of digestion and cleanses the heart.

The powder of Vacha, Nagara, Shati and Ela is added with whey. This recipe is taken along with Prasanna, Arista or Asava (a type of alcoholic preparations).

The patient should take the paste of Devadaru ,Sunthi, Pippali, Marica, Pathya, Palasa, Citraka, Sati and Kustha along with the cow's urine.

He may also take alkali preparations which are digestive stimulants (described in Cikitsa 15: 168:193)

He is given Basti prepared of Bilva, Shyonaka,Gambhari, Patala, Gani-Karika, Salaparni, Prsniparni, Brhati, Kantakari and Goksura along with cow's urine. [The enema recipe containing this Dashamula is described in siddhi 3:35-36]

Alternatively, he may also take Madhu Tailika type of medicated enema (to be described later in Siddhi 12:18:13) added with cow's urine and adequate quantity of salt. [15-20]

Etiology, signs and Treatment of adhmana

अल्पवीर्या महादोषे रूक्षे क्रूराशये कृतः|बस्तिर्दोषावृतो रुद्धमार्गं रुन्ध्यात् समीरणम्||२१||
स विमार्गोऽनिलः कुर्यादाध्मानं मर्मपीडनम्|विदाहं गुरुकोष्ठस्य मुष्कवङ्क्षणवेदनाम्||२२||
रुणद्धि हृदयं शूलैरितश्चेतश्च धावति|श्यामाफलादिभिः कुष्ठकृष्णालवणसर्षपैः||२३||
धूममाषवचाकिण्वक्षारचूर्णगुडैः कृताम्|कराङ्गुष्ठनिभां वर्तिं यवमध्यां निधापयेत्||२४||
अभ्यक्तस्विन्नगात्रस्य तैलाक्तां स्नेहिते गुदे|अथवा लवणाङ्गारधूमसिद्धार्थकैः कृताम्||२५||
बिल्वादिना निरूहः स्यात् पीलुसर्षपमूत्रवान्|सरलामरदारुभ्यां सिद्धं चैवानुवासनम्||२६||

If enema of mild potency is given to a person who has excessively aggravated Doshas, whose body is un-unctuous and who has costive bowel, then it gets occluded by Doshas, and gets clogged in the channel thereby causing obstruction to the movement of vata. This vata then moves through a diverted path thereby causing exceedingly painful Adhmana (flatulence), Vidaha (burning sensation), Guru-Kosthata (heaviness of the gastro- intestinal tract) and pain in the testicles as well as groins. It causes impediment in the functioning of the heart by causing cardiac pain, and moves about irregularly in different directions.

A varti (medicated suppository) of the size of thumb, and sharp of barley seed is prepared of Shyama, etc. (nine drugs viz Shyama, Trivrt, Chaturangula, Tilvaka, Mahavrksa, Saptala, sankhini,Danti and Dravanti-vide kalpa 1: 6),Phala etc., (six drugs, viz, Phala, Jimutaka, Iksvaku, Dhamargava, Kutaja and Salt, Sarsapa, powder of dhuma (kitchen soot), Masa, Vacha, Kinva (yeast) and Ksara (alkali) and jaggery.

Alternatively, this Varti (suppository) can be prepared by adding salt, kitchen soot and Siddharthaka (to Shyama, etc., and Phala etc. described above).

These suppositories may be smeared with oil and inserted into the lubricated anus of the patient who is precisely given massage and fomentation therapies.

The patient may be given Niruha with a recipe containing bilva etc., (vide verse no. 11) and added with pilu, sarsapa and cow's urine.

Oil cooked with Sarala and Devadaru may be used for giving anuvasana basti or unctuous types of enema to the patient. [21-26]

Etiology, signs and Treatment of Hikka

मृदुकोष्ठेऽबले बस्तिरतितीक्ष्णोऽतिनिर्हरन्|कुर्यादि्धिक्कां, हितं तस्मै हिक्काघ्नं बृंहणं च यत्||२७||

बलास्थिरादिकाश्मर्यत्रिफलागुडसैन्धवैः|सप्रसन्नारनालाम्लैस्तैलं पक्त्वाऽनुवासयेत्||२८||

कृष्णालवणयोरक्षं पिबेदुष्णाम्बुना युतम्|धूमलेहरसक्षीरस्वेदाश्चान्नं च वातनुत्||२९||

If a very strong recipe of Basti is administered to a person having laxed bowel and weakness, then it causes elimination of morbid matter in excess quantity as a result of which the patient suffers from Hikka (hiccup).

For this is given Anuvasana Basti or unctuous types of medicated enema with oil cooked by adding Bala, Sthira etc., Kasmarya, Haritaki, Bibhitaka, Amalaki, Guda, Saindhava, Prasanna and sour Aranala.

The patient may take one Aksa (12 g) of powder of Krshna (pippali) and rock-salt along with hot water.

He is given vata-alleviating dhuma (smoking therapy), linctus, meat-soup, medicated milk, fomentation therapy and suitable food. [27-29]

Aetiology, signs and treatment of Hrt-Prapti

अतितीक्ष्णः सवातो वा न वा सम्यक् प्रपीडितः| घट्टयेद्धृदयं बस्तिस्तत्र काशकुशेत्कटैः||३०||

स्यात् साम्ललवणस्कन्धकरीरबदरीफलैः| शृतैर्बस्तिर्हितः सिद्धं वातघ्नैश्चानुवासनम्||३१||

If the enema recipe is of exceedingly strong nature, if the enema fluid is injected along with air, or if appropriate pressure is not applied over the receptacle of enema-fluid during administration, then this afflicts the heart.

In this case the decoction of Kasa, Kusa, Itkata, drugs belonging to Amla (sour) and Lavana (saline) Skanadha (group) Karira and fruit of Badari is used for enema (Niruha). The patient may also be given Anuvasana or an unctuous type of enema prepared with vata-alleviating drugs (like Dashamula). [30-31]

Aetiology, signs and treatment of urdhva-Gamana (Upward movement)

वातमूत्रपुरीषाणां दत्ते वेगान्निगृह्णतः|अति वा पीडितो बस्तिर्मुखेनायाति वेगवान्||३२||

मूर्च्छाविकारं तस्यादौ दृष्ट्वा शीताम्बुना मुखम्| सिञ्चेत् पार्श्वोदरं चाधः प्रमृज्याद्वीजयेच्च तम्||३३||

केशेष्वालम्ब्य चाकाशे धुनुयात्रासयेच्च तम्| गोखराश्वगजैः सिंहै राजप्रेष्यैस्तथोरगैः||३४||

उल्काभिरेवमन्यैश्च भीतस्याधः प्रवर्तते| वस्त्रपाणिग्रहैः कण्ठं रुन्ध्यान्न म्रियते यथा||३५||

प्राणोदाननिरोधादि्ध प्रसिद्धतरमार्गवान्| अपानः पवनो बस्तिं तमाश्वेवापकर्षति||३६||

ततः क्रमुककल्काक्षं पाययेताम्लसंयुतम्| औष्ण्यातैक्ष्यात् सरत्वाच्च बस्तिं सोऽस्यानुलोमयेत्||३७||

पक्वाशयस्थिते स्विन्ने निरूहो दाशमूलिकः| यवकोलकुलत्थैश्च विधेयो मूत्रसाधितः||३८||

बिल्वादिपञ्चमूलेन सिद्धो बस्तिरुरःस्थिते| शिरःस्थे नावनं धूमः प्रच्छाद्यं सर्षपैः शिरः||३९||

If after the administration of enema the patient suppresses the natural urges for voiding flatus, urine and stool, and if excessive pressure is applied over the enema- receptacle during the administration of this therapy, then because of forceful flow the enema fluid comes out through the oral cavity.

If on account of this there is fainting, the following remedial measures are undertaken:

• In the beginning the face of the patient is sprinkled with cold water.

• His sides of the chest and abdomen are squeezed downwards;

• He is fanned;

• He is pulled up to the mid-air by holding his hair, and shaken;

• He is frightened by means of infuriated bull, ass, horse, elephant, lion, and executions of the king, serpents, fire-works and such other fearful objects. Being terrified in this manner, the enema fluid will start flowing downwards.

• The throat of the patient is squeezed with the help of a piece of cloth or by hand, taking care not to asphyxiate the patient, which may otherwise lead to his death. By the obstruction to the path of prana and udana caused in the above said manner, the Apana vata becomes predominant in the passage, and instantaneously draws the fluid downwards to the normal course.

• Thereafter, one Aksa (12 g) of the paste of Kramuka (Puga phala) added with sour juice is given to the patient to drink, because of hot, sharp and mobile attributes, the recipe helps in the downward movement of the enema-fluid.

• If the enema fluid is located in the Pakvasaya (colon), then the patient is given fomentation therapy and thereafter, Niruha type of enema is given with a recipe containing Dashamula (Bilva, Shyonaka, Gambhari, Patala, Ganikarika, Shalaparni, Prsniparni, Brhati, Kantakari and Goksura),Yava, Kola and Kulattha cooked by adding cow's urine;

• If the enema- fluid is located in the chest region, then Niruha Basti prepared by cooking Panacamula (Bilva, Shyonaka, Gambhari, patala and ganikarika) is administered and

• If the enema fluid gets located in the head (upper part of the body) then the patient is given Navana (inhalation therapy) and Dhuma (smoking therapy) after anointing his head with the mustard paste. [32-39]

Etiology, signs and Treatment of Pravahika (gripping Pain)

स्निग्धस्विन्ने महादोषे बस्तिर्मृद्वल्पभेषजः|उत्क्लिश्याल्पं हरेद्दोषं जनयेच्च प्रवाहिकाम्||४०||

स बस्तिपायुशोफेन जङ्घोरुसदनेन वा|निरुद्धमारुतो जन्तुरभीक्ष्णं सम्प्रवाहते||४१||

स्वेदाभ्यङ्गान्निरूहांश्च शोधनीयानुलोमिकान्| विदध्याल्लङ्घयित्वा तु वृतिं कुर्यादिवरिक्तवत्||४२||

If a mild recipe of enema is administered in a small dose to patient who is oleated and fomented, and whose body is afflicted with excessively aggravated Doshas, then after excitation this enema eliminates morbid material (Doshas) only in small quantity thereby causing Pravahika (dysentery).

The patient having obstructed vata passes stool frequently because of the inflation of the bladder (basti) and anus, and asthenia of calf region as well as thighs.

In such cases, after fasting, the patient is given fomentation, massage and Niruha type of enema with recipes containing drugs which are Shodaniya or purificatory (like Trivrt etc.), and Anulomaniya or inducing downward movement of vata (like milk, sugarcane juice) in nature. He should resort to regimens as prescribed for a person who has undergone purgation therapy. [40-42]

Aetiology, signs and treatment of shirorti (headache)

दुर्बले क्रूरकोष्ठे च तीव्रदोषे तनुमृदुः| शीतोऽल्पश्चावृतो दोषैर्बस्तिस्तद्विहतोऽनिलः||४३||

मार्गैर्गात्राणि सन्धावन्नूर्ध्वं मूर्धिन विहन्यते| ग्रीवां मन्ये च गृह्णाति शिरः कण्ठं भिनति च||४४||

बाधिर्यं कर्णनादं च पीनसं नेत्रविभ्रमम्| कुर्यादभ्यञ्जनं तैललवणेन यथाविधि||४५||

युञ्ज्यात् प्रधमनैनैस्यैर्धूमैरस्य विरेचयेत्| तीक्ष्णानुलोमिकेनाथ स्निग्धं भुक्तेऽनुवासयेत् [६] ||४६||

If the enema recipe which is thin, mild and cooling in nature is administered in a small dose to a patient who is weak, who has costive bowel and who is afflicted with exceedingly aggravated Doshas, then the enema fluid gets occluded by doshas. The vata, thus pressed, moves fast through the channels to different parts of the body, causes stiffness of the neck and temples and gets stuck up in the head and throat, causing deafness, tinnitus, coryza and agitation of the eyes.

The patient is given following therapies:

• Massage with oil mixed with salt in appropriate manner

• Elimination of Doshas by Pradhamana nasya (inhalation therapy given by blowing drugs into the nostrils) and vairechanika dhuma (dosha purging smoking therapy)

• Enema prepared with drugs which are Tikshna (sharp) and Anulomika (causing downward movement of vata) is given after food to the patient who has been oleated [43-46]

Aetiology, signs and treatment of Angarti (Pain in Limbs)

स्नेहस्वेदैरनापाद्य गुरुस्तीक्ष्णोऽतिमात्रया| यस्य बस्तिः प्रयुज्येत सोऽतिमात्रं प्रवर्तयेत्||४७||

सुतेषु तस्य दोषेषु निरूढस्यातिमात्रशः| स्तब्धोदावृतकोष्ठस्य वायुः सम्प्रतिहन्यते||४८||

विलोमनसमुद्भूतो रुजत्यङ्गानि देहिनः| गात्रवेष्टननिस्तोदभेदस्फुरणजृम्भणैः ||४९||

तं तैललवणाभ्यक्तं सेचयेदुष्णवारिणा| एरण्डपत्रनिष्क्वाथैः प्रस्तरैश्चोपपादयेत्||५०||

यवान् कुलत्थान् कोलानि पञ्चमूले तथोभये| जलाढकद्वये पक्त्वा पादशेषेण तेन च||५१||

कुर्यात् सबिल्वतैलोष्णलवणेन निरूहणम्| तं निरूढं समाश्वस्तं द्रोण्यां समवगाहयेत्||५२||

ततो भुक्तवतस्तस्य कारयेदनुवासनम्| यष्टीमधुकतैलेन बिल्वतैलेन वा भिषक् ||५३||

If without oleation and fermentation therapies, the patient is given enema, ingredients of which are Guru (heavy) and Tikshna (sharp) in large doses, and then there will be excessive elimination.

When the Dosha is eliminated in excessive quantity by Niruha Basti, then because of stiffness and occlusion in the gastro-intestinal tract vata gets impeded. By its upward movement, it causes pain in the limbs of a person in the form of cramps, pricking pain, breaking pain, throbbing pain and Jrmbhana (stretc.hing pain).

To this patient, a massage with oil added with salt is given, and his body is sprinkled with warm water. He is given fomentation with the decoction of the leaves of Eranda and Prastara type of fomentation (vide Sutra 14: 47: 48)

Yava, Kulattha, Kola and both the type of Panacamula (Dashamoola), is added with two adhakas (512 tolas) of water, and boiled till one fourth of the liquid remains. To this decoction, warm Bilva Taila and salt is added. This recipe may be used for NiruhaBasti. Thereafter, the patient is comforted and given a tub bath.

After he has taken food, the physician should be given anuvasana or unctuous types of enema with Yastimadhu Taila or Bilva Taila. [47-53]

Aetiology, Signs and Treatment of Parikartika (Sawing Pain)

मृदुकोष्ठाल्पदोषस्य रूक्षस्तीक्ष्णोऽतिमात्रवान्| बस्तिर्दोषान्निरस्याशु जनयेत् परिकर्तिकाम्||५४||

त्रिकवङ्क्षणबस्तीनां तोदं नाभेरधो रुजम्| विबन्धोऽल्पाल्पमुत्थानंबस्तिनिर्लेखनादभवेत्||५५||

स्वादुशीतौषधैस्तत्र पय इक्ष्वादिभिः शृतम्| यष्ट्याह्वतिलकल्काभ्यां बस्तिः स्यात् क्षीरभोजिनः||५६||

ससर्जरसयष्ट्याह्वजिङ्गिनीकर्दमाञ्जनम्| विनीय दुग्धे बस्तिः स्यात् व्यक्ताम्लमृदुभोजिनः||५७||

If enema with un-unctuous and sharp ingredients is given to a patient who has laxed bowel and who has less of aggravated Doshas, then it immediately eliminates Doshas to cause partikartika (sawing pain), pricking pain in the lumbar region, groins and the region of urinary bladder and pain in the lower abdomen below the umbilical region. Because of the scraping effect of enema, the patient suffers from constipation and frequent voiding of stool in small quantities.

Milk is boiled by adding sweet and cooling ingredients like sugarcane, etc. To this medicated milk, the paste of Yastimadhu and Tila is added. Enema is given with this recipe keeping the patient on a milk diet.

Milk is added with Sarjarasa, Yastimadhu, Jingini, Kardama (mud) and Anjana (solid extract of Daruharidra). This recipe is added with sour juice and used as enema for the patient who is on a soft diet. [54-57]

Aetiology, Signs and Treatment of Parisrava (Anal Exudation)

पित्तरोगेऽम्ल उष्णो वा तीक्ष्णो वा लवणोऽथवा|बस्तिर्लिखति पायुं तु क्षिणोति विदहत्यपि||५८||

स विदग्धः स्रवत्यस्रं पित्तं चानेकवर्णवत्|सार्यते बहुवेगेनमोहं गच्छति चासकृत्||५९||

आर्द्रशाल्मलिवृन्तैस्तु क्षुण्णैराजं पयः शृतम्|सर्पिषा योजितं शीतं बस्तिमस्मै प्रदापयेत्||६०||

वटादिपल्लवेष्वेष कल्पो यवतिलेषु च|सुवर्चलोपोदिकयोः कर्बुदारे च शस्यते||६१||

गुदे सेकाः प्रदेहाश्च शीताः स्युर्मधुराश्च ये| रक्तपित्तातिसारघ्नी क्रिया चात्र प्रशस्यते||६२||

If a patient suffering from Paittika diseases is given enema with ingredients which are sour, hot, sharp or saline, then this causes seeping of the anus resulting in ulceration and burning sensation. From this inflamed anus there is exudation of blood and Pitta having variegated colour. Because of forceful exudation the patient faints frequently.

To this patient, cold enema of goat's milk boiled by adding pounded green stalks of Salmali, and added with ghee is given.

This enema may also be prepared with the following recipes:

Leaves of vata, etc.:

Yava and Tila

Sauvarcala (Sunisannaka) and Upodika and

Karbudara (Kancanara)

The anal region of the patient is sprinkled or anointed with drugs which are cooling and sweet. Therapies prescribed for Raktapitta (vide Chikitsa 3) atisara (vide Chikitsa 19) are useful in this condition. [58-62]

Drugs for mild and strong enema

तीक्ष्णत्वं मूत्रपील्वग्निलवणक्षारसर्षपैः| प्राप्तकालं विधातव्यं क्षीराद्यैर्मार्दवं तथा||६३||

When required, the recipe of enema can be made strong by adding ingredients like cow's urine, Pilu (a fruit of Uttarapatha), Agni (Citraka), salt, Alkalies and mustard seed. By adding milk, etc., the enema recipe can be made milder in action when required. [63]

Importance of Basti

आपादतलमूर्धस्थान् दोषान् पक्वाशये स्थितः| वीर्येण बस्तिरादत्ते खस्थोऽर्को भूरसानिव||६४||

Basti (medicated enema) lodged in the colon, by its potency, draws [and eliminates] morbid Doshas located in the entire body - extending right from the toes to the head, just like the sun situated in the sky absorbs all the moisture (lit. juice) from the earth. [64]

Elimination of Morbid Matter Excluding Nutrients

यद्वत् कुसुम्भसम्मिश्रात्तोयाद्रागं हरेत् पटः| तद्वद्द्रवीकृताद्देहान्निरूहो निर्हरेन्मलान्||६५||

Just like a piece of cloth soaked in the water mixed with the powder of Kusumbha (a vegetable dye) sucks up only the colour (the colour pigments), the Niruha (evacuative) type of medicated enema eliminates only the morbid material (faeces, doshas) from the body of a person in whom the morbid material has been liquefied following proper administration of oleation and fomentation therapies. [65]

तत्र श्लोकः:-

इत्येता व्यापदः प्रोक्ता बस्तेः साकृतिभेषजाः| बुद्ध्वा कात्स्न्र्येन तान् बस्तीन्नियुञ्जन्नापराध्यति||६६||

To sum up: - Thus, the complications of Basti along with their signs and treatment are described. The physician administering Basti (medicated enema) after comprehension of this therapy does not commit any error. [66]

इत्यग्निवेशकृते तन्त्रे चरकप्रतिसंस्कृतेऽप्राप्ते दृढबलसम्पूरिते सिद्धिस्थाने बस्तिव्यापत्सिद्धिर्नाम सप्तमोऽध्यायः||७||

Thus, ends the seventh chapter of Siddhi- Sthana dealing with "the SuccessfulTreatment of Complications of Basti therapy" in Agnivesha's work as redacted by Charaka, and because of its non –availability, supplemented by Drdhabala.

33

Siddhisthana Chapter 8 Prasrita Yogiya Siddhi

अथातः प्रासृतयोगीयां सिद्धिं व्याख्यास्यामः॥१॥

इति ह स्माह भगवानात्रेयः॥२॥

Now we shall explore the chapter on the "Successful administration of enema with Recipes having ingredients in Prastra unit". Thus, said Lord Atreya. [1-2]

Dialogue

अथेमान् सुकुमाराणां निरूहान् स्नेहनान् मृदून्| कर्मणा विप्लुतानां च वक्ष्यामि प्रसृतैः पृथक्॥३॥

Hereafter, I (refers to Lord Atreya) shall explain unctuous and mild recipes of Niruha-Basti (evacuative type of medicated enema), ingredients of which are to be taken in the unit quantity of Prasrta (two Palas) for persons of tender health and for those who are exhausted because of hard work. [3]

Recipe of Niruha for Promotion of Complexion etc.

क्षीराद्द्वौ प्रसृतौ कार्यौ मधुतैलघृतात्त्रयः| खजेन मथितो बस्तिर्वातघ्नो बलवर्णकृत्॥४॥

Two Prasrtas of milk and three Prasrtas of honey, oil and ghee (taken together) is stirred with a stirrer. Basti of this recipe eliminates Vata, and promotes strength as well as complexion. [4]

Recipe of Niruha for Vata

एकैकः प्रसृतस्तैलप्रसन्नाक्षौद्रसर्पिषाम्| बिल्वादिमूलक्वाथाद्द्वौ कौलत्थाद्द्वौ स वातनुत्॥५॥

Enema with the recipe containing one Prasrta each of oil, Prasanna (a type of alcohol), honey and ghee, and two Prasrtas each of the decoctions of Bilva, etc., (Bilva, Shyonaka, Gambhari, Patala, Ganikarika, Salaparni, Prsniparni,Brhati, Kantakari and Goksura) as well as Kulattha cures Vata. [5]

Second Recipe of Niruha for Vata

पञ्चमूलरसात् पञ्च द्वौ तैलात् क्षौद्रसर्पिषोः| एकैकः प्रसृतो बस्तिः स्नेहनीयोऽनिलापहः॥६॥

Five Prasrtas of the decoction of Panchamula (Bilva, Shyonaka, Gambhari, Patala and Ganikarika), two Prastas of Til oil and one Prasthas each of honey as well as ghee is used in Basti (enema) for oleation and cure for Vata diseases. [6]

Recipe of Niruha for Promotion of Semen

सैन्धवार्धाक्ष एकैकः क्षौद्रतैलपयोघृतात्| प्रसृतो हपुषाकर्षो निरूहः शुक्रकृत् परम्॥७॥

The recipe of Niruha containing half aksa (tola) rock-salt, one prasrta each of honey, till-oil, milk and ghee, and one karsa (tola) of Hapusa is excellent for the promotion of semen. [7]

Pancha-Tikta Niruha

पटोलनिम्बभूनिम्बरास्नासप्तच्छदाम्भसः। चत्वारः प्रसृता एको घृतात् सर्षपकल्कितः॥८॥

निरूहः पञ्चतिक्तोऽयं मेहाभिष्यन्दकुष्ठनुत् ।९।

Four Prasrtas of the decoction of Patola, Nimba, Bhunimba, Rasna and Saptacchada and one Prasrta of ghee are added with the paste of Sarsapa. This recipe is called Pancha-Tikta Niruha. Administration of this Basti cures Meha (obstinate urinary disorders including diabetes), Abhisyanada (conjunctivitis) and Kustha (obstinate skin diseases including leprosy). [8-1/2 9]

Recipe of Niruha for Helminthiasis

विडङ्गत्रिफलाशिग्रुफलमुस्ताखुपर्णिजात्॥९॥ कषायात् प्रसृताः पञ्च तैलादेको विमथ्य तान्।

विडङ्गपिप्पलीकल्को निरूहः क्रिमिनाशनः॥१०॥

Five Prasthas of the decoction of Vidanga, Haritaki, Bibhitaka, Amalaki, Sigru, Madanapala, Musta and Akhuparni (Danti) is added with one Prasrta of oil, and the paste of Vidanga and Pippali. The recipe is stirred (emulsified) and used for Niruha (evacuative) type of medicated enema which cures helminthiasis. [9 ½- 10]

Recipe of Niruha for Virility

पयस्येक्षुस्थिरारास्नाविदारीक्षौद्रसर्पिषाम्। एकैकः प्रसृतो बस्तिः कृष्णाकल्को वृषत्वकृत्॥११॥

Basti with the recipe containing one Prasrta each (of the decoction) of Payasya, sugarcane [juice], Sthira, Rasna and Vidari, one Prasrta each of honey and ghee, and the paste of Krsna (Pippali) promotes virility (semen).[11]

Recipe of Niruha for Bhedana

चत्वारस्तैलगोमूत्रदधिमण्डाम्लकाञ्जिकात्। प्रसृताः सर्षपैः कल्कैर्विट्सङ्गानाहभेदनः॥१२॥

Basti (enema) with four prasrta of til-oil, cow's urine, whey and sour conjee, added with the paste of sarsapa causes bhedana (disintegration) and elimination of arrested stool (vit –sanga) of a constipated patient. [12]

The recipe of niruha for Dysuria

श्वदंष्ट्राश्मभिदेरण्डरसातैलात् सुरासवात्।प्रसृताः पञ्च यष्ट्याह्वकौन्तीमागधिकासिताः॥१३॥

कल्कः स्यान्मूत्रकृच्छ्रे तु सानाहे बस्तिरुत्तमः।

The recipe containing five prasrta of decoction of Svadamstra, Ashmabheda and Eranda, till oil and Surasva (alcoholic preparation), and added with the paste of yastimadhu, Kaunti, Magadhika and sita is used for enema which is excellent for curing Mutrakrcchra (dysuria) and Anaha (constipation). [13 – ½ 14]

एते सलवणाः कोष्णा निरूहाः प्रसृतैर्नव॥१४॥

Thus, nine recipes of Niruha with ingredients having the unit quantity described in the form of Prasrta, are elaborated above (in verse no. 4 – ½ 14). These recipes, when warm are to be used along with salt. [14 ½]

Administration of Repeated Basti

मृदुबस्तिजडीभूते तीक्ष्णोऽन्यो बस्तिरिष्यते।तीक्ष्णैर्विकर्षिते स्वादु प्रत्यास्थापनमिष्यते [१] ॥१५॥

If a mild enema (Niruha) gets stagnated, then another strong basti having sharp ingredients is to be administered. If, because of strong enema, the patient becomes excessively depleted, then another Niruha or Asthapana basti containing sweet drugs (like Ghrta, etc.) is given to him. [15]

Recipe for burning sensation in Anus

वातोपसृष्टस्योष्णैः स्युर्गुददाहादयो यदि। द्राक्षाम्बुना त्रिवृत्कल्कं दद्याद्दोषानुलोमनम्॥१६॥

तद्धि पित्तशकृद्वातान् हत्वा दाहादिकाञ्जयेत्। शुद्धश्चापि पिबेच्छीतां यवागूं शर्करायुताम्॥१७॥

If the administration of hot Basti to a Vata afflicted person gives rise to burning sensation in the anus, and such other complications (like fainting and morbid thirst), then he is given Draksha decoction mixed with the paste of Trivrt which causes downward movement of Doshas. By causing elimination of bile, stool and flatus, this recipe cures daha (burning sensation), etc.

After the body is cleansed [of more morbid matter], the patient should take cold Yavagu (thick gruel) mixed with sugar. [16-17]

Treatment of Diminished Stool

अथवाऽतिविरिक्तः स्यात् क्षीणविट्कः स भक्षयेत्| माषयूषेण कुल्माषान् पिबेन्मध्वथवा सुराम्||१८||

Alternatively, if because of excessive purgation, the patient suffers from excessive loss of faecal matter, then he should eat Kulmasha (food containing half steamed barley) along with the soup of masha or he should drink honey or sura type of alcohol. [18]

Treatment of Six Types of Diarrhoea

सामं चेत् कुणपं शूलैरुपविशेदरोचकी| स घनातिविषाकुष्ठनतदारुवचाः पिबेत्||१९||

शकृद्वातमसृक् पित्तं कफं वा योऽतिसार्यते| पक्वं, तत्र स्ववर्गीयैर्बस्तिः श्रेष्ठं भिषग्जितम्||२०||

If the patient voids Ama, which has the smell of a dead body and which is associated with colic pain as well as anorexia, then he should drink the decoction of Ghana, Ativisha, Kustha, Nata, Devadaru and Vaca.

If the patient excessively voids stool, flatus, blood, pitta or kapha which are pakva (cooked), then enema prepared with groups of drugs appropriate to each of these morbidities is the best remedy. [19-20]

Number of diarrhoeas

षण्णामेषां दिवसंसर्गात् त्रिंशद्भेदा भवन्ति तु| केवलैः सह षट्त्रिंशदिवद्यात् सोपद्रवानपि||२१||

The above mentioned six types of diarrhoea may get manifested in the form of the combination of two types thus making thirty more varieties of diarrhoea which are manifested along with their complications. [21]

Complications of diarrhoea

शूलप्रवाहिकाध्मानपरिकर्त्यरुचिज्वरान्| तृष्णोष्णदाहमूर्च्छादींश्चैषां विद्यादुपद्रवान्||२२||

Colic pain (sula), gripping pain (pravahika), flatulence (adhmana), sawing pain (parikartika), anorexia (aruci), fever (jvara), burning sensation (Daha), fainting (murccha), etc., are the complications of diarrhoea. [22]

Treatment of Diarrhoea with Ama

तत्रामेऽन्तरपानं स्यात् व्योषाम्ललवणैर्युतम्| पाचनं शस्यते बस्तिरामे हि प्रतिषिध्यते||२३||

If there is diarrhoea of ama type (containing mucus or uncooked product of digestion), then the recipe for pachana (carminative drugs described in the verse no. 19) along with Sunthi, Pippali, Maricha and sour as well as saline drugs is useful. Administration of enema in ama condition is prohibited. [23]

Treatment of diarrhoea along with fecal matter

वातघ्नैर्ग्राहिवर्गीयैर्बस्तिः शकृति शस्यते|२४|

Enema prepared with Vata alleviating and grahi (astringent group of drugs is useful if the diarrhoea is associated with faecal matter. [1/2 24]

Treatment of diarrhoea with flatus

स्वाद्वम्ललवणैः शस्तः स्नेहबस्तिः समीरणे||२४||

If the diarrhoea is associated with the voiding of flatus, then, sneha or Anuvasana-Basti (unctuous enema) prepared of [fat cooked with] sweet, sour and saline drugs is useful. [24 ½]

Treatment of Diarrhoea with Blood, Pitta and kapha

रक्ते रक्तेन, पित्ते तु कषायस्वादुतिक्तकैः| सार्यमाणे कफे बस्तिः कषायकटुतिक्तकैः||२५||

If the diarrhoea is associated with the voiding of blood then enema of blood is useful.

If there is diarrhoea with the voiding of Pitta, then enema prepared with astringent, sweet and bitter drugs is useful. If there is diarrhoea associated with the voiding of kapha, then enema prepared of astringent, pungent and bitter drugs is useful. [25]

Treatment of diarrhoea caused by two Factors:

शकृता वायुना वाऽऽमे तेन वर्चस्यथानिले| संसृष्टेऽन्तरपानं स्याद् व्योषाम्ललवणैर्युतम्||२६||

पित्तेनामेऽसृजा वाऽपि तयोरामेन वा पुनः| संसृष्टयोर्भवेत् पानं सव्योषस्वादुतिक्तकम्||२७||

तथाऽऽमे कफसंसृष्टे कषायव्योषतिक्तकम्| आमेन तु कफे व्योषकषायलवणैर्युतम्||२८||

वातेन विशि पित्ते वा विट्पित्ताभ्यां तथाऽनिले| मधुराम्लकषायः स्यात् संसृष्टे बस्तिरुत्तमः||२९||

शकृच्छोणितयोः पित्तशकृतो रक्तपित्तयोः| बस्तिरन्योन्यसंसर्गे कषायस्वादुतिक्तकः||३०||

कफेन विशि पित्ते वा कफे विट्पित्तशोणितैः| व्योषतिक्तकषायः स्यात् संसृष्टे बस्तिरुत्तमः||३१||

स्याद्बस्तिर्व्योषतिक्ताम्लः संसृष्टे वायुना कफे| मधुरव्योषतिक्तस्तु रक्ते कफविमूर्च्छिते||३२||

मारुते कफसंसृष्टे व्योषाम्ललवणो भवेत्| बस्तिर्वातेन पित्ते तु कार्यः स्वाद्वम्लतिक्तकः||३३||

Pachana (carminative recipe) added with Sunthi, Pippali, Maricha, sour ingredients and salt is given, if the diarrhoea is caused by the combination of two factors as follows:

• More of Ama and less of faecal matter

• More of Ama and less of flatus

• More of faecal matter less of Ama and

• More of flatus and less of Ama

Pachana (carminative recipe) added with Sunthi, Pippali, Maricha, and Sweet as well as bitter drugs are given if the diarrhoea is caused by the two factors as follows:

Less of Pitta and more of Ama

Less of blood and more of ama

Less of Ama and more of Pitta and

Less of Ama and more of Blood

Pachana (carminative recipe) added with astringent drugs, Sunthi, Pippali, Maricha and bitter drugs is given to the patient if the diarrhoea is caused by two factors viz., more of Ama and less of Kapha.

Pachana(carminative recipe) added with Sunthi, Pippali and Maricha, and astringent drugs as well as salt is given to the patient if the diarrhoea is caused by two factors, viz., less of Ama and more of Kapha.

Enema-recipe containing sweet, sour and astringent drugs is useful if the diarrhoea is caused by two factors as follows:

• Less of Vata and more of faecal matter an

• Less of Vata and more of Pitta

• More of Vata and less of faecal matter and

• More of Vata and less of pitta

Enema recipe containing astringent, sweet and bitter drugs is given if the diarrhoea is caused by two factors as follows:

• Less of faecal matter and less of blood

• More of blood and less of faecal matter

• More of Pitta and less of faecal matter

• More of faecal matter and less of Pitta:

• More of blood and less of less of Pitta and

More of pitta and less of blood

Enema –recipe containing Sunthi, Pippali and Maricha and bitter as well as astringent drugs is very useful if the diarrhoea is caused by two factors as follows:

• Less of kapha and more of faecal matter

• Less of kapha and more of Pitta

• More of kapha and less of faecal matter
• More of kapha and less of Pitta and
• More of Kapha and less of blood

Enema- recipe containing Sunthi, Pippali and Maricha, and bitter as well as sour drugs is useful if the diarrhoea is caused by two factors, viz., more of Kapha and less of Vata.

Enema-recipe containing Sunthi, Pippali and Maricha and sweet as well as bitter drugs is useful if the diarrhoea is caused by two factors, viz., more blood and less of kapha.

Enema-recipe containing sweet, sour and bitter drugs is given if the diarrhoea is caused by two factors, viz., less of Vata and more of Pitta. [26-33]

Treatment of diarrhoea caused by More Than Two factors

त्रिचतुःपञ्चसंसर्गानेवमेव विकल्पयेत्|
युक्तिश्चैषातिसारोक्ता सर्वरोगेष्वपि स्मृता||३४||

When the diarrhoea is caused by the combination of three, four or five factors, the corresponding therapeutic measures are combined and administered.

The methodology of selecting treatment entered above with reference to diarrhoea is applicable to all the diseases. [34]

Treatment of diarrhoea caused by all six factors

युगपत् षड्रसं षण्णां संसर्गे पाचनं भवेत् | निरामाणां तु पञ्चानां बस्तिः षाड्रसिको मतः||३५||

When all the six morbid factors are combined to cause diarrhoea then a recipe of Pachana (carminative) consisting of drugs of all the six tastes is given. When five out of the six morbid factors (excluding Ama) are combined to cause diarrhoea, then basti (enema) having ingredients of all the six tastes is given.

Medicated Ghee for diarrhoea

उदुम्बरशलाटूनि जम्ब्वाम्रोदुम्बरत्वचः| शङ्खं सर्जरसं लाक्षां कर्दमं च पलांशिकम्||३६||
पिष्ट्वा तैः सर्पिषः प्रस्थं क्षीरादिगुणितं पचेत्| अतीसारेषु सर्वेषु पेयमेतद्यथाबलम्||३७||

One Pala each of Udumbara-Salatu (unripe fruits cut into slices and dried), barks of Jambu, Amra as well as Sankha (conch-shell), Sarjarasa, Laksha and Kardama are made into a paste. Along with this paste, one Prastha of ghee is cooked by adding double the quantity of milk. In accordance with the strength of the patient, this medicated ghee is given as a potion for all the type of diarrhoea. [36-37]

Medicated gruels for Diarrhoea

कच्छुराधातकीबिल्वसमङ्गारक्तशालिभिः| मसूराश्वत्थशुङ्गैश्च यवागूः स्याज्जले शृतैः||३८||
बालोदुम्बरकट्वङ्गसमङ्गाप्लक्षपल्लवैः | मसूरधातकीपुष्पबलाभिश्च तथा भवेत्||३९||
स्थिरादीनां बलादीनामिक्ष्वादीनामथापि वा| क्वाथेषु समसूराणां यवाग्वः स्युः पृथक् पृथक्||४०||
कच्छुरामूलशल्यादितण्डुलैरुपसाधिताः| दधितक्रारनालाम्लक्षीरेष्विक्षुरसेऽपि वा||४१||
शीताः सशर्कराक्षौद्राः सर्वातिसारनाशनाः| ससर्पिर्मरिचाजाज्यो मधुरा लवणाः शिवाः||४२||

Following recipes of Yavagu (thick gruel) are useful for the patient suffering from diarrhoea:

A decoction is prepared of kacchura (Kapikacchu), Dhataki, Bilva, Samanga, red variety of Sali rice, masura and roots of asvattha by boiling with water. (The procedure prescribed for Sadanga Paniya is to be followed in this connection-vide commentary on Charaka: Chikitsa 3: 145). Yavagu (thick gruel) is prepared with this decoction.

Similarly, Yavagu may be prepared with the decoction of unripe Udumbara (made into slices), Katvanga (aralu), Samanga, leaves of Plaksa, Masura, Dhataki-flower and Bala

Yavagu may be prepared with the decoction of the drugs of Sthiradi-group along with Masura

Yavagu may be prepared with the decoction of drugs of Baladi- group along with Masura

Yavagu may be prepared with the decoction of drugs of Iksvadi group along with Masura and

Yavagu may be prepared with the root of Kacchura (Kapikacchu) and rice of Sali, etc., and added with curd, butter-milk, and sour Kanji, milk and sugarcane juice. Intake of this gruel, when cold and added with sugar and honey, cures all the types of diarrhoea.

The above-mentioned gruels are auspicious (for curing diarrhoea) when added with ghee, Maricha, ajaji, sweet ingredients and salt. [38- 42]

भवन्ति चात्र श्लोकाः-

स्निग्धाम्ललवणमधुरं पानं बस्तिश्च मारुते कोष्णः| शीतं तिक्तकषायं मधुरं पित्ते च रक्ते च||४३||

तिक्तोष्णकषायकटुश्लेष्मणि सङ्ग्राहि वातनुच्छकृति| पाचनमामे पानं पिच्छासृग्बस्तयो रक्ते||४४||

अतिसारं प्रत्युक्तं मिश्रं द्वन्द्वादियोगजेष्वपि च| तत्रोद्रेकविशेषाद्दोषेषूपक्रमः कार्यः||४५||

Thus, it is said:

In diarrhoea caused by Vata, the patient should drink Pachana (carminative recipe), and use lukewarm basti (enema) containing unctuous, sour, saline and sweet ingredients.

In diarrhoea caused by Pitta and Rakta (vitiated Blood), the patient is given Pachana (carminative recipe) containing cooling, bitter, astringent and sweet ingredients.

In diarrhoea caused by vitiated faecal matter, the patient should take recipes (in the form of enema, etc.) which causes constipation and which alleviates or Vata.

In diarrhoea caused by Ama (uncooked product of digestion), the patient should drink Pachana (carminative recipe).

In diarrhoea caused by vitiated blood, the patient is given Piccha-basti (medicated enema containing mucilaginous material) and enema of blood.

In this way, various methods of treating diarrhoea are described.

If the diarrhoea is caused by more than one factor, then the respective therapies are given in a combined form.

Among these combined factors, the principle of treatment is followed to correct the predominant ones first. [43-45]

तत्रश्लोकः-

प्रासृतिकाःसव्यापत्क्रियानिरुहास्तथाऽतिसारहिताः| रसकल्पघृतयवाग्वश्चोक्तागुरुणाप्रसृतसिद्धौ||४६||

To sum up:

In this chapter "One the successful Treatment with Recipes Described with Prasrta as the Unit Quantity of its Ingredients" the Teacher has described the following topics:

Recipes of Niruha- basti ingredients of which are described in the unit quantity of Prasrta (vide verse nos. 4-14)

Complications arising out of mild recipe for enema etc. and their treatment (vide verse no 15-180)

Recipes for Niruha basti, and those containing ingredients of different attests for the treatment of diarrhoea (vide verse nos. 19-35)

Recipe of medicated ghee for the treatment of diarrhoea (vide verse nos. 36-37).

Recipes of medicated gruel for the treatment of diarrhoea (vide verse nos. 38-42) [46]

इत्यग्निवेशकृते तन्त्रे चरकप्रतिसंस्कृतेऽप्राप्ते

दृढबलसम्पूरिते सिद्धिस्थाने प्रासृतयोगीयसिद्धिर्नामाष्टमोऽध्यायः||८||

Thus, ends the eight chapter of Siddhi-section dealing with the "Success in Treatment with Recipes Ingredient of which are Described in the Unit Quantity of Prasrta" in Agnivesha's work as redacted by Charaka, and because of its non-availability, supplemented by Drdhabala.

34

Siddhisthana Chapter 9 Tri Marmiya Siddhi

Prologue

अथातस्त्रिमर्मीयां सिद्धिं व्याख्यास्यामः||१||

इति ह स्माह भगवानात्रेयः||२||

Now, we shall expound the chapter dealing with "perfection in the treatment of diseases affecting three vital organs. Thus said lord Atreya. [1-2]

Dialogue

सप्तोत्तरं मर्मशतमस्मिञ्छरीरे स्कन्धशाखासमाश्रितमग्निवेश!| तेषामन्यतमपीडायां समधिका पीडा भवति, चेतनानिबन्धवैशेष्यात्|

तत्र शाखाश्रितेभ्यो मर्मभ्यः स्कन्धाश्रितानि गरीयांसि, शाखानां तदाश्रितत्वात्; स्कन्धाश्रितेभ्योऽपि हृद्वस्तिशिरांसि, तन्मूलत्वाच्छरीरस्य||३||

Oh! Agnivesha, (addressed by preceptor Atreya), there are one hundred and seven vital spots (marmas) located in the trunk and limbs of the body. Affliction of any one of these produces excruciating pain because of the specific association of consciousness in these parts.

Amongst these vital spots, the ones located in the Sakhas (limbs of the body) are important because these limbs are dependent upon the trunk.

Amongst vital organs in the trunk, the ones located in the heart, urinary bladder and head are the most important because these organs constitute every basic substratum of the body. [3]

Heart, head and urinary bladder

तत्र हृदयेदश धमन्यः प्राणापानौमनो बुद्धिश्चेतना महाभूतानि च नाभ्यामरा इव प्रतिष्ठितानि, शिरसि इन्द्रियाणि इन्द्रियप्राणवहानि च स्रोतांसि सूर्यमिव गभस्तयः संश्रितानि, बस्तिस्तु स्थूलगुदमुष्कसेवनीशुक्रमूत्रवाहिनीनां नाडी(ली)नां मध्ये मूत्रधारोऽम्बुवहानां सर्वस्रोतसामुदधिरिवापगानां प्रतिष्ठ , बहुभिश्च तन्मूलैर्मर्मसञ्ज्ञकैः स्रोतोभिर्गगनमिव दिनकरकरैर्व्याप्तमिदं शरीरम्||४||

As the spokes of a wheel are attached to the centre (Nabhi), similarly the ten vessels, Prana-vayu, Apana-vayu, Manas (mind), Buddhi (wisdom) consciousness and Maha-bhutas are attached to (associated with) the heart.

Head is the abode of senses, sensory channels and channels carrying elan vitae as the sun is the abode of its rays.

Just as all the rivers on the earth flow into the ocean, the urinary bladder, located in the midst of sthula-guda (rectum), muska (testicles), sevani (perennial sutures) and seminal vessels as well as urinary channels, is the receptacle of urine into which all the channels of the body carrying liquid elements converge.

From the base of these three, viz., heart, head and urinary bladder, which are called Marmas (vital organs), the entire body is pervaded with channels (Srotas) just like the entire sky is pervaded with the rays of the sun. [4]

Injury to vital organs

• 447 •

तेषां त्रयाणामन्यतमस्यापि भेदादाश्वेव शरीरभेदः स्यात्, आश्रयनाशादाश्रितस्यापि विनाशः; तदुपघातातु घोरतरव्याधिप्रादुर्भावः; तस्मादेतानि विशेषेण रक्ष्याणि बाह्याभिघाद्वातादिभ्यश्च||५||

Serious injury to any one of these vital organs (heart, head and urinary bladder) causes destruction of the body since the destruction of the substratum leads to the destruction of the superstructure. Partial injury to vital organs leads to affliction by serious diseases. Therefore, these three vital organs are specially protected from external injury and afflictions by vataetc. [5]

Ailments caused by injury to vital organs

तत्र हृद्यभिहते कासश्वासबलक्षयकण्ठशोषक्लोमाकर्षणजिह्वानिर्गममुखतालुशोषापस्मारोन्मादप्रलापचित्तनाशादयः स्युः; शिरस्यभिहते मन्यास्तम्भार्दितचक्षुर्विभ्रममोहोद्वेष्टनचेष्टानाशकासश्वाससहनुग्रहमूकगद्गदत्वाक्षिनिमीलन-गण्डस्पन्दनजृम्भणलालास्रावस्वरहानिवदनजिह्मत्वादीनि,   बस्तौ   तु वातमूत्रवर्चोनिग्रहवङ्क्षणमेहनबस्तिशूलकुण्डलोदावर्तगुल्मानिलास्थीलोपस्तम्भनाभिकुक्षिगुदश्रोणिग्रहादयः ; वाताद्युपसृष्टानां त्वेषां लिङ्गानि चिकित्सिते सक्रियाविधीन्युक्तानि||६||

Injury to the heart gives rise to cough, asthma, loss of strength, dryness of throat, klomakarsana (pain as if there is stretching of the Kloman or lungs), protraction of the tongue, dryness of mouth as well as palate, epilepsy, insanity, delirium, unconsciousness etc.,

Injury to the head gives rise to Manya-stambha (torticollis), Ardita (facial paralysis), Caksu-vibhrama (agitation of eyes), Moha (unconsciousness), Udvestana (cramps), cesta –nasa (loss of motor activities), Cough, Asthma, Hanu-graha (lock-jaw), Mukatva (dumbness), gadgadatva (lulling speech), aksi-nimilana (closure of the eye-lids), Ganda-spandana (twitching of cheeks), Jrmbhana (yawning), Laha-srava (excessive salivation), Svara-hani (aphasia), asana-jihmatva (twisting of the face)., etc

Injury to the urinary bladder gives rise to retention of flatus, urine as well as faeces, pain in the groin, phallus as well as urinary bladder, Kundala (spiraling spansm in the bladder), Udavarta (upward movement of wind in the abdomen), gulma (phantom tumour), Vatasthila (hard tumour caused by vayu), Upastambha (spasticity of the bladder), stiffness of umbilicus, pelvis, anus as well as hips. Etc.

The signs, symptoms and treatment of different varieties of the above-mentioned ailments caused by the affliction of vital organs by vayu, etc., are already described in (the twenty sixth chapter of) chikitsa-section.

Involvement of vatain ailments of vital organs

किन्त्वेतानि विशेषतोऽनिलाद्रक्ष्याणि, अनिलो हि पित्तकफसमुदीरणे हेतुः प्राणमूलं च, स बस्तिकर्मसाध्यतमः, तस्मान्न बस्तिसमं किञ्चित् कर्म मर्मपरिपालनमस्ति| तत्र षडास्थापनस्कन्धान् विमाने द्वौ चानुवासनस्कन्धाविह च विहितान् बस्तीन् बुद्ध्या विचार्य महामर्मपरिपालनार्थं प्रयोजयेद्वातव्याधिचिकित्सां च||७||

These marmas (vital organs, viz, heart, head and urinary bladder) are to be protected from aggravated vatabecause it is this aggravated vatawhich is responsible for the excitation (aggravation) of pitta and kapha, and the elan vitae is dependent upon its vayu. This vatais best treated by basti (medicated enema-therapy). Therefore, there is none other than basti therapy which can safeguard the vital organs.

Therefore, after intelligent consideration, basti-recipes prepared of six groups of drugs for niruha (vide vimana 8: 139-144), two groups of drugs for anuvasana (vide vimana 8:150) and therapeutic measures prescribed for the treatment of vata-vyadhi (diseases caused by aggravated vayu- as described in 28th chapter chikitsa-section) is employed to protect these vital organs. [7]

Recipes for treatment of ailments of vital organs

भूयश्च हृद्युपसृष्टे हिङ्गुचूर्णं लवणानामन्यतमचूर्णसंयुक्तं मातुलुङ्गस्य रसेनान्येन वाम्लेन हृद्येन वा पाययेत्, स्थिरादिपञ्चमूलीरसः सशर्करः   पानार्थं,   बिल्वादिपञ्चमूलरससिद्धा   च   यवागूः,   हृद्रोगविहितं   च   कर्म;   मूर्ध्नि   तु वातोपसृष्टेऽभ्यङ्गस्वेदनोपनाहस्नेहपानन्तःकर्मावपीडनधूमादीनि; बस्तौ तु कुम्भीस्वेदः, वर्तयः, श्यामादिभिर्गोमूत्रसिद्धो निरूहः, बिल्वादिभिश्च   सुरासिद्धः,   शरकाशेक्षुदर्भगोक्षुरकमूलशृतक्षीरैश्च   त्रपुसैर्वारुखराश्वाबीजयवर्षभकवृद्धिकल्कितो   निरूहः, पीतदारुसिद्धतैलेनानुवासनं,   तैल्वकं   च   सर्पिर्विरेकार्थं,

शतावरीगोक्षुरकबृहतीकण्टकारिकागुडूचीपुनर्नवोशीरमधुकदि्वसारिवालोध्रश्रेयसीकुशकाशमूलकषायक्षीरचतुर्गुणं
बलावृषभकखराश्वोपकुञ्चिकावत्सकत्रपुसैर्वारुबीजशितिवारकमधुकवचाशतपुष्पाश्मभेदकवर्षाभूमदनफलकल्कसिद्धं
तैलमुत्तरबस्तिर्निरूहो वा शुद्धस्निग्धस्विन्नस्य बस्तिशूलमूत्रविकारहर इति||८||

If the heart gets afflicted by vayu, then [in addition to basti] the following measures are employed:

The patient should drink the juice of matulunga or any other sour drink which is pleasing to the heart by adding the powder of hingu and any of the salts;

Decoction of ksudra-pancamula (salaparni, prsniparni, brhati, kantakari and goksura) added with sugar may also be used as a drink.

He may take yavagu (thick gruel) prepared with the decoction of bilva, syonaka, gambhari, patala and ganikarika.

He may give other therapeutic measures prescribed for the treatment of heart- diseases (vide chikitsa 2-81-103).

If the head is afflicted by vayu, then [in addition to basti], the following therapeutic measures are employed:

Massage

Fomentation

Application of hot poultices

Unctuous potions

Inhalation therapy

Avapida (administration of medical powders through the nostrils by applying pressure) and

Smoking and such other therapies

If the urinary bladder is afflicted by vayu, then the following therapeutic measures are employed:

Kumbhi-sveda (types of fomentation therapy vide sutra 14:5-58)

Vartis (medicated suppositaries)

Niruha type of enema prepared of cow's urine boiled with shyama, etc., (shyama, trivrt, chaturangula, tilvaka, maha-vrksa, saptala, sankhini, danti and dravanti- vide vimana 8:136)

[Niruha type of enema] prepared of alcohol boiled with bilva etc., (bilva, syonaka, gambhari, patala, ganikarika) or root of bilva, trivrt, devadaru, yava, kola and kulattha (vide siddhi 7:11)

niruha basti containing milk boiled with the root of sara, kasa, iksu, darbha and goksura, and added with the paste of trapusa, ervaruka, seeds of kharasva (aja-moda), yavu, rsabhaka and vrddhi.

Anuvasana-basti with the oil cooked with pittadaru (daruharidra; some physician interprete this term "pitta-daru-siddha-tailena" as extracted from the heart- wood of sarala);

Purgation with tilvaka sarpis (vide kalpa 9:14-15)

Uttara-basti (urethral douche) or niruha with the medicated oil cooked by adding the following:

Decoction of shatavari, goksuraka, brhati, kantakarika, guduchi, punarnava, usira, madhuka, two varieties of sariva (anantamula and shyama) lodhra, sreyasti (rasna) and roots of kusa as well as kasa

The above mentioned decoction and four times of milk and paste of bala, vrsa (vasaka), rasabhaka, kharasva (ajamoda), upakuncika (krsana-jiraka), vatsaka, seeds of trapusa as well as ervaruka, sitivaraka (salinaca), madhuka, vaca, satapuspa, asmabhedaka, (pasanabheda), varsabhu and madana phala and after the patient has been subjected to purgation, oleation and fomentation therapies, niruha basti is given for the cure of pain in the bladder and urinary disorders. [8]

Summary of the topics

भवन्ति चात्र श्लोकाः:-

हृदये मूर्ध्नि बस्तौ च नृणां प्राणाः प्रतिष्ठिताः| तस्मात्तेषां सदा यत्नं कुर्वीत परिपालने||९||

आबाधवर्जनं नित्यं स्वस्थवृत्तानुवर्तनम्| उत्पन्नार्तिविघातश्च मर्मणां परिपालनम्||१०||

Thus, it is said:

Prana of human beings are located in the heart, head and urinary bladder. Therefore, efforts should always be made to protect these vital organs.

The measures to be taken for or the protection of these vital organs (heart, head and urinary bladder) are as follows:

Avoidance of the cause of injury to those organs

Constantly following the rules and regimens for svastha-vrtta (maintenance of positive health and prevention of diseases) and

Prompt treatment of the diseases of these vital organs immediately after their onset. [9]

Description of additional diseases of vital organs

अत उर्ध्वं विकारा ये त्रिमर्मीये चिकित्सिते| न प्रोक्ता मर्मजास्तेषां कांश्चिद्वक्ष्यामि सौषधान्||११||

Hereafter, I (refers to lord Atreya) shall describe some diseases along with their treatment, originating from these vital organs which were left out in the twenty sixth chapter of Chikitsa-section. [11]

Apatantraka and apatanaka (convlusions)

क्रुद्धः स्वैः कोपनैर्वायुः स्थानादूर्ध्वं प्रपद्यते| पीडयन् हृदयं गत्वा शिरः शङ्खौ च पीडयन्||१२||

धनुर्वन्नमयेद्गात्राण्याक्षिपेन्मोहयेत्तथा| (नमयेच्चाक्षिपेच्चाङ्गान्युच्छ्वासं निरुणद्धि च)|

कृच्छ्रेण चाप्युच्छ्वसिति स्तब्धाक्षोऽथ निमीलकः ||१३||

कपोत इव कूजेच्च निःसज्ञः सोऽपतन्त्रकः| दृष्टिं संस्तम्भ्य सज्ञां च हत्वा कण्ठेन कूजति||१४||

हृदि मुक्ते नरः स्वास्थ्यं याति मोहं वृते पुनः| वायुना दारुणं प्राहुरेके तमपतानकम्||१५||

There are specific factors for the aggravation of vayu. Being provoked by these factors, it spreads upwards from its natural habitat (seats) to affect the heart. From there, it moves further upwards to the head, and afflicts the two temples (sankha). As a result of this, it bends the limbs [of the body] like a bow, causes convulsions and fainting [after causing bending and convulsions, it obstructs the expiration] eyes remain either fixed or closed. He breathes like the cooing of a pigeon, and becomes unconscious. This aliment is called apatantraka.

This aggravated vayu, after keeping the eyes fixed and causing unconsciousness, makes the patient moan with a cooing sound coming out of the throat. After the affliction of the heart by this vatais relieved, the patient's normal health is restored. If the affliction of the heart by this aggravated vatatakes place again, then the patient becomes unconscious again. Some physicians call this serious ailment caused by the [exceedingly] aggravated vata (in association of aggravated kapha) as apatanaka. [12-15]

Treatment of apatantraka and apatanaka

श्वसनं कफवाताभ्यां रुद्धं तस्य विमोक्षयेत्| तीक्ष्णैः प्रधमनैः सज्ञां तासु मुक्तासु विन्दति||१६||

मरिचं शिग्रुबीजानि विडङ्गं च फणिज्झकम्| एतानि सूक्ष्मचूर्णानि दद्याच्छीर्षविरेचनम्||१७||

तुम्बुरूण्यभया हिङ्गु पौष्करं लवणत्रयम्| यवक्वाथाम्बुना पेयं हृद्ग्रहे चापतन्त्रके ||१८||

हिङ्ग्वम्लवेतसं शुण्ठीं ससौवर्चलदाडिमम्| पिबेद्वातकफघ्नं च कर्म हृद्रोगनुद्दिधतम्||१९||

शोधना बस्तयस्तीक्ष्णा न हितास्तस्य कृत्स्नशः| सौवर्चलाभयाव्योषैः सिद्धं तस्मै घृतं हितम्||२०||

If the breath of the patient gets obstructed by kapha and vayu, this obstruction is corrected, and he should be made capable of breathing freely by the administration of strong pradhamana therapy (a type of inhalation therapy for which drugs in powder form are blown into the nostrils). After the obstruction to breath (in the channel carrying consciousness) is removed, then the patient gets back consciousness.

For Shiro-virechana (elimination of morbid matter from the head), fine powder of marica, seeds of sigru, vidanga and phanijihaka is used.

If there is hrd-graha (cardiac spasm) in apatantraka, then the patient is given the powder of tumburu, abhaya, hingu, puskaramula and three type of salt along with the decoction of yava (prepared according to the method prescribed for sadanga –paniya – vide commentary on chikitsa 3:145-147)

The patient suffering from cardiac spasm and apatantraka should take the decoction of hingu, amlavetasa, sunthi, sauvarcala and dadima.

Therapies which alleviate vataand kapha, and which are curative of heart diseases are useful in the treatment of apatantraka (including apatanaka).

Cleansing enema (niruha basti) of strong nature should not be given in full quantity (but can be given in small dose because in large doses they may provoke aggravated vayu).

For such patients (of apatantraka and apatanaka), medicated ghee prepared by cooking with sauvarcala, abhaya, sunthi, pippali and marica is useful. [16-20]

Etiology, pathogenesis, signs and treatment of tandra

मधुरस्निग्धगुर्वन्नसेवनाच्चिन्तनाच्छ्रमात् शोकाद्व्याध्यनुषङ्गाच्च वायुनोदीरितः कफः||२१||

यदासौ समवस्कन्द्य हृदयं हृदयाश्रयान्| समावृणोति ज्ञानादींस्तदा तन्द्रोपजायते||२२||

हृदये व्याकुलीभावो वाक्चेष्टेन्द्रियगौरवम्| मनोबुद्ध्यप्रसादश्च तन्द्राया लक्षणं मतम्||२३||

कफघ्नं तत्र कर्तव्यं शोधनं शमनानि च| व्यायामो रक्तमोक्षश्च भोज्यं च कटुतिक्तकम्||२४||

When the vataprovoked by the intake of sweet, unctuous and heavy food, fatigue and grief and by constant suffering from chronic diseases, incites / aggravates kapha, then this kapha getting lodged in the heart occludes the jnana (knowledge) etc, located therein giving rise to tandra (drowsiness).

The symptoms of tandra – When with kapha, the vitiated vataenters the hrdaya, the hrdaya gets disturbed, there would appear heaviness in the speech, body activities and sense organs, the pleasantness of the mind and intellect (consciousness) would disappear

This ailment is treated with the following:

Therapies for the alleviation and elimination of kapha

Physical exercise

Bloodletting and

Food ingredients which are pungent and bitter in taste [21-24]

Enumeration of urinary diseases

मूत्रौकसादो जठरं कृच्छ्रमुत्सङ्गसङ्क्षयौ| मूत्रातीतोऽनिलाष्ठीला वातबस्त्युष्णमारुतौ||२५||

वातकुण्डलिका ग्रन्थिर्विड्घातो बस्तिकुण्डलम्| त्रयोदशैते मूत्रस्य दोषास्ताँल्लिङ्गतः शृणु||२६||

The following are the thirteen urinary diseases:

• Mutraukasada (passage of dense urine)

• Mutra-jathara (abdominal swelling because of urinary retention);

• Mutra-krcchra (dysuria)

• Mutra-utsanga (retention of residual urine in the bladder)

• Mutra-sanksaya (anuria)

• Mutratita (delayed micturation)

• Vatasthila (stone like growth in the bladder because of aggravated vayu)

• Vata-basti (affliction of bladder by vayu)

• Usna-maruta (burning micturition)

• Vata-kudalika (spiral movement of vatain the bladder)

• Granthi (tumour)

• Vid-vighata (fecal fistula) and

• Basti-kundala (spiral distension of bladder)

The signs of the mentioned urinary disorders will be described hereafter which you (addressed by lord atreya to agnives) may listen to. [25-26]

Pathology, signs and treatment of mutraukasada

पित्तं कफो द्वावपि वा बस्तौ संहन्यते यदा| मारुतेन तदा मूत्रं रक्तं पीतं घनं सृजेत्||२७||

सदाहं श्वेतसान्द्रं वा सर्वैर्वा लक्षणैर्युतम्| मूत्रौकसादं तं विद्यात् पित्तश्लेष्महरैर्जयेत्||२८||

When, either vayu, pitta or kapha, or both pitta and kapha in the bladder get considered, then the patient voids urine which is either red or yellow, thick and associated with burning sensation. The urine may also be white and dense and may be associated with all the signs (relating to all the three Doshas).

This ailment is called mutraukasada, and it treated with therapies for the alleviation of pitta and kapha. [27-28]

Etiology, signs and treatment of mutra –jathara

विधारणात् प्रतिहतं वातोदावर्तितं यदा| पूरयत्युदरं मूत्रं तदा तदनिमित्तरुक्||२९||

अपक्तिमूत्रविट्सङ्गैस्तन्मूत्रजठरं वदेत्| मूत्रवैरेचनीं तत्र चिकित्सां सम्प्रयोजयेत्||३०||

हिङ्गुद्विरुत्तरं चूर्णं त्रिमर्मीये प्रकीर्तितम्| हन्यान्मूत्रोदरानाहमाध्मानं गुदमेढ्रयोः||३१||

When because of the suppression of the manifested urge for urination, the retarded flow of urine moves upwards, and fills up the abdominal cavity, then the patient suffers from the following:

Pain without any appreciable reason

Indigestion and

Retention of urine and stool

This condition is called mutra-jathara (abdominal swelling by urine).

The patient is treated with diureties, Hingu dviruttara- churna (or dviruttara-hingvadi churna) described in chikitsa 26-20 cures mutrodara (or mutra-jathara) constipation and distension of rectum as well as phallus. [29-31]

Etiology of mutra-krcchra

मूत्रितस्य व्यवायातु रेतो वातोद्धतं च्युतम्| पूर्वं मूत्रस्य पश्चाद्वा स्रवेत् कृच्छ्रं तदुच्यते||३२||

If a person having the manifested urge for urination enters into sexual act, the semen excited by vatagets discharged from its location. It is ejaculated before or after the passage of urine which is painful, and it is called mutrakrcchra. [32]

Etiology and signs of mutra-utsanga

खवैगुण्यानिलाक्षेपैः किञ्चिन्मूत्रं च तिष्ठति| मणिसन्धौ स्रवेत् पश्चात्तदरुग्वाऽथ चातिरुक्||३३||

मूत्रोत्सङ्गः स विच्छिन्नमुच्छेषगुरुशेफसः |

If the urinary tract (urethra) is vitiated, then because of the spasm caused by vayu, a part of the urine remains accumulated in the sphincter of glans penis. Subsequently the residual urine [flows out with interruptions] with either severe pain or without pain flows from the heavy phallus. This condition is called mutrotsanga (dribbling of the residual urine). [33 – ½ 34]

Etiology and signs of mutra sanksaya

वाताकृतिर्भवेद्वातान्मूत्रे शुष्यति सङ्क्षयः||३४||

If the urinary secretion gets dried up (becomes less in quantity) because of aggravated vayu, then signs and symptoms of vataare manifested, and this condition is called mutra-sanksaya (diminution of urine-flow) [34 ½]

Etiology and signs of mutratita

चिरं धारयतो मूत्रं त्वरया न प्रवर्तते| मेहमानस्य मन्दं वा मूत्रातीतः स उच्यते||३५||

The person with the habit of holding up urination for a long time becomes incapable of passing urine immediately after the urge, and the flow of urine becomes slow, this condition is called mutratita (delayed urination). [35]

Etiology and signs of vatasthila

आध्मापयन् बस्तिगुदं रुद्ध्वा वायुश्चलोन्नताम्| कुर्यातीव्रार्तिमष्ठीलां मूत्रविण्मार्गरोधिनीम्||३६||

vatacausing obstruction in the bladder and rectum, and distension of these organs, produces hard tumour (asthila) which is mobile and elevated, which is exceedingly painful and which obstructs the urinary and fecal passages. This ailment is called vatasthila]

Etiology and signs of vata- basti

मूत्रं धारयतो बस्तौ वायुः क्रुद्धो विधारणात्| मूत्ररोधार्तिकण्डूभिर्वातबस्तिः स उच्यते||३७||

In the person who habitually suppresses the manifested urge for urination, vatagets aggravated because of obstruction thereby giving rise to retention of urine, pain and itching. This ailment is called vata- basti (affliction of bladder by vayu). [37]

Etiology and signs of usna-vata

उष्मणा सोष्मकं मूत्रं शोषयन् रक्तपीतकम्| उष्णवातः सृजेत् कृच्छ्राद्बस्त्युपस्थार्तिदाहवान्||३८||

Vayu, in association with pitta, dries up the urine. It is associated with pitta, and thereafter, becomes red and yellow in colour, burning sensation in the bladder and phallus. This is called usna-vata (affliction of the bladder and phallus). This is called usna-vata (affliction of urine by vatain association with pitta) [38]

Etiology and signs of vata- kundalika

गतिसङ्गादुदावृत्तः स मूत्रस्थानमार्गयोः| मूत्रस्य विगुणो वायुर्भग्नव्याविद्धकुण्डली||३९||
मूत्रं विहन्ति संस्तम्भभङ्गगौरववेष्टनैः| तीव्ररुङ्मूत्रविट्सङ्गैर्वातकुण्डलिकेति सा||४०||

Because of the obstruction in the urinary passage, the vitiated vatamoves upwards, and afflicts the bladder as well as urinary channel as a result of which urination takes place in broken, curved and spiral manner. This ailment is called vata-kundalika (spiralmovement of vatain bladder). It is characterised by morbidities of urinary tract like stiffness, breaking pain, heaviness, twisting, excruciating pain and retention of urine as well as faeces. [39-40]

Etiology and signs of rakta-granthi – tumor, fibroid

रक्तं वातकफाद्दुष्टं बस्तिद्वारे सुदारुणम्|
ग्रन्थिं कुर्यात् स कृच्छ्रेण सृजेन्मूत्रं तदावृतम्||४१|| अश्मरीसमशूलं तं रक्तग्रन्थिं प्रचक्षते|

Blood vitiated by vataand kapha produces serious type of tumour in the neck of the bladder. Because of this occlusion, the patient voids urine with difficulty and experiences pain like that which is felt because of calculi in the urinary passage. This is called rakta-granthi – tumour, fibroid (blood tumour in bladder) [41- ½ 42]

Etiology and signs of vid-vighata

रूक्षदुर्बलयोर्वातेनोदावृत्तं शकृद्यदा||४२||
मूत्रस्रोतः प्रपद्येत विट्संसृष्टं तदा नरः| विड्गन्धं मूत्रयेत् कृच्छ्रादिवड्विघातं विनिर्दिशेत्||४३||

When the faeces gets occluded by vatato enter the urinary passage in an un-unctuous and weak person, then he voids foul smelling urine mixed with faecal matter with difficulty. This condition is called vid-vigraha (recto-vesical fistula). [42 ½-43]

Etiology and signs of basti-kundala

द्रुताध्वलङ्घनायासादभिघातात् प्रपीडनात्| स्वस्थानादवस्तिरुद्वृत्तः स्थूलस्तिष्ठति गर्भवत्||४४||
शूलस्पन्दनदाहार्तो बिन्दुं बिन्दुं स्रवत्यपि| पीडितस्तु सृजेद्धारां संस्तम्भोद्वेष्टनार्तिमान्||४५||
बस्तिकुण्डलमाहुस्तं घोरं शस्त्रविषोपमम्| पवनप्रबलं प्रायो दुर्निवारमबुद्धिभिः||४६||
तस्मिन् पित्तान्विते दाहः शूलं मूत्रविवर्णता| श्लेष्मणा गौरवं शोफः स्निग्धं मूत्रं घनं सितम्||४७||
श्लेष्मरुद्धबिलो बस्तिः पित्तोदीर्णो न सिध्यति| अविभ्रान्तबिलः साध्यो न तु यः कुण्डलीकृतः||४८||
स्यादवस्तौ कुण्डलीभूते ह्यन्मोहः श्वास एव च|४९|

Because of fast-wayfaring, fasting, exhaustion, trauma, and compression, the urinary bladder gets displaced upwards, and becomes enlarged to appear like a gravid uterus.

Being afflicted with colic pain, throbbing pain and burning sensation, the patient passes urine in drops. When pressed in the bladder region, the urine comes out in a jet. The patient suffers from stiffness, cramps and pain. This ailment is called basti-kundala (spiral distension of bladder). This is a serious condition like injury by weapons or poison. This is generally dominated by aggravated vayu, and cannot be handled by less intelligent physicians.

Associated with vitiated pitta, this ailment gives rise to burning sensation, colic pain and discoloration of urine. Associated with kapha, this ailment gives rise to heaviness, oedema and unctuousness, density as well as white coloration of the urine.

If the urinary passage is clogged by kapha, and if pitta is aggravated, then the ailment is incurable. If the passage is not blocked or twisted, then the ailment is curable. Twisting of the bladder is characterised by cardiac distress and asthma. [44- ½ 49]

Line of treatment of urinary morbidities

दोषाधिक्यमवेक्ष्यैतान् मूत्रकृच्छ्रहरैर्जयेत्||४९||

बस्तिमुतरबस्तिं च सर्वेषामेव दापयेत्|५०|

After ascertaining the predominance of various Doshas in the above-mentioned urinary disorders, the patient is treated with therapies prescribed for curing mutra-krcchra (vide chikitsa 26:45-58). Basti (medicated enema) and uttata basti (urethral douche) are administered in all the above mentioned ailments. [49 ½- ½ 50]

Netra (nozzle or catheter)

पुष्पनेत्रं तु हैमं स्याच्छलक्ष्णमौतरबस्तिकम्||५०||

जात्यश्वहनवृन्तेन समं गोपुच्छसंस्थितम्| रौप्यं वा सर्षपच्छिद्रं द्विकर्णं द्वादशाङ्गुलम्||५१||

The netra (nozzle of catheter) for uttara-basti (urethral douche) is prepared of gold or silver, and it is smooth. Its tip is of the size of the flower-stalk of jati or asvahana (karavira), and in shape it is tapering like the cow's tail. It must have a hole in the middle which should allow a mustard seed to pass through. It should have two rings, and its length must be twelve angulas (one angula or finger-breadth= ¾ th of an inch approximately) [50 ½ -51]

Dose of recipe for douche

तेनाजबस्तियुक्तेन स्नेहस्यार्धपलं नयेत्| यथावयोविशेषेण स्नेहमात्रां विकल्प्य वा||५२||

The nozzle or catheter is tied to a goat's bladder containing half pala of the unctuous recipe which is to be administered. The exact dose in which this unctuous recipe is to be administered is determined on the basis of the age of the patient. [52]

Methods of administering urethral douche

स्नातस्य भुक्तभक्तस्य रसेन पयसाऽपि वा| सृष्टविण्मूत्रवेगस्य पीठे जानुसमे मृदौ||५३||

ऋजोः सुखोपविष्टस्य हृष्टे मेढ्रे घृताक्तया| शलाकयाऽन्विष्य गतिं यद्यप्रतिहता व्रजेत्||५४||

ततः शेफःप्रमाणेन पुष्पनेत्रं प्रवेशयेत्| गुदवन्मूत्रमार्गेण प्रणयेदनु सेवनीम्||५५||

हिंस्यादतिगतं बस्तिमूने स्नेहो न गच्छति| सुखं प्रपीड्य निष्कम्पं निष्कर्षेन्नेत्रमेव च||५६||

प्रत्यागते द्वितीयं च तृतीयं च प्रदापयेत्|

The patient who has taken bath, who has taken food along with meat soup or milk and who has voided stool as well as urine is made to sit over a knee-high soft seat in a straight and comfortable position with his erected phallus. The passage of the urethra is determined with the help of a ghee smeared probe. If the probe passes through the urethra without any difficulty, then the nozzle of the cateter is inserted up to the length of the phallus following the direction of perineal suture in the manner prescribed for the insertion of the enema –nozzle in the anus (for basti or medicated enema).

If the catheter is inserted beyond the prescribed limit, it will cause injury to the bladder. If it is inserted less than that limit, the unctuous recipe will not enter the bladder.

Gentle pressure is applied over the douche, receptable without shaking it. Therafter, the catheter is withdrawn. After the injected fluid has come out, the process is repeated for the second and third time. [53- ½ 57]

Retention of douche-fluid

अनागच्छन्नुपेक्ष्यस्तु रजनीव्युषितस्य च||५७||
पिप्पलीलवणागारधूमापामार्गसर्षपैः| वार्ताकुरसनिर्गुण्डीशम्पाकैः ससहाचरैः||५८||
मूत्राम्लपिष्टैः सगुडैर्वर्तिं कृत्वा प्रवेशयेत्| अग्रे तु सर्षपाकारां पश्चार्धं माषसम्मिताम्||५९||
नेत्रदीर्घां घृताभ्यक्तां सुकुमारामभङ्गुराम्| नेत्रवन्मूत्रनाड्यां तु पायौ चाङ्गुष्ठसम्मिताम्||६०||
स्नेहे प्रत्यागते ताभ्यामानुवासनिको विधिः| परिहारश्च सव्यापत् ससम्यग्दत्तलक्षणः||६१||

If the fluid does not come out then the physician should wait for one night. Thereafter, a varti (medicated suppository) is inserted into the urethra. For this varti, pippali - long pepper fruit - Piper longum, salt, house-soot, apamarga – Achyranthes aspera, sarsapa, juice of vartaku, nirgundi, sampaka – amaltas – Cassia fistula and sahacara is triturated with cow's urine and sour juice. By cooking with jaggery syrup, varti is prepared (cooking with jaggery syrup is done in such a way that the suppository becomes hard and smooth). The tip of the varti is the size of sarshapa (mustard) in the front and that of a Masha (black gram) at the back. The length of this varti is similar to the length of the netra (nozzle or catheter). Smeared with ghee, this tender and unbreakable suppository is inserted into the urethra. Simultaneously, the suppository of the size of the thumb is inserted into the anus of the patient.

After the return of sneha (unctuous recipe used for douche) by these two vartis or suppositories (one inserted in the urethra and the other in the anus), the patient is given regimens which are prescribed to be given after the administration of the anuvasana or unctuous type of medicated enema.

Prohibitions (parihara), complications (vyapat) and signs of appropriate administration (samyak_ yoga_laksana) of uttara-basti are the same as those described in respect of anuvasana-basti. [58-61]

Urethral douche for women

स्त्रीणामार्तवकाले तु प्रतिकर्म तदाचरेत्| गर्भासना सुखं स्नेहं तदाऽऽदत्ते ह्यपावृता||६२||
गर्भं योनिस्तदा शीघ्रं जिते गृह्णाति मारुते| बस्तिजेषु विकारेषु योनिविभ्रंशजेषु च||६३||
योनिशूलेषु तीव्रेषु योनिव्यापत्स्वसृग्दरे| अप्रसवति मूत्रे च बिन्दुं बिन्दुं स्रवत्यपि||६४||
विदध्यादुत्तरं बस्तिं यथास्वौषधसंस्कृतम् |६५|

In the case of a woman, this uttara-basti (urethral douche) is administered during her menstrual period because [the cervix of] the uterus remains open during this time, and readily receives the unctuous fluid given in the form of douche. This therapy subdues the (local) vataas a result of which the uterus becomes capable of conception.

The douche prepared with appropriate drugs is administered to the women for the following ailments:

Diseases of the urinary bladder

Prolapsed of uterus

Excruciating pain in the uterus

Gynecic disorders

Menorrhagia

Anuria and

Dribbling of urine [62-1/2 65]

Nozzles of Utrara-Basti for Females

पुष्पनेत्रप्रमाणं तु प्रमदानां दशाङ्गुलम्||६५|| मूत्रस्रोतःपरीणाहं मुद्गस्रोतोऽनुवाहि च|
अपत्यमार्गे नारीणां विधेयं चतुरङ्गुलम्||६६|| द्व्यङ्गुलं मूत्रमार्गे तु बालायास्त्वेकमङ्गुलम्|

The Puspa-Netra (nozzle or catheter) for women should be ten Angulas in length. In circumference, it is of the size of their urethral canal. The hole in the middle of the nozzle or catheter is spacious enough to allow the passage of the seed of Mudga (green gram).

For giving douche in the gential organ of an adult woman, the nozzle is inserted up to four Angulas (finger breadth), and for douche in their urethral passage, it is inserted up to two Angulas. In the case of young girls, the catheter is inserted up to one Angula in their urethral passage. [65½ -1/2 67]

Method of administering Uttara-Basti to Females

उतानायाः शयानायाः सम्यक् सङ्कोच्य सक्थिनी||६७|| अथास्याः प्रणयेन्नेत्रमनुवंशगतं सुखम्|
द्विस्त्रिश्चतुरिति स्नेहानहोरात्रेण योजयेत्||६८|| बस्तौ , बस्तौ प्रणीते च वर्तिः पीनतरा भवेत्|त्रिरात्रं कर्म कुर्वीत स्नेहमात्रां विवर्धयेत्||६९||
अनेनैव विधानेन कर्म कुर्यात् पुनस्त्र्यहात्||७०|

Uttara-Basti is given to a female when she is lying in the bed on her back with thighs lifted up and flexed.the catheter (nozzle) is inserted comfortably in the direction of her spinal (vertrbral) column. Two, three or four unctuous recipes should thus be administered into the bladder during the course of a day and night.

For women, the (varti) suppository to be inserted into the urethra [in the case of retention of unctuous fluid] is thicker.

In the aforesaid manner, douching is done for three nights by gradually increasing the dose of unctuous recipe. After a gap of three days, this douching therapy is repeated following the above mentioned procedure. [67 ½- ½ 70]

Diseases of Head

अतः शिरोविकाराणां कश्चिद्भेदः प्रवक्ष्यते||७०||

Hereafter we shall describe some diseases of the head (Shiro-Roga). [70 ½]

Sankhaka

रक्तपित्तानिला दुष्टाः शङ्खदेशे विमूर्च्छिताः| तीव्ररुग्दाहरागं हि शोफं कुर्वन्ति दारुणम्||७१||
स शिरो विषवद्वेगी निरुध्याशु गलं तथा| त्रिरात्राज्जीवितं हन्ति शङ्खको नाम नामतः||७२||
परं त्र्यहाज्जीवति चेत् प्रत्याख्यायाचरेत् क्रियाम्| शिरोविरेकसेकादि सर्वं वीसर्पनुच्च यत्||७३||

The vitiated blood, Pitta and Kapha, interact in the region of temples to cause a serious type of oedema associated with excruciating pain, burning sensation and inflammation. This disease called Sankhaka with the velocity of poison, causes immediate obstruction in the head as well as throat leading to the death of the patient within three nights.

If the patient survives after three critical days, the physician, while appropriately informing about the difficulty in curing the patient, should administer all therapies like Shirovirechana and effusion including those prescribed for the treatment of Visarpa (erysipelas).[70 ½- 73]

Etiology, Signs and Treatment of Ardhavadhedaka (Hemicrania)

रूक्षात्यध्यशनात् पूर्ववातावश्यायमैथुनैः| वेगसन्धारणायासव्यायामैः कुपितोऽनिलः||७४||
केवलः सकफो वाऽर्धं गृहीत्वा शिरसस्ततः| मन्याभ्रूशङ्खकर्णाक्षिललाटार्धेऽतिवेदनाम्||७५||
शस्त्रारणिनिभां कुर्यातीव्रां सोऽर्धावभेदकः| नयनं वाऽथवा श्रोत्रमतिवृद्धो विनाशयेत्||७६||
चतुःस्नेहोत्तमा मात्रा शिरःकायविरेचनम्| नाडीस्वेदो घृतं जीर्णे बस्तिकर्मानुवासनम्||७७||
उपनाहः शिरोबस्तिर्दहनं चात्र शस्यते| प्रतिश्याये शिरोरोगे यच्चोदिद्दिष्टं चिकित्सितम्||७८||

The vatagets aggravated by the intake of un-unctuous ingredients, food in excess quantity, intake of food before the previous meal is digested, exposure to the east wind as well as fog, excessive sexual indulgence, suppression of the manifestating natural urges, fatigue and physical work. This Vata, alone or in association with Kapha causes seizure of half of the head thereby causing excruciating pain in the sterno-mastoid region, eye-brows, temples, ears, and forehead of that half side. The patient experiences excruciating pain as if caused by the injury of a weapon or Arani (churning rod used for producing sacrificial fire), i.e by the fire itself. This ailment is called Ardhavadhedaka (hemicrania). If exceedingly aggravated, this ailment may even destroy the eyes and ears of the patient.

For the treatment of this ailment the therapies to be used are as follows:

• Catuh –sneha (four types of of fat, viz, oil, ghee, muscle-fat and bone-marrow) to be taken in heavy dose;

• Shiro-virechana (inhalation therapy for the elimination of morbid matter from the head)

• Kaya-Virechana (enemies and purgation therapy for the elimination of morbid from the body)

- Nadi-sveda (a type of fomentation therapy- vide Sutra 14:43)
- Jirna-Ghrta (ten years old ghee)
- Niruha and Anuvasana types of medicated enema
- Upanaha (Application of hot poultice)
- Shiro- basti (Keeping medicated oil over head with the help of a cap with open ends)
- Dahana (cauterization) and
- Therapies prescribed for Pratisyaya and Shiro-Roga (head- diseases) [74-78]

Etiology, signs and Treatment of Suryavarta

सन्धारणादजीर्णाद्यैर्मस्तिष्कं रक्तमारुतौ| दुष्टौ दूषयतस्तच्च दुष्टं ताभ्यां विमूर्च्छितम्||७९||

सूर्योदयेंऽशुसन्तापाद्द्रवं विष्यन्दते शनैः| ततो दिने शिरःशूलं दिनवृद्ध्या विवर्धते||८०||

दिनक्षये ततः स्त्याने मस्तिष्के सम्प्रशाम्यति| सूर्यावर्तः स तत्र स्यात् सर्पिरौतरभक्तिकम्||८१||

शिरःकायविरेकौ च मूर्ध्नी त्रिस्नेहधारणम् | जाङ्गलैरुपनाहश्च घृतक्षीरैश्च सेचनम् [३] ||८२||

बर्हितित्तिरिलावादिशृतक्षीरोत्थितं घृतम्| स्यान्नावनं जीवनीयक्षीराष्टगुणसाधितम्||८३||

Because of vega-sandharana (suppression of the manifestation of natural urges), Ajirna (indigestion) etc., Rakta (blood) and Maruta (Vayu) being vitiated, afflict the mastiska (brain). The brain / cerebrum thus get afflicted by these two vitiated factors. Because of the effect of sun-rays after the sun-rise, the morbid matter in the cerebrum which is in liquid form gets exudates slowly. Therefore, during day time, as the day advances, the headache becomes more and more intense. When the sun goes down, the liquefied morbid material becomes thicker and thicker on density in the brain as a result of which the headache gets alleviated. This ailment is called Suryavarta.

For the cure of this ailment, therapeutic measures to be given are as follows:

- The patient is given a potion of ghee after meals.
- Shiro-virechana (inhalation therapy for the elimination of morbid matter from the head)
- Kaya-virechana (emesis and purgation for the elimination of morbid matter from the body)
- Shiro-basti is given with three types of fat (oil, ghee and muscle-fat)
- Upanaha (hot poultice) prepared of the meat of animals inhabiting arid zone forests;
- Sprinkling of the head with ghee and milk and
- Milk should be made with the meat of peacock, partridge, quails, etc., and ghee is taken out of this milk. This ghee is added with eight times of milk, and the paste of drugs belonging to Jivaniya-Group (vide sutra 4: 9: 1) with this medicated ghee, (inhalation therapy) is given to the patient. [79-83]

Etiology, signs and symptoms of Ananta-Vata

(उपवासातिशोकातिरूक्षशीताल्पभोजनैः)|

दुष्टा दोषास्त्रयो मन्यापश्चाद्घाटासु [२] वेदनाम्||८४|| तीव्रां कुर्वन्ति सा चाक्षिभ्रूशङ्खेष्ववतिष्ठते|

स्पन्दनं गण्डपार्श्वस्य नेत्ररोगं हनुग्रहम्||८५|| सोऽनन्तवातस्तं हन्यात् सिराकार्वतनाशनैः|

Because of fasting, excessive grief, intake of food which is exceedingly un-unctuous and cold, and intake of extremely small quantity of food, all the three Doshas (vayu, pitta and Kapha) get vitiated to cause acute pain in the sterno-mastoid (region of jugular veins), in the back and at the back of the neck (ghata). This pain (thereafter) gets localised in the eyes, eye-brows and temples. The patient gets throbbing pain in the sides of cheeks, eye-diseases and lockjaw. This ailment is called Ananta-vata. It can be cured by venesection and by therapies prescribed for the treatment of Suryavarta (vide verse nos. 79-83). [84-1/2 86]

Etiology, signs and treatment of Sirah-kampa

वातो रूक्षादिभिः क्रुद्धः शिरःकम्पमुदीरयेत्||८६|| तत्रामृताबलारास्नामहाश्वेताश्वगन्धकैः|

स्नेहस्वेदादि वातघ्नं शस्तं नस्यं च तर्पणम्||८७||

Being aggravated by the use of ununctuous and such other ingredients, vatacauses trembling of the head (Sirah Kampa). For the treatment of this ailment, oleation, fomentation, Nasya (inhalation) and Tarpana (demulcent nasal medication) therapies prepared with Vayu- alleviating drugs like Amrta, Bala, Rasna, Maha-Sveta and Asvagandha are useful.[86 ½ - 87]

Importance of inhalation therapy

नस्तःकर्म च कुर्वीत शिरोरोगेषु शास्त्रविद्| द्वारं हि शिरसो नासा तेन तद् व्याप्य हन्ति तान्||८८||

For the treatment of the diseases of the head, the expert physician should administer Nasta-Karma (inhalation therapy) because the nose is the gateway of the head. The inhalation therapy given through the nasal passage spreads into the different parts of the head, and cures diseases located there. [88]

Varieties of Inhalation Therapy

नावनं चावपीडश्च ध्मापनं धूम एव च| प्रतिमर्शश्च विज्ञेयं नस्तःकर्म तु पञ्चधा||८९||

स्नेहनं शोधनं चैव द्विविधं नावनं स्मृतम्| शोधनः स्तम्भनश्च स्यादवपीडो द्विधा मतः ||९०||

चूर्णस्याध्मापनं तद्दि देहस्रोतोविशोधनम्| विज्ञेयस्त्रिविधो धूमः प्रागुक्तः शमनादिकः||९१||

प्रतिमर्शो भवेत् स्नेहो निर्दोष उभयार्थकृत्| एवं तद्रेचनं कर्म तर्पणं शमनं त्रिधा||९२||

Inhalation therapy is of five types as follows:

1. Navana (inhalation of drug in the form of nasal drops) - This is of two types, viz., snehana (drops for oleation) and Sodhana (drops for elimination of morbid material from the head);

2. Avapida (insufflations of drugs in thin paste from through the nasal passage) - This is of two types, viz. Sodhana (insufflations of drugs for the elimination of morbid matter) and Stambhana (insufflations of drugs for the stoppage of excessive secretion);

3. Dhmapana (insufflations of drugs in powder form through the Nasal passage) - It cleanses the channels of the body;

4. Dhuma (inahalation of drugs in the form of smoke) - it is of three types, viz., Samana or Prayogika (smoke used for the alleviation of Doshas) Snaihika (smoke used for oleation of different parts of the head), and Virechana (smoke used for the alimentation of morbid material from the head) and

5. Prati-Marsa (application of medicated oil in the nostrils). It is harmless and it serves both the purposes (i.e oleation and elimination of morbid matter from the head).

The inhalation therapy (as a whole) can be reclassified into three categories as follows:

Rechana (which causes elimination of morbid matter from the head)

Tarpana (which provides nourishment to the organs located in the head) - It includes Snehana action also and

Samana (which alleviates the aggravated Doshas in the head) - It includes Stambhana action also. [89-92]

Inhalation therapy for different ailments

स्तम्भसुप्तिगुरुत्वाद्याः श्लैष्मिका ये शिरोगदाः| शिरोविरेचनं तेषु नस्तःकर्म प्रशस्यते||९३||

ये च वातात्मका रोगाः शिरःकम्पार्दितादयः| शिरसस्तर्पणं तेषु नस्तःकर्म प्रशस्यते ||९४||

रक्तपित्तादिरोगेषु शमनं नस्यमिष्यते| ध्मापनं धूमपानं च तथा योग्येषु शस्यते ||९५||

(दोषादिकं समीक्ष्यैव भिषक् सम्यक् च कारयेत्)|९६|

In the case of head-diseases associated with stiffness, numbness, heaviness etc., caused by the aggravated kapha inhalation therapy of sira-Virechana type of (which causes elimination of morbid matter from the head) is useful.

In sirah-Kampa (trembling of head), Ardita (facial paralysis) etc., caused by aggravated vayu, inhalation therapy which causes tarpana (nourishment by oleation) of the head is useful.

In diseases like Rakta-Pitta (an ailment characterised by bleeding from different parts of the body) and such other diseases, Samana (which causes alleviation of Doshas) type of inhalation therapy is useful.

Inhalation therapy through Adhmapana (Insufflation) and Dhumapana (inhalation of smoke) is used in appropriate conditions.

After appropriate examination of Doshas, etc., involved in the causation of the diseases, the physician should administer suitable inhalation therapy. [93- ½ 96]

Drugs for Virechana and Tarpana Nasya

फलादिभेषजं प्रोक्तं शिरसो यदि्विरेचनम्||९६|| तच्चूर्णं कल्पयेतेन पचेत् स्नेहं विरेचनम्|

यदुक्तं मधुरस्कन्धे भेषजं तेन तर्पणम्||९७||

In Vimana 8:15 (seven categories of) drugs whose fruits, (Leaves, roots, rhizomes, flowers, excludes and barks) are useful for Shiro-virechana are described. These drugs can be used for pradhmana and Avapida types of inhalation therapy in powder form. Oil may be cooked by adding the powder of these drugs. This medicated oil may be used for inhalation therapy of Virechana type (which eliminates the morbid matter from the head).

Oil may be cooked by adding drugs belonging to Madhura skandha (sweetGroup) described in Vimana 8:139). This medicated oil may also be used for Tarpana type of inhalation therapy. [96-97]

Methods of administering Avapida Nasya

साधयित्वा भिषक् स्नेहं नस्तः कुर्यादि्विधानवित्|९८|

प्राक्सूर्ये मध्यसूर्ये वा प्राक्कृतावश्यकस्य च||९८|| उतानस्य शयानस्य शयने स्वास्तृते सुखम्|

प्रलम्बशिरसः किञ्चित् किञ्चित् पादोन्नतस्य च||९९|| दद्यान्नासापुटे स्नेहं तर्पणं बुद्धिमान् भिषक्|

अनवाक्शिरसो नस्यं न शिरः प्रतिपद्यते||१००|| अत्यवाक्शिरसो नस्यं मस्तुलुङ्गेऽवतिष्ठति|

अत एवंशयानस्य शुद्ध्यर्थं स्वेदयेच्छिरः||१०१|| संस्वेद्य नासामुन्नम्य वामेनाङ्गुष्ठपर्वणा|

हस्तेन दक्षिणेनाथ कुर्यादुभयतः समम्||१०२|| प्रणाड्या पिचुना वाऽपि नस्तःस्नेहं यथाविधि|

कृते च स्वेदयेद्भूय आकर्षेच्च पुनः पुनः||१०३|| तं स्नेहं श्लेष्मणा साकं तथा स्नेहो न तिष्ठति|

स्वेदेनोत्क्लेशितः श्लेष्मा नस्तःकर्मण्युपस्थितः ||१०४|| भूयः स्नेहस्य शैत्येन शिरसि स्त्यायते ततः|

श्रोत्रमन्यागलाद्येषु विकाराय स कल्पते||१०५|| ततो नस्तःकृते धूमं पिबेत् कफविनाशनम् |

हितान्नभुङि्नवातोष्णसेवी स्यान्नियतेन्द्रियः||१०६|| विधिरेषोऽवपीडस्य कार्यः प्रध्मापनस्य तु|

In the morning or noon time, after the patient has completed his daily acts of ablutions, he is made to lie comfortably in supine position on a well spread bed with his head slightly hanging down, and legs slightly raised. A wise physician should give him Tarpana (nourishing) type of medicated oil through his nostrils.

If the head is not kept in a lower position then the recipe for inhalation therapy will not reach the desired destination in the head. If the head is lowered in excess then the recipe gets lodged in the brain (mastulunga). Therefore, the patient should maintain the aforesaid position while lying down.

As a preparatory measure for cleaning, fomentation therapy is applied over the head of the patient. Thereafter, the physician with the thumb of his left hand should raise the tip of the nose, and with his right hand, should appropriately pour the recipe of medicated oil through a Pranadi (pipette) or Picu (cotton swab) in equal quantities in each of the nostrils.

After this, fomentation therapy is applied over the head once again, and the recipe of medicated oil along with Slesma (Phlegm or mucous matter) is drained out frequently till no trace of medicated oil is left.

Because of fomentation, the Slesma (Mucous matter) gets excited and by the administration of inhalation therapy, it gets dislodged, if a part of the medicated oil is left behind then because of its cooling effort, the localised mucous matter gets concealed in the head. This may give rise to diseases of the ears, manya (sides of the neck), throat etc.

After the administration of the inhalation therapy, the patient is given Dhuma-Pana (smoking therapy) which is curative of Kapha.

The patient should take wholesome food, and stay in a warm apartment free from drought. He should observe sensual restraint.

This is the procedure to be followed for the administration of Avapida and Adhumapana types of Nasya. [98 ½- ½ 107]

Pradhaman Type of Inhalation therapy

तत् षडङ्गुलया नाड्या धमेच्चूर्णं मुखेन तु||१०७|| विरिक्तशिरसं तूष्णं पाययित्वाऽम्बु भोजयेत्|
लघु त्रिष्वविरुद्धं च निवातस्थमतन्द्रितः||१०८|| विरेकशुद्धो दोषस्य कोपनं यस्य सेवते|
स दोषो विचरंस्तत्र करोति स्वान् गदान् बहून्||१०९|| यथास्वं विहितां तेषु क्रियां कुर्यादिवचक्षणः|
अकालकृतजातानां रोगाणामनुरूपतः||११०||

As per Pradhamana types of inhalation therapy, the recipe in powder form is blown by the physician through his mouth into the nostrils of the patient with the help of tubes which are six Angulas in breadth. After the morbid matter is eliminated from the head of the patient, the physician should make him drink warm water and give him food ingredients which are light and in harmony with all the three Doshas. Thereafter, the patient is made to stay in a breeze free house.

After the body is cleansed of morbid matter, intake of unwholesome (dosa-aggravating) regimen causes the aggravated Doshas to circulate all over the body giving rise to several diseases peculiar to that Doshas. In that case, the wise physician should administer therapies specifically required for the same aggravated Dosa. Complications arising out of untimely administration of inhalation therapy are treated on the same line specifically suggested for each of these complications. [107 ½- 110]

Complications arising out of Kapha and Their Treatment

अजीर्णे भोजने भुक्ते तोये पीतेऽथ दुर्दिने| प्रतिश्याये नवे स्नाते स्नेहपानेऽनुवासने||१११||
नावनं स्नेहनं रोगान् करोति श्लैष्मिकान् बहून्| तत्र श्लेष्महरः सर्वस्तीक्ष्णोष्णादिर्विधिर्हितः||११२||

Several Kaphaja types of ailments are manifested when virechana or snehana (Oleating) type of inhalation therapy is administered in the following conditions:

During indigestion

After-the intake of food

After drink water

In a cloudy day

During corzya of recent origin

After bath

After the intake of Sneha (potion of ghee) and

After and Anuvasana (Unctuous) type of enema

For the treatment of such ailments all the Kapha-alleviating, therapeutic measures containing ingredients which are Tiksna (sharp) hot, etc are useful. [111-112]

Complications Caused by vayu, and their treatment

क्षामे विरेचिते गर्भे व्यायामाभिहते तृषि| वातो रूक्षेण नस्येन क्रुद्धः स्वाञ्जनयेद्गदान्||११३||
तत्र वातहरः सर्वो विधिः स्नेहनबृंहणः| स्वेदादिः, स्याद्घृतं क्षीरं गर्भिण्यास्तु विशेषतः||११४||

Several Vatika types of ailments are manifested by the aggravated vataif Ruksa (non unctuous) type of inhalation therapy is administered in the following conditions:

• If the patient is emaciated

• If the patient has taken purgation therapy

• If the patient (woman) is pregnant

• If the patient is afflicted with hard work and

• If the patient is thirsty

For the treatment of these ailments, all the Snehana (oleation), Brmhana), (Nourishing), Svedana (fomentation) and such other therapies which alleviate vataare useful. In the case of pregnant women, ghee and milk is specially given. [113-114]

Timira and its treatment

ज्वरशोकातितप्तानां तिमिरं मद्यपस्य तु| रूक्षैः शीताञ्जनैर्लेपैः पुटपाकैश्च साधयेत्||११५||

Inhalation therapy given to a patient who is exceedingly afflicted with fever as well as grief, and who is alcoholic gives rise to Timira (Cataract). For the treatment of this Timira, the patient is given Sitanjana, Lepa (application of ointment over the eyes) and Puta-paka (juice of the paste of herbs covered with mud and cooked over fire) with ununctuous ingredients. [115]

Pratimarsa type of inhalation therapy

स्नेहनं शोधनं चैव द्विविधं नावनं मतम्| प्रतिमर्शस्तु नस्यार्थं करोति न च दोषावान्||११६||

नस्तः स्नेहाङ्गुलिं दद्यात् प्रातर्निशि च सर्वदा| न चोच्छिङ्घेदरोगाणां प्रतिमर्शः स दाढर्यकृत्||११७||

Navana type of inhalation therapy is of two types viz Snehana (which causes oleation) and Sodhana (which causes elimination of Doshas). Pratimarsa (application of oil in the nostrils) type of inhaliation therapy performs both these actions, and it is harmless.

For Pratimarsa, the finger is dipped into the medicated oil and then applied in the inner wall of the nostrils. It is not necessary to be snuffed deeply as is done in the case of other forms of inhalation therapy. It can be used in the morning or at night, in all the seasons. Even a healthy person can use this type of inhalation therapy for promoting good function [of the organs in the head] [116-117]

Epilogue

तत्र श्लोकौ-

त्रीणि यस्मात् प्रधानानि मर्माण्यभिहतेषु च| तेषु लिङ्गं चिकित्सां च रोगभेदाश्च सौषधाः||११८||

विधिरुत्तरबस्तेश्च नस्तःकर्मविधिस्तथा| सव्यापद्भेषजं सिद्धौ मर्माख्यायां प्रकीर्तितम्||११९||

In this chapter dealing with the success in the treatment of three vital organs, the topics discussed are as follows:

Reasons for which three organs (viz., heart, head and urinary bladder) are the most important ones; (vide verse nos. 3-5)

Signs and symptoms of the afflictions of these three vital organs, and their treatment; (vide verse nos. 6-8)

Virities of the diseases of these vital organs, and medicaments to be used for the treatment of these ailments and (vide verse nos. 9 ½- 49)

Method of administration of Uttara-Basti (urethral and vaginal douche) and Nasta-Karma (inhalation therapy), their complications, and treatment of these complications. (Vide verse nos. 49 ½- 117) [118-119]

इत्यग्निवेशकृते तन्त्रे चरकप्रतिसंस्कृतेऽप्राप्ते दृढबलसम्पूरिते सिद्धिस्थाने त्रिमर्मीयसिद्धिर्नाम नवमोऽध्यायः||९||

Thus, ends the ninth chapter of Siddhi- srhana dealing with the "Successful Treatment of Ailments Caused by the Afflictions of three Vital Organs" in Agnivesha's work as redacted by Caraka, and because of its non-availability supplemented by Drdhabala.

35

Siddhisthana Chapter 10 Basti Siddhi

Prologue

अथातो बस्तिसिद्धिं व्याख्यास्यामः||१||

इति ह स्माह भगवानात्रेय||२||

We shall now explore the chapter on "Effective Recipes of medicated Enema". Thus, said Lord Atreya. [1-2]

Dialogue

सिद्धानां बस्तीनां शस्तानां तेषु तेषु रोगेषु|

शृण्वग्निवेश ! गदतः सिद्धिं सिद्धिप्रदां भिषजाम्||३||

O! Agnivesha, listen to the discourses on effective and useful recipes of Basti (medicated enema) for various diseases which bestow success upon the successful physicians. [3]

Importance of Basti Therapy

बलदोषकालरोगप्रकृतीः प्रविभज्य योजिताः सम्यक् स्वैः स्वैरौषधवर्गैः स्वान् स्वान् रोगान्नियच्छन्ति||४||

कर्मान्यद्बस्तिसमं न विद्यते शीघ्रसुखविशोधित्वात्| आश्वपतर्पणतर्पणयोगाच्च निरत्ययत्वाच्च||५||

If Basti is administered appropriately keeping in view the strength of the patient, Doshas involved in the causation of diseases, nature of the diseases, physical constitution of the patient and the properties of different groups of drugs prescribed for different diseases, it would cure these ailments.

No therapeutic measure other than Basti, cleanses the body quickly and easily, causes depletion and nourishment instantaneously, and is free from any adverse effect. [4-5]

Superiority of Basti in Comparison to Purgation

सत्यपि दोषहरत्वे कटुतीक्ष्णोष्णादि भेषजादानात्| दुःखोद्गारोत्क्लेशाहृद्यत्वकोष्ठरुजा विरेके स्युः||६||

अविरेच्यौ शिशुवृद्धौ तावप्राप्तप्रहीनधातुबलौ| आस्थापनमेव तयोः सर्वार्थकृदुत्तमं कर्म||७||

बलवर्णहर्षमार्दवगात्रस्नेहान्नृणां ददात्याशु|८|

The purgation (including emesis) therapy no doubt, causes elimination of Doshas; but it involves intake of recipes, ingredients of which are pungent, sharp, hot etc., these ingredients cause unpleasantness, eructation, nausea, cardiac discomfort and pain in the gastrointestinal tract.

Infants have immaturity of tissues and less strength. There is diminution of tissues and reduction of strength in old people. For both these categories of patients, viz, infants and old persons, purgation therapy is contraindicated. Asthapana type of medicated enema can, however, be given to both these types of patients which are excellent both for the elimination of Doshas and nourishment of the body, this basti therapy instantaneously promotes strength, complexion, sense of exhilaration and tenderness as well as unctuousness of the body. [6- ½ 8]

Three types of Basti

अनुवासनं निरूहश्चोत्तरबस्तिश्च स त्रिविधः||८|| शाखावातार्तानां सकुञ्चितस्तब्धभग्नरुग्णानाम् |
विट्सङ्गाध्मानारुचिपरिकर्तिरुगादिषु च शस्तः||९|| उष्णार्तानां शीताञ्छीतार्तानां तथा सुखोष्णांश्च|
तद्योग्यौषधयुक्तान् बस्तीन् सन्तर्क्य विनियुज्यात्||१०||

Basti is of three types and are as follows:

Anuvasana (enema given with oil and such other unctuous ingredients);

Niruha (enema given with decoction, etc., added with oil etc) and

Uttara –Basti (urethral and vaginal douche)

These different forms of medicated enema are useful in the following categories of ailments:

Afflictions of the exterior (limbs) of the body by the aggravated Vata;

For those who are suffering from contractures, stiffness, fractures and pain and

Obstruction to the passage of faeces, flatulence, anorexia, sawing pain, aching pain etc

For the patients afflicted with diseases caused by heat, cooling recipes are used for enema. For those afflicted with diseases caused by cold, lukewarm recipes of enema are administered.

After determining the exact requirement of the patient, enema is administered with recipes containing appropriate, viz hot or cold ingredients. [8 ½ - 10]

Contra –indications

बस्तीन्न बृंहणीयान् दद्याद् व्याधिषु विशोधनीयेषु| मेदस्विनो विशोध्या येऽपि नराः कुष्ठमेहार्ताः||११||
न क्षीणक्षतदुर्बलमूर्च्छितकृशशुष्कदेहानाम्| युञ्जादिवशोधनीयान् दोषनिबद्धायुषो ये च||१२||

Nourishing types of medicated enema should not be given in the following conditions:

• Diseases requiring elimination of aggravated Doshas

• Patients with adiposity even if they are otherwise suitable for elimination therapies and

• Patients suffering from Kustha (obstinate skin diseases including leprosy) and Meha - urinary tract disorders, diabetes (obstinate urinary diseases including diabetes)

• Shodhana Basti - Eliminative (evacuative) type of medicated enema should not be given to the patients suffering from consumption, phthisis, weakness, fainting and emaciation as well as dryness of the body. This type of enema is also contraindicated for patients whose life is sustained because of the retention of faeces. [11-12]

Different types of ingredients for various ailments

वाजीकरणेऽसृक्पित्तयोश्च मधुघृतपयोयुक्ताः| शस्ताः सतैलमूत्रारनाललवणाश्च कफवाते||१३||
युञ्जाद्द्रव्याणि बस्तिष्वम्लं मूत्रं पयः सुरां क्वाथान्| अविरोधाद्धातूनां रसयोनित्वाच्च जलमुष्णम्||१४||

• For aphrodisiac effects, for the treatment of diseases caused by Rakta (vitiated blood) and pitta, the recipe of enema containing honey, ghee and milk is useful.

• Recipes of enema containing Til oil, cow's urine, Aranala (vinegar) and salt are useful for the diseases caused by aggravated Kapha and Vata.

• In the recipe of enema, ingredients like Amla (sour drinks), cow's urine, cow's milk, alcohol and decoctions which are not antagonistic to Dhatus (Doshas and tissue elements responsible for the causation of the diseases) are appropriately added. Similarly, water which is the source of nourishment (rasa-Yoni) is added to the recipe when it is warm. [13-14]

Ingredients for Avapa

सुरदारुशताह्वैलाकुष्ठमधुककपिप्पलीमधुस्नेहाः| ऊर्ध्वानुलोमभागाः ससर्षपाः शर्करा लवणम्||१५||
आवापा बस्तीनामतः प्रयोज्यानि येषु यानि स्युः| युक्तानि सह कषायैस्तान्युत्तरतः प्रवक्ष्यामि||१६||

Suradaru (Devadaru), Satahva, Ela – Cardamom, Kustha, Madhuka, Pippali - Long pepper fruit - Piper longum, madhu (honey), sneha (fats like oil and ghee), drugs which are urdhvabhagahara (cause upward motion in the gastrointestinal tract), Sarsapa, sugar and salt - these are to be used (individually or all together) added as avapa (ingredients which are added later to the recipe in small quantity) in recipes for enema.

From amongst these ingredients which are to be added along with type of Decoction and to which type of enema-recipe will be described later. [15-16]

Strong and mild enemas

चिरजातकठिनबलेषु व्याधिषु तीक्ष्णा विपर्यये मृदवः| सप्रतिवापकषाया योज्यास्त्वनुवासननिरूहाः||१७||

For chronic, obstinate and serious types of diseases, recipes containing Prativapa (ingredients added later) and decoctions of strong action ingredients are used for Anuvasana (unctuous types of enema) and Niruha (evacuative type of enema). For other types of diseases (which are of recent origin, which are easily amenable to therapeutics and which are of mild nature) ingredients having only mild effects are used. [17]

Enema Recipes for Vata, Pitta and Kapha

अर्धश्लोकैरतः सिद्धान् नानाव्याधिषु सर्वशः| बस्तीन् वीर्यसमैर्भागैर्यथार्हालोडनाञ्छृणु||१८||

बिल्वोऽग्निमन्थः श्योनाकः काश्मर्यः पाटलिस्तथा| शालपर्णी पृश्निपर्णी बृहत्यौ वर्धमानकः||१९||

यवाः कुलत्थाः कोलानि स्थिरा चेति त्रयोऽनिले| शस्यन्ते सचतुःस्नेहाः पिशितस्य रसान्विताः||२०||

नलवञ्जुलवानीरशतपत्राणि शैवलम्| मञ्जिष्ठा सारिवाऽनन्ता पयस्या मधुयष्टिका||२१||

चन्दनं पद्मकोशीरं तुङ्गं ते पैत्तिके त्रयः| सशर्कराक्षौद्रघृताः सक्षीरा बस्तयो हिताः||२२||

अर्कस्तथैव चालर्क एकाष्ठीला पुनर्नवा| हरिद्रा त्रिफला मुस्तं पीतदारु कुटन्नटम्||२३||

पिप्पल्यश्चित्रकश्चेति त्रयस्ते श्लेष्मरोगिषु | सक्षारक्षौद्रगोमूत्रा नातिस्नेहान्विता हिताः||२४||

Now, listen to the comprehensive description of effective enema-recipes for different diseases, each one of which is described in half (one line) of the following verses. These recipes contain drugs which are harmonious in potency and proportion. In addition, Alodanas or Avapas (ingredients which are added later to the recipe) for each group are also described.

Ingredients for Vata

Bilva – Bael – Aegle marmelos, Agni-Mantha, Syonaka, Kasmarya and Patali – Stereospermum suaveolens
Salaparni, Prsniparni, Brhati, Kantakari - Yellow berried nightshade (whole plant) – Solanum xanthocarpum and Vardhamanaka (Eranda - Castor) and
yava, Kulattha, Kola and Sthira.
These three recipes are to be used as enema for Vatika diseases along with four types of fat (oil, ghee, muscle-fat and bone-marrow) and, meat-soup).

Ingredients for Pitta

Nala, Vanjula (vetsa), vanira (a type of Vetasa), Shatapatra and Saivala,
Manjistha, Sariva, Ananta, Payasya and yastimadhu and
Chandana, Padmaka, usira and tunga (punnaga).
The above mentioned three recipes prepared with milk are to be used as enema for Paittika type of diseases, along with sugar, honey and ghee.

Ingredients for Kapha

Arka, Alarka (mandara), ekasthika (Patha) and Punarnava Haridra, Haritaki, Bibhitaka, Amalaki, Musta, Pitadaru and Kutannata (Kaivarta or Tagara) and Pippali and Chitraka.

Enema –recipes for colon-cleansing

फलजीमूतकेक्ष्वाकुधामार्गवकवत्सकाः | श्यामा च त्रिफला चैव स्थिरा दन्ती द्रवन्त्यपि||२५||

प्रकीर्या चोदकीर्या च नीलिनी क्षीरिणी तथा| सप्तला शङ्खिनी लोध्रं फलं कम्पिल्लकस्य च||२६||

चत्वारो मूत्रसिद्धास्ते पक्वाशयविशोधनाः| (व्यस्तैरपि समस्तैश्च चतुर्योगा उदाहृताः)||२७||

The following four recipes are to be boiled with cow's urine and used as enema for cleansing colon:
Phala, Jimuta, Iksvaku, Dhamargava and Vatsaka.
Syama, Haritaki, Bibhitaka, Amalaki, Sthira, Danti and Dravanti (a type of Danti); Prakirya (Karanja), Udakriya,

Nilini (Nila-Vuhna or Nilanjanika) and Ksirini.

Saptala, Sankhini, Lodhra and fruit of Kampillaka

The four recipes illustrated above can be used separately or jointly. [25-27]

Enema- recipe for Promotion of semen and Muscle-tissue

काकोली क्षीरकाकोली मुद्गपर्णी शतावरी| विदारी मधुयष्ट्याह्वा शृङ्गाटककशेरुके||२८||

आत्मगुप्ताफलं माषाः सगोधूमा यवास्तथा| जलजानूपजं मांसमित्येते शुक्रमांसलाः ||२९||

The following (four) enema- recipes help in the promotion of semen and muscle- tissue

Kakoli, Ksira-kakoli, Mudgaparni and satavari

Vidari, Madhuyasti, Srngataka and kaseruka

Fruit (seed) of Atmagupta, Masa, Godhuma and Yava and meat of aquatic and marshy land inhabiting animals [28-29]

Enema- recipe for Astringent Action

जीवन्ती चाग्निमन्थश्च धातकीपुष्पवत्सकौ| प्रग्रहः खदिरः कुष्ठं शमी पिण्डीतको यवाः||३०||

प्रियङ्गू रक्तमूली च तरुणी स्वर्णयूथिका| वटाद्याः किंशुकं लोध्रमिति साङ्ग्राहिका मताः||३१||

The following (four) enema- recipes help in producing astringent action:

Jivanti, Agnimantha, flower of Dhataki and Vatsaka

Pragraha, Khadira, Kustha, Sami, Pinditaka (madanaphala) and Yava;

Priyangu, Rakta-Muli (Samanga),Taruni (Aramataruni) or Nava Mallika and Svarna, Yuthika and Vata, etc (trees having latex), Kimsuka and lodhra [30-31]

Enema- recipes for Arresting Excessive Secretion

परिस्रावे शृतं क्षीरं सवृश्चीरपुनर्नवम्| आखुपर्णिकया वाऽपि तण्डुलीयकयुक्तया||३२||

The following (two) enema - recipes arrest excessive secretion from the body:

Milk boiled with Vrscira and punarnava and

Milk boiled with Akhuparni and Tanduliyaka [32]

Enema- recipes for Burning –Syndrome

कालङ्कतककाण्डेक्षुदर्भपोटगलेक्षुभिः| दाहघ्नः सघृतक्षीरो द्वितीयश्चोत्पलादिभिः||३३||

The following enema- recipes cure daha (burning syndrome):

Milk or ghee cooked with kalankataka, kandeksu (Brhadiksu) and Darbha, Potagala (Hoggala) and Iksu and

Milk or ghee cooked with Utpala and such other drugs (flowers of aquatic plants like Nalina and Saugandhika) [33]

Enema recipes for sawing pain

कर्बुदाराढकीनीपविदुलैः क्षीरसाधितैः| बस्तिः प्रदेयो भिषजा शीतः समधुशर्करः||३४||

परिकर्ते तथा वृन्तैः श्रीपर्णीकोविदारजैः| (देयो बस्तिः सुवैद्यैस्तु यथाविदिविदितक्रियैः)||३५||

Milk cooked with Karbudara, Adhaki, Nipa and Vidula (Vetasa) is cooled, and added with honey as well as sugar. The physician should give enema with this recipe to cure Parikarika (sawing pain).

A wise and expert physician should be give the enema of milk cooked with the stalks of Sriparni and Kovidara which is cooled, and added with honey as well as sugar to cure Parikartika (swaging / cutting pain) [34-35]

Enema- recipe for Gripping Pain

बस्तिः शाल्मलिवृन्तानां क्षीरसिद्धो घृतान्वितः| हितः प्रवाहणे तद्वद्वेष्टैः शाल्मलिकस्य च||३६||

Milk is cooked with the stalks of Salmali, and added with ghee. This recipe when given as enema cures Pravahana (gripping pain).

Similarly, milk is cooked with the gum of Salmali, and added with ghee. Enema given with this recipe cures Pravahana(Gripping pain). [36]

Enema- recipe for correcting over-action of Basti

अश्वावरोहिकाकाकनासाराजकशेरुकैः|

सिद्धाः क्षीरेऽतियोगे स्युः क्षौद्राञ्जनघृतैर्युताः||३७|| न्यग्रोधाद्यैश्चतुर्भिश्च तेनैव विधिना परः|३८|

For correcting the complications caused by over-action (atiyoga) of Basti (medicated enema), the following two recipes for enema are useful:

Milk boiled with asvavarohika (Asvagandha, Asvakarna or iksuraka), Karkanasa and Rajakaseruka, and added with honey, Rasanjana (Daruharidra Ghana Kvatha) and ghee and

Milk boiled with Nyagrodha, (Udumbara, Asvatha and Plaksa), and added with honey, Rasanjana and ghee. [37- ½ 38]

Enema- recipe for correcting Haemorrhage

बृहती क्षीरकाकोली पृश्निपर्णी शतावरी||३८|| काश्मर्यबदरीदूर्वास्तथोशीरप्रियङ्गवः|

जीवादाने शृतौ क्षीरे द्वौ घृताञ्जनसंयुतौ||३९|| बस्ती प्रदेयौ भिषजा शीतौ समधुशर्करौ|

गोऽव्याजामहिषीक्षीरैर्जीवनीययुतैस्तथा||४०|| शशैणदक्षमार्जारमहिषाव्यजशोणितैः|

सद्यस्कैर्मृदितैर्बस्तिर्जीवादाने प्रशस्यते||४१||

For arresting haemorrhage, the following (three) recipes of enema are useful:

Milk boiled with Brhati, Ksirakakoli,Prsniparni and satavari and added with ghee, Anjana (Daruharidra Ghana Kvatha), honey and sugar. This is administered when cool

Milk boiled with Kasmarya, Badari, Durva, Usira and Priyangu and added with ghee, Anjana, honey and sugar. This should be administered when cool and

Milk of cow, sheep, goat or buffalo is added with the paste of Jivaniya group of drugs and the fresh blood of rabbit, deer, cock, cat, buffalo, sheep or goat. [38 ½ - 41]

Enema- recipes for Rakta-Pitta and Prameha

मधूकमधुकद्राक्षादूर्वाकाश्मर्यचन्दनैः| तेनैव विधिना बस्तिर्देयः सक्षौद्रशर्करः||४२||

मञ्जिष्ठासारिवानन्तापयस्यामधुकैस्तथा| शर्कराचन्दनद्राक्षामधुधात्रीफलोत्पलैः|

रक्तपित्ते, प्रमेहे तु कषायः सोमवल्कजः||४३||

The recipe containing madooka, madhuka, Draksa, Durva, Kasmarya and Chandana is prepared in the above-mentioned manner by adding honey and sugar. This medicated enema [is useful for the treatment for rakta-pitta (an ailment characterised by bleeding from different parts of the body).]

Following the above-mentioned procedure, enema is prepared of manjistha, Sariva, ananta, payasya, madhuka, sarkara (sugar), Chandana, Draksa, Madhu (honey), fruits of Dhatri and Utpala which is useful for the treatment of rakta- pitta.

For Prameha, enema with the decoction of soma-valka is useful. [42-43]

Enema- recipe for other Ailments

गुल्मातिसारोदावर्तस्तम्भसङ्कुचितादिषु| सर्वाङ्गैकाङ्गरोगेषु रोगेष्वेवंविधेषु च||४४||

यथास्वैरौषधैः सिद्धान् बस्तीन् दद्यादिवचक्षणः| पूर्वोक्तेन विधानेन कुर्वन् योगान् पृथग्विधान||४५||

For Gulma (tumour), Atisara (diarrhoea), Udavarta (upward movement of wind in abdomen), Stambha (stiffness of Limbs), Sankucita (contraction of limbs), sarvanga-roga (paralysis of the whole body), ekanga-Roga (paralysis of one limb) and for such other diseases, an expert physician should give basti (medicated enema) of effective recipes containing different types of drugs appropriate to each of these conditions prepared according to the methods described before. [44-45]

Epilogue

तत्र श्लोकाः:-

त्रिकास्त्रयोऽनिलादीनां चतुष्काश्चापरे त्रयः| पक्वाशयविशुद्ध्यर्थं वृष्याः साङ्ग्राहिकास्तथा||४६||

परिस्रावे तथा दाहे परिकर्ते प्रवाहणे| सातियोगे मतौ द्वौ द्वौ जीवादाने तथा त्रयः||४७||

द्वौ रक्तपित्ते मेहे च एकत्रिंशच्च सप्त ते| सुलभाल्पौषधक्लेशा बस्तयो गुणवत्तमाः||४८||

To sum up:

In this chapter, thirty-seven excellent recipes containing small number of ingredients which are easily available and which have less of adverse effects are described as follows:

1-3. three recipes of enema for vatika diseases {vide verse nos. 19-20]

4-6. three recipes of enema for Paittika diseases [vide verse nos 21-22]

7-9. three recipes of enema for Kaphaja diseases {vide verse nos. 23-24]

10-13. four recipes of enema for cleansing the colon [vide verse nos. 25-27]

14-17. four recipes of enema for the promotion of virility (including those for promotion of seminal power) [vide verse nos. 28-29]

18-21. four recipes of enema with astringent effect [vide verse nos. 30-31]

22-23. two recipes of enema for arresting excessive secretion; [vide verse no 32]

24-25. Two recipes of enema for curing burning syndrome; [vide verse nos. 33]

26-27. two recipes of enema for curing sawing pain [vide verse nos. 34-35]

28-29. two recipes of enema for curing gripping pain [vide verse nos. 36]

30-31. two recipes of enema for correcting over-action (Ati-yoga) of Basti (medicated enema therapy) [vide verse nos. 37 – ½ 38]

32-34. three recipes of enema for arresting haemorrhage. [vide verse nos. [38 ½ -41]

35-36. two recipes of enema for correcting rakta-Pitta (an ailment characterised by bleeding from different parts of the body) and [vide verse nos. 42-43]

37. one recipe of enema for correcting meha (obstinate urinary including diabetes) [vide verse no. 43] [46-48]

Colophon

इत्यग्निवेशकृते तन्त्रे चरकप्रतिसंस्कृतेऽप्राप्ते दृढबलसम्पूरितेसिद्धिस्थाने बस्तिसिद्धिर्नाम दशमोऽध्यायः||१०||

Thus, ends tenth chapter of siddhi- section dealing with "Effective Recipes of Medicated Enema" of Agnivesha's work as redacted by Charaka, and because of its non-availability supplemented by Drdhabala.

36

Siddhisthana Chapter 11 Phala matra Siddhi

Prologue

अथातः फलमात्रासिद्धिं व्याख्यास्यामः||१||

इति ह स्माह भगवानात्रेयः||२||

We shall now explore the chapter dealing with the "determination of appropriateness of medicaments, etc., for enema, and its veterinary dosage to achieve success". Thus, said Lord Atreya [1-2]

Seminar to resolve disputes

भगवन्तमुदारसत्त्वधीश्रुतिविज्ञानसमृद्धमत्रिजम्| फलबस्तिवरत्वनिश्चये सविवादा मुनयोऽभ्युपागमन्||३||

भृगुकौशिककाप्यशौनकाः सपुलस्त्यासितगौतमादयः| कतमत् प्रवरं फलादिषु स्मृतमास्थापनयोजनास्विति||४||

To resolve dispute over the most useful ingredient amongst madana-phala (randia dumetorum), etc., for athapana-basti, and to determine the excellence of basti with those of madanaphala etc., in specific ailments, sages like bhrgu, kausika, kapya, Saunaka, pulastya and asita Gautama came to Lord Atreya, who is richly endowed with liberal mind. Wisdom, memory and mundane knowledge.[3-4]

Opinion of Saunaka about excellence of jimutaka

कफपित्तहरं वरं फलेष्वथ जीमूतकमाह शौनकः|

Saunaka said, "amongst the fruits, jimutaka is the foremost in efficacy (for medicated for enema) because of its effects to eliminate kapha and pitta. [5½]

Opinion of vamaka on excellence of katu- tumbi

मृदुवीर्यतयाऽभिनत्ति तच्छकृदित्याह नृपोऽथ वामकः||५|| कटुतुम्बममन्यतोत्तमं वमने दोषसमीरणं च तत्|

Tthe king Vamaka said, "because of low potency this (fruits of jimutaka) is less effective in disintegrating and voiding of stool. On the other hand katu- tumbi which is the best as emetic is considered to be excellent because of its action to eliminate the doshas (through enema). [5 ½ - 6½]

Opinion of Gautama on excellence of dhamargava

तदवृष्यमशैत्यतीक्ष्णताकटुरौक्ष्यादिति गौतमोऽब्रवीत्||६||

कफपित्तनिबर्हणं परं स च धामार्गवमित्यमन्यत |

Gautama said "(katutumbi) is non-aphrodisiac (avrsya) because of its sharp, pungent and un-unctuous effects. Dhamargava which is excellent for eliminating kapha and pitta may be considered to be best for basti (medicated enema)." [6 ½- 7½]

Opinion of badisa on excellence of kutaja

तदमन्यत वातलं पुनर्बंडिशो ग्लानिकरं बलापहम्||७||
कुटजं प्रशशंस चोत्तमं न बलघ्नं कफपित्तहारि च|

Badisa said, "it (dhamargava) is the aggravator of vata, it causes depression (glani), and it reduces strength (for which it is not suitable for basti or enema). On the other hand, kutaja is considered as excellent [for enema] because it does not reduce strength, and it alleviates kapha as well as pitta" [7 ½- 8½]

Opinion of kapya on excellence of krita-vedhana

अतिविज्जलमौर्ध्वंभागिकं पवनक्षोभि च काप्य आह तत्||८||
कृतवेधनमाह वातलं कफपित्तं प्रबलं हरेदिति|

Kapya said, "it (kutaja) is very viscid, it causes elimination of doshas through the upward tract (emesis), and it causes aggravation of vata (pavana- ksobhi) [for which it is not suitable for basti or enema]. On the other hand, kutaja is considered as excellent [for enema] because it does not reduce strength, and it alleviates kapha as well pitta". On the other hand, krta-vedhana which is vatala (promoter of vata) and which (instantaneously) eliminates excessively aggravated kapha and pitta (is the best drug for basti or medicated enema). [8 1/2- 91/2]

Refutation by Bhadra –Saunaka

तदसाध्विति भद्रशौनकः कटुकं चातिबलघ्नमित्यपि||९||

BhadraSaunaka said, 'the statement [regarding the utility of krta-vedhana in enema therapy] is not correct because it is pungent, and it reduces strength in excess. [9 1/2]

Atreya's concluding statement

इति तद्वचनानि हेतुभिः सुविचित्राणि निशम्य बुद्धिमान् | प्रशशंस फलेषु निश्चयं परमं चात्रिसुतोऽब्रवीदिदम्||१०||
फलदोषगुणान् सरस्वती प्रति सर्वैरपि सम्यगीरिता| न तु किञ्चिददोषनिर्गुणं गुणभूयस्त्वमतो विचिन्त्यते [४] ||११||
इह कुष्ठहिता गरागरी हितमिक्ष्वाकु तु मेहिने मतम्| कुटजस्य फलं हृदामये प्रवरं कोठफलं च पाण्डुषु||१२||
उदरे कृतवेधनं हितं, मदनं सर्वगदाविरोधि तु| मधुरं सकषायतिक्तकं तदरूक्षं सकटूष्णविज्जलम्||१३||
कफपित्तहृदाशुकारि चाप्यनपायं पवनानुलोमि च| फलनाम विशेषतस्त्वतो लभतेऽन्येषु फलेषु सत्स्वपि||१४||

Having heard to the (above mentioned) interesting statement, the wise teacher Atreya admired the effort of the speakers, and thereafter, delivered the final judgement regarding the best among the fruits for enema as follows:
in your statements, all of you have appropriately described the beneficial effects and shortcomings of different fruits [for use in cncma therapy]. There is no drug which is absolutely free from shortcomings or which is absolutely free from good effects. Therefore, we should, (while selecting the appropriate drug for enema), think of a drug which possesses more of good attributes [for a particular ailment].

In the present context (of basti or medicated enema), jimutaka (garagari) is useful for the treatment of kustha (obstinate skin diseases including leprosy); katutumbi (iksvaku) is for meha (obstinate urinary diseases including diabetes); fruit of kutaja for heart diseases; kotha-phala - dhamargava is for pandu (anemia) and krta-vedhana is useful for udara (obstinate abdominal diseases including ascites).

Madana-phala is, however, not contra-indicated in any diseases. It is sweet and slightly astringent as well as bitter in taste. It is sweet and slightly pungent, hot and viscid. It eliminates kapha and pitta, it acts (eliminates doshas) instantaneously, it is harmless, and it causes downward movement of vata. Therefore, the term "phala" (lit, fruit) specifically indicates madanaphala (fruit of madana) even though there are several other fruits which are in medicine. [10-14]

Query about action of basti

गुरुणेति वचस्युदाहृते मुनिसङ्घेन च पूजिते ततः | प्रणिपत्य मुदा समन्वितः सहितः शिष्यगणोऽनुपृष्टवान्||१५||
सर्वकर्मगुणकृद्गुरुणोक्तो बस्तिरूर्ध्वमथ नैति नाभितः| नाभ्यधो गुदमतः स शरीरात् सर्वतः कथमपोहति दोषान् ||१६||

The above statement of the teacher was duly honoured by the assembly of sages. Thereafter, all the disciples bowed before him happiness and enquired about the following:

the teacher has described the basti (medicated enema) to possess actions and attributes for curing all the diseases. But it does not reach above the level of umbilicus because the rectum through which it is administered is located below this umbilicus. Then, how is it possible for basti (medicated enema) to eliminate morbid material (doshas) from all over the body? [15-16]

Preceptor's reply

तद्गुरुरब्रवीदिदं शरीरं तन्त्रयतेऽनिलः सङ्गविघातात् | केवल एव दोषसहितो वा स्वाशयगः प्रकोपमुपयाति||१७||

तं पवनं सपित्तकफविट्कं शुद्धिकरोऽनुलोमयति बस्तिः| सर्वशरीरगश्च गदसङ्घस्तत्प्रशमात् प्रशान्तिमुपयाति||१८||

The body is sustained by vata because of its ability to cause detachment (vighat) of any adhesion (sanga). vata alone or along with other doshas (generally) gets aggravated in its own habitat / seat (i.e colon). Basti (medicated enema), by its purificatory action, causes downward movement of that vata along with pitta, kapha and faeces. Because of the alleviation of this vata, all the diseases pervading the whole body get alleviated. [17-18]

Enema therapy for animals

अथाधिगम्यार्थमखण्डितं धिया गजोष्ट्रगोश्वाव्यजकर्म रोगनुत्|

अपृच्छदेनं स च बस्तिमब्रवीद्विधिं च तस्याह पुनः प्रचोदितः||१९||

After having understood the aforesaid concept in its entirety by intelligence, the disciple (agnivesa) enquired about the cure of diseases affecting elephants, camels, cattle, horses, sheep and goats.

The preceptor (Atreya) described basti (medicated enema) [as the excellent therapy for the treatment of their diseases].

After further query, the preceptor explained the procedure of administering enema to these animals as follows (to be discussed in subsequent verse nos. 20-26) [19]

Enema – receptacles for different animals

आजोरणौ सौम्य गजोष्ट्रयोः कृते गवाश्वयोर्बस्तिमुशन्ति माहिषम्|

अजाविकानां तु जरद्गवोद्भवं वदन्ति बस्तिं तदुपायचिन्तकाः||२०||

For giving enema to the elephant and camel, the urinary bladder of goat and sheep is used as enema-receptacle (basti) for giving enema to cows and horses, the urinary bladder of old ox (jaradgava) is used as enema-receptacle.

O! Blessed on (addressed to the disciple agnivesa), this is the option of veterinary physicians proficient in the administration of medicated enema to animals. [20]

Enema-nozzle for different animals

अरत्निमष्टादशषोडशाङ्गुलं तथैव नेत्रं हि दशाङ्गुलं क्रमात्|

गजोष्ट्रगोश्वाव्यजबस्तिसन्धौ चतुर्थभागोपनयं हितं वदेत्||२१||

The length of enema – nozzles for different animals is as follows:

elephants: one aratni (length of the fore arm)

camels: 18 angulas (one angula= ¾th of an inch);

cattle and horses :16 angulas and

sheep and goats :10 angulas

it is stated to insert one fourth of this length of the nozzle into the anus of the animals while administering enema. [21]

Dose of enema- recipe for different animals

प्रस्थस्त्वजाव्योर्हि निरूहमात्रा गवादिषु द्वित्रिगुणं यथाबलम्|

निरूहमुष्ट्रस्य तथाऽऽढकद्वयं गजस्य वृद्धिस्त्वनुवासनेऽष्टमः||२२||

The dose of the fluids to be used as niruha (evacuative enema) for different animals is as follows:

goats and sheep: one prastha (64 tolas)

cattle (cows, buffalo and horses): two to three prasthas depending upon their physique;

camels: two adhakas (one adhakas= 25 tolas) and

elephants: four adhakas.

For anuvasana (unctuous types of medicated enema), the quantity of oil, etc., to be used for these animals is one-eight of the quantity prescribed above for niruha (evacuative type of medicated enema). (22)

Enema- recipe for all animals in general

कलिङ्गकुष्ठे मधुकं च पिप्पली वचा शताह्वा मदनं रसाञ्जनम्|
हितानि सर्वेषु गुडः ससैन्धवो द्विपञ्चमूलं च विकल्पना त्वियम्||२३||

the recipe containing [the decoction of] ingredients like kalinga, kustha, madhuka, pippali, vaca, satahva, madana and rasanjana and added with jaggery, rock-salt and two varieties of dasamula (bilva, syonaka, gambhari, patala, ganikarika, salaparni, prsniparni, brhati, kantakari and goksura) is useful for all the types of veterinary enema. [23]

Additional ingredients for elephants

गजेऽधिकाऽश्वत्थवटाश्वकर्णकाः सखादिरप्रग्रहशालतालजाः|

The recipes described above (in verse no. 23) is added with [the decoction of] ingredients like asvattha,vata, asva-karna, khadira, pragraha (syonaka), sala and fruits of tala. Enema, along with these additional ingredients, is useful for curing diseases of elephants. [2/4 24]

Additional ingredients for cows

तथा च पण्यौँ धवशिग्रुपाटली मधूकसाराः सनिकुम्भचित्रकाः||२४||
पलाशभूतीकसुराह्वरोहिणीकषाय उक्तस्त्वधिको गवां हितः|

The decoction of mudgaparni, masaparni, dhava, sigru, patali, madhuka-sara (heart- wood of madhuka), nikumbha, citraka, palasa, bhutika (ajamoda), surahva (devadaru) and rohini (katurohini) is used in addition (to the drugs described in the verse no. 23 as enema for cattle – diseases. [24 2/4- 2/4 25]

Additional ingredients for horses

पलाशदन्तीसुरदारुकतृणद्रवन्त्य उक्तास्तुरगस्य चाधिकाः||२५||

The decoction of palasha, danti, suradaru, kattrna and dravanti, in addition (to the decoction of drugs described in the verse no. 23) is used for enema to cure diseases of horses. [25 2/4]

Additional ingredients for asses and camels

खरोष्ट्रयोः पीलुकरीरखादिराः शम्याकबिल्वादिगणस्य च च्छदाः|

The decoction of pilu, karira, khadira, samyaka and leaves of drugs belonging to bilvadi group is used in addition (to the decoction of drugs described in the verse no. 23) as enema for the diseases of asses and camels. [2/4 26]

Additional ingredients for goats and sheep

अजाविकानां त्रिफलापरूषकं कपित्थकर्कन्धु सबिल्वकोलजम्||२६||

The decoction of haritaki, bibhitaka, amalaki, parusaka, kapittha, karkanadu, bilva and kola is used in addition (to the decoction of drugs described in the verse no. 23) as enema for the diseases of goats and sheep. [26 2/4]

Query about always exposed to diseases

अथाग्निवेशः सततातुरान् नरान् हितं च पप्रच्छ गुरुस्तदाह च|
सदाऽऽतुराः श्रोत्रियराजसेवकास्तथैव वेश्या सह पण्यजीविविभिः||२७||

Thereafter, Agnivesha enquired from the preceptor about the persons who are eternally sick, and also about their treatment. The preceptor replied that the persons who are eternally exposed to sickness are the following:

srotriyas (people belonging to the priest class)

raja- sevakas (servants of the king)
vesyas (courtesans) and
panya-jivins (merchants) [27]

Priests
दिवजो हि वेदाध्ययनव्रताह्निकक्रियादिभिर्देहहितं न चेष्टते [२] |
The priests (brahmins) are always engaged in the study of the vedas, observance of different types of sacred vows (vratas), performance of daily rituals (ahnika-kriya), etc., they, thus, fail to attend to regimens which are useful for their health. [2/4 28]

King's servants
नृपोपसेवी नृपचित्तरक्षणात् परानुरोधाद्बहुचिन्तनाद्भयात् [३] ||२८||
King's servants are always preoccupied with such acts as would cause the gratification of the king's mind. They cater to the requirements of other subordinates of the kings's, and they are exposed to excessive worry and fear; [thus they fail to their regiments which are useful for their health]. [28 2/4]

Courtesans
नृचित्तवर्तिन्युपचारतत्परा मृजाभि(वि)भूषानिरता पणाङ्गना|
Depending upon the whims and the moods of men (clients), the courtesan devotes herself to their entertainment constantly by keeping her body clean, and by using various cosmetics as well as ornaments. Thus they fail to attend to their regimens which are useful for health]. [2/4 29]

Merchants
सदासनादत्यनुबन्धविक्रयक्रयादिलोभादपि पण्यजीविनः||२९||
Merchants lead to a sedentary life being excessively attached to greediness involved in their profession of selling and purchasing goods. [thus, they fail to attend to regimens which are useful for their health] [29 2/4]

Common causes of their diseases
सदैव ते ह्यागतवेगनिग्रहं समाचरन्ते न च कालभोजनम्|
अकालनिर्हारविहारसेविनो भवन्ति येऽन्येऽपि सदाऽऽतुराश्च ते||३०||
All above mentioned four categories of persons become eternally sick because of the following:
they are always involved in –
suppression of the manifested natural urges
not taking timely food
untimely voiding of stools, urine etc
untimely indulgence in different regimens
other persons (apart from priests, king's servants, courtesans and merchants) who resort to the above mentioned irregularities also become perpetually sick. [30]

Use of phala-varti for treatment of their sickness
समीरणं वेगविधारणोद्धतं विबन्धसर्वाङ्गरुजाकरं भिषक्| समीक्ष्य तेषां फलवर्तिमादितः सुकल्पितां स्नेहवर्तीं प्रयोजयेत्||३१||
Because of the suppression of natural urges, vata gets aggravated to cause constipation and pain all over the body. The physician, having ascertained this, should, in the beginning, give phala-varti (medicated suppository) well prepared with unctuous material. [31]

Niruha and anuvasana-basti
पुनर्नवैरण्डनिकुम्भचित्रकान् सदेवदारुत्रिवृतानिदिग्धिकान्| महान्ति मूलानि च पञ्च यानि विपाच्य मूत्रे दधिमस्तुसंयुते||३२||

सतैलसर्पिर्लवणैश्च पञ्चभिर्विमूर्च्छितं बस्तिमथ प्रयोजयेत्| निरूहितं धन्वरसेन भोजितं निकुम्भतैलेन ततोऽनुवासयेत्||३३||

Punarnava, eranda, nikumbha, citraka, devadaru, trivrt, nidigdhika and maha-mula (bilva,syonaka, gambhari, patala and ganikarika) is cooked by adding cow's urine, curd and whey. To this, oil, ghee and five types of salt (saindhava, samudra, vida, sauvarcala and audbhida) is added. With this recipe, niruha type of enema is given, after this, the patient is given food prepared by cooking with the meat-soup of animals living in arid zone.

There after, he is given anuvasana or unctuous types of enema with nikumbha-taila. [32-33]

Other recipes for basti

बलां सरास्नां फलबिल्वचित्रकान् द्विपञ्चमूलं कृतमालकात् फलम्| यवान् कुलत्थांश्च पचेज्जलाढके रसः स पेष्यैस्तु कलिङ्गकादिभिः||३४|| सतैलसर्पिर्गुडसैन्धवो हितः सदातुराणां बलवर्णवर्धनः| तथाऽनुवास्ये मधुकेन साधितं फलेन बिल्वेन शताह्वयाऽपि वा||३५||

Bala, rasana, phala (madanaphala), bilva, citraka, two varieties of pancamula, (bilva, syonaka, gambhari, patala, ganikarika, salaparni, prsniparni, brhati, kantakari and goksura), fruit of krtamala (aragvadha), yava and kulattha is boiled by adding one adhaka (25 tolas) of water, to this decoction, the paste of kalinga, etc., (vide verse no.23 for details of these drugs), oil, ghee, jaggery and rock-salt is added. Enema with this recipe is useful for persons who are perpetually sick (vide verse no. 27). This enema promotes their strength and complexion. Similarly, for these patients, oil cooked with either madhuka, phala (madana-phala), bilva or satahva may be used for anuvasana or unctuous types of enema. [34-35]

Enema – recipes for infants

सजीवनीयस्तु रसोऽनुवासने निरूहणे चालवणः शिशोर्हितः| न चान्यदाश्वङ्गबलाभिवर्धनं निरूहबस्तेः शिशुवृद्धयोः परम्||३६||

Anuvasana (unctuous types of medicated enema) prepared of the decoction of drugs belonging to jivaniya- group (jivaka, rsabhaka, meda, mahameda, kakoli, ksirakakoli, mudgaparni,masaparni, jivanti and madhuka-vide sutra 4:9:1), and niruha (evacuative type of medicated enema) prepared of these very drugs without adding salt are useful for children.

There is no therapy other than niruha-basti which effectively and rapidly promotes the growth of limbs and physical strength of both infants and old persons. [36]

तत्र श्लोकः-

फलकर्म बस्तिवरता नेत्रं यद्बस्तयो गवादीनाम्| राततातुराश्च दिष्टाः फलमात्रायां हितं चैषाम्||३७||

To sum up:-

in this chapter entitled" phala- matra-siddhi" the topics discussed are as follows:

action of various types of fruits [vide verse nos. 5-14]

excellence of basti – therapy [vide verse nos. 15-18]

the nozzle for giving enema to animals [vide verse nos. 19-22]

enema – recipes for cattle etc., [vide verse nos. 23-26]

categories of persons who are perpetually sick and [vide verse nos. 27-30]

therapies useful for these perpetually sick persons [vide verse nos. 31-36] [37]

Colophon

इत्यग्निवेशकृते तन्त्रे चरकप्रतिसंस्कृतेऽप्राप्ते दृढबलसम्पूरिते सिद्धिस्थाने फलमात्रासिद्धिर्नामैकादशोऽध्यायः||११||

Thus, ends the eleventh chapter of siddhi-section dealing with the "determination of appropriateness of madana-phala, etc., for enema. And its veterinary dose to achieve success ". In Agnivesha's work as redacted by Charaka, and because of its non- availability, supplemented by drdhabala.

37

Siddhisthana Chapter 12 Uttara Basti Siddhi

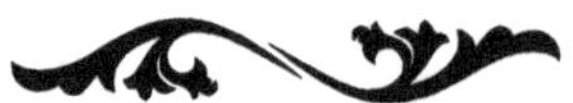

अथात उत्तरबस्तिसिद्धिं व्याख्यास्यामः||१||

इति ह स्माह भगवानात्रेयः||२||

We shall now explore the chapter dealing with the "Successful application of excellent recipes for Uttara Basti". Thus said Lord Atreya [1-2]

Post- therapeutic Management of Patients

अथ खल्वातुरं वैद्यः संशुद्धं वमनादिभिः| दुर्बलं कृशमल्पाग्निं मुक्तसन्धानबन्धनम्||३||

निर्हृतानिलविण्मूत्रकफपित्तं कृशाशयम्| शून्यदेहं प्रतीकारासहिष्णुं परिपालयेत्||४||

यथाऽण्डं तरुणं पूर्णं तैलपात्रं यथैव च| गोपाल इव दण्डी गाः सर्वस्मादपचारतः||५||

Just as we need to handle a fresh egg with tenderness and delicacy, just like we need to handle a brimful oil pot with care, and just like the cattle need to be protected by a cowherd having a staff in his hand, the physician too should similarly protect his patient carefully from the unwholesome (diets, regimens etc.) factors. This is because after having administered with the purificatory therapies, the body of the patient would undergo certain changes as follows –

• The body of the patient becomes weak and emaciated;

• His digestive power becomes weak

• The ligaments and his joints become loose;

• The (gastro- intestinal tract, bladder and other) viscera become empty (emaciated) because of the elimination of flatus, feces, urine, kapha (phlegm) and Pitta (bile).

• The body becomes empty

• The patient becomes intolerant to adverse situations (like loud speech and other strong therapeutic measures) [3-5]

Post therapeutic Diet

अग्निसन्धुक्षणार्थं तु पूर्वं पेयादिना भिषक्| रसोत्तरेणोपचरेत् क्रमेण क्रमकोविदः||६||

स्निग्धाम्लस्वादुहृद्यानि ततोऽम्ललवणौ रसौ| स्वादुतिक्तौ ततो भूयः कषायकटुकौ ततः||७||

अन्योऽन्यप्रत्यनीकानां रसानां स्निग्धरूक्षयोः| व्यत्यासादुपयोगेन प्रकृतिं गमयेद्भिषक्||८||

After the administration of purificatory therapy, the physician who is adept in handling post-therapeutic measures should first of all give to the patient (gradually lighter to heavier) the diet beginning with Peya (thin gruel) and ending with Rasa (meat–soup) for the stimulation of Agni (power of digestion and metabolism).

The patient is given unctuous, soul, sweet and pleasing (Hrudya) food. Then he is given dietetic articles having sour and saline tastes. Later on, he is given articles/foods having sweet and bitter tastes. Thereafter, he is given foods predominant in astringent and pungent tastes.

The patient is given ingredients having mutually contradictory tastes, and mutually contradictory properties like unctuousness and un-unctuousness alternatively till the normal diet (Prakriti) are restored. [6 -8]

Restoration of normal health

सर्वक्षमो ह्यसंसर्गो रतियुक्तः स्थिरेन्द्रियः| बलवान् सत्त्वसम्पन्नो विज्ञेयः प्रकृतिं गतः||९||

[After the intake of Peya, etc., and ingredients having different tastes as well as attributes], the patient is to be considered as the one having his normal health restored as indicated by the following factors:

• Ability to take and digest various ingredients/foods having all the different tastes.

• Non-obstruction to his natural urges

• Restoration of zest for life

• Sharp functioning of the senses

• Return of strength

• Endowment of strong will power [9]

Ashta Mahadoshakara Bhavas - Eight Impediments

एतां प्रकृतिमप्राप्तः सर्ववर्ज्यानि वर्जयेत्| महादोषकराण्यष्टाविमानि तु विशेषतः||१०||

उच्चैर्भाष्यं रथक्षोभमविचङ्क्रमणासने| अजीर्णाहितभोज्ये च दिवास्वप्नं समैथुनम्||११||

तज्जा देहोर्ध्वसर्वाधोमध्यपीडामदोषजाः| श्लेष्मजाः क्षयजाश्चैव व्याध्यः स्युर्यथाक्रमम्||१२||

Till the health, as characterized by the above-mentioned characteristic features (signs) is restored, the patient should avoid all the prohibited activities. He should especially avoid eight factors which are exceedingly harmful. These are as follows:

Avoidable factor and effect of not avoiding

1 Uccaih Bhasya or loud speech causes pain in the upper part of the body

2 Ratha-ksobha or jolts by riding wooden cart (conveyance) causes pain in all over the body

3 Ati-Cankramana or long wayfaring causes pain in the lower part of the body

4 Ati- Asana or constant sitting causes pain in the middle part of the body

5 Ajirna or indigestion gives rise to diseases caused by Ama or uncooked material

6 Ahita-bhojana or intake of unwholesome food gives rise to diseases caused by different Doshas

7 Diva-Svapna or sleep during day time gives rise of diseases caused by kapha

8 Maithuna and sexual intercourse gives rise to diseases caused by Ksaya or diminution of tissue elements [10-20]

Details off impediments

तेषां विस्तरतो लिङ्गमेकैकस्य च भेषजम्|

यथावत्सम्प्रवक्ष्यामि सिद्धान् बस्तींश्च यापनान्||१३||

Now, I (refers to Atreya) shall appropriately explain in detail the signs, treatment and effective Yapana type of Bastis (medicated enemas) for each of these impediments. [13]

Complications of loud and excessive speech

तत्रोच्चैर्भाष्यातिभाष्याभ्यां शिरस्तापशङ्खकर्णनिस्तोदश्रोत्रोपरोध मुखतालुकण्ठशोषतैमिर्यपिपासाज्वरतमक हनुग्रहमन्यास्तम्भनिष्ठीवनोरःपार्श्वशूलस्वरभेदहिक्काश्वासादयः स्युः (१)|

Speaking loudly or speaking in excess [before the restoration of normal health after the purificatory therapy] gives rise to complications as follows:

• Burning sensation in the head

• Pricking pain in the temples and ears

• Auditory dysfunction (deafness)

• Dryness of mouth, palates and throat

• Fainting

• Thirst, fever, Tamaka (a feeling as if entering into darkness), spasticity of jaws, torticollis and ptyalism;

• Pain in the chest and sides of the chest
• Hoarseness of voice
• Hiccup and asthma and Such other complications [14 (1)]

Complications of Jolting by conveyance

रथक्षोभात् सन्धिपर्वशैथिल्यहनुनासाकर्णशिरःशूलतोदकुक्षिक्षोभाटोपान्त्रकूजनाध्मानहृदयेन्द्रियोपरोध-
स्फिक्पार्श्ववङ्क्षणवृषणकटीपृष्ठवेदनासन्धिस्कन्धग्रीवादौर्बल्याङ्गाभितापपादशोफप्रस्वापहर्षणादयः (२)।

Jolting caused by riding conveyance [before the restoration of normal health after purificatory therapy] gives rise to complications as follows:
Looseness of big and small joints
Colic and pricking pain in jaws, nose, ears and head
Irritation in the pelvic region, meteorism, gurgling noise in intestines and flatulence;
Obstruction in the functioning of the heart and sense organs,
Pain in the hips, sides of the chest, groin, scrotum, waist and back
Weakness of joints, shoulders and neck
Burning sensation in limbs
Oedema, numbness and tingling sensation in feet and
Such other complications [14] (2)

Complications of long wayfaring:

अतिचङ्क्रमणात् पादजङ्घोरुजानुवङ्क्षणश्रोणीपृष्ठशूलसक्थिसादनिस्तोद-
पिण्डिकोद्वेष्टनाङ्गमर्दासाभितापसिराधमनीहर्षश्वासकासादयः (३)।

Long wayfaring [before the restoration of health after the purificatory therapy] gives rise to complications as follows:
Pain in the feet, calf region, thighs, knees, groins, waist and back
Asthenia and pricking pain in legs (Sakthi)
Cramps in the calf region
Malaise
Burning sensation in the shoulders
Swelling of the veins and arteries
Asthma and cough and
Such other complications [14 (3)]

Complications of Constant Sitting

अत्यासनाद्रथक्षोभजाः स्फिक्पार्श्ववङ्क्षणवृषणकटीपृष्ठवेदनादयः (४)।

Constant sitting [before the restoration of health after shodhana] gives rise to complications like pain in the hips, sides of the chest, groins, scrotum, waist and back which are described earlier in respect of jolting by conveyance, and such other complications. [14 (4)]

Complications of Indigestion and Adhyasana

अजीर्णाध्यशनाभ्यां तु मुखशोषाध्मानशूलनिस्तोदपिपासागात्रसादच्छर्द्यतीसारमूर्च्छाज्वरप्रवाहणामविषादयः(५)।

Indigestion and Adhyasana (intake of food before the previous meal is digested) [before the restoration of normal of normal health of after purificatory therapy] give rise to following complications:
Dryness of the mouth, flatulence, colic pain and pricking pain
Thirst, prostration of the body, vomiting, diarrhoea, fainting, fever and gripping pain
Ama Visha or poisoning effect caused by Ama (product of indigestion) and
Such other complications [14 (5)]

Complications of Unwholesome food and Irregular meal

विषमाहिताशनाभ्यामनन्नाभिलाषदौर्बल्यवैवर्ण्यकण्डूपामागात्रसादवातादिप्रकोपजाश्च ग्रहण्यर्शोविकारादयः (६)|

Intake of irregular meals and unwholesome food [before the restoration of normal health after purificatory therapy] produces complications as follows:

Lack of desire for taking food

Weakness, discoloration of the skin, itching, scabies and prostration of the body; and

Sprue, piles and such other diseases caused by the aggravation of vayu. [14 (6)]

Complications of Day-sleep

दिवास्वप्नादरोचकाविपाकाग्निनाशस्तैमित्यपाण्डुत्वकण्डूपामादाहच्छर्द्यङ्गमर्दहृत्स्तम्भजाड्यतन्द्रानिद्रा-
प्रसङ्गग्रन्थिजन्मदौर्बल्यरक्तमूत्राक्षितातालुलेपाः (७)|

Sleep during the day time [before the restoration of normal health after purificatory therapy] produces complications as follows:

Anorexia, indigestion and suppression of the power of digestion

Staimitya (feeling as if the body is covered with wet leather)

Anaemia, itching, scabies, burning sensation, vomiting and malaise

Impairment of the cardiac functions, stiffness, drowsiness and continuous sleep

Appearance of nodules

Weakness

Reddish coloration of urine and eyes and

Coating over the palate [14 (7)]

Complications of sexual intercourse

व्यवायादाशुबलनाशोरुसादशिरोबस्तिगुदमेढ्रवङ्क्षणोरुजानुजङ्घापादशूलहृदयस्पन्दननेत्रपीडाङ्गशैथिल्य-
शुक्रमार्गशोणितागमनकासश्वासशोणितष्ठीवनस्वरावसादकटीदौर्बल्यैकाङ्गसर्वाङ्गरोगमुष्कश्वयथु-
वातवर्चोमूत्रसङ्गशुक्रविसर्गजाड्यवेपथुबाधिर्यविषादादयः स्युः; अवलुप्यत इव गुदः, ताड्यत इव मेढ्रम्, अवसीदतीव मनो, वेपते हृदयं,
पीड्यन्ते सन्धयः, तमः प्रवेश्यत इव च (८)|

Sexual intercourse [before the restoration of health after shodhana] produces complications as follows;

Instantaneous loss of strength, Prostration of thighs, Colicky pain in the head, region of urinary bladder, anus, phallus, groins, thighs, knees, calf regions and feet, Palpitation of heart, Pain in the eyes, Asthenia of the limbs , Bleeding through the seminal passage, Cough, asthma, haemoptysis and asthenia of the voice;

Weakness of lumbar region, Paralysis of the part of the body or the whole body, Oedema in the scrotum, Retention of flatus, stool and urine, Excessive discharge of semen, Numbness, trembling, deafness and Vishada (depression), A feeling as if the anus is being cut, Pain in the phallus as if it is being cut, A feeling as if the mind is shrinking, Trembling of the heart,Pain in joints hearts

A feeling as if entering into darkness [14- (8)]

इत्येवमेभिरष्टभिरपचारैरेते प्रादुर्भवन्त्युपद्रवाः||१४||

Thus, the above-mentioned complications arise because of the eight types of impediments [described in the verse no. 11] [14]

Management of complications caused by loud speech & excessive speech

तेषां सिद्धिः- तत्रोच्चैर्भाष्यातिभाष्यजानामभ्यङ्गस्वेदोपनाहधूमनस्योपरिभक्तस्नेहपानरसक्षीरादिर्वातहरः सर्वो विधिर्मौनं च (१)|

Now the successful treatment of these complications [arising out of impediments during the period of convalescence] will be discussed.

Complications caused by loud speech and excessive speech can be cured by all the alleviating measures including the following:

Massage and fomentation therapies
Upanaha (application of hot poultices)
Dhuma (smoking therapy)
Nasya (inhalation therapy)
Upari-Bhakta sneha-pana (intake of medicated ghee after the meal)
Intake of meat soup, milk etc., and
Observation of silence [15 (1)]

Management of complications caused by conveyance jolting, etc.,

रथक्षोभातिचङ्क्रमणात्यासनजानां स्नेहस्वेदादिवातहरं कर्म सर्व निदानवर्जनं च (२)|

Complications because of jolting by conveyance, long wayfaring and excessive sitting can be cured by all vayu alleviating therapies like oleation, fomentation, etc., the patient should avoid the causative factors. [15 (2)]

Management of complications caused by Indigestion & Adhyasana

अजीर्णाध्यशनजानां निरवशेषतश्छर्दनं रूक्षः स्वेदो लङ्घनीयपाचनीयदीपनीयौषधावचारणं च (३)|

Complications arising out of indigestion and adhyasana (taking food before the previous meal is digested) can be cured by the following:

Administration of emetic therapy in order to completely take out the undigested material [from the stomach]
Ruksa sveda (dry or ununctuous fomentation) and
Administration of medications which are Langhaniya (producing lightening effect on the body), Pachaniya (carminative) and Dipaniya (digestive stimulant) [15 (3)]

Management of complications caused by irregular meal & unwholesome food

विषमाहिताशनजानां यथास्वं दोषहराः क्रियाः (४)|

Complications arising out of irregular and intake of unwholesome food can be cured by appropriate therapies for the alleviation of respective Doshas which are aggravated. [15 (4)]

Management of complications caused by Day sleep

दिवास्वप्नजानां धूमपानलङ्घनवमनशिरोविरेचनव्यायामरूक्षाशनारिष्टदीपनीयौषधोपयोगः प्रघर्षणोन्मर्दनपरिषेचनादिश्च श्लेष्महरः सर्वो विधिः (५)|

Complications arising out of day sleep can be cured by all the Kapha- alleviating measures including the following:
Dhuma-Pana (smoking)
Langhana (fasting or lightening therapy)
Vamana (emetic therapy)
Shiro- virechana (therapy for the elimination of morbid matter from the head)
Vyayama (physical exercise)
Ruksa Ashana (intake of ununctuous food)
Arista (intake of alcoholic preparations)
Administration of drugs which are dipaniya (digestive stimulant) and
Pragharsana (friction massage), unmardana (kneading the body) and Parisecana (hot affusion) etc.,

Management of Complications caused by sexual Intercourse

मैथुनजानां जीवनीयसिद्धयोः क्षीरसर्पिषोरुपयोगः, तथा वातहराः स्वेदाभ्यङ्गोपनाहा वृष्याश्चाहाराः स्नेहाः स्नेहविधयो यापनाबस्तयोऽनुवासनं च; मूत्रवैकृतबस्तिशूलेषु चोतरबस्तिर्विदारीगन्धादिगणजीवनीयक्षीरसंसिद्धं तैलं स्यात्||१५||

Complications caused by sexual intercourse can be cured by the following:
Administration of milk and ghee cooked by adding drugs belonging to Jivaniya- group of herbs (Jivaka, Rsabhaka, Meda, Mahameda, Kokoli, Ksirakakoli, Mudgaparni, Mashaparni, Jivanti and Madhuka- Vide Sutra 4: 9:1)

Administration of fomentation, massage and upanaha (application of hot poultice) which are best in alleviating vata

Intake of food which promotes virility

Intake of unctuous foods and application of unctuous therapies:

Yapana and Anuvasana types of medicated enema and

If there are urinary morbidities, and pain in the region of urinary bladder, then Uttara-Basti is given with oil cooked by adding milk boiled with Vidarigandhadi and Jivaniya Gana groups of drugs. [15]

Mustadya Yapana – Basti

यापनाश्च बस्तयः सर्वकालं देयाः; तानुपदेक्ष्यामः-
मुस्तोशीरबलारग्वधरास्नामञ्जिष्ठाकटुरोहिणीत्रायमाणापुनर्नवाबिभीतकगुडूचीस्थिरादिपञ्चमूलानि पलिकानि खण्डशः क्लृप्तान्यष्टौ च मदनफलानि प्रक्षाल्य जलाढके परिक्वाथ्य पादशेषो रसः क्षीरद्विप्रस्थसंयुक्तः पुनः शृतः क्षीरावशेषः पादजाङ्गलरसस्तुल्यमधुघृतः शतकुसुमामधुककुटजफलरसाञ्जनप्रियङ्गुकल्कीकृतः ससैन्धवः सुखोष्णो बस्तिः शुक्रमांसबलजननः क्षतक्षीणकासगुल्मशूलविषमज्वरब्रध्न(वर्ध्म)- कुण्डलोदावर्तकुक्षिशूलमूत्रकृच्छ्रासृग्जोविसर्पप्रवाहिकाशिरोरुजा-जानूरुजङ्घाबस्तिग्रहाश्मर्युन्मादार्शःप्रमेहाध्मानवातरक्तपित्तश्लेष्मव्याधिहरः सद्यो बलजननो रसायनश्चेति (१)।

Yapana type of Basti (medicated enema for the promotion of longevity) can be administered at all times. The recipes for this type of medicated enema will be described hereafter.

One Pala each of Musta, Usira, Bala, Aragvadha, Rasna, Manjistha, Katurohini, Trayamana, Punarnava, Bibhitaka, Guduchi, Shalaparni, Brhati, Kantakari and Gokshura are cut into small pieces. To this, eight fruits of madana are added. The whole recipe should then be washed well and cooked by adding one adhaka (25 Tolas) of water till one fourth of water remains. To this decoction, two prasthas (128 Tolas) of cow's milk is added and boiled again till two prasthas of the liquid remains. To this liquid, half prastha of the soup of the meat of animals inhabiting desert like zone, ghee taken in quantity equal to honey (as prescribed in earlier enema- recipes) and the paste of Shatakusuma (Shatapuspa), Madhuka, fruit of kutaja, rasanjana, Priyangu as well as a little of saindhava (rock-salt) is added. This recipe, when luke-warm, is used for enema.

This medicated enema has the following therapeutic effects –

It promotes semen, muscle, tissue and strength

It cures Kshata-ksina (consumption), cough, Gulma (phantom tumour), colic pain, irregular fever, Bradhna or vardhana (inguinal swelling), Kundala (circular movement of wind), Udavarta (upward movements of wind in the abdomen), pain in the pelvic region, dysuria, Asrg-rajah (menorrhagia), Visarpa (erysipelas), Pravahika (dysentery) and headache.

It cures stiffness of knee joints, thighs, calf regions and the region of urinary bladder.

It cures asmari (calculus in the urinary tract and in other parts of the body), insanity, piles, prameha (obstinate urinary disorders including diabetes), flatulence, vatarakta (gout) and diseases caused by aggravated pitta as well as kapha.

It instantaneously promotes strength and

It rejuvenates the body [16 (1)]

Erandamuladya Yapana Basti

एरण्डमूलपलाशात् षट्पलं शालिपर्णीपृश्निपर्णी बृहती कण्टकारिका गोक्षुरको रास्नाश्वगन्धा गुडूची वर्षाभूरारग्वधो देवदार्विति पलिकानि खण्डशः क्लृप्तानि फलानि चाष्टौ प्रक्षाल्य जलाढके क्षीरपादे पचेत्।
पादशेषे कषायं पूतं शतकुसुमाकुष्ठमुस्तपिप्पलीहपुषाबिल्ववचावत्सकफलरसाञ्जनप्रियङ्गुयवानिप्रक्षेपकल्कितं मधुघृततैलसैन्धवयुक्तं सुखोष्णं निरूहमेकं द्वौ त्रीन् वा दद्यात्।
सर्वेषां प्रशस्तो विशेषतो ललितसुकुमारस्त्रीविहारक्षीणक्षतस्थविरचिरार्शसामपत्यकामानां च (२)।

Six Palas of the root and leaves of Eranda and one Pala each of Shalaparni, Prsniparni, Brhati, Kantakari, Gokshura, Rasna, Ashvagandha, Guduchi, Varsabhu (punarnava), Aragvadha and Devadaru is cut into pieces, washed well and cooked by adding one adhaka of water and one fourh adhaka of milk till one fourth of the liquid remains. To this decoction, the paste of Shata-Kusuma (Shatapuspa), Kustha, Musta, Pippali, Hapusa, Bilva, Vacha, fruit of Vatsaka, Rasanjana, Priyangu and Yavani is added. By adding honey, ghee, oil and rock- salt, this recipe, when luke-warm, is given in the form of Niruha (evacuative) once, twice of three times.

This medicated enema is useful for all, especially for the following types of persons:

Pleasure- loving people

Those having tender health

Those indulging excessively in sex

Emaciated persons and those suffering from phthisis

Old persons

Persons suffering from chronic piles and

Persons desirous of progeny [16(2)]

Sahacaradya Yapana-basti

तद्वत् सहचर बला दर्भमूल सारिवा सिद्धेन पयसा (३) |

Following the above-mentioned procedure, enema recipe can be prepared of milk boiled with Sahacara, Bala, root of Darbha and Sariva. [16 (3)]

Brhatyadi Yapana-Basti

तथा बृहती कण्टकारी शतावरी च्छिन्नरुहाश्रृतेन पयसा मधुक मदन पिप्पलीकल्कितेन पूर्ववद्वस्तिः (४) |

Milk is boiled by adding Brhati, Kantakari, Shatavari and Chinnaruha. To this milk, the paste of Madhuka, Madana and Pippali is added. Following the above-mentioned procedure (described in Para 16-2) enema of this recipe is given. [16 (4)]

Baladya Yapana Basti – First recipe

तथा बलातिबला विदारी शालिपर्णी पृश्निपर्णी बृहती कण्टकारिका दर्भमूल परूषक काश्मर्य बिल्वफल यव सिद्धेन पयसा मधुक मदन कल्कितेन मधु घृत सौवर्चलयुक्तेन कास ज्वर गुल्म प्लीहार्दितस्त्रीमद्यक्लिष्टानां सद्योबलजननो रसायनश्च (५)|

Milk boiled with bala, Vidari, Shaliparni, Prsniparni, Brhati, kantakarika, root of Darbha, Parusaka, Kashmarya, fruit of Bilva and Yava is added with the paste of madhuka and Madana along with honey, ghee as well as sauvarcala.

Enema with this recipe instantacously promotes strength, and rejuvenates the body of persons suffering from cough, fever, gulma (phantom tumour), pliha (splenic disorders) and ardita (facial paralysis). This recipe also instantaneously promotes the strength, and rejuvenates the body of persons who are afflicted with excessive sexual indulgence and alcoholism. [16 (5)]

Baladya Yapana – Basti – second Recipe

बलातिबला रास्नारग्वध मदन बिल्व गुडूची पुनर्नवैरण्डाश्वगन्धा सहचर पलाश देवदारु द्विपञ्चमूलानि पलिकानि यव कोलकुलत्थ द्विप्रसृतं शुष्कमूलकानां च जलद्रोणसिद्धं निरुह प्रमाणावशेषं कषायं पूतं मधुक मदन शतपुष्पा कुष्ठ पिप्पली वचा वत्सकफल रसाञ्जन प्रियङ्गु यवानी कल्किकृतं गुड घृत तैल क्षौद्रक्षीरमांस रसाम्ल काञ्जिक सैन्धवयुक्तं सुखोष्णं बस्तिं दद्याच्छुक्रमूत्रवर्चःसङ्गेऽनिलजे गुल्म हृद्रोगाध्मान ब्रध्न पार्श्व पृष्ठ कटीग्रह सञ्ज्ञानाश बलक्षयेषु च (६)|

One Pala each of Bala, Atibala, Rasna, Aragvadha, Madana, Bilva (fruit), Guduchi, Punarnava, Eranda, Ashwagandha, Sahacara, Palasa, Devadaru, Bilva (root), Shyonaka, Gambhari Patala, Ganikarika, Shalaparni, Prsniparni, Brihati, Kantakari, and Gokusura, and two prasta each of Yava, Kola, Kulattha as well as Suska Mulaka is boiled by adding one drona of water till five Prasthas (vide commentary) of liquid remains. To this strained decoction the paste of Madhuka, Madana, Shatapuspa, Kustha, Pippali, Vacha, fruit of Vatsaka, Rasanjana, Priyangu and Yavani is added. By adding Jaggery, ghee, oil, honey, milk, meat soup, sour vinegar (amla Kanjika) and Saindhava. This recipe, when lukewarm, is used for enema.

This enema cures the following ailments:

Retention of semen, urine and stool caused by the aggravated vayu and

Gulma (phantom tumour),

hrdroga (heart diseases),

flatulence,

Bradhna (inguinal swellings),

stiffness of the sides of the chest, back and lumbar region,

unconsciousness and

diminution of strength [16 (6)]

Hapusadya Yapana Basti

हपुषार्धकुडवो द्विगुणार्धक्षुण्णयवः क्षीरोदक सिद्धः क्षीरशेषो मधु घृत तैल लवणयुक्तः सर्वाङ्ग विसृत वातरक्त सक्त विण्मूत्रस्त्रीखेदितहितो वातहरो बुद्धि मेधाग्नि बल जननश्च (७)|

Half Kuduva of Hapusa and one Kudava of half crushed grains of Yava is boiled by adding water and milk till the quantity left over is equal to the quantity of milk. This is added with honey, ghee, oil and rock–salt [and administration for enema].

This medicated enema has the following effects

It cures Vatarakta (gout) afflicting the entire body

It cures retention of stool and urine

It cures afflication by ailments caused by excessive sexual intercourse with women;

It alleviates vayu and

It promotes wisdom, intellect, Agni, (power of digestion and metabolism) and strength. [16 (7)]

Laghupancamuladya Yapana Basti

ह्रस्व पञ्च मूली कषायः क्षीरोदक सिद्धः पिप्पली मधुक मदन कल्कीकृतः सगुड घृत तैल लवणः क्षीण विषमज्वर कर्शितस्य बस्तिः (८) |

Decoction of Laghupancamula (Shalaparni, Prsniparni, Brhati, Kantakari and Gokshura) prepared by boiling with milk and water is added with the paste of Pippali, Madhuka and Madana. Added with jaggery, ghee, oil and rock-salt, this recipe is administered as enema.

Enema with this recipe is useful for consumption and for persons emaciated because of Vishama-Jvara (irregular fever). [16 (8)]

Baladya Yapana Basti - Third Recipe

बलातिबलापामार्गात्मगुप्ताष्टपलार्ध क्षुण्ण यवाञ्जलि कषायः सगुड घृत तैल लवणयुक्तः पूर्ववद्बस्तिःस्थविर दुर्बल क्षीण शुक्र रुधिराणां पश्यतगः (९)|

Eight Palas of Bala, Atibala, Apamarga and Atmagupta, and one anjali of half crushed barley are made into a decoction [by boiling with milk and water]. To this decoction, jaggery, ghee, oil and rock-salt is added, and used for enema as before. This enema is exceedingly wholesome for old and weak persons, and for persons having diminished semen and blood. [16 (9)]

Baladya Yapana basti - Fourth Recipe

बला मधुक विदारी दर्भमूल मृद्वीका यवैः कषायमाजेन पयसा पक्त्वा मधुक मदन कल्कितं समधु घृत सैन्धवं ज्वरार्तेभ्यो बस्तिं दद्यात् (१०) |

The decoction of Bala, madhuka, Vidari, root of Darbha, Mrdvika and Yava is boiled by adding goat's milk. This decoction is mixed with the paste of Madhuka and madana. This recipe is added with honey, ghee and rock-salt.

Enema with this recipe is useful for persons suffering from fever. [16 (10)]

Shaliparnyadya Yapana Basti

शालिपर्णी पृश्निपर्णी गोक्षुरक मूल काश्मर्य परूषक खर्जूरफल मधूकपुष्पैरजाक्षीर जल प्रस्थाभ्यां सिद्धः कषायः पिप्पली मधूकोत्पलकल्कितः सघृत सैन्धवः क्षीणेन्द्रिय विषमज्वर कर्शितस्य बस्तिः शस्तः (११) |

Roots of Shaliparni, Prsniparni and Gokshura, Kashmarya, Parusaka, fruits of Kharjura and flowers of madhuka are added with one prastha each of goat's milk and water, and cooked. In this decoction, the paste of Pippali, Madhuka and Utpala is mixed. Added with ghee and rock-salt, this recipe is used as enema.

This medicated enema is useful for weakened sense faculties and emaciation caused by Vishama Jvara (Irregular fever). [16 (11)]

Sthiradi Yapana Basti

स्थिरादि पञ्चमूलीपञ्चपलेन शालि षष्टिक यव गोधूम माष पञ्चप्रसृतेन छागं पयः शृतं पादशेष कुक्कुटाण्ड रस सम मधु घृत शर्करा सैन्धव सौवर्चल युक्तो वस्तिर्वृष्यतमो बलवर्णजननश्च |

इति यापना बस्तयो द्वादश||१६||

Five Palas of Sthiradi Panchamula (Shalaparni, Prsniparni, Brhati, Kantakari and Gokshura), and five Prasrtas of Shali, Shashtika, Yava, Godhuma and Masha are boiled by adding goat's milk and reduced to one-fourth. In this decoction equal quantity of the sap of hen's egg is mixed. By adding honey, ghee, sugar, rock-salt and Sauvarcala to this recipe, enema is given.

This medicated enema is exceedingly aphrodisiac, and it promotes strength as well as complexion.

Thus, ends the description of twelve recipes for Yapana type of basti (medicated enema for promotion of longevity). [16]

Extension of Recipe No Twelve

कल्पश्चैष शिखि गोनर्द हंस सारसाण्ड रसेषु स्यात्||१७||

The above-mentioned enema recipe can also be prepared by substituting the sap of hen's egg with that of the eggs of Sikhi (pea-hen), Gonarda (hill-partridge), Hamsa (swan) or Sarasa (crane). [17]

Tittiradya Yapana Basti

सतित्तिरिः समयूरः सराजहंसः पञ्चमूली पयः सिद्धः शतपुष्पा मधुक रास्ना कुटज मदनफल पिप्पली कल्को घृत तैल गुड सैन्धव युक्तो बस्ति बल वर्ण शुक्र जननो रसायनश्च (१) |

Pancha mula (Shalaparni, Prsniparni, Brhati, Kantakari and Gokshura) is boiled with milk. To this milk, soup of the meat of Tittiri, Mayura and rajahamsa, and the paste of Shatapuspa, madhuka, rasna, Kutaja, madanaphala and Pippali is added. This recipe is mixed with ghee, oil, jaggery and rock-salt and used for enema.

Enema with this recipe promotes strength complexion and semen. This rejuvenates the body. [18 (1)]

Dvipanchamuladya Yapani Basti

द्विपञ्चमूली कुक्कुट रस सिद्धं पयः पादशेषं पिप्पली मधुक रास्ना मदन कल्कं शर्करा मधु घृतयुक्तं स्त्रीष्वतिकामानां बलजननो बस्तिः (२) |

Drugs belonging to two types of DwiPanchamula (Bilva, Shyonaka, Gambhari, Patala, Ganikarika, Shalaparni, Prsniparni, Brhati, Kantakari and Gokshura) and chicken soup are boiled by adding milk till one fourth of the liquid remains. To this liquid, the paste of Pippali, madhuka, rasna and madana is added. By adding sugar, honey and ghee, this recipe is used for enema.

Enema with this recipe promotes the strength of the persons who are addicted to excessive sexual indulgence. [18 (2)]

Mayuradya Yapana Basti

मयूरमपितपक्षपादास्यान्त्रं स्थिरादिभिः पलिकैः सजले पयसि पक्त्वा क्षीरशेषं मदन पिप्पली विदारी शतकुसुमा मधुक कल्कीकृतं मधु घृत सैन्धव युक्तं बस्तिं दद्यात् स्त्रीष्वति प्रसक्त क्षीणेन्द्रियेभ्यो बलवर्णकरम् (३) |

The gall-bladder, feather, legs, beak and intestines of the peacock are removed. The meat of this peacock is added with one pala each of Shalaparni, Prsniparni, Brhati, Kantakari and Gokshura, and cooked by adding water and milk till the remaining liquid is equal to the quantity of milk. To this liquid, the paste of Madana, Pippali, Vidari, Shata-Kusuma (Shatapushpa) and Madhuka is added. By further adding honey, ghee and rock-salt, this recipe is used for

enema.
Enema with this recipe promotes the strength and complexion of persons who has diminished functioning of their sensory faculties and motor organs because of over indulgence in sex. [18 (3)]

Extension of recipe no Fifteen

कल्पश्चैष विष्किर प्रतुद प्रसहाम्बुचरेषु स्यात्, अक्षीरो रोहितादिषु च मत्स्येषु (४) |

The above-mentioned enema – recipe can be prepared by substituting peacock – meat with meat of animals and birds of the following categories:

Viskira (Gallinaceous brids)

Pratuda (pecker birds)

Prasaha (animals and birds who eat by snatching their food) and

Vaicara (birds moving in the water)

Similarly, different types of fish like Rohiita can be used in place of the meat of peacock. But while preparing enema recipes with fish, milk should not be added. [18 (4)]

Godhadya Yapana Basti

गोधानकुल मार्जार मूषिक शल्लक मांसानां दशपलान् भागान् सपञ्चमूलान् पयसि पक्त्वा तत्पयःपिप्पलीफल कल्क सैन्धव सौवर्चल शर्करा मधु घृत तैल युक्तो बस्तिर्बल्यो रसायनः क्षीणक्षतस्य सन्धानकरो मथितोरस्करथ गज हय भग्न वातबलासक प्रभृत्युदावर्त वातसक्तमूत्र वर्चश्शुकाणां हिततमश्च (५)|

Drugs belonging to the group of Panchamula (Bilva, Syonaka, Gambhari, Patala and Ganikarika) and ten palas of the meat of iguana (godha), mongoose (nakula), cat (marjara) and mouse (musika) are cooked by adding milk. To this liquid (containing milk), the paste of pippali and Phala (Madanaphala) should be added. This should further be added with rock-salt, Sauvarcala, sugar, honey, ghee and oil, and used for enema.

Enema with this recipe is exceedingly useful for the following:

Promotion of strength

Rejuvenation of the body

Healing the phthisis lesion

Curing ailments caused by the compression of the chest

Correcting fractures caused by riding ratha (wooden cart) elephant and horse

Curing vata-balasaka (an ailment caused by the simultaneous aggravation of vayu and kapha) and such other diseases and

Curing Udavarta (upward movement of wind in the abdomen) and retention of urine, stool as well as semen caused by the aggravation of vayu. [18 (5)

Kurmadya Yapana Basti and Ten Other Extension Recipes

कूर्मादीनामन्यतम पिशित सिद्धं पयो गो वृषनागहयनक्र हंस कुक्कुटाण्डरस मधु घृत शर्करा सैन्धवेक्षुरकात्मगुप्ताफल कल्क संसृष्टो बस्ति वृद्धानामपि बलजननः (६) |

The meat of any Kurma (tortoise) group of aquatic animals, is boiled with milk. This milk should be added with the soup of the testicles of bull, elephant and horse, the sap of the eggs of crocodile, swan and hen, honey, ghee, sugar and rock-salt. To this, the paste of Iksuraka as well as the fruit of atmagupta is added, and used for enema.

Enema with these recipes promotes strength even in old person. [18 (6)]

Karkata Rasadya Yapana-basti

कूर्मादीनामन्यतमपिशितसिद्धं   पयो   गोवृषनागहयनक्रहंसकुक्कुटाण्डरसमधुघृतशर्करासैन्धवेक्षुरकात्मगुप्ताफलकल्कसंसृष्टो बस्तिर्वृद्धानामपि बलजननः (६) |

Soup of the meat of Karkataka (crab) added with the sap of the egg of Cataka, honey, ghee and sugar is used as enema. Enema with these recipes is exceedingly aphrodisiac. If milk boiled with Uccataka, Iksuraka, Kokilaksa and

Atmagupta is taken after the administration of these enemas, then the person becomes capable of having sexual intercourse with many (lit hundred) women. [18 (7)]

Go Vrsadya Yapana Basti

गोवृष बस्त वराह वृषण कर्कट चटक सिद्धं क्षीरमुच्चटकेक्षुरकात्मगुप्ता मधु घृत सैन्धव युक्तः किञ्चिल्लवणितो बस्तिः (८) |

Milk boiled with the testicles of Go-Vrsa (bull), goat and Pig, Karkataka and Cataka is added with the paste of Uccata, Iksuaka (Kokilaksa) and Atmagupta, honey, ghee, rock–salt and small quantity of sea-salt and used for enema.

Enema with this recipe is exceedingly aphrodisiac and it enables a person to indulge in sex with many women. [18 (8)]

Dashamuladya Yapana Basti

दशमूल मयूर हंस कुक्कुट क्वाथात् पञ्चप्रसृतं तैल घृत वसा मज्ज चतुष्प्रसृतयुक्तं शतपुष्पा मुस्त हपुषा कल्कीकृतः सलवणो बस्तिः पाद गुल्फोरुजानु जङ्घा त्रिक वङ्क्षण बस्ति वृषणानिल रोगहरः (९)|

To five Prasthas of the decoction of Dashamula (Bilva, Synonaka, Gambhari, Patala, Ganikarika, Shalaparni, Prsniparni, Brhati, Kantakari and Gokshura) and meat of peacock, swan as well as domestic fowl, four prasrtas of oil, ghee, vasa (muscle–fat and majja (bone marrow) is added. This liquid is added with the paste of Shatapuspa, Musta and Hapusa. By adding salt (rock-salt) this recipe is used for enema.

This enema cures Vatika diseases afflicting feet, ankle joints, thighs, knee-joints, calf region, lumbar region, groins, urinary bladder region and testicles. [18 (9)]

Extension of recipe No Twenty

मृग विष्किरानूप बिलेशयानामेतेनैव कल्पेन बस्तयो देयाः (१०) |

Following the above-mentioned procedure, enema is given with the meat of the following categories of animals and birds:

Mrga (animals inhabiting dry land/forests)

Viskira (gallinaceous birds)

Anupa (animals inhabiting marshy land) and

Bilesaya (animals living in the burrows in earth) [18 (10)]

Madhvadya Yapana – Basti

मधु घृत द्विप्रसृतस्तुल्योष्णोदकः शतपुष्पार्धपलः सैन्धवार्धाक्षयुक्तो बस्तिर्वृष्यतमो मूत्रकृच्छ्रपित्तवातहरः (११) |

Two Prasrtas of madhu (honey) and Ghrta (ghee) is added with two Prasrtas of warm water. To this, half pala [of the paste] of Shatapuspa and half aksa of rock salt should be added. It cures mutrakrccha (dysuria) and diseases caused by pitta as well as vayu. [18 (11)]

Sadyo Ghrtadya Yapana Basti

सद्योघृत तैल वसा मज्ज चतुष्प्रस्थं हपुषार्धपलं सैन्धवार्धाक्षयुक्तो बस्तिर्वृष्यतमो मूत्रकृच्छ्र पित्तव्याधिहरो रसायनः (१२)|

Four Prasthas of freshly collected ghee, oil, vasa (muscle fat) and Majja (bone-marrow) is added with [the paste of] half pala Hapusa, and half aksa of rock-salt and used for enema

This enema is exceedingly aphrodisiac. It cures Mutrakrcchra (dysuia) and diseases caused by pitta. It rejuvenates the body. [18 (12)]

Madhutailadya Yapana basti

मधुतैल चतुःप्रसृत शतपुष्पार्धपलं सैन्धवार्धाक्षयुक्तो बस्तिर्दीपनो बृंहणो बलवर्णकरो निरुपद्रवो वृष्यतमो रसायनः क्रिमि कुष्ठोदावर्त गुल्मार्शो ब्रध्न प्लीह मेहहरः (१३) |

Four prastas of madhu (honey) and taila (oil) are added with [the paste of] half pala of Shatapuspa, and half aksa of rock-salt.

Enema with this recipe produces the following effects:

Stimulates the power of digestion (dipana)

Nourishes the body (Brmhana)

Promotes strength and complexion (bala-varnakara)

Produces no harmful effects (nirupadrava)

Promotes virility exceedingly (Vrsyatama)

Rejuvenates the body (Rasayana)

Cures krimi (parasitic infestation), Kustha (obstinate skin diseases including leprosy), Udavarta (upward movement of wind in the abdomen), Gulma (phantom tumour), Arsas (piles), Bradhna (inguinal swelling), Phiha (splenic disorder) and Meha (obstinate urinary disorders including diabetes) [18 (13)]

Madhughrtadya Yapana basti – First Recipe

तद्वन्मधुघृताभ्यां पयस्तुल्यो बस्तिः पूर्वकल्केन बलवर्णकरो वृष्यतमो निरुपद्रवो बस्ति मेढ्र पाक परिकर्तिका मूत्रकृच्छ्र पित्तव्याधिहरो रसायनश्च (१४) |

Similarly, Madhu (honey) and Ghrta (ghee) added with equal quantity of milk is mixed with the paste of drugs described above (in recipe no. 23)

Enema with this recipe has the following effects:

It promotes strength and complexion (Bala-Varnakara)

It produces aphrodisiac effects (Vrshyatama)

It causes no adverse effects (Nirupadrava)

It cures inflammation of urinary bladder and phallus (basti–medhra-paka), sawing pain (Parikaritika), dysuria (mutra-krcchra) and diseases caused by Pitta and

It rejuvenates the body (Rasayana) [18 (14)]

Madhu-Ghrtadya Yapana Basti - Second Recipe

तद्वन्मधुघृताभ्यां मांसरसतुल्यो मुस्ताक्षयुक्तः

पूर्ववद्बस्तिर्वात बलास पादहर्ष गुल्म त्रिकोरुजानूरुनिकुञ्चन बस्ति वृषण मेढ्र त्रिक पृष्ठशूलहरः (१५) |

Similarly, honey (Madhu) and ghee (ghrta) is added with equal quantity of meat-soup and [the paste of] one aksa of Musta. This enema recipe prepared according to earlier procedure (recipe no.23) cures vata-balasa (an ailment caused by aggravated vayu and kapha), padaharsa (tingling sensation in the feet), gulma (phantom tumour), contraction (stiffness) of lumbar region, thighs and knee-joints, and pain in the region of the urinary bladder, scrotum, phallus, lumbar region and back. [18 (15)]

Suradya Yapana Basti

सुरा सौवीरक कुलत्थ मांसरस मधु घृत तैल सप्तप्रसृतो मुस्त शताह्वा कल्कितः सलवणो बस्तिः सर्ववातरोगहरः (१६) |

Seven Prasrtas of Sura (a type of alcohol), Sauviraka (vinegar), Kulattha-soup, meat-soup, honey, ghee and oil is added with the paste of Musta and Shatahva. This recipe added with salt may be used for enema which cures all the vatika diseases. [18 (16)]

Dvi-Panchamuladya Yapana Basti

द्विपञ्चमूल त्रिफला बिल्व मदनफल कषायो गोमूत्र सिद्धः कुटज मदनफल मुस्त पाठा कल्कितः सैन्धवयावशूक क्षौद्र तैलयुक्तो बस्तिः श्लेष्म व्याधि बस्त्याटोप वातशुक्रसङ्ग पाण्डुरोगाजीर्ण विसूचिकालसकेषु देय इति||१८||

Two types of Panchamula (roots of Bilva, Shyonaka, Gambhari, Patala, Ganikarika, Shalaparni, Prsniparni, Brhati, Kantakari and Gokshura), Triphala (Haritaki, Bibhitaka and Amalaki), Bilva (fruit) and Madanaphala is boiled by adding cow's urine. To this decoction, the paste of Kutaja, Madanaphala, Musta and Patha is added. By adding rock-salt, yava-ksara (an alkali preparation of barley), honey and oil, this is used for enema.

This enema is used for treatment of diseases caused by Kapha, Bastyatopa (flatulence in the region of the urinary bladder), retention of flatus and semen, anaemia, indigestion, visucika (choleric diarrhoea) and alasaka (intestinal torpor). [18]

Recipes of Anuvasana Basti
Shatavaryadi Sneha Basti

अत ऊर्ध्वं वृष्यतमान् स्नेहान् वक्ष्यामः|

शतावरी गुडूचीक्षुविदार्यामलक द्राक्षा खर्जूराणां यन्त्रपीडितानां रसप्रस्थं पृथगेकैकं तद्वद्घृत तैल गो महिष्यजाक्षीराणां द्वौ द्वौ दद्यात्,

जीवकर्षभक मेदा महामेदा त्वक्क्षीरी शृङ्गाटक मधूलिका मधुकोच्चटा पिप्पली पुष्करबीज नीलोत्पल कदम्बपुष्प- पुण्डरीक केशरकल्कान्

पृषततरक्षुमांसकुक्कुटचटकचकोरमताक्षबर्हिजीवञ्जीवकुलिङ्गहंसाण्डरसवसामज्जादेश्च प्रस्थं दत्वा साधयेत्|

ब्रह्म घोष शङ्ख पटहभेरी निनादैः सिद्धं सितच्छत्रकृतच्छायं गजस्कन्धमारोपयेद्भगवन्तं वृषध्वजमभिपूज्य, तं स्नेहं त्रिभागमाक्षिकं मङ्गलाशीः स्तुतिदेवतार्चनैर्बस्तिं गमयेत्|

नृणां स्त्रीविहारिणां नष्टरेतसां क्षतक्षीण विषमज्वरार्तानां व्यापन्नयोनीनां वन्ध्यानां रक्तगुल्मिनीनां मृतापत्यानामनार्तवानां च स्त्रीणां क्षीणमांसरुधिराणां पथ्यतमं रसायनमुत्तमं वलीपलितनाशनं विद्यात् (१)|१९|

Now we shall describe oleating recipes having excellent aphrodisiac effects.

One Prastha each of the juice of Shatavari, Guduchi, Iksu, Vidari, Amalaki, Draksha and Kharjura is taken out separately with the help of instruments (mechanically). To this, two Prasthas each of ghee, oil, cow's milk, buffalo-milk and goat–milk is added. This should then be added with the paste of Jivaka, Rsabhaka, Meda, Mahameda, Tvak-Ksiri (vamsalocana), Srngataka, Madhulika, Madhuka, Uccata, and Pippali, seeds of Pushkara, Nilotpala, and flower of kadamba, pundarika and Kesara. The recipe is cooked by adding one prastha of the meat-soup of Prasta and Taraksu, and the sap of the eggs of Kukkuta, Cakora, Mattaksa (kokila), Barhi, Jivajivaka, Kulinga and Hamsa, vasa (muscle-fat), Majja (bone-marrow) etc.

After having worshiped Lord Siva, this cooked Sneha (medicated fat) is placed on the back of an elephant with a white umbrella held over it. While chanting Vedic mantras and blowing conch-shell accompanied with the beating sound of Pataha (hand- drum) as well as Bheri (kettle Drum).

To this medicated fat, honey one-third in quantity thereof is added. With auspicious benedictions, prayers and worshiping of the Gods, this recipe is administered as enema.

This enema–recipe is exceedingly wholesome for the following:

Persons indulging in sexual act in excess

Persons suffering from loss of semen

Patients suffering from Kshata-Ksina (Phthisis) and Vishama-Jvara (irregular fever)

Women suffering from gynecological disorders, sterility and rakta-gulma (uterine tumour)

Women whose offspring succumb to death before or after delivery

Women suffering from amenorrhoea and

Persons having diminished muscle-tissue and blood

It is excellent Rasayana (rejuvenating therapy), and it cures the appearance of wrinkles on the skin (vali) and graying of hair (Palita). [19 (1)]

Baladya Sneha-basti

बला गोक्षुरक रास्नाश्वगन्धा शतावरी सहचराणां शतं शतमापोथ्य जलद्रोणशते प्रसाध्यं, तस्मिन् जल द्रोणावशेषे रसे वस्त्रपूते विदार्यामलक स्वरसयोर्बस्त महिष वराह वृष कुक्कुट बर्हि हंस कारण्डवसारसाण्डरसानां घृत तैलयोश्चैकैकं प्रस्थमष्टौ प्रस्थान् क्षीरस्य दत्वा चन्दन मधुक मधूलिका त्वक्क्षीरी बिसमृणाल नीलोत्पल पटोलात्मगुप्तान्नपाकि ताल मस्तक खर्जूर मृद्वीकातामलकी- कण्टकारी जीवकर्षभक क्षुद्रसहा महासहा शतावरी मेदा पिप्पली ह्रीबेर त्वक्पत्र कल्कांश्च दत्वा साधयेत्|

ब्रह्मघोषादिना विधिना सिद्धं बस्तिं दद्यात्|

तेन स्त्रीशतं गच्छेत्; न चात्रास्ते विहाराहार यन्त्रणा काचित्|

एष वृष्यो बल्यो बृंहण आयुष्यो वली पलितनुत् क्षतक्षीण नष्टशुक्र विषमज्वरार्तानां व्यापन्नयोनीनां च पथ्यतमः (२)|१९|

One hundred Palas of each of bala, Gokshuraka, Rasna, Ashwagandha, Shatavari and Sahacara is crushed into small pieces and boiled by adding remains. This liquid should then be filtered out by a cloth. This is cooked by adding the following ingredients:

One Prastha (768 g) each of the juice of Vidari and Amalaki

One Prastha each of the meat-soup of goat, buffalo, pig and bull

One Prastha each of saps of the eggs of domestic fowl, pea-hen, swan, Karandava and Sarasa

One prastha each of ghee and oil

Eight Prasthas of milk and

Paste of Chandana, Madaka, madhulika, Tvak-Ksiri (vamsa- locana), Bisa-Mrnala, Nilotpala, Patola, Atmagupta, Anna-Paki, (Odana- Paki), tala-mastaka, Kharjura, Mrdvika, Tamalak, Kantakari, Jivaka, Rsabhaka, Ksudrasaha (mudgaparni), mahasaha (Mashaparni), Shatavari, Meda, Pippali, Hribera, Tvak and Patra.

Following the procedure of the recitation of Vedic mantras and such other rituals described earlier (in respect of recipe no.27), enema with this recipe is given.

By this enema a person becomes capable of having sexual intercourse with many (lit. Hundred) women). This enema does not involve any restriction of diet or regimen on the part of the patient. It promotes virility, strength, corpulence and longevity. It cures wrinkles (vali) on the skin and graying of hairs (palita). It is exceedingly wholesome for patients suffering from phthisis, loss of semen, Vishama-Jvara (irregular fever) and Gynecic disorders. [19(2)]

Sahacaradya Sneha- Basti

सहचर पल शतमुदक द्रोण चतुष्ट्ये पक्त्वा द्रोणशेषे रसे सुपूते विदारीक्षुरस प्रस्थाभ्यामष्टगुणक्षीरं घृत तैल प्रस्थं बला मधुक मधूक चन्दन मधूलिका सारिवा मेदा महामेदा काकोलि क्षीरकाकोली पयस्यागुरु मञ्जिष्ठा व्याघ्रनख- शटी सहचर सहस्रवीर्या वराङ्ग लोध्राणामक्षमात्रैर्द्विगुणशर्करैः कल्कैः साधयेत्‌।

ब्रह्मघोषादिना विधिना सिद्धं बस्तिं ददयात्‌।

एष सर्वरोगहरो रसायनो ललितानां श्रेष्ठोऽन्तःपुरचारिणीनां क्षत क्षय वात पित्त वेदना श्वास कास हरस्त्रिभागमाक्षिको वली पलितनुद्वर्ण रूप बल मांस शुक्र वर्धनः (३)॥

One hundred Palas (4.8 kg) of Sahacara is added with four Dronas of water, and cooked till one drona of the liquid remains. This decoction should then be strained out, and cooked by adding the following Ingredients:

One Prastha each of the juice of vidari and sugarcane

Sixteen Prasthas of milk

One Prastha each of ghee and oil

Paste of one Aksa each of Bala, madhuka, Madhuka, Chandana, Madhulika, Sariva, Meda, Mahameda, kakoli, Ksirakakoli, Payasya, Aguru, Manjistha, Vyaghranakha, Salt, Sahacara, Sahasravirya, (durva), Varanga (Guda- Tvak) and Lodhra, and two Aksas, of sugar.

This recipe is administered as enema while reciting Vedic Mantras and performing other sacred rituals. This enema has the following effects:

It is a panacea for all diseases

It rejuvenates the body

It is the best therapy for delicate women living in harems

It cures Kshata-Ksina (Phthisis), pain caused by Vayu and Pitta, Asthma, and cough and

When used by adding honey, one third in quantity of the recipe, it cures wrinkles (vali), graying of hair (palita) and promotes colour, complexion, beauty strength, muscle tissues and semen. [19 (3)]

Augmenting Potency of Basti Recipes

इत्येते रसायनाः स्नेह बस्तयः सति विभवे शतपाकाः सहस्रपाका वा कार्या वीर्यबलाधानार्थमिति॥१९॥

If the patient is affluent enough, then the above-mentioned rejuvenating Sneha-Bastis (unctuous enema) is prepared by cooking for the hundred times (Shata-paka) or one thousand times (Sahasra-paka) for promotion of their potency and strength. [19]

Recapitulation

भवन्ति चात्र-

इत्येते बस्तयः स्नेहाश्चोक्ता यापनसञ्ज्ञिताः|

स्वस्थानामातुराणां च वृद्धानां चाविरोधिनाः||२०||

अतिव्यवायशीलानां शुक्रमांसबलप्रदाः|

सर्वरोगप्रशमनाः सर्वेष्वृतुषु यौगिकाः||२१||

नारीणामप्रजातानां नराणां चाप्यपत्यदाः|

उभयार्थकरा दृष्टाः स्नेहबस्तिनिरूहयोः||२२||

The above-mentioned oleating enema recipes are called Yapana Bastis. These are not contra-indicated either for healthy persons or for patients or for old persons. They promote semen and muscular tissue of persons, excessively indulging in sex. These are panaceas for all diseases, and are suitable for administration in all the seasons. These recipes are suitable for both, Sneha-basti (unctuous enema) and Niruha- Basti (evacuative enema). [20-22]

Prohibitions

व्यायामो मैथुनं मद्यं मधूनि शिशिराम्बु च|

सम्भोजनं रथक्षोभो बस्तिष्वेतेषु गर्हितम्||२३||

While using the above mentioned Yapana-Bastis, the patient should avoid physical exercise, sexual intercourse, intake of alcohol, intake of different types of honey and cold water, eating full meal and jolting by conveyances. [23]

Summary

तत्र श्लोकाः -

शिखिगोनर्दहंसाण्डैर्दक्षवद्बस्तयस्त्रयः| विंशतिर्विष्किरैस्त्रिंशत्प्रतुदैः प्रसहैर्नव||२४||

विंशतिश्च तथा सप्तविंशतिश्चाम्बुचारिभिः| नव मत्स्यादिभिश्चैव शिखिकल्पेन बस्तयः||२५||

दश कर्कटकाद्यैश्च कूर्मकल्केन बस्तयः| मृगैः सप्तदशैकोनविंशतिर्विष्किरैर्दश ||२६||

आनूपैर्दक्षशिखिवद्भूशयैश्च चतुर्दश| एकोनत्रिंशदित्येते सह स्नेहैः समासतः||२७||

प्रोक्ता विस्तरशो भिन्ना द्वे शते षोडशोत्तरे|

Thus, in brief, twenty-nine Yapana-Bastis including three sneha bastis are described above. In addition, the following extended categories of enema recipes are also described.

(1) to (3) three Bastis with the eggs of Sikhi (Peahen), Gonarda (bird Indian crane) and Hamsa (swan) which are to be prepared in the same way like the method described for the egg of hen in para no. 16(12). [Vide para no. 17]

(4) to (118) twenty recipes with the meat of Viskiras (gallinaceous birds), thirty recipes with Pratudas (pecker birds), 29 recipes with Prasthas (animals who eat by snatching food), 27 recipes with aquatic animals, and nine recipes with fish, etc., which are to be prepared on the line suggested for the enema recipe with the meat of peacock in para 18 (3). [Vide para no. 18 (4)

(119) to (128) ten recipes with the meat of Karkata, etc. which are to be prepared on the line suggested for Kurma in Para no. 18(6)

(129) to (187) seventeen recipes with the meat of mrgas (animals dwelling in dry land forests), nineteen recipes with the meat of Viskiras (gallinaceous birds), nine recipes with the meat of anupas (marshy land inhabiting animals), and fourteen recipes with bhusayas (animals living in burrows on the earth) which are to be prepared on line suggested for the recipes of domestic fowl and peacock in para no 18(9). [Vide para no.18 (10)]

Thus, when classified in detail, the 29 original recipes and 187 extended recipes make for 216 recipes in total. [24-27 ½]

Augmenting Potency of recipes

एते माक्षिकसंयुक्ताः कुर्वन्त्यतिवृषं नरम्||२८||

नातियोगं न वाऽयोगं स्तम्भितास्ते च कुर्वते|२९|

Use of above-mentioned enema recipes by adding honey makes a person exceedingly virile. When fortified (with honey), they do not allow any over action (atiyoga) or under action (ayoga). [28 ½- ½ 29]

Management of Non-eliminated recipes

मृदुत्वान्न निवर्तन्ते यस्य त्वेते प्रयोजिताः||२९||
समूत्रैर्बस्तिभिस्तीक्ष्णैरास्थाप्यः क्षिप्रमेव सः|३०|

If, because of mild nature, the administered enema recipes described above do not get eliminated, then immediately Asthapana-Basti (evacuative enema) containing cow's urine and other sharp ingredients is given. [29 ½ - ½ 30]

Adverse effects of excessive use of Yapana-bastis, and their management

शोफाग्निनाश पाण्डुत्व शूलार्शःपरिकर्तिकाः||३०||
स्युज्र्वरश्चातिसारश्च यापनात्यर्थसेवनात्|३१|
अरिष्टक्षीरसीध्वाद्या तत्रेष्टा दीपनी क्रिया||३१||
युक्त्या तस्मान्निषेवेत यापनान्न प्रसङ्गतः|

Excessive use of these Yapana-Bastis gives rise to oedema, loss of the power of digestion, anemia, colic pain, piles, parikartika (sawing pain), fever and diarrhea.

For the treatment of these ailments, the patient is given aristas (medicated wines), milk, sidhu (a type of alcohol) etc. and therapies for the promotion of digestion.

Therefore, Yapana-Basti is used judiciously and should not be used continuously (as a matter of habit). [30 ½- ½ 32]

Impediments and their management

इत्युच्चैर्भाष्यपूर्वाणां व्यापदः सचिकित्सिताः||३२||
विस्तरेण पृथक् प्रोक्तास्तेभ्यो रक्षेन्नरं सदा|३३|

Different factors (e.g., loud speech) which cause impediments and their management are separately described earlier in detail (in verse/para nos. 10-15).

The patient should always be guarded against these impeding factors. [32 ½- ½ 33]

Definition of Siddhi- Sthana

कर्मणां वमनादिनामसम्यक्करणापदाम्||३३||
यत्रोक्तं साधनं स्थाने सिद्धिस्थानं तदुच्यते|३४|

The section (sthana) describing the succcssful (siddhi) administration of elimination therapy (emesis, etc.) the complications arising out of their mal-administration, and management of these complications is called Siddhi-Sthana". [33 ½- ½ 34]

Merits achieved by study

इत्यध्यायशतं विंशमात्रेयमुनिवाइ्मयम्||३४||
हितार्थं प्राणिनां प्रोक्तमग्निवेशेन धीमता|३५|
दीर्घमायुर्यशः स्वास्थ्यं त्रिवर्गं चापि पुष्कलम्||३५||
सिद्धिं चानुत्तमां लोके प्राप्नोति विधिना पठन्|३६|

Thus, this treatise comprising one hundred and twenty chapters which expound the statements of the sage Atreya was propounded by Agnivesha, endowed with therapeutic wisdom for the benefit of all the living beings.

The systematic study of this treatise endows a person with longevity, fame, health, abundance, fulfilment of the three basic desires of life and unsurpassable professional accomplishment in this world. [34 ½ - ½ 36]

Pratisamskarta or Redactor

विस्तारयति लेशोक्तं सङ्क्षिपत्यतिविस्तरम्||३६||
संस्कर्ता कुरुते तन्त्रं पुराणं च पुनर्नवम्| अतस्तन्त्रोत्तममिदं चरकेणातिबुद्धिना||३७||

संस्कृतं तत्त्वसम्पूर्णं त्रिभागेनोपलक्ष्यते|

A redactor expands the concised statements and abbreviates the very prolix ones in an old work, and thus, puts it in a new (revised) form.

Therefore, Charaka, possessed with excellent wisdom redacted this illustrious treatise, which however, is incomplete in as much as (almost) one-third of this redacted text was missing (not available at the time of Drdhabala). [36 ½ - ½ 38]

Drdhabala and His Supplementations

तच्छङ्करं भूतपतिं सम्प्रसाद्य समापयत्||३८||

अखण्डार्थं दृढबलो जातः पञ्चनदे पुरे| कृत्वा बहुभ्यस्तन्त्रेभ्यो विशेषोञ्छशिलोच्चयम्||३९||

सप्तदशौषधाध्यायसिद्धिकल्पैरपूरयत्| इदमन्यूनशब्दार्थं तन्त्रदोषविवर्जितम्||४०||

षड्विंशता विचित्राभिर्भूषितं तन्त्रयुक्तिभिः|४१|

Drdhabala, born in Panchanadapura (present Punjab) supplemented these (non- available) chapters after propitiating God Shiva, the protector of all creatures, to make the work complete.

By culling matter from several important treatises, he compiled and restored 17 chapters of Cikitsa-sthana and all the chapters of Siddhi as well as kapla-sthanas.

This text is not deficient in words (shabda) or their implications (artha) concerning medical science, and it is decorated with 2 relevant Tantra-yuktis (canons of scientific exposition). [38 ½- ½ 41]

Tantra-Yuktis (Canons of Expositions)

तत्राधिकरणं योगो हेत्वर्थोऽर्थः पदस्य च||४१||

प्रदेशोद्देशनिर्देशवाक्यशेषाः प्रयोजनम्| उपदेशापदेशातिदेशार्थापत्तिनिर्णयाः||४२||

प्रसङ्गैकान्तनैकान्ताः सापवर्गो विपर्ययः| पूर्वपक्षविधानानुमतव्याख्यानसंशयाः||४३||

अतीतानागतावेक्षास्वसञ्ज्ञोह्यसमुच्चयाः| निदर्शनं निर्वचनं सन्नियोगो विकल्पनम्||४४||

प्रत्युत्सारस्तथोद्धारः सम्भवस्तन्त्रयुक्तयः|४५|

Tantra-Yuktis or canons of compositions are as follows:

Adhikarana or subject matter: (the central theme the author intends to expound in a treatise while the author composes a treatise) For example, in Sutra 1:7, it is stated that this Ayurvedic treatise is presented in order to prevent and cure diseases which are impediment to the path of an individual willing to perform righteous tasks on the context of duties. Here the diseases, the treatise, etc., constitute the Adhikarana or the central theme).

Yoga or union: Justifying a statement by putting together different words in order to explain the point from various angles. For example - origin of the embryo from maternal factors etc., has been explained on the basis of logical terms like Pratijna, Hetu, Udaharana, Upanaya and Nigamana in Sarira 3: 10-114)

Hetvartha or extension of Argument: When a statement is made in a particular context that is applicable to other situations as well it is called as hetvartha. For example, in Sutra 12: 5, habitual intake of homologous matter is stated to increase dhatus. The term "dhatu" in this context implies doshas as well besides tissue elements. The statement made here is in the context of Vayu Dosa. The same Principle is applicable to other situations like the augmentation of the quantity of Rasa, etc.

Padartha or implication of words: One, two or many words individually or jointly may carry specific (technical) meanings. For example, the term "Dravya" stands for five Mahabhutas and Atman, and the two terms "Ayusah Vedah" (science of life) stands for the treatise on Ayurveda)

Pradesha or partial enunciation: When there are many objectives of a topic and all of these cannot be explained in one place, then in a given situation, only a partial statement is made [in the form of a sample]. For example, in Sutra 27:329 while explaining the properties of various types of Anupanas, they in their entirety cannot be explained, and only a part of these, including some of the commonly used ones are described).

Uddesha or concise statement: Making a concise statement having wider implications. For example, the scope of Ayurveda is described in Sutra 1: 24 as hetu, linga, usadhi jnanam, i.e the knowledge of the etiology, signs and symptoms and medicines i.e., treatment or management of healthy persons and patients)

Nirdesha or amplication: The above-mentioned concise statement has been implied later. The explanation of Hetu linga usadhi jnana is provided later in Sutra 1: 44- 53)

Vakya Sesha or supply of ellipsis: Sometimes, in order to make the statement lighter or smaller in size, certain parts of it are omitted, and this ellipsis has to be inferred with reference to the context. For example, in the statement "pravrttihetun Bhuvanam" (vide Sutra 16: 28), the verb "Asti" has to be inferred though it is not specifically mentioned in the text. Without this verb the sentence is incomplete. Similarly, while describing the soup (rasa) of the meat (mamsa) of animals inhabiting dry land forests (jangala), only Jangalajaih Rasaih is mentioned (vide Siddhi 1:9). In this statement, the term "Mamsa" has to inserted to make the meaning complete. Since it is not mentioned in the text, it has to be inferred.

Prayojana or object: It is the purpose for which a treatise is composed. For example, the purpose of composing Charaka Samhita is to provide information regarding measures to be adopted for achieving equilibrium of Doshas and Dhatus (vide Sutra 1:53)

Upadesa or Authoritative instruction: The preceptor's instructions are included in a treatise. For example, first of all oleation (sneha) therapy is administered, and only thereafter, fomentation (Sveda) therapy is given to the patient (vide Sutra 13: 99)

Apadesha or reasoning a statement: When a statement is made, the reason for making such a statement is provided, for example, among the pollutions of vayu (air), jala (water), Desa (land) and kala (time), the latter ones are more serious than the former ones because the latter ones are more unavoidable (vide Vimana 3:10) this unavoidability (duspariharyatva) is the reason for making the statement.

Atidesha or indication: A specific statement might indicate non- specified objects. For example, in Sutra 9: 34, it is stated. "The regimens not specified in this chapter are also to be adopted if these are wholesome".

Arthapatti or implication: Statement may imply an unspecified object. For example, it is stated in Sutra 7:61, "one should not take curd at night". By implication, curd can be taken during the day time.

Nirnaya or decision: The conclusion drawn after proper examination. For example, it is stated in sutra 10:3, "Sixteen aspects of treatment, four each relating to the physician, drug, attendant and patient, described earlier are sine Qua non for good health provided these are applied appropriately". This proper application (yukti-yukta) represents the decision (Nirnaya) after proper examination)

Prasanga or restatement: Statement made earlier is repeated in view of context. For example, the statement regarding the wrong utilization, etc., of senses made in Sutra11: 37 is repeated in sutra1: 118: 126 because of contextual propriety.

Ekanta or Categorical statement: A statement made for explaining another view-point without upholding it. For example, the death of pressers for want of medicines, it is stated that even the diseases of these persons are not (always) amenable to therapeutic measures- vide Sutra 10: 5)

Apavarga or exception: A statement made regarding exceptions to general rules. For example, as a general rule intake of stale food is prohibited. But in case of meat etc., the stale (dried) ones are not prohibited. In fact, as exceptions to the general rule, these are permitted (vide Sutra 8:20)

Viparyaya or reconfirmation of implied opposite action: A statement made to reconfirm the implied meaning. For example, it is stated that the factors responsible for the causation of the diseases are not wholesome for the patient. By implication, factors having opposite attributes are wholesome for the patient. But this is reconfirmed in another statement made subsequently- vide Nidana 3:7)

Purva-Paksa or amplification of earlier statements: Sometimes a statement in general made earlier is partially modified. For example, having stated that all types of fish are not be taken with milk, the statement is amplified by the statement that cilicima type of fish especially should not be taken with milk- vide Sutra 26: 84)

Vidhana or correct interpretation: Sometimes a statement made earlier is further explained in order to bring out its correct implications.

According to some, this term "Vidhana" means description in correct order. For example, tissue elements are described in their appropriate sequence, rasa, rakta etc. Vide Chikitsa 15: 16)

Anumata or Confession: Non-contradiction, a different view. For example, the author has quoted another view regarding the method to be followed for the extraction of the dead foetus, and has not contradicted it. By implication, the author has accepted it Vide sarira 8: 31)

Vyakhyana or explanation: Explaining a topic to make it comprehensible by people having different intellectual quotients. For example, the condition of the foetus during the first month of pregnancy is described in detail- vide Sarira 4: 9)

Samsaya or doubt: Description of different view-points on a selected topic leaving the concluding uncertain. For example, the cause of procreation is described differently by various authors as mother (ovum), father (sperm), Svabhava (nature), Paranirmana (supernatural force) or Yaddrccha (accidental, not predetermined) vide Sutra 11: 6)

Atitaveksana or retrospective reference: Sometimes, the text refers to the description of a given topic made earlier. For example, while describing the treatment of Jvara (fever), a reference is made to the fomentation therapy details of which were described earlier – Chikitsa 3: 29)

Anagataveksana or prospective reference: Sometimes while describing a topic, a reference is made to a recipe which is to be described later. For example, while describing the treatment of fever, Tikta-Sarpis is described to be used. Details of this recipe are however described later)

Svasanjna or use of technical terms: Sometimes, the author uses certain technical terms which are generally not found elsewhere. For example, Jentaka, Holaka etc., Vide Sutra 14: 39:40)

Uhya or deduction: Sometimes, regarding a statement made in the text, the physician is advised to use his own power of discretion. For example, while describing ingredients of a recipe, the physician is advised to ignore the inappropriate ones according to his own desecration depending on as specific situation- vide Vimana 8: 149)

Samuccaya or specification: Sometimes, the term "Ca", is used repeatedly after each item which imply all these items are to be taken together. For example, the term "Ca" is used after Varna (complexion), Svara (voice) etc., in Indriya 1:3 to emphasise that all these items are to be considered together to determine the span of life of a person.

Nidarsana or illustration: Sometimes, a topic is illustrated with similes in order to make it understandable by intelligent and non-intelligent people alike. For example, it is stated that the use of a drug with which the physician is well acquainted works like ambrosia – vide Sutra 1:124)

Nirvachana or citation of analogy: Sometimes, an example is given in order to facilitate easy comprehension of a topic for the annihilation of beings which cannot be comprehended because such factors are unpredictable. This is based on the analogy of time. Time is always in the process of quick movement. It automatically goes on changing or destroying itself – Sutra 16: 32.

Nidarsana (item no. 30) facilitates comprehension of a topic by both intelligent and non-intelligent physicians whereas Nirvachana is exclusively for intelligent physicians.

The term "Nirvachana" can also be explained as a definition. For example, the disease "Visarpa" is defined as the ailment which moves (sarpati) in different direction (Vividha) vide Chikitsa 21:11)

Sanniyoga or injuction: Chakrapani has used the word "Niyoga in the place of Sanniyoga mentioned in the text.

Sometimes a statement is made in order to emphasise absolute necessity. For example, it is stated that the patient (undergoing jentaka therapy) should not leave the bench even if he gets tired owing to excessive heat – vide Sutra 14: 46)

Vikalpa or option

Pratyutsara or rebuttal: Sometimes the author quotes different views, each rebooting the other. For example, Varyovida is stated to hold the view that the diseases are caused by rasa- dhatu, and this view is refuted by Hiranyaksa who holds the view that these are caused by six basic elements, viz, five mahabhutas and the conscious elements – vide Suta 25: 13- 15

Uddhara or reaffirmation: Sometimes the author establishes his own view after refuting another scholar's view. For example, the statement that diseases are caused by the unwholesomeness of such factors, the wholesomeness of which is conducive to procreation- vide Sutra 25:29)

Sambhava or Possibility: Sometimes the place of origin or the infrastructure of manifestation is to be judged from the ailment. For example, the description of Piplu, Vyanga, Nilika etc., implies their location in the face). [41 ½ - ½ 45]

Availability of Tantra-Yuktis

तन्त्रे समासव्यासोक्ते भवन्त्येता हि कृत्स्नशः||४५||

एकदेशेन दृश्यन्ते समासाभिहिते तथा|४६|

All these Tantra-yuktis or canons of exposition are adopted in their entirety in treatises which are composed in both aphoristic and expository styles. However, in treatises which are composed excessively in aphoristic style, such canons are found only partially. [45 ½ - ½ 46]

Importance of Tantra-Yuktis

यथाऽम्बुजवनस्यार्कः प्रदीपो वेश्मनो यथा||४६||

प्रबोधनप्रकाशार्थास्तथा तन्त्रस्य युक्तयः|४७|

As the sun causes blossoming of the lotus pond (lit forest) and as the lamp enlightens the (dark) house: similarly, the knowledge of these Tantra-Yuktis serves the purpose of awakening (blossoming and enlightening of the physician). [46 ½ -1/2 47)

Assistance of Tantra-Yuktis in understanding other treatises

एकस्मिन्नपि यस्येह शास्त्रे लब्धास्पदा मतिः||४७||

स शास्त्रमन्यदप्याशु युक्तिज्ञत्वात् प्रबुध्यते|

अधीयानोऽपि शास्त्राणि तन्त्रयुक्त्या विना भिषक्|

नाधिगच्छति शास्त्रार्थानर्थान् भाग्यक्षये यथा||४८||

The physician who has a good grasp even of only one treatise can also understand other treatises quickly because of his proficiency in tantra-yuktis or canons of composition. As a person fails to acquire wealth [in spite of his best efforts] when fortune deserts him, similarly one who is not conversant with tantra-yuktis (canons of exposition) does not understand the real implications of treaties even if he has studied many of them. [47 ½ - 48]

Proper and improper understanding of treatises

दुर्गृहीतं क्षिणोत्येव शास्त्रं शस्त्रमिवाबुधम्|

सुगृहीतं तदेव ज्ञं शास्त्रं शस्त्रं च रक्षति||४९||

(तस्मादेताः प्रवक्ष्यन्ते विरतरेणोत्तरे पुनः|

तत्त्वज्ञानार्थमस्यैव तन्त्रस्य गुणदोषतः) ||५०||

Just like a badly handled weapon destroys the person himself, similarly badly understood treatise causes harm to the user himself. On the other hand, just like a properly handled weapon protects the user from the enemy, similarly the treatise well understood becomes a source of protection against the opponents.

Therefore, to enable the physician to critically analyse the merits and demerits, and comprehend the real implications of statements in this treatise (Ayurveda), these tantra-yuktis or canons of exposition will be explained in detail in the Uttara Tantra or supplementary section of this work. [49-50]

Merits of studying this treatise

इदमखिलमधीत्य सम्यगर्थान् विमृशति योऽविमनाः प्रयोगनित्यः|

स मनुजसुखजीवितप्रदाता भवति धृतिस्मृतिबुद्धिधर्मवृद्धः||५१||

After studying this text in its entirety with appropriate meaning, the physician who has reflected upon the statements made in it with concentration of mind, who has applied the text constantly in practice, and who has developed the power of reflection, recollection, description and righteousness becomes bestowed of happiness and life (longevity) to human beings. [51]

Epilogue

यस्य द्वादशसाहस्री हृदि तिष्ठति संहिता| सोऽर्थज्ञः स विचारज्ञश्चिकित्साकुशलश्च सः||५२||
रोगांस्तेषां चिकित्सां च स किमर्थं न बुध्यते| चिकित्सा वह्निवेशस्य सुस्थातुरहितं प्रति||५३||
यदिहास्ति तदन्यत्र यन्नेहास्ति न तत्क्वचित्| अग्निवेशकृते तन्त्रे चरकप्रतिसंस्कृते||५४||
सिद्धिस्थानेऽष्टमे प्राप्ते तस्मिन् दृढबलेन तु| सिद्धिस्थानं स्वसिद्ध्यर्थं समासेन समापितम्) ||५५||

The physician who has in his memory this treatise containing twelve thousand (verses and prose paragraphs] is definitely the knower of its implications. He has the power of discrimination and he is proficient in the treatment of diseases. Such a person cannot fail to diagnose and initiate its [appropriate] treatment.

The therapeutic measures described in Agnivesa's work are useful both for healthy persons [to maintain their positive health and prevent occurrence of diseases] and patients [to cure found elsewhere.

The treatise of Agnivesha as redacted by Charaka has reached up to its [final] eighth section called Siddhi-sthana. For the accomplishment of this Siddhi-sthana, the final touch in brief is given by Drdhabala. [52- 55]

Colophon

इत्यग्निवेशकृते तन्त्रे चरकप्रतिसंस्कृतेऽप्राप्ते दृढबलसम्पूरिते सिद्धिस्थाने उत्तरबस्तिसिद्धिर्नाम द्वादशोऽध्यायः||१२||
इति चरकसंहितायां अष्टमं सिद्धिस्थानं सम्पूर्णम्|
समाप्तेयं चरकसंहिता|

Thus, ends the twenty chapter of Siddhi- section dealing with "Measures to Attain Perfection in the administration of Uttara- Basti (important recipes of Enema)" in Agnivesha 's work as reducted by Charaka, and Because of its non-availability, supplemented by Drdhabala.

Thus ends Charaka Samhita.